HPV and Other Infectious Agents in Cancer

HPV AND OTHER INFECTIOUS AGENTS IN CANCER

OPPORTUNITIES FOR PREVENTION AND PUBLIC HEALTH

Hans Krueger
Gavin Stuart
Richard Gallagher
Dan Williams

Preface by
Jon F. Kerner

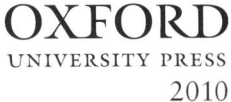

UNIVERSITY PRESS
2010

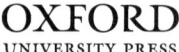
UNIVERSITY PRESS

Oxford University Press, Inc., publishes works that further
Oxford University's objective of excellence
in research, scholarship, and education.

Oxford   New York
Auckland   Cape Town   Dar es Salaam   Hong Kong   Karachi
Kuala Lumpur   Madrid   Melbourne   Mexico City   Nairobi
New Delhi   Shanghai   Taipei   Toronto

With offices in
Argentina   Austria   Brazil   Chile   Czech Republic   France   Greece
Guatemala   Hungary   Italy   Japan   Poland   Portugal   Singapore
South Korea   Switzerland   Thailand   Turkey   Ukraine   Vietnam

Copyright © 2010 by Oxford University Press, Inc.

Published by Oxford University Press, Inc.
198 Madison Avenue, New York, New York 10016
www.oup.com

Oxford is a registered trademark of Oxford University Press.

All rights reserved. No part of this publication may be reproduced,
stored in a retrieval system, or transmitted, in any form or by any means,
electronic, mechanical, photocopying, recording, or otherwise,
without the prior permission of Oxford University Press.

Library of Congress Cataloging-in-Publication Data

HPV and other infectious agents in cancer: opportunities for prevention and public health / Hans
Krueger ... [et al.].
p. ; cm.
Includes bibliographical references and index.
ISBN 978-0-19-973291-3
1. Viral carcinogenesis.   2. Oncogenic viruses.   3. Papillomaviruses.
4. Papillomavirus diseases.   I. Krueger, Hans.
[DNLM: 1. Oncogenic Viruses.   2. Alphapapillomavirus.
3. Neoplasms—prevention & control.   4. Neoplasms—virology.
5. Tumor Virus Infections—prevention & control. QW 166 H872 2010]
RC268.57.H68 2010
616.99'4071—dc22
2009022868

9 8 7 6 5 4 3 2 1

Printed in the United States of America
on acid-free paper

Preface

The role of viruses in the etiology of cancer has been a focus of scientific inquiry for much of the twentieth century; the more recent development of vaccines against the hepatitis B virus and some types of human papillomavirus has provided an important public health opportunity for preventing the development of liver and cervical cancers, respectively. A fuller appreciation of this topic is a priority in cancer control. Thus, the National Infectious Agents Committee of the Canadian Partnership Against Cancer's Primary Prevention Action Group, in partnership with Canadian Cancer Society, sponsored the development and publication of this volume.

Despite significant improvements in cancer prevention, treatment, and survival, more and more Canadians are diagnosed with cancer. This story is repeated in many jurisdictions in the world. One driver of such trends is an aging population, but cancer is not only a disease of the elderly. For example, cancer is the leading cause of death in middle-aged adults in Canada. In the 35- to 64-year age group, cancer causes more deaths than heart disease, stroke, injury, and infectious diseases combined.

Over a decade ago, facing the reality of a growing burden of cancer within Canadian society, cancer community stakeholders from across the country identified a need to create a coordinated, national plan for cancer control. The Canadian Strategy for Cancer Control (CSCC) was the volunteer network that drafted such a plan and successfully advocated for its funding. With that funding in place, the work begun by the

CSCC is being refined and driven forward by the Canadian Partnership Against Cancer (CPAC).

Networks of expert groups are leading efforts across all priority areas of cancer control, supported by CPAC since it began operations on April 1, 2007. One of these eight expert groups is the Primary Prevention Action Group, which in turn includes three subcommittees focused on advancing efforts that are central to the prevention of cancer: the National Committee on Environmental and Occupational Exposure, the National Committee on Skin Cancer Prevention, and the National Committee on Infectious Agents.

This volume was supported by the Partnership through funding by Health Canada and by the Canadian Cancer Society's National Cancer Institute of Canada. Given the sponsorship and concerns of this book, and active cooperation in medical research across the border, there will sometimes be a Canadian or U.S. focus to the information presented. But as also will become clear in the book, researching the infection/cancer connection was an international project from the start, and continues to be so.

Although infectious agents have been the focus of etiological and applied research for many decades, the relative interest and the level of research investment on infectious agents in Canada, the United States, and the rest of the developed world has waxed and waned over that time frame. Above and beyond the complexity of the science to understand how viral and bacteriological agents increase the risk for developing cancer, an explanation for the uneven research investment on infectious agents and cancer in the developed world is the fact that the infection-related burden is disproportionately found in developing countries.

Moreover, within the developed world, many of the cancers linked to infectious agents (e.g., cervical cancer) disproportionately burden the most vulnerable populations (e.g., low income, ethnic minorities). These underserved populations often have few, if any, voices to advocate for more research investment in addressing the cancers that contribute to the cancer health disparities they experience.

Particularly in the developing world, where resources available for early detection and the treatment of disease are extremely limited, controlling a complex set of diseases like cancer must perforce focus on prevention and palliation. The relatively recent developments of clinical prevention approaches for liver cancer (vaccination against hepatitis B virus) and cervical cancer (vaccination against specific types of HPV) hold great promise for cancers that are a much larger public health burden for vulnerable populations worldwide. Thus, this book goes beyond an update of the biological and clinical data relevant to infections that cause cancer by focusing on prevention as a theme of the knowledge synthesis provided.

As suggested earlier, the primary prevention perspective is the particular value that the present book seeks to add to the several published reviews of infectious causes of cancer. It is important to organize the proven and potential interventions so that classic primary prevention categories are clearly delineated. In this way, health care planners worldwide can more easily see where their proposed strategies fit on the prevention spectrum, thereby promoting comprehensive prevention approaches and clear resource allocation decisions.

This book hopefully will assist those in Canada, the United States, and around the world interested in building on the knowledge gained from research to expand cancer prevention partnership initiatives and enhance the strategies that can be put into practice to prevent cancers linked to infectious agents.

Jon F. Kerner, Ph.D.
Chair, Primary Prevention Action Group
Senior Scientific Advisor for Cancer Control
and Knowledge Translation
Canadian Partnership Against Cancer

ACKNOWLEDGMENTS

The authors originally researched and reviewed the topics found in this book as part of a project funded by the Canadian Partnership Against Cancer (CPAC) and the Canadian Cancer Society (CCS) through the National Cancer Institute of Canada. Overall leadership for the project was provided by the National Infectious Agents Committee (NIAC), a working group under the umbrella of the Primary Prevention Action Group (PPAG) of CPAC. The sponsorship of both CPAC and CCS was instrumental in the early drafting of this work. This project began under the visionary cancer prevention leadership of Ms. Barbara Kaminsky, then chair of the PPAG. More recently, Dr. Jon Kerner, the current chair of the PPAG, has continued the support for this project, as reflected in his Preface.

Two highly experienced members of NIAC were generous and helpful in reviewing and making suggestions about draft versions of chapters in this book, namely, Drs. Anthony B. Miller and Morris Sherman of the University of Toronto.

As the book came to fruition, many support roles were played by the skilled staff members of H. Krueger & Associates Inc., including Ms. Laura Powe, Ms. Celia Kinney, Ms. Alicia Krueger, Mr. Sam Dueckman, and Ms. Marianne Chomiak. This book truly could not have been completed without their tireless labors.

Finally, the authors are grateful for the enthusiastic and comprehensive support offered by Oxford University Press in New York, especially through our editor Ms. Tracy O'Hara and her assistant, Ms. Anna Bierhaus. Ms. O'Hara's early encouragement reassured us that the original report deserved a broader audience, and inspired us to review many hundreds of new journal articles in order to provide a final package of information that was as up-to-date as possible and highly applicable to jurisdictions beyond Canada. We are excited to see how many other readers will "catch the bug" of the themes herein and ultimately be helped by our treatment of an important and growing area of cancer prevention.

Hans Krueger
Gavin Stuart
Richard Gallagher
Dan Williams

Contents

1 Introduction—Infection and Cancer: An Expanding Paradigm ... 3
2 Human Papillomavirus: Structure, Transmission, and Occurrence ... 21
3 Human Papillomavirus: Infection, Natural History, and Carcinogenesis ... 57
4 Human Papillomavirus: Associations with Cervical Cancer ... 79
5 Human Papillomavirus: Associations with Noncervical Cancer ... 129
6 Human Papillomavirus: Detection of Infection and Disease ... 213
7 Human Papillomavirus: Prevention of Infection and Disease ... 259
8 Hepatitis Viruses ... 287
9 *Helicobacter pylori* ... 341
10 Epstein-Barr Virus ... 385
11 Human Herpesvirus Type 8 ... 429
12 Human T-cell Lymphotropic Virus Type 1 ... 471
13 Conclusion—Infection and Cancer: A Paradigm Shift ... 505
Index ... 537

HPV and Other Infectious Agents in Cancer

1

INTRODUCTION—INFECTION AND CANCER: AN EXPANDING PARADIGM

Major advances in the prevention, diagnosis, and treatment of human cancers came along with a better understanding of their etiology, pathogenesis, and natural history. Thus, it is mandatory to properly validate any suspected causal link between viruses and human tumors. Unfortunately, it is not a trivial task.[1]

If informed that more than 25% of the annual cancer burden in the developing world could be prevented, with the added clarification that smoking cessation was *not* the specific agenda under consideration, many people would be hard pressed to identify the anticipated intervention category. Perhaps an equal number of people would be surprised to discover that the actual target in mind—infectious agents—indeed play such a substantial role in the development of cancer.

The recent licensing and deployment of vaccines preventing infection with certain types of the human papillomavirus (HPV) has had an enormous impact within the media and among cancer control professionals. The vaccines prevent a specific viral infection that is a necessary cause of cervical carcinoma. To be described as a "necessary" cause means that, among other pieces of evidence, essentially 100% of tumors demonstrate the presence of the virus. This combination of facts and events has finally brought before a general audience a phenomenon heretofore restricted to the world of cancer researchers, that is, the existence of infectious agents that cause cancer.

The subtitle for this Introduction was originally intended to be "An *Emerging* Paradigm"; but that wording would have created the wrong impression. It is true that a belief in the contagious nature of cancers, which arose in classical times and persisted for centuries, actually fell out of favor.[2] But the hypothesis of HPV involvement in cervical cancer already dates back to 1975[3]; indeed, scientific confirmation of the general concept of infectious agency in human cancers was achieved almost a half century ago.[4] Thus, it no longer represents a new or emerging topic; the field is a fully established part of oncology and cancer prevention, and one that continues to expand at a remarkable rate.

Notably, if animal hosts are included, the history of this topic is even longer.[5] For example, at about the beginning of the twentieth century, Peyton Rous discovered that solid tumors could be passed like an infection between Plymouth Rock fowls. Using special filters, the agent involved was proven to be subcellular; eventually, the causative agent was isolated and named the Rous sarcoma virus, with molecular confirmation following at a later date.[6,7] Research suggesting an infectious basis for leukemia in animals was pursued even earlier, led by Ellermann and Bang.[8] Similarly, the proof of the infectious nature of benign tumors such as warts may be traced back to animal studies at the end of the nineteenth century[9]; by 1907, the same result had been achieved for human warts, specifically through the cell-free transmission experiments of Ciuffo.[10] Of course, certain HPV types are now known to be the agents involved with warts and other skin lesions in humans. While there was substantial resistance to applying the results of animal studies to humans, and serious doubts about what was once known as the "virus theory of cancer," the role of infectious agents is now globally recognized.[11]

Given that the Canadian Partnership against Cancer and the National Cancer Institute of Canada sponsored the research for this book, there will sometimes be a Canadian focus to the information presented. But researching the infection–cancer connection was an international project from the start, and continues to be so. A hundred years ago, Rous was pursuing the topic in a U.S. institute, Ellermann and Bang in Denmark, and Ciuffo in Italy. Most famously, the examination in a British laboratory of Burkitt lymphoma cells, cultured from patients living in the middle of sub-Saharan Africa, has proven to be a milestone in medical history.[12,13] The 1964 discovery of the Epstein-Barr virus (EBV) in those cells by Epstein and colleagues properly launched the scientific field related to infections and cancer.[14,15] Since that seminal event, the range of infections investigated for their cancer-causing potential is truly remarkable.

It is clear today that EBV (and its related diseases) is a relatively modest part of the infection–cancer connection, even though the virus accounts for about 1% of cancers worldwide. In fact, epidemiologists suggest that nearly one-fifth of global cancer incidence is causally linked to one or another of the implicated infections. The most quoted review of this topic pegged the proportion of global cancer incidence attributable to infections at 17.8% in 2002, or some 1.9 million cases.[16] In this light, how can one account for the relatively low profile of the topic of infections and cancer? One explanation is the fact that the infection-related burden is disproportionately found in developing countries, by a factor of almost 4 to 1. It is also true that the science is very complex and difficult to communicate to a lay audience. The ultimate reason, however, for the slow increase in public awareness and public health concern is the dramatic paradigm shift that is required in standard thinking about cancer risk factors and cancer prevention. The nature of this paradigm shift will be revisited in the concluding chapter.[17]

PURPOSE OF THE BOOK

Infectious agents actually intersect in a number of ways with the arena of cancer. For example, clinicians are often challenged by controlling primary or reactivated infections that occur in cancer patients, especially following cancer treatments.[18,19] Also, viruses are now being adapted for use in innovative therapies against cancer.[20,21] However, the focus of the present book, the infectious causes of cancer, is manifestly different than either of these topics. There are three goals that guided the literature review and commentary:

- To raise the consciousness of key players in cancer prevention regarding the importance of and potential for decreasing cancer incidence by directly addressing infectious causes
- To provide an up-to-date presentation of the biology, cancer pathology, and prevention options related to selected infectious agents
- To suggest directions for future research, practice, and policy

While other writers—indeed, world-class experts—have reviewed the basic science and clinical implications of individual agents, few have attempted to pull the entire picture together. A notable exception is *Infections Causing Human Cancers*,[22] a monograph survey by a pioneer in the field, Harald zur Hausen. He was one of the key investigators of the role of HPV in cervical carcinoma, the research that won him a portion of the 2008 Nobel Prize in Medicine.[23] Prior to zur Hausen's monograph in 2006, the best-known treatment was a 2000 volume edited by J Goedert.[24]

A large volume of research information has been published since zur Hausen's monograph (indeed, a new journal specific to the field, called *Infectious Agents and Cancer*, was launched after his textbook was completed). Substantial review articles have been recently published, each of which have covered the same agents selected for the present book.[25-27] However, this book seeks to go beyond an update of the biological and clinical information by offering insights on the current and emerging prevention possibilities relevant to infections that cause cancer. In short, the unique perspective of this synthesis project is the prevention theme.

INFECTIOUS AGENTS OF INTEREST

The mention of "selected infectious agents" in the purpose statement immediately raises the issue of selection criteria. As will be clear later in this Introduction, the sheer scope of the topic required some focusing, lest hundreds of pages turn into thousands. Three main questions shaped the table of contents:

- Is the infection strongly established as a cause of cancer?
- Is there a compelling prevention priority because of the burden of related cancers measured globally and/or in the United States, Canada, and other parts of the developed world?
- And, even if one or other of the preceding criteria were not convincing, is there another overriding feature of interest, such as what the infection teaches us about carcinogenesis?

Each of these points can be expanded. The question related to causation will be further explored below; the other two criteria will be revisited in the book's concluding chapter.

CRITERION OF CAUSATION

The term "cause" has been used rather freely so far in this Introduction. In fact, causation (or etiology) is a complex phenomenon biologically, clinically, and philosophically. This is especially the case when the etiology theme is embedded within the general complexity of cancer, not to mention the bewildering world of infectious agents.[28] The causal pathways of cancer are still being worked out at both risk factor and molecular levels. Cancer is a disruption of cellular processes usually involving DNA mutations and usually manifesting as uncontrolled cell growth; it is a notoriously complicated disease entity. This is because cancer involves multiple factors or influences—either endogenous (or originating within the host) and exogenous (or environmental)—manifesting along a multistep development pathway. And, for any of the 100 human cancers that have been delineated, a full research program involves looking at the transformation steps, the risk factors, and how and where the factors interact with each other at each step.

Figure 1.1 provides a simple schematic of the developmental stages of cancer when an infectious cause is involved.

The diagram pictures the situation where at least some cases of a particular cancer are directly initiated by an infection. In other words, certain cellular changes created by the infection lead to the transformation that ultimately generates a malignancy. This role of infection may be deemed as *direct* causation of cancer. Of special interest is the situation where all cases of a certain cancer have the same direct cause; as suggested earlier, the agent in this situation is referred to as a necessary cause.

One of the reasons for the intense focus on HPV in the past decade is the discovery that it was a necessary cause of cervical cancer. Cervical cancer is a malignancy of great concern to women and health care providers. The fact that all cases of an important cancer could be traced to a known infection, and the promise that this cancer could be reduced by known infection control measures, has generated understandable excitement. Contrary to some perceptions, however, this is neither the first nor the only discovery of a necessary infectious agent of cancer. As will become clear in later chapters, both human herpesvirus type 8 (HHV-8) and human T-cell lymphotropic virus type 1 (HTLV-1) are also responsible for essentially 100% of cases of a particular cancer.

HTLV-1 is especially interesting, as it represents the forerunner of a new trend in cancer taxonomy. Instead of defining a category of cancer and then looking for causes and other risk factors, some very specific cancers are now being defined at histological and even molecular levels

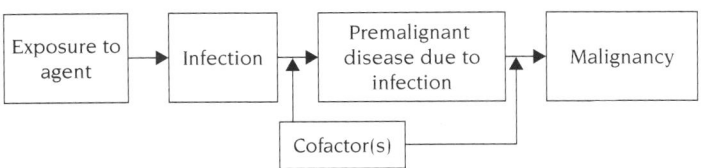

Figure 1.1. Carcinogenesis related to infection.

according to the infectious cause detected. Thus, the type of lymphoma considered to be caused by HTLV-1 is basically equated with the lymphoma cases in which the virus is present; this yields an attributable risk of 100%, and makes HTLV-1 a necessary causal agent *by definition*. This microscopic and especially molecular approach to defining cancer is destined to be repeated, with particular implications for the expanding profile of infectious agents of cancer.

The direct causes of cancer do not cover the whole picture, however. As is suggested in Figure 1.1, cofactors can also be involved in carcinogenesis. In fact, cofactors appear to always play a role in human malignancy. One piece of circumstantial evidence supporting this conclusion is the fact that there is no situation in human biology where the presence of a direct causal agent always leads to cancer; this is another way of saying that there is no known example of a single *sufficient* cause of cancer. Some other factor is always involved, either as another direct cause of critical cellular changes, or as a promoter of cancer development at the start or at some later stage of carcinogenesis. One of the fascinating aspects of this phenomenon is that quite often the cofactor involved with infection-related cancers is *another* infection. Indeed, interactions between microbial agents will be a frequent subtopic in the subsequent chapters of this book. One of the more studied mechanisms involves HIV and HHV-8, but evidence has been accumulating for other important interactions, including HHV-8 and HPV.[29]

The most important causal pathways involving infections are schematized in Figure 1.2.

The various scenarios illustrated in Figure 1.2 suggest that unveiling all the details of the infection–cancer topic could be a daunting task. New information is regularly emerging that implicates infections in cancer, not only as direct causes, but as influences of biological conditions related to carcinogenesis. The conditions include those conducive to a primary infection itself, to the type of infectious process that is carcinogenic, or to the process of moving cancer precursors toward full malignancy.

While all of these roles involving infection may be thought of as causative, the main focus of this book will be on *direct* causes; the one exception to this guideline may be the bacterium *Helicobacter pylori* (see Chapter 9). Apart from the benefit of reducing the scope of the discussion, the rationale for mostly limiting the focus to direct causes is that the selected infections may offer the clearest, most productive, and possibly most efficient targets for prevention of cancer. In other words, controlling direct causes related to infection promises to produce a predictable and potentially dramatic decrease in cancer incidence.

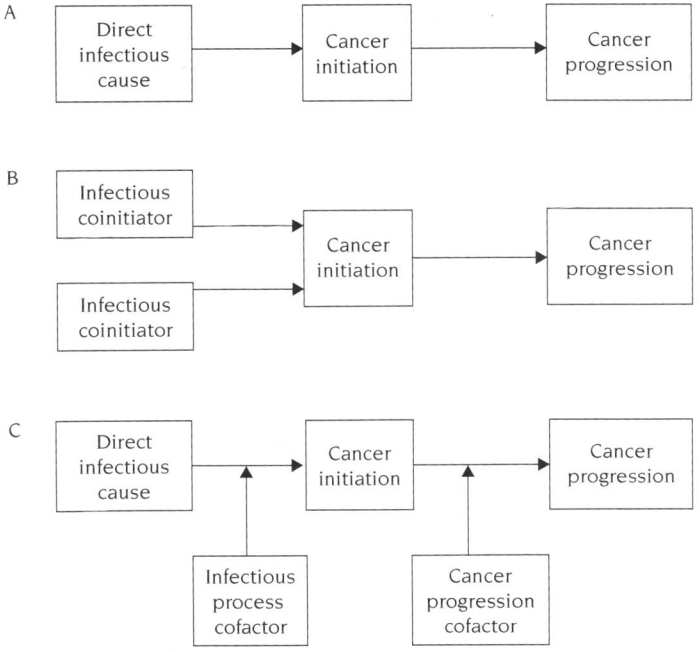

Figure 1.2. Causal pathways in infection and cancer.

INCLUDED INFECTIONS

The criteria indicated above generated the following inventory of infectious agents of cancer as an outline for the book:

- Human papillomavirus
- Hepatitis B and C viruses
- *Helicobacter pylori*
- Epstein-Barr virus
- Human herpesvirus type 8
- Human T-cell lymphotropic virus type 1

This table of contents presupposes that the best way to approach the topic is from the point of view of the infection. Another possibility would be to organize the discussion around the related cancers, and then to highlight the infectious cause(s) within the spectrum of risk factors that may be involved. The closest the book came to this approach was amalgamating the discussions of hepatitis B and C viruses in one chapter, driven by their common etiologic link with liver cancer. In fact, a subset of the scientific literature does approach the topic of infectious agents from

Table 1.1. Investigational Infectious Agents with Cancer Association

Viruses	Bacteria	Fungi	Protozoa	Worms and Flukes
Human herpesvirus 1	Borrelia burgdorferi	Epidermophyton floccosum	Plasmodium spp. (Malaria)	Clonorchis sinensis
Human herpesvirus 2	Campylobacter jejuni	Microsporum canis	Trichomonas vaginalis	Opisthorchis felineus
Human cytomegalovirus	Helicobacter bilis	Fonsecaea pedrosoi	Cryptosporidium parvum	Opisthorchis viverrini
Human herpesvirus 6	Helicobacter heimannii			Schistosoma haematobium
Adenovirus	Helicobacter hepaticus		Toxoplasma gondii	Schistosoma japonicum
Human adenovirus 5	Escherichia coli			Schistosoma mansoni
BK polyomavirus	Salmonella typhi			Taenia solium
JC polyomavirus	Lawsonia intracellularis			Strongyloides stercoralis
Merkel cell polyomavirus	Bartonella spp.			
Simian virus 40	Chlamydia pneumoniae			
B19 virus	Chlamydia psittaci			
Human mammary tumour virus	Chlamydia trachomatis			
Melanoma-associated retrovirus	Mycoplasma spp.			
Mouse mammary tumour virus	Mycobacterium tuberculosis			
Human T-cell lymphotropic virus 2	Streptococcus infantarius (or bovis)			
Hepatitis delta virus				
Measles virus				
Torque teno virus				

the starting point of a particular cancer of interest.[30] But, in addition to the complication of navigating through a large number of cancers and the maze of noninfectious causal factors, a discussion consistently oriented toward cancer would too often require dealing with multiple infectious agents for the same malignancy. For example, gastric lymphomas are caused by both *H. pylori* and EBV. Similarly, the same agent would keep emerging for different types of cancers; EBV, which causes a remarkable range of malignancies, again provides a good example of that scenario. In the end, allowing the infectious agent to drive the discussion seemed like the most straightforward approach, especially given that the prevention agenda of this book is meant to focus precisely on *the agent*.

The de facto "table of contents" for the book is dominated by viruses, a feature that also marks the broader inventory of infectious causes of cancer that have ever been investigated (as summarized in Table 1.1). This imbalance is not surprising, given that viruses are, in their essence, genetic disrupters, and thus natural engines of cancer.

Table 1.2. Infectious Agents and Associated Cancers Canada, 1995–2004

Infectious Agent	Main Associated Cancers	Males	Females
Human papillomavirus (HPV)	Cervix	—	8.36
	Anus	1.27	1.29
	Vulva/Vagina	—	3.20*
	Penis	0.82	—
	Oropharyngeal	0.51	0.16
	Larynx	6.19	1.16
	Esophageal	5.94	1.79
	Non-melanoma Skin	1.16	0.85
Hepatitis B/C virus (HBV, HCV)	Liver	4.75	1.40
Helicobacter pylori	Stomach	12.23	5.36
Epstein-Barr virus (EBV)	Hodgkin's disease	3.04	2.44
	Nasopharyngeal carcinoma	0.91	0.38
	Burkitt lymphoma	rare	rare
Human herpesvirus type 8 (HHV-8)	Kaposi sarcoma	0.65	0.06
HumanT cell lymphotrophic virus type I (HTLV-1)	Adult T cell leukemia/lymphoma	rare	rare

Age standardized cancer incidence per 100,000.
Standardized to 1991 population.
*Used the rate for "other female genital organs."
Source: Public Health Agency of Canada—Cancer Surveillance Online.

The list of included infections fulfills a criterion implied earlier; in short, the selected agents generate the majority of infection-related cancers known in the world.[31] As an illustration of the overall burden, Table 1.2 details the Canadian incidence rates for the cancers actually caused by the infections that are the focus of the book.

EXCLUDED INFECTIONS

Possibly the most noticeable omission from the selected agents is human immunodeficiency virus (HIV), the causal agent for acquired immunodeficiency syndrome (AIDS). HIV/AIDS is associated with a short list of so-called AIDS-defining cancers, as well as a longer list of other (non-defining) cancers.[32] The "defining" rubric means that, when the cancer is ruled in and other causes of immunosuppression are ruled out, the patient is clinically defined as having AIDS. The cancers in question, along with various nonmalignant conditions, show up preferentially in HIV-positive individuals. Indeed, detecting one of the defining conditions can permit a diagnosis of AIDS even in the absence of positive HIV serology.[33]

Not including HIV among the infections of interest essentially means acknowledging that the virus is not a *direct* cause of cancer. In fact, evidence suggests that HIV is probably an indirect cause, in the sense described earlier. Thus, it promotes other infections and infectious processes that may lead to cancer; HIV accomplishes this specifically by causing the immunosuppression that permits persistent coinfections and ultimately the development of cancer. What is sometimes missed in this story is the fact that *all* of the AIDS-defining cancers are *directly caused* by such coinfections.[34] This includes Kaposi sarcoma (caused by HHV-8), non-Hodgkin's lymphoma (the varieties caused by EBV), and invasive cervical cancer (which is, of course, HPV-related). This fact alone clearly positions HIV as an important collateral topic in the field of infections and cancer, even though it does not warrant a separate chapter in this book.

The categorization of HIV as essentially an *indirect* cause of cancer is consistent with the work of other authorities. For example, zur Hausen does not include HIV as a chapter in his 2006 monograph on the infectious agents of cancer.[35] A major 2008 review article on infections and cancer adopted the same perspective, concluding that "HIV...is not carcinogenic per se."[36]

HIV, though, is only the "tip of the iceberg" in terms of agents that could be considered as part of a more encyclopedic treatment of the topic. The basic scientific research and academic publishing on infections and cancer has been steadily expanding. Table 1.1 summarizes the list of investigational infectious agents pursued by researchers in recent decades. (More details, including the suggested cancer associations and a bibliography, are provided in the Conclusion.)

While dominated by viruses and bacteria, the agents of interest come from all parts of the microbial spectrum. There are many intriguing research areas suggested by the list in Table 1.1, including the potential involvement of a range of human herpesviruses.[37] Finding a role for multiple herpesviruses in cancer may not be surprising, as there is no clear biological reason why carcinogenesis should be restricted to just two herpesvirus types, EBV and HHV-8. Similarly, it does not seem plausible that the story of bacteria and cancer would start and end with merely one species of *Helicobacter*. Nonetheless, based on the reasoning already laid out, the seven selected agents appear to be the most defensible candidates for the present review, especially in the context of compelling prevention priorities.

Having refined the criteria and argued for the agents to include, it must be admitted that some of the exclusions are mostly a matter of scoping. The most obvious omission of this sort would be certain species of *Schistosoma*, flukes with proven links to hepatocellular carcinoma and urinary bladder cancer. This certainly is a genus of persistent concern in endemic regions, and it may even have growing implications for countries with high levels of immigration from endemic regions. *Schistosoma* would clearly be the logical candidate for another category of infectious agents to consider, though other flukes, worms, and protozoa might try to squeeze onto the list as well.[38]

PREVENTION PERSPECTIVE

As suggested above, the prevention perspective is the particular value that the present book seeks to add to the discussion of infectious causes of cancer. In particular, the critical role of primary prevention has been highlighted. It seemed important to organize the proven and potential interventions so that classic primary prevention categories were well delineated. In this way, health care planners can easily see where their proposed maneuvers fit on the prevention spectrum, thereby promoting comprehensive decisions and clear communication.

Figure 1.3 situates the prevention categories logically along the idealized pathogenetic pathway suggested earlier in this Introduction.

14   HPV and Other Infectious Agents in Cancer

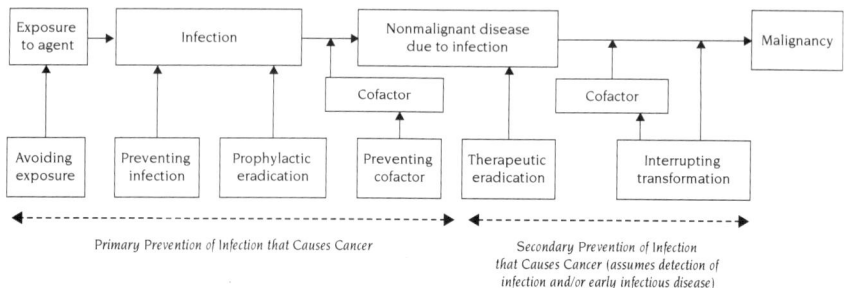

Figure 1.3. Prevention options in infection-related carcinogenesis.

The qualifiers "primary" and "secondary" are so inconsistently applied in the world of prevention as to render them almost useless. The terms are employed in a very precise way in Figure 1.3: primary prevention of infection that causes cancer (and thus prevention of the related cancer) and secondary prevention of infection that causes cancer (and thus prevention of the related cancer). Both of these categories are defined *from the perspective of infection*, which in fact is the focus of this book. Thus, secondary prevention in this context builds on the reality that an infection (and possibly early infectious disease) is established, and indeed detected, in an individual. This is what "secondary" logically means in the specific context of the book; it refers to prevention that is appropriate when primary prevention measures against the infection have "failed."

It is important to acknowledge that this definition is different than what secondary prevention denotes when the perspective is shifted to the cancer itself. In fact, the classic secondary approaches to cancer prevention (detecting and treating precursors or early malignancies) are *not* the main agenda of the book (and therefore are not reflected in Figure 1.3). This is notwithstanding the fact that infection can play a role in secondary prevention of cancer as well. For instance, there is evidence that clearing infections at late stages of carcinogenesis can sometimes be beneficial as an adjunct to therapy or surgery, specifically by promoting remission and/or preventing recurrence.

To sum up, the terms primary and secondary are specifically used in this book to distinguish two important overarching prevention contexts: first, the clinical situation before known infection and early infectious disease are in place; and, second, the scenario where infection is already established and indeed detected. Each of these two contexts incorporates multiple prevention categories, which will in turn be applied to each infectious agent throughout the book. The six prevention categories are identified in Figure 1.3. They each have a clear connection to infection per se; they intersect with the carcinogenic pathway at distinct points, all of which *precede* the emergence of frank malignancy.

The prevention perspective has informed other components of the book. For instance, given the direct link between transmission routes and exposure prevention, that part of the natural history of each target infection has been thoroughly described. Unfortunately, transmission is sometimes a poorly elucidated subject, which in turn limits the development and application of related primary prevention measures. Given this particular knowledge gap, the ongoing drive toward other types of primary prevention (especially vaccination) is even more understandable.

At the other end of the pathogenetic pathway, where the focus is on interrupting transformation, it is important to recognize that the methods of interest still relate directly to infection, rather than to medical or surgical interventions for premalignant disease. The idea is to review any therapies that act directly on the infectious processes that lead to cancer. This explains why the overview of each infection includes a section on disease mechanisms. Finally, given that detection of the agent is a prerequisite implied by the meta-category of "secondary prevention of infection that causes cancer," a synopsis of detection methods relevant to each agent has been provided.

The taxonomy of prevention approaches suggested above will become clearer once it is applied to the first agent covered in the book, human papillomavirus (see Chapter 7). It will become apparent that the last two categories, therapeutic eradication/suppression and interrupting malignant transformation, sometimes coincide with treatments for the various premalignancies and early cancer stages preceding invasive cervical cancer. The practical overlap between prevention and treatment modalities simply underlines the fact that the objective of therapy is a "moving target" throughout the natural history of HPV disease. Thus, one passes from primary prevention related to controlling HPV infection per se, through intermediate stages of premalignant development that call for other types of management, and finally to the point where advanced precursors or early cancer is clearly in place. For the purposes of this book, the very end of this disease succession is considered to be the target of classic secondary prevention maneuvers well known to oncologists. As such, these approaches are not the main focus of the book. However, given the dominant position that HPV-related disease holds in the contemporary discussion of infections and cancer, some background on screening for cervical lesions will be offered as a convenience (see Chapter 6); screening, of course, is the normal precursor to classic secondary preventive treatments such as ablation.[39]

PLAN OF THE BOOK

The main thrust of each chapter of the book is a standard literature review. Academic journals were consulted using established search procedures applied to Medline (e.g., simply coordinating terms such as "HPV" and "cancer"). High-quality review articles by recognized experts provided a foundation, but individual studies were also consulted, especially to fill in more recent results on matters of interest (e.g., "EBV" coordinated with "transmission"). Apart from a few instances, there was no lack of information on the selected infectious agents. As already noted, the infection–cancer connection has become a prolific area of research and publishing. The intention was to comprehensively cover the most recent literature published, up to early 2009.

The knowledge gleaned from journal articles and selected gray literature sources was organized into similar chapter sections for each infection, as follows:

- The virus (or bacterium, in the case of *H. pylori*)
- Evidence of associated cancers
- Transmission and occurrence of the agent
- Disease mechanisms
- Detection methods
- Prevention approaches

The one deviation from this pattern involved the coverage of HPV. The sheer volume of literature related to this virus and its many related cancers, recently augmented by burgeoning research on the development and implementation of a prophylactic vaccine, necessitated a much fuller review. To avoid a single unwieldy chapter, eventually six were developed for this agent alone. These were combined as Chapters 2–7 of the book, with the rest of the infectious agents covered in Chapters 8–13. This may give the book an unbalanced appearance. However, the value of in-depth coverage of HPV will soon become clear. Such an approach allowed this virus to serve as a paradigm for both the biological understanding of and the comprehensive prevention responses to each of the infectious agents covered in the book. Since HPV continues to be a key driver of the intensifying interest in infectious agents and cancer, it is only appropriate that the book begins with a comprehensive consideration of this now-famous virus.

NOTES

1. Elgui de Oliveira D. DNA viruses in human cancer: an integrated overview on fundamental mechanisms of viral carcinogenesis. *Cancer Letters.* 2007; 247(2):182–96.
2. Epstein MA. Historical background. *Philosophical Transactions of the Royal Society of London. Series B, Biological Sciences.* 2001; 356(1408): 413–20.
3. Syrjanen S, Syrjanen K. The history of papillomavirus research. *Central European Journal of Public Health.* 2008; 16(suppl): S7–13.
4. Young LS, Rickinson AB. Epstein-Barr virus: 40 years on. *Nature Reviews.* 2004; 4(10): 757–68.
5. Bertout J, Thomas-Tikhonenko A. Infection & neoplastic growth 101: the required reading for microbial pathogens aspiring to cause cancer. *Cancer Treatment and Research.* 2006; 130: 167–97.
6. Martin GS. The road to Src. *Oncogene.* 2004; 23(48): 7910–7.
7. Varmus HE, Vogt PK, Bishop JM. The classic: integration of deoxyribonucleic acid specific for Rous sarcoma virus after infection of permissive and nonpermissive hosts: (RNA tumor viruses/reassociation kinetics/duck cells). 1973. *Clinical Orthopaedics and Related Research.* 2008; 466(9): 2031–8.
8. Elgui de Oliveira D. DNA viruses in human cancer: an integrated overview on fundamental mechanisms of viral carcinogenesis. *Cancer Letters.* 2007; 247(2): 182–96.
9. Aaltonen LM, Rihkanen H, Vaheri A. Human papillomavirus in larynx. *Laryngoscope.* 2002; 112(4): 700–7.
10. zur Hausen H. Papillomaviruses in the causation of human cancers—a brief historical account. *Virology.* 2009; 384(2): 260–5.
11. van Helvoort T. A dispute over scientific credibility: the struggle for an independent institute for cancer research in pre-World War II Berlin. *Studies in History and Philosophy of Biological and Biomedical Sciences.* 2000; 31(2): 315–54.
12. Pagano JS. Epstein-Barr virus: the first human tumor virus and its role in cancer. *Proceedings of the Association of American Physicians.* 1999; 111(6): 573–80.
13. Coakley D. Denis Burkitt and his contribution to haematology/oncology. *British Journal of Haematology.* 2006; 135(1): 17–25.
14. Epstein MA, Achong BG, Barr YM. Virus particles in cultured lymphoblasts from Burkitt's lymphoma. *The Lancet.* 1964; 1(7335): 702–3.
15. Some authorities mark the beginning of the human infection-cancer story to the characterization of hepatitis B virus in 1963. See Kuper H, Adami HO, Trichopoulos D. Infections as a major preventable cause of human cancer. *Journal of Internal Medicine.* 2000; 248(3): 171–83.
16. The total is composed of 7.7% of cancers in the developed world (390,000) and 26.3% in the developing (1.5 million). See Parkin DM. The global health burden of infection-associated cancers in the year 2002. *International Journal of Cancer.* 2006; 118(12): 3030–44.
17. Sobol RE. The rationale for prophylactic cancer vaccines and need for a paradigm shift. *Cancer Gene Therapy.* 2006; 13(8): 725–31.
18. Segal BH, Freifeld AG, Baden LR et al. Prevention and treatment of cancer-related infections. *Journal of the National Comprehensive Cancer Network.* 2008; 6(2): 122–74.

19 Ljungman P, de la Camara R, Cordonnier C et al. Management of CMV, HHV-6, HHV-7 and Kaposi-sarcoma herpesvirus (HHV-8) infections in patients with hematological malignancies and after SCT. *Bone Marrow Transplantation.* 2008; 42(4): 227–40.
20 Liu TC, Kirn D. Systemic efficacy with oncolytic virus therapeutics: clinical proof-of-concept and future directions. *Cancer Research.* 2007; 67(2): 429–32.
21 Sorensen MR, Thomsen AR. Virus-based immunotherapy of cancer: what do we know and where are we going? *APMIS.* 2007; 115(11): 1177–93.
22 zur Hausen H. *Infections Causing Human Cancer.* Heidelberg: Wiley-VCH; 2006.
23 Shared with two of the discoverers of the human immunodeficiency virus (HIV).
24 Goedert JJ. *Infectious Causes of Cancer: Targets for Intervention.* New Jersey: Humana Press Inc.; 2000.
25 Carrillo-Infante C, Abbadessa G, Bagella L et al. Viral infections as a cause of cancer (review). *International Journal of Oncology.* 2007; 30(6): 1521–8.
26 McLaughlin-Drubin ME, Munger K. Viruses associated with human cancer. *Biochimica et Biophysica Acta.* 2008; 1782(3): 127–50.
27 de Martel C, Franceschi S. Infections and cancer: established associations and new hypotheses. *Critical Reviews in Oncology/Hematology.* 2009; 70(3): 183–94.
28 Franco EL, Correa P, Santella RM et al. Role and limitations of epidemiology in establishing a causal association. *Seminars in Cancer Biology.* 2004; 14(6): 413–26.
29 Underbrink MP, Hoskins SL, Pou AM et al. Viral interaction: a possible contributing factor in head and neck cancer progression. *Acta Oto-Laryngologica.* 2008; 128(12): 1361–9.
30 For example, Al-Daraji WI, Smith JH. Infection and cervical neoplasia: facts and fiction. *International Journal of Clinical and Experimental Pathology.* 2009; 2(1): 48–64; Hjalgrim H, Engels EA. Infectious aetiology of Hodgkin and non-Hodgkin lymphomas: a review of the epidemiological evidence. *Journal of Internal Medicine.* 2008; 264(6): 537–48; Selgrad M, Malfertheiner P, Fini L et al. The role of viral and bacterial pathogens in gastrointestinal cancer. *Journal of Cellular Physiology.* 2008; 216(2): 378–88; Burnett-Hartman AN, Newcomb PA, Potter JD. Infectious agents and colorectal cancer: a review of Helicobacter pylori, Streptococcus bovis, JC virus, and human papillomavirus. *Cancer Epidemiology, Biomarkers and Prevention.* 2008; 17(11): 2970–9; Hengge UR. Role of viruses in the development of squamous cell cancer and melanoma. *Advances in Experimental Medicine and Biology.* 2008; 624: 179–86; Verma V, Shen D, Sieving PC et al. The role of infectious agents in the etiology of ocular adnexal neoplasia. *Survey of Ophthalmology.* 2008; 53(4): 312–31.
31 Parkin DM. The global health burden of infection-associated cancers in the year 2002. *International Journal of Cancer.* 2006; 118(12): 3030–44.
32 AIDS-defining cancers classically comprise Kaposi sarcoma, high-grade non-Hodgkin's lymphoma, and invasive cervical cancer. Non AIDS-defining cancers (i.e., with increased incidence in HIV-infected adults) include: anal cancer, Hodgkin's disease, head and neck cancer, testicular cancer, lung cancer, colon cancer, basal cell carcinoma of the skin, squamous cell carcinoma of the skin, and melanoma. See Cooley TP. Non-AIDS-defining cancer in HIV-infected people. *Hematology/Oncology Clinics of North America.* 2003; 17(3): 889–99.

33 Bower M, Mazhar D, Stebbing J. Should cervical cancer be an acquired immunodeficiency syndrome—defining cancer? *Journal of Clinical Oncology*. 2006; 24(16): 2417–19.
34 Boshoff C, Weiss R. AIDS-related malignancies. *Nature Reviews: Cancer*. 2002; 2(5): 373–82.
35 zur Hausen H. *Infections Causing Human Cancer*. Heidelberg: Wiley-VCH; 2006.
36 de Martel C, Franceschi S. Infections and cancer: established associations and new hypotheses. *Critical Reviews in Oncology/Hematology*. 2009; 70(3): 183–94.
37 See, for example, Leite JL, Stolf HO, Reis NA et al. Human herpesvirus type 6 and type 1 infection increases susceptibility to nonmelanoma skin tumors. *Cancer Letters*. 2005; 224(2): 213–9.
38 Mayer DA, Fried B. The role of helminth infections in carcinogenesis. *Advances in Parasitology*. 2007; 65: 239–96.
39 Ablation refers to the removal or destruction of a body part or tissue or its function. Ablation may be performed by surgery, hormones, drugs, lasers, radiation, heat, freezing, or other methods.

2

HUMAN PAPILLOMAVIRUS: STRUCTURE, TRANSMISSION, AND OCCURRENCE

Papillomaviruses have proved to be the most complex group of human pathogenic viruses....[1]

These are the words Harald zur Hausen used to characterize research progress on the human papillomavirus (HPV) up to 1999, a story that has only continued to expand and accelerate in the decade since.

HPV is a ubiquitous microbe found in a majority of epithelial tissues in males and females, and sometimes in tumors. The biological, clinical, and economic implications of this pathogen are profound. Indeed, since the recognition of its close association with cervical precursor lesions in the 1970s, HPV has emerged as the most important human tumor virus.[2] This virus has always been with us, as have the diseases with which it is associated. In short, there is no era in history when human beings have not been afflicted by cervical cancer and genital warts.[3]

The motivation to pursue primary prevention initiatives related to HPV is not hard to find. Demographic changes in the high-risk region of Latin America and the Caribbean suggest that actual burden of new cervical cancer cases will still increase by 75% in the next 20 years.[4] Furthermore, the present impact of disease is substantial even in areas with well-established secondary prevention programs. The annual incidence of cervical cancer in the United States is over 10,000, with an estimated 4,000 women dying from the disease each year.[5]

As a family, papillomaviruses demonstrate both exquisite simplicity and extreme complexity, leading researchers to ponder the following related questions: How can one of the smallest of all viruses, with DNA coding for very few proteins (only eight in the case of HPV), manage to have such a devastating disease impact on humans and a wide range of other vertebrates, even to the point of causing death? Even more importantly, how can the burden of such afflictions be avoided?

COMPLEX CONNECTIONS TO CANCER

The topic of human papillomavirus (HPV) and cancer is a highly dynamic area of research because it represents not only a significant story but a very complex one. At least three dimensions of complexity can be identified.

First, the virus exhibits remarkable genetic variation. In fact, HPV is an umbrella term for a wide array of viral types, subtypes, and variants. More than 150 HPV types have been identified so far, and at least 50 others are presumed to exist.[6,7] Furthermore, the distribution of types varies geographically, possibly calling for approaches to disease control tailored for different regions.

Second, the connections to disease, and especially to cancer, are diverse. Approximately 40 known viral types infect the human genital tract; of these, up to half appear to be oncogenic. Classically, the types that cause high-grade cervical intraepithelial neoplasia (CIN) and cervical cancer have been labeled as high risk. These types also cause a pathologically distinct group of oropharyngeal tumors. Other HPVs are associated with cutaneous tumors, in particular epidermodysplasia verruciformis and nonmelanoma skin cancers. Still other viral types, usually described as low risk (as oncogenic agents), have been implicated in benign diseases such as genital warts. Finally, some types play a role in both malignant and benign disease.

Third, subtle yet powerful strategies are employed by the virus to evade the human immune system, infect cells, and produce new viruses (or, in some cases, effect neoplastic transformation). In fact, much more remains to be discovered about the molecular processes involved, including a full explanation for why only a small percentage of infections, even those with viral types of known oncogenic properties, lead to cancer.

There are also a number of simpler aspects of HPV. For instance, the majority of cancer-causing forms are related genetically to two main types, HPV-16 and HPV-18.[8,9] Indeed, these two types together may account for 70–75% of cervical cancer cases (an increase from earlier estimates of 50%).[10–12] Of the two, HPV-16 is the most pathogenic, conferring (in the words of a 2007 report) "by far the highest risk of high-grade CIN lesions and cervical cancer."[13]

The information about HPV-16 is especially pertinent because of the central importance of cervical cancer in the HPV story. But new parts of that story are now ranging well beyond the cervical cancer theme, a fact that has not been well reflected in some recent textbooks on HPV.[14] In addition to several other serious malignancies, HPV-related benign diseases must also be included in any comprehensive discussion. Indeed, the first licensed prophylactic vaccine not only targets HPV-16 and 18 but also HPV-6 and 11, the principal known causal agents of benign genital warts.

In short, contrary to popular impression, HPV is not solely about cervical cancer. Academic and clinical investigations continue to be propelled by the growing evidence of HPV as a causal agent for a wide array of tumors and other diseases. Table 2.1 summarizes the current understanding of the etiologic links to various HPV types (see Chapters 4 and 5 for additional details).[15]

Table 2.1. Known Clinical Burden of HPV Infection

	Proportion of Cases Due to HPV Infection	Proportion of HPV-Related Cases by HPV Type			
		16	18	6	11
Cancers					
Cancer of the cervix	100%	55%	13%		
Ano-genital cancers					
Cancer of the vulva	44%	67%	9%		
Cancer of the vagina	57%	51%	8%		
Cancer of the penis	47%	68%	3%	7%	
Cancer of the anus	78%	78%	6%	1%	1%
Head and neck cancers					
Cancer of the larynx	25%	65%	19%		
Oral cancers	30%	73%	28%		
Cancer of the tonsils	41%	87%	2%		
Sinonasal cancers	22%	100%	0%		
Cancer of the ocular surface	78%	50%	50%		
Total—Cancers	58%	62%	11%	<1%	<1%
Nonmalignant Diseases					
Genital warts	100%			90%	
Recurrent respiratory papillomatosis	76%			60%	40%
Sinonasal papilloma	33%			Primary	
Conjunctival papilloma	92%			85%	
Total—Nonmalignant diseases	100%	0%	0%	>90%	

Two things are immediately apparent from the table: the great variety of malignant and benign diseases that are associated with HPV, and the variable propensity of different types of the virus to cause any one condition (e.g., HPV-16 causing about four times the amount of cervical cancer as HPV-18). What will become evident on closer examination of the biological evidence is a very important common feature: most, if not all, of the diseases related to HPV are marked by the singular affinity of the virus for epithelial tissue. This will be explored in greater detail in Chapter 3.

While the cancers in Table 2.1 cannot be discounted in terms of morbidity and mortality, few could be characterized as common within the spectrum of human malignancies. One exception is cervical cancer, which is the second most frequent female cancer worldwide (only exceeded by breast cancer). Considerable energy has been devoted to finding a connection between HPV and other tumors with a high population burden; this has included investigations related to cancer of the lung, female breast, prostate, and colorectum, among other sites. Although most of the data related to such tumors remain equivocal, there is certainly potential to increase the list of HPV-related cancers in the future. This possibility becomes more pointed when one realizes the importance of epithelial tumors (i.e., carcinoma) in the total spectrum of cancer, and recalls that HPV specifically targets epithelial cells. Malignancies of epithelial tissue are in fact the most common form of cancer, and are responsible for 95% of cancer mortality.[16,17] While admittedly only a tiny fraction of this toll has been explicitly linked to HPV, given the "skill" demonstrated by the virus in exploiting epithelial cells, it is likely that the final chapter on HPV infection and associated disease has yet to be written.

EVOLVING RESEARCH

The scholarly literature associated with HPV in relation to cancer has been accelerating in recent years. The difficulty in trying to keep up with the literature is underlined by the current definitive textbook on the biology of infections and cancer, which covers material published up to early 2005.[18] A comprehensive review of the research on HPV and cancer in the subsequent 3 years would involve over 3,000 new articles. This number is multiplied several times over when other infectious agents are brought into the discussion. With respect to HPV alone, the challenge for a review project such as the current book has only intensified with the volume of reports on the vaccines aimed at combating the virus and its associated diseases.

As noted in the Introduction, a similar pattern will be followed in dealing with each of the oncogenic agents covered in this book: discussing the biology of the virus and its transmission, occurrence, and disease-causing mechanisms; reviewing the connection to specific malignancies; and examining the basic approaches to cancer prevention.

In the case of HPV, the sheer volume of information requires six chapters. Such an extensive review is justifiable given the current level of scientific interest and policy implications surrounding HPV and cancer prevention, including the very current topic of prophylactic vaccines.

Following the present chapter, which overviews the basic structure, transmission and occurrence of the virus, material will be grouped under the following chapter headings:

- Infection, Natural History, and Carcinogenesis
- Associations with Cervical Cancer
- Associations with Noncervical Cancers
- Detection of Infection and Disease
- Prevention of Infection and Disease

THE VIRUS

The International Committee on the Taxonomy of Viruses has formally classified papillomaviruses as a distinct viral family, the Papillomaviridae.[19] The name is derived from the common macroscopic feature of papillomavirus infection, that is, papilloma,[20] the small protuberances seen, for instance, in the case of epithelial warts.

In addition to the demonstrated pathogenic connection to human beings, papillomaviruses infect and cause disease in a range of vertebrate animals. Although papillomas are the classic attribute, benign diseases such as warts only constitute the beginning of the pathology story. Papillomavirus infection was linked to cancer from as early as 1934, when an association was observed in rabbits. The first published analysis of oncogenic HPV in humans emerged in 1972. The causal role of high-risk HPV infections in cervical cancer was finally confirmed by epidemiological studies during the 1990s.[21]

By any normal measures, a papillomavirus would have to be considered a simple entity. The complete virion comprises a protein coat (capsid) surrounding the single, circular, supercoiled, double-stranded DNA molecule. With all components assembled, each roughly spherical[22] virion has a diameter measuring about 55 nm, making them one of the smaller viruses. The particles in other viral families typically range up to six times larger.

Research on papillomavirus has gradually revealed more information on its structure and activity. The genome of HPV is organized into coding and noncoding regions. The coding segments are referred to as open reading frames (ORFs), a technical name for what is commonly understood as a gene. Eight early ORFs (labeled E1–E8) and two late ones (L1 and L2) have been identified in the coding region of papillomavirus.[23] The early ORFs encode proteins that interact with the host genome to produce new viral DNA, whereas late ORFs are activated only after viral DNA replication. The protein products are referred to by the same labels as the ORFs; the ones characterized so far include six nonstructural regulatory proteins (E1, E2, E4, E5, E6, and E7) and two structural capsid proteins (L1 and L2). E1 and E2 are especially involved with genome replication, whereas E4–E7 contribute to the initial destabilization of the host cell.[24] Two of the early viral proteins (E6 and E7) are also important in HPV-associated malignant transformation.

The various types of papillomavirus appear to be highly specific to different animal species. The one common feature is the tropism for epithelial tissues, in fact, for a particular type of epithelium found in certain body sites. It seems that HPV characteristically infects keratinocytes in stratified squamous epithelium. The mechanism by which keratinocyte differentiation interacts with HPV expression is not fully understood. What is known is the fact that the viruses replicate in the nucleus of the infected epithelial cell.

The prophylactic HPV vaccines currently in production prevent infection by inducing neutralizing antibodies against the capsid proteins L1 and L2. This approach allows a vaccinated host to offer an efficient immune response upon exposure to a new HPV infection. However, because infected and even transformed cells generally do not express L1 or L2 at an early stage, therapeutic HPV vaccines require a different strategy. They are designed to treat established infections and malignancies by targeting early nonstructural antigens related to, notably, E6 and E7.[25] The topic of vaccines will be revisited in the final chapter on HPV and cancer.

As of 2006, over 100 human and about 22 nonhuman genotypes were fully described; undoubtedly, this inventory will continue to increase.[26] Virology is the only domain in biology where taxonomy is driven completely by genomic analysis. Papillomavirus classification is based on the most conserved genetic elements, which generally excludes the E5, E6, and E7 segments; the latter elements demonstrate high divergence rates and, in fact, are absent from some papillomaviruses. Types, subtypes, and variants within the Papillomaviridae family have been classified based on the sequence of the L1 gene, though alternate paradigms are being proposed.[27] Within the overall family, related types are grouped as species and genera.

HPV types that are most closely related (i.e., forming a "species" group) tend to be associated with similar lesions in the human body. The 16 known genera are identified by Greek letters, with the most clinically important being the α-papillomaviruses. The types included in the latter category include all those associated with genital and other mucosal lesions in humans.[28]

An HPV type is defined as an isolate whose L1 gene sequence is at least 10% different from that of any other type, whereas a subtype is 2–10% different.[29] At the end of the scale, variants of HPV types differ by less than 2% of the original isolate. As HPV has not changed very much over its existence, the majority of genetic divergence is covered under the variant designation. Studies throughout the world have found that there are 20–100 common variants for each HPV type. As would be expected, variants demonstrate maximal divergence when they are sampled from ethnic groups that have long been isolated from one another (e.g., tribes of aboriginal peoples).[30] HPV variants can also be used to track patterns of migration and contact between people groups.[31]

As already noted, certain types of HPV (e.g., HPV-16 and -18) are designated high-risk or oncogenic, whereas others (e.g., HPV-6 and -11) are designated low-risk or nononcogenic.[32] Some HPV types are still being investigated in terms of their oncogenicity; when a type is suspected of having some capacity to promote cancer development, the label "intermediate risk" is occasionally used by epidemiologists. Variants of oncogenic types demonstrate differing levels of risk for cancer development. Geographic regions with a high prevalence of high-risk variants can coincide with an increased incidence of certain cancers.[33,34] This sort of geographical variation may have implications for disease control strategies such as vaccination.[35]

HPV TYPES AND LESIONS

Causation is difficult to establish with certainty in epidemiological studies.[36] In the case of HPV, however, there appears to be irrefutable evidence that certain HPV types are a necessary causal factor in cervical cancer and genital warts. The connection between HPV and epithelial disease is so strong that circumstantial evidence may be enough to "convict" HPV of pathogenesis in some new epithelial tissue. In other words, though it should not be deemed conclusive, detecting HPV DNA in affected epithelial cells is enough to create strong suspicion of an etiologic link. More caution is required when drawing conclusions from indirect assays such as serum antibodies for HPV, because immunological evidence of infection in the past offers a more tenuous causal connection with current disease.

The intensity of research into the basic structure, variation, and occurrence of HPV has been matched by studies of basic disease connections. Evidence of pathogenesis has been found for virtually every one of the 100-plus viral types distinguished and named according to the traditional method (HPV-1, HPV-2, etc.), as well for several novel types.[37] Over 300 studies from a 25-year period have detailed such results, and only a handful of more recent HPV types have not yet been definitively associated with disease.[38] To the knowledge of the authors, only one type, HPV-12, has ever been described as having no disease connection, and even this claim was subsequently proven false.[39] It is a good assumption that novel or newly characterized HPV types will also be linked to disease in the near future.

A summary of the literature reviewed is presented in Table 2.2, indicating the HPV types and selected diseases to which they have been linked. The clearly oncogenic types and other broad disease categories are indicated by shading. Several observations may be made about the disease association data:

- The classic HPV numbering system represents the approximate order of discovery and pathogenic characterization. It is apparent that the earliest disease associations detected for the virus involved benign skin warts
- The uncovering of HPV types connected with mucosal lesions, including cancer, has intensified in recent years
- Several HPV types have been numbered as discrete forms, only to be confirmed as subtypes at a later point. In fact, while HPV variants are numerous, formal subtypes (where genomic variation from a known type is more than 2% but less than 10%) are rare phenomena in the world of HPV. Beyond those indicated in Table 2.2, only two other examples have been reported: HPV-68a/b and -38a/b[40,41]
- There is essentially a balance between HPV types that target mucosal tissues and those that favor cutaneous tissues
- Reviewing the information in the full table found at www.krueger.ca, it is apparent that the mucosal HPV types "cross over" to infect cutaneous sites more often than the reverse, and that there is a special propensity for oncogenic types 16 and 18 to appear and cause lesions in many epithelial sites
- Some HPV types exhibit high specificity for particular tissues and have very distinct biological functions. Examples seen in Table 2.2 include the so-called butcher's warts (associated with HPV-7), the unique connection of HPV-6 with benign and (rarely) malignant lesions in the external auditory canal, and the strong link between HPV-1 and -60 and palmoplantar warts

Table 2.2. HPV Types and Associated Lesions

HPV Type	Typical Lesions	HPV Type	Typical Lesion(s)
1	Verruca plantaris; verruca palmaris (palmoplantar warts)	51	Cervical carcinoma
2	Verruca (skin wart)	52	Cervical carcinoma
3	Verruca plana (flat wart)	53	Cervical carcinoma
4	Verruca (skin wart)	54	*Mucosal lesions*
5	Epidermodysplasia verruciformis; skin cancer	55	(subtype of HPV-44)
6	Condyloma acuminatum (genital wart); recurrent respiratory papillomatosis; special connection: external auditory canal papilloma	56	Cervical carcinoma
7	Verruca (skin wart); special connection: Butcher's wart (hand lesion)	57	Verruca (skin wart)
8	Epidermodysplasia verruciformis; skin cancer	58	Cervical carcinoma
9	Skin cancer	59	Cervical carcinoma
10	Verruca plana (flat wart)	60	Verruca plantaris; verruca palmaris (palmoplantar warts)
11	Condyloma acuminatum (genital wart); recurrent respiratory papillomatosis	61	Cervical lesions
12	Epidermodysplasia verruciformis	62	Cervical lesions
13	Focal epithelial hyperplasia (oral lesion)	63	Skin lesions

(Continued)

Table 2.2. (Continued)

HPV Type	Typical Lesions	HPV Type	Typical Lesion(s)
14	Epidermodysplasia verruciformis	64	(subtype of HPV-34)
15	Skin cancer	65	Verruca (skin wart)
16	Cervical, anogenital, and oral carcinoma	66	Cervical carcinoma
17	Epidermodysplasia verruciformis	67	Cervical lesions
18	Cervical, anogenital, and oral carcinoma; special connection: Cervical adenocarcinoma	68	Cervical carcinoma
19	Skin cancer	69	*Cervical lesions*
20	Epidermodysplasia verruciformis; skin cancer	70	Cervical carcinoma
21	Epidermodysplasia verruciformis	71	Cervical lesions
22	*Skin cancer*	72	Oral lesions
23	Skin cancer	73	Cervical carcinoma
24	Epidermodysplasia verruciformis; skin cancer	74	Condyloma acuminatum (genital wart)
25	Epidermodysplasia verruciformis; skin cancer	75	*Verruca (wart)*
26	*Condyloma acuminatum (genital wart)*	76	*Verruca (wart)*
27	Verruca (skin wart)	77	*Verruca (wart)*
28	Verruca plana (flat wart)	78	*Verruca (wart)*
29	*Verruca (skin wart)*	79	Condyloma acuminatum (genital wart)
30	Cervical lesions	80	*Verruca (wart)*
31	Cervical carcinoma	81	Mucosal lesions
32	Focal epithelial hyperplasia (oral lesion)	82	Cervical carcinoma

33	Cervical carcinoma	83	Mucosal lesions
34	Cervical lesions	84	Condyloma acuminatum (genital wart)
35	Cervical carcinoma	85	Cervical lesions
36	Epidermodysplasia verruciformis	86	Anal lesions
37	Epidermodysplasia verruciformis; skin cancer	87	Mucosal lesions
38	Skin cancer	88	*Skin lesions*
39	Cervical carcinoma	89	Anal lesions
40	Verruca (skin wart)	90	Cervical lesions
41	Verruca (skin wart)	91	Anal lesions
42	Cervical lesions	92	Skin lesions
43	Cervical lesions	93	*Skin cancer*
44	Cervical lesions	94	*Verucca plana*
45	Cervical carcinoma	95	*Pigmented wart*
46	(subtype of HPV-20)	96	*Skin cancer*
47	Epidermodysplasia verrucifor mis	97-100	Disease uncharacterized
48	*Skin lesions*	101	*Cervical lesions*
49	Verruca (skin wart)	102	Disease uncharacterized
50	Epidermodysplasia verruciformis	103	*Cervical lesions*

Legend
Mucosal Carcinoma — HPV Type
Other Mucosal Lesions — HPV Type
Skin Cancer or Precursor — HPV Type
Other Skin Lesions — HPV Type

Note: Italics indicates limited evidence.

The use of genomic information to drive viral classification has been described. The strong link between genetic categories and disease associations is displayed in Figure 2.1.[42] The distinctive genome-disease connections raise the possibility that simply locating a novel HPV type within a known genus and species would allow for sound predictions concerning the tissue tropism and pathology of the new virus.

Genus	Species	Prototype	Other types →									
α-papillomavirus	1	HPV-32	HPV-42									
	2	HPV-10	HPV-3	HPV-28	HPV-29	HPV-78	HPV-94					
	3	HPV-61	HPV-62	HPV-72	HPV-81	HPV-83	HPV-84	HPV-86	HPV-87	HPV-89		
	4	HPV-2	HPV-27	HPV-57								
	5	HPV-26	HPV-51	HPV-69	HPV-82							
	6	HPV-53	HPV-30	HPV-56	HPV-66							
	7	HPV-18	HPV-39	HPV-45	HPV-59	HPV-68	HPV-70	HPV-85				
	8	HPV-7	HPV-40	HPV-43	HPV-91							
	9	HPV-16	HPV-31	HPV-33	HPV-35	HPV-52	HPV-58	HPV-67				
	10	HPV-6	HPV-11	HPV-13	HPV-44	HPV-74						
	11	HPV-34	HPV-73									
	13	HPV-54										
	14	HPV-90										
	15	HPV-71										
β-papillomavirus	1	HPV-5	HPV-8	HPV-12	HPV-14	HPV-19	HPV-20	HPV-21	HPV-24	HPV-25	HPV-36	HPV-47	HPV-93
	2	HPV-9	HPV-15	HPV-17	HPV-22	HPV-23	HPV-37	HPV-38	HPV-80			
	3	HPV-49	HPV-75	HPV-76								
	4	HPV-92										
	5	HPV-96										
γ-papillomavirus	1	HPV-4	HPV-65	HPV-95								
	2	HPV-48										
	3	HPV-50										
	4	HPV-60										
	5	HPV-88										
μ-papillomavirus	1	HPV-1										
	2	HPV-63										
υ-papillomavirus	1	HPV-41										

Legend
Mucosal carcinoma — **HPV Type**
Other mucosal lesions — HPV Type
Skin cancer or precursor — **HPV Type**
Other skin lesions — HPV Type

Figure 2.1. Disease characteristics of HPV genera and species. *Source:* de Villiers et al., *Virology*, 2004. Used by permission.

TRANSMISSION OF THE VIRUS

HPV is the most common sexually transmitted infection in the world, demonstrating a lifetime risk of infection among women of up to 80%.[43,44]

The primary mode of anogenital HPV transmission appears to be sexual intercourse. Studies show that the number of recent sexual partners is significantly associated with the incidence of HPV infection.[45,46] Generally, the highest risk of testing positive for HPV is in the first few years after the initiation of intercourse. HPV positivity (and thus infectiousness) tends to decline with age, a result of the transient nature of most HPV infections following effective suppression by the host immune system. This basic age-specific pattern, while generally observed across developed countries, does not hold true in every region of the world (see the next section on "Occurrence of the Virus").

Concordance of HPV genotypes found in sexual couples offers strong direct evidence of transmission. For example, a recent case study from Italy discovered the same five types in the male and female partner, HPV-6, -16, -53, -73, and -84.[47] Transmission appears to operate in both directions in the context of heterosexual intercourse. Infection with HPV is frequent in male sexual partners of women with cervical lesions.[48] Likewise, men with low-risk HPV-related genital warts or high-grade penile neoplasms spread HPV efficiently to their sexual partners. Flat, subclinical penile lesions have recently been shown to be a more frequent manifestation of high-risk HPV infection in men. These lesions may represent a substantial reservoir of HPV and thus a source of transmission to sexual partners.[49] Anal cancer has been associated with both high-risk HPV infection and the practice of receptive anal intercourse in individuals of both sexes, providing strong evidence that penetrative sexual activity is involved in viral transmission.[50] Other aspects of anogenital infection in men will be discussed in Chapter 5.

Other modes of sexual transmission under investigation include nonpenetrative activities (including oral-genital contact).[51] In this regard, women who have sex with women have been cautioned against being too complacent about their HPV status, even if one or the other partner has had no sexual contact with men.[52]

The specific mechanism of transmission of oral HPV infection in either gender has not yet been elucidated. Sexual transmission generally does not seem to be a satisfactory explanation, given that the oral HPV types found in sexual partners are generally not concordant.[53] An obvious suspect route such as oral-genital contact has not been clearly linked to oral HPV infection in the past.[54] However, newer data have revived the possibility of penile-oral transmission.[55] Direct mouth-to-mouth transmission cannot be ruled out; this potential route recently surfaced in a case report of a married couple where each partner had head and neck cancer caused by a genetically identical strain of HPV-16.[56] A recent prospective study of spouses in Finland detected only one statistically significant association: persistent oral HPV infection in an individual led to a 10-fold increase in the risk of persistent oral infection in their spouse.[57] This topic will be revisited in the discussion of HPV and head and neck cancers in Chapter 5.

Compounding the mystery of oral transmission, it seems that individual women can harbor different types of HPV in their genital and oral mucosa simultaneously. Despite these findings, skin-to-hand-to-mouth transfer (so-called autoinoculation) has been posited as one possible route of oral HPV infection.

All of the topics related to sexual transmission remain contentious. Indeed, it is difficult to track the full story concerning any type of HPV transmission given the phenomena of subclinical infection, high rates of viral clearance, and the often long latency period prior to the development of any disease symptoms. Adding to the complexity is the fact that HPV can remain infectious within shed (and even desiccated) epithelial cells for up to 1 week. Given the current knowledge about the natural history of the virus, it is not surprising that the evidence for nonsexual transmission of HPV has remained equivocal. For example, though limited research has shown that the virus may be transmitted via fomites (substances or articles such as swabs, exam tables, and sex toys that may hold and convey infection) or via routine skin-to-skin contact, the implication of such findings continues to be debated.[58] The conclusion of one older study suggested that normal sterilization routines ought to provide sufficient protection in medical settings.[59] Furthermore, no research supporting indirect or routine forms of contact transmission has demonstrated a linkage to subsequent genital lesions.[60] Nonetheless, the detection of HPV in adults with no sexual experience, and in infants and younger children (see the major section below), provides a strong caution against conceptually limiting HPV infection to a venereal context.[61-64]

The most intensely investigated alternate route for passing on and acquiring HPV is vertical transmission between mother and baby, primarily during labor and delivery.[65-67] But, as Arena et al. acknowledged, "the data reported in the literature on the relationship between HPV and pregnancy are highly discordant."[68] One of the challenges involved in such research is distinguishing between infection and contamination.[69] Although earlier studies have demonstrated evidence of vertical transmission, more recent research has concluded that this route of viral spread is at best associated with low pathogenicity.[70] Even when the virus is found in newborns, it often seems to clear after only a few months.[71] On a related front, a report was published detailing fetal HPV infection contracted through intrauterine exposure.[72] Recently, research has intensified on this potentially important route of transmission, combined with a call for more surveillance of the consequences of fetal exposure to HPV.[73]

In sum, the argument for vertical transmission may be restricted currently to plausibility. To paraphrase Cason and Mant, if many genital pathogens are known to be transmitted from mother to baby, why should this not be true for HPV?[74] However, parents should be reassured that perinatal transmission, if it exists at all, appears to be a rare occurrence.[75]

For completeness, it should be noted that the possibility of HPV transmission by blood transfusion has also been investigated.[76] The studies are partly inspired by HPV DNA being detected in the peripheral blood of cervical cancer patients; in fact, the presence of high-risk viral DNA in the blood has been proposed as an auxiliary biomarker for cervical neoplasms.[77] It is important to recognize that the detection of

HPV DNA is not synonymous with finding active viruses in blood cells. Much more research is required to draw a final conclusion about a reservoir for HPV in the bloodstream, both in terms of potential routes of nonsexual transmission and options for the detection of infection.

Although the full details related to transmission are still being worked out, one critical conclusion is clear: anogenital HPV infection is "easily transmitted" by sexual contact.[78] In fact, a 2006 Canadian Simulation Study demonstrated that HPV transmissibility is severalfold higher than for other sexually transmitted viral infections, including human immunodeficiency virus and herpes simplex virus type 2.[79]

OCCURRENCE OF THE VIRUS

The licensing of the first of many possible HPV prophylactic vaccines in the United States, Canada, and other parts of the world has naturally intensified interest in the overall prevalence of HPV infection, as well as the population distribution of viral types. One research objective involves establishing "a baseline against which postvaccine prevalence can be compared."[80] This sort of project is being pursued in multiple jurisdictions.[81] Epidemiological information is also required to facilitate more accurate studies of cost-effectiveness. The discussion of HPV prevalence comprises two different large topics. One is the occurrence of the virus in the general population, that is, among individuals where disease has not been detected. The prevalence of the virus and the distribution of types in abnormal or diseased tissue will become the key focus in later chapters.

Important information was derived from more than 1,900 U.S. females in a study by Dunne et al. published in 2007. The results were stratified by nonmodifiable and modifiable risk factors, as shown in Table 2.3.[82]

The data in this study that reinforce the concept of sexual transmission of the virus are especially compelling; for example, there is a clear dose–response association between infection rates and the number of sex partners. This aspect of the HPV story helps to inform the various behavior-based, sexual health strategies aimed at reducing exposure and subsequent disease. The results also suggest the need to deploy prevention efforts (such as vaccination) at younger ages (i.e., prior to sexual debut). As well, creating a prevention program across the whole population appears to be vital. It may not be as effective to specifically target high-risk groups, given that there are relatively high rates of HPV infection among women who have only had one sexual partner. This conclusion is reinforced by a 2006 U.S. study that indicated that

Table 2.3. Prevalence of Any HPV Infection, by Risk Factors in U.S. Females

Risk Factor	Sample Size	HPV Prevalence, % (95% C.I.)
Overall	1,921	26.8 (23.3–30.9)
Age		
14–19	652	24.5 (19.6–30.5)
20–24	189	44.8 (36.3–55.3)
25–29	174	27.4 (21.9–34.2)
30–39	328	27.5 (20.8–36.4)
40–49	324	25.2 (19.7–32.2)
50–59	254	19.6 (14.3–26.8)
Marital status		
Married	676	17.3 (14.0–21.5)
Widowed, divorce, separated	231	41.2 (32.3–52.4)
Never married	882	31.1 (28.1–34.5)
Living with partner	132	46.1 (35.2–60.4)
Education		
< High school	383	35.0 (29.4–41.7)
High school or equivalent	380	29.7 (23.4–37.6)
> High school	754	24.7 (20.9–29.1)
Poverty index		
Below poverty	503	37.5 (29.9–47.1)
At or above poverty	1,322	24.4 (21.1–28.4)
Ever had sex		
Yes	1,477	28.1 (24.6–32.1)
No	283	5.2 (2.4–11.2)
Age at first sexual intercourse		
<16	519	33.6 (27.5–41.1)
≥16	953	26.2 (22.6–30.3)
Number of lifetime sex partners		
0	283	5.2 (2.4–11.2)
1	349	11.5 (7.8–16.9)
2	185	24.3 (16.5–35.7)
3–5	430	32.0 (26.9–38.2)
≥6	499	35.5 (29.7–42.0)

Source: Dunne et al., *JAMA*, 2007. Used by permission.

more than 14% of the women (aged 18–25) reporting only one lifetime vaginal sex partner still demonstrated evidence of an HPV infection.[83] Finally, it is important to note that a small percentage (5.2%) of the cohort in Dunne et al. who reported not having vaginal, anal, or oral sex still demonstrated HPV infection, underlining the argument made earlier for nonvenereal transmission routes.

Predictors or correlates of HPV (and especially high-risk HPV) infection continue to be investigated. The goal is to see whether there are factors beyond age and sexual history that influence the risk of acquiring the virus, which in turn might identify groups requiring a special prevention focus. Recent U.S. research has offered consistent evidence on the importance of socioeconomic status. In a study by Kahn et al., women living below the poverty line were twice as likely to have a high-risk HPV infection compared with women above the poverty line.[84] Another study, based in Hawaii, also demonstrated that cervical HPV acquisition decreased with income.[85]

Geographical Variation: General HPV Prevalence

An interesting geographical comparison was provided in a 2005 pooled analysis of studies from different regions (Table 2.4).[86] The great

Table 2.4. Prevalence of Any HPV Infection, by Geographic Area in Cytologically Normal Women

Region	Age-Standardized HPV
Country, City	Prevalence, % (95% C.I.)
Sub-Saharan Africa	
Nigeria, Ibadan (2004)	25.6 (22.4–28.8)
Asia	
India, Ambilikai (2005)	14.2 (12.0–16.4)
Vietnam, Ho Chi Minh (2003)	10.6 (0.7–2.4)
Thailand, Lampang (2003)	7.2 (5.3–9.2)
Korea, Busan (2003)	13.3 (4.7–21.9)
Thailand, Songkla (2003)	3.6 (1.9–5.4)
Vietnam, Hanoi (2003)	1.6 (0.7–2.4)
Subtotal	*8.7 (7.9–9.5)*
South America	
Colombia, Bogota (2002)	13.9 (12.1–15.7)
Argentina, Concordia (2003)	16.3 (13.7–18.9)
Chile, Santiago (2004)	11.9 (9.6–14.3)
Subtotal	*14.3 (13.1–15.5)*
Europe	
Netherlands, Amsterdam (2000)	7.7 (4.1–11.3)
Italy, Turin (2005)	9.2 (7.5–11.0)
Spain, Barcelona (2003)	1.4 (0.5–2.2)
Subtotal	*5 (4.2–6.2)*
All areas	10.5 (9.9–11.0)

Source: Clifford et al., *The Lancet*, 2005. Used by permission.

variability in HPV infection prevalence presents challenges for a prevention strategy based on a single vaccine product for all parts of the world.

As indicated earlier, the advent of HPV vaccines has intensified interest in understanding the baseline epidemiology in various countries. For example, recent studies have shown that the population-wide prevalence of all HPV types in the cervix is 26.4% in Denmark, which is very similar to the U.S. results found by Dunne et al.[87] Some research is not population-based but has focused on high-risk types and/or women with normal cervical cytology, which can make comparisons between reports challenging. An instance of this approach was a meta-analysis of nine studies from India that indicated that 12% of women with normal cervical cytology were positive for high-risk HPV types.[88]

Geographical Variation: Type-Specific Prevalence

The distribution of different viral types in a population is of greater relevance than general HPV prevalence when considering the utility of prophylactic vaccines. While the HPV profile among actual cancer patients may ultimately be even more relevant (see Chapters 4 and 5), models of vaccine efficacy typically start with an assessment of viral epidemiology in the general female population and/or cytologically normal women. Figure 2.2, adapted from the two recent studies examined previously in

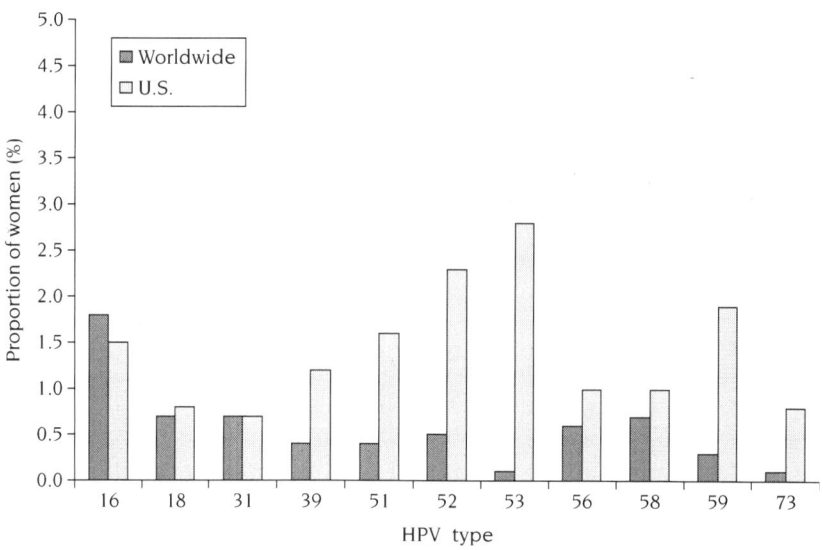

Figure 2.2. HPV infection rates, by oncogene HPV type: cytologically normal women, worldwide and U.S. *Source:* Dunne et al., *JAMA*, 2007; Clifford et al., *The Lancet*, 2005.

this chapter, provides the distribution of oncogenic HPV types pooled from different regions of the world compared with data specific to the United States.[89,90]

The information suggests substantial geographic variation in the occurrence of HPV types among different populations. Support for the idea of variation in different parts of the world can also be found when the data for HPV-positive women is stratified in more geographical detail (Table 2.5).

Data from specific countries offers further granularity to the picture.[91–93] For example, a 2005 paper described prevalence rates for selected oncogenic HPV types among Taiwanese women (Table 2.6).[94] The main difference when compared with the United States is the fact that there is a more even distribution across the HPV types, which may in turn have implications for optimum vaccine development among such

Table 2.5. Prevalence of HPV Infections, by Type and Region in Cytologically Normal Women

	Proportion of Infected Women (%)			
HPV Type	Europe	South America	Asia	Sub-Saharan Africa
16	21	15	14	8
18	5	5	5	4
31	9	5	4	7
33	3	4	6	2
35	4	3	3	8
42	5	5	7	11
45	4	5	2	6
52	2	4	5	4
56	4	4	6	6
58	4	7	4	6
81	2	4	5	7

Source: Clifford et al., *The Lancet*, 2005. Used by permission.

Table 2.6. Occurrence of HPV Types, by Age Group [Taiwanese Women (N=1320) Prevalence among Age Groups (%)]

Age	HPV 16	HPV 18	HPV 58	HPV 52	HPV 51	HPV 56
21–30	9.33	8.77	8.14	8.06	7.94	7.16
31–40	6.13	5.85	5.77	5.17	5.88	3.86
41–50	3.42	3.11	3.03	3.01	2.21	2.01
51–65	2.96	2.55	3.08	1.98	1.74	2.58
Total	4.92	4.70	3.26	3.11	2.95	2.88

Source: Jeng et al., *Clinical and Investigative Medicine*, 2005. Used by permission.

populations. This analysis is strengthened by the evidence for substantially higher attribution of cancer burden in Taiwan related to globally rare types such as HPV-52 and -58 (see Chapter 4).

These data also offer a good illustration of the natural clearance that typically occurs with different types of HPV infection. Although prevalence rates are certainly high in younger women, for a large proportion of people, the infection (regardless of viral type) resolves over time, with no development of disease symptoms.[95,96] In general, an estimated two-thirds of HPV infections clear within 1 year, and more than 90% clear within 3 years.[97,98]

Time Trends Within a Population

A modest amount of research, mostly based in Nordic countries, has examined the changing prevalence of HPV infection over time.[99] Countries such as Finland and Sweden have had population-based invitational screening programs in place for five decades, augmented by a national registration system.[100] This provides basic data for HPV time trend analysis.

In the past, prevalence information has been derived indirectly from clinical diagnoses, cytology programs, or serological (antibody) studies.[101,102] There are problems with the indirect methods of HPV analysis. For example, a 1986 study of cellular changes observed in smears from an STD clinic suggested a dramatic increase in HPV infection over 5 years, but the trend largely disappeared upon reanalysis with a newer classification scheme.[103] Direct DNA detection of HPV in tissues of interest is now commonly employed to facilitate more valid point and trend results. However, older research still offers some useful insights.

While other countries demonstrate stable or decreasing trends,[104] there was a 60% increase in cervical cancer incidence in Finland between 1991 and 1995. The growing rate of moderate-to-severe dysplasia has been sustained over a much longer period.[105] Likewise, an increase in cervical adenocarcinoma between 1958 and 1996 has been observed across the Swedish population.[106] Explanations for these effects are sought in terms of a combination of screening uptake variation and changes in background risks, especially HPV infection. In fact, there has been a major increase over time in HPV seroprevalence in Nordic countries.[107] In Finland, research has shown that the seroprevalence of HPV-16 among women aged 23–31 years increased from 17% in 1983–1985 to 24% in 1995–1997; the trend was traced as far back as 1974 among women under age 23.[108] A similar increase was found in Sweden between 1969 and 1989.[109] In contrast, DNA analysis of cervical samples in a 1990 Australian study indicated no significant change in HPV-16 prevalence over a 15-year period.[110] It is clear that developing current information about HPV prevalence trends in different populations would assist in calibrating prevention efforts.

Age-Specific Prevalence

Before considering modifiable risk factors related to HPV infection and carcinogenesis in Chapter 3, it is useful to underline the role of a non-modifiable factor, namely, age. One "classic" pattern was already seen in the U.S. data developed by Dunne et al. that were reported earlier, that is, a decline in HPV prevalence with age.[111] The same inverse relationship with age was recently revealed for high-risk HPV infection in Finland.[112] A 2006 study of age and HPV occurrence in women from different parts of the world often uncovered a comparable picture (e.g., see the Netherlands data in Figure 2.3).[113] But at least three other age-specific patterns were also found: (1) a high prevalence that remains relatively constant across age groups, (2) a consistently low prevalence across age groups, and (3) a U-shaped curve where prevalence increases again in older cohorts. Each of these profiles is illustrated by a specific national population in Figure 2.3.

Variations in age-specific profiles were confirmed in the largest review to date of HPV prevalence research. Smith et al. (2008) examined 375 studies covering in excess of 346,000 women from 70 countries worldwide; more than one-third of the studies offered age-stratified information, mostly drawn from Europe and North America.[114] The greatest

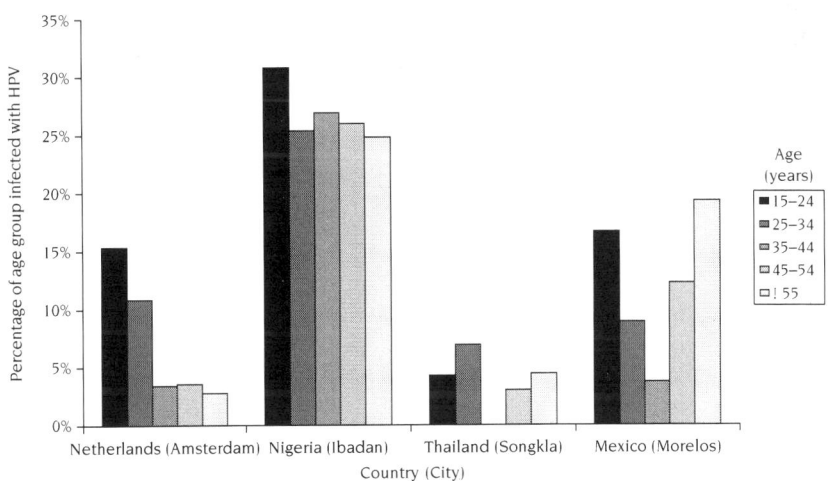

Figure 2.3. HPV prevalence patterns, by geographical area: age-specific percentage of infected women. *Source:* Franceschi et al., *International Journal of Cancer,* 2006.

inconsistency in the age-specific pattern was seen in older women, with a decrease or plateau compared with younger groups, and occasionally a rise in prevalence (creating the U-shaped curve that was illustrated by Mexico in Figure 2.3). Reasons for the latter pattern are not well understood, though some research has pointed to molecular selection pressures producing increased rates of viral persistence if HPV is not cleared by menopause.[115] Perhaps the most notable result revealed by Smith et al. across the globe was the consistent peak in HPV prevalence in younger women (<25 years of age). This has implications for primary prevention strategies, including the timing of vaccination programs. Focused research has indicated that cumulative incidence of HPV in sexually active adolescents is very high.[116] This information provides a key rationale for administering HPV vaccines before adolescence.

Studies have shown that the age-specific prevalence patterns also vary across individual HPV types.[117] Two interrelated phenomena have been posited as potential causes of prevalence differences across age groups for high-risk types such as HPV-16 and -18. First, some HPV types are attracted to specific tissues (e.g., high-risk types to the so-called transformation zone of the cervix, where HPV-related cancer mostly originates); furthermore, there is a known process of microanatomical changes in the cervix during the life span of females that in turn affects the degree of HPV tropism.[118] The occurrence of high-risk HPV in older women continues to be a focus of research,[119] especially in light of the fact that "catch-up" vaccination has not been licensed for women beyond age 26.

INFECTION IN INFANTS AND CHILDREN

The approval and licensing of an HPV vaccine for girls as young as 9, with routine distribution to females at around age 12 in order to cover individuals before sexual debut, has raised questions about the occurrence of HPV infection in the young. Although mostly transmitted by sexual intercourse, HPV infection has been detected in infants and children (as well as in adults with no reported sexual experience). As noted earlier, this offers strong support for the assertion that HPV infection is not just a venereal phenomenon. In particular, though sexual abuse must always be considered as a source, other forms of transmission to children appear to exist.

Indirect evidence for HPV infection in children may be inferred from the occurrence of pediatric diseases related to HPV.[120] One example is juvenile recurrent respiratory papillomatosis (RRP), a disease marked by wart-like growths in the aerodigestive tract; in severe cases, RRP can be fatal. Juvenile RRP typically presents in children younger than age 5, with about 25% of cases occurring in infancy. Incidence is rare at 1–4 per 100,000 children, with boys and girls being equally affected.[121,122] Most importantly for the purposes of this book, the disease has been shown to be caused by HPV-6 and 11.[123,124] The most likely transmission route in such cases is a vertical one, with the virus being passed during vaginal delivery.[125] Reinforcing this suggestion, adverse outcomes for RRP in a child were recently shown to be associated with an adverse HPV-related gynecological history in the mother.[126] Other factors indirectly related to HPV infection, such as primary or secondary immunodeficiency, have been suggested with respect to RRP, but the evidence is inconsistent.[127]

This sort of indirect indication of HPV infection also arises with the demonstrated cases of anogenital disease in children; thus, in one 1999 study in New England, 1.75% of 10 to 14-year-olds were found to have squamous intraepithelial lesions in the anogenital region.[128]

In terms of actual presence of the virus in young people, there is strong evidence of substantial HPV prevalence in females once they reach the teen years. The 2007 study of females in the United States detailed earlier offers a good example; the data indicated that almost 25% of adolescent females are infected with HPV, a phenomenon that is presumably traceable to sexual debut.[129]

The story may be extended to prepubescent age groups, specifically in terms of cutaneous lesions. HPV-related skin warts are in fact relatively common in young children. A 2003 Swedish study showed that the prevalence of cutaneous HPV infections in children 1 month to 4 years of age varied between 50% and 70%. Among positive cases, a total of 73 HPV types were isolated.[130] HPV has also been implicated in the development of psoriasis in children.[131]

Recent evidence indicates that the incidence of anogenital warts in prepubescent children is increasing. Aside from the well-known causative agents HPV-6 and 11, HPV-1 and 2 have been commonly detected in these lesions.[132,133] In several patient series, the proportion thought to have acquired HPV from sexual abuse was limited to 3–35%.[134] This again leaves the doorway of nonvenereal transmission wide open.

The often high prevalence of HPV DNA (as detected by nasopharyngeal aspirates or oral swabs) among newborns is well-established, as is the concordance of HPV types with the mother. However, there are also indications that the majority of neonatal cases represent transient infections.[135] The limited data for preadolescent children after the perinatal period are more heterogeneous, at least with respect to DNA detection in susceptible tissues. A Finnish study of 324 infants demonstrated 10% oral and 1.5% genital infections with high-risk HPV types persisting

Table 2.7. HPV Detection in Finnish Children

	HPV DNA Prevalence (%)	
Sample Subset/Age	Genital	Oral
Parents	13–25	8–34
Children/birth	15	10
Children/6 months	18	21
Children/24 months	10	10

Source: Rintala et al., *Journal of Clinical Microbiology*, 2005.

over the first 26 months of life.[136] A prospective investigation of 76 families by the same researchers demonstrated even higher rates of genital infection with high-risk HPV types in children (Table 2.7).[137]

A Finnish study from 10 years earlier obtained similar results for a group that included older children, with HPV DNA found in 31.6% of the oral scrapings from 98 individuals with a mean age of 4.0 ± 2.8 years. HPV-16/18 were the dominant types detected.[138] This contrasts sharply with smears collected from two body sites in a much larger sample of Danish children in 1997; the anal HPV detection rate was 1.6% and the oral only 0.25%.[139]

The specific assay methodology may account for conflicting data among children. A UK study in 2000 demonstrated that high-risk mucosal HPV infection may be substantial in children, but the often low levels of DNA require sensitive, type-specific detection methods. Using such strategies, about 52% of oral swabs from the 267 children in their sample tested positive for HPV-16 DNA; the prevalence ranged from less than 40% in 1-year-olds to more than 60% in 9-year-olds.[140] A U.S. study from the following year examined oral samples from 268 healthy young people.[141] Intriguingly, HPV was only detected in children younger than 7 and older than 12, but due to the small sample size, the difference in HPV positivity across age groups was not statistically significant. Overall, the prevalence of HPV in the oral cavities of children under 7 years of age was 8.7%. Again, HPV-16/18 predominated. The presence of HPV, including high-risk types, in oral mucosa of young children was confirmed in a 2003 study of 3- to 5-year-old Japanese girls and boys, with even higher rates of infection than found in previous studies.[142]

HPV serology offers another means of assessing HPV prevalence in children. This indirect approach, where antibodies for HPV are detected in the bloodstream, has limitations; most seriously, the presence of circulating antibodies does not prove that there is current HPV infection or disease.[143] A further obstacle is the fact that detection is HPV type-specific.[144]

Table 2.8. Studies of HPV-16 Seroprevalence in Children, by Geographical Area

Year	First Author	Sample Size	Age	Location	HPV Seroprevalence (%)
1997	Luxton	35	0–10	UK	5.7
1997	Marais	155	1–12	South Africa	2.5
1997	Mund	66	1–10	Germany	1.5
1998	Cubie	1,192	11–13	Scotland	7.6
1999	af Geijersstam	1,031	0–13	Sweden	3
1999	Manns	100	2–5	Jamaica	3
2000	Marais	115	2–12	South Africa	6.1
2005	Dunne	1,316	6–11	U.S.	2.4
2007	Chen	238	1–12	Taiwan	0.84

Sources: Dunne et al., *Journal of Infectious Diseases*, 2005; Chen et al., *Journal of Clinical Virology*, 2007.

Seroprevalence studies in the last decade have mostly focused on one key type, HPV-16. Dunne and colleagues offered a helpful summary of this research in 2005, augmented with their own research update. The information is provided in Table 2.8, where more recent data from a Taiwanese study have also been included.[145,146]

In summary, both the direct and indirect evidence suggests that HPV infection is found in prepubescent children; in fact, the virus can be quite common in young girls, well before the lowest age of consensual sexual activity.[147] The full explanation for HPV detection in children is still being worked out. Substantial clearance of any high-risk viral types from the mucosal tissues of newborns and infants appears to be common, but the possibility of latent infections persisting in oral and anogenital "reservoirs" in young people still must be considered. More epidemiological research is especially required in the key cohort of children below age 12 in order to fully understand the implications for newly launched immunization programs. A key issue is the fact that the positive efficacy of licensed HPV vaccines is largely limited to females who are HPV-naive to virus types targeted by the vaccine.

NOTES

1. zur Hausen H. Papillomaviruses in human cancers. *Proceedings of the Association of American Physicians*. 1999; 111(6): 581–7.
2. Syrjanen K. PL8 The causal role of genital human papillomavirus (hpv) infections in cervical carcinogenesis. *Oral Diseases*. 2006; 12(suppl 1): 2.

3 Bernard HU. The clinical importance of the nomenclature, evolution and taxonomy of human papillomaviruses. *Journal of Clinical Virology.* 2005; 32(suppl 1): S1-6.
4 Parkin M, Almonte M, Bruni L et al. Burden and trends of type-specific human papillomavirus infections and related diseases in the Latin America and Caribbean region. *Vaccine.* 2008; 26(suppl 11): L1-15.
5 Wiley D, Masongsong E. Human papillomavirus: the burden of infection. *Obstetrical and Gynecological Survey.* 2006; 61(6 suppl 1): S3-14.
6 Prado JC, Calleja-Macias IE, Bernard HU et al. Worldwide genomic diversity of the human papillomaviruses-53, 56, and 66, a group of high-risk HPVs unrelated to HPV-16 and HPV-18. *Virology.* 2005; 340(1): 95-104.
7 Syrjanen K. PL8 The causal role of genital human papillomavirus (hpv) infections in cervical carcinogenesis. *Oral Diseases.* 2006; 12(suppl 1): 2.
8 Munoz N, Bosch FX, de Sanjose S et al. Epidemiologic classification of human papillomavirus types associated with cervical cancer. *New England Journal of Medicine.* 2003; 348(6): 518-27.
9 Bosch FX, Manos MM, Munoz N et al. Prevalence of human papillomavirus in cervical cancer: a worldwide perspective. International biological study on cervical cancer (IBSCC) Study Group. *Journal of the National Cancer Institute.* 1995; 87(11): 796-802.
10 Clifford GM, Smith JS, Plummer M et al. Human papillomavirus types in invasive cervical cancer worldwide: a meta-analysis. *British Journal of Cancer.* 2003; 88(1): 63-73.
11 Goldie SJ, Grima D, Kohli M et al. A comprehensive natural history model of HPV infection and cervical cancer to estimate the clinical impact of a prophylactic HPV-16/18 vaccine. *International Journal of Cancer.* 2003; 106(6): 896-904.
12 Harper DM, Franco EL, Wheeler C et al. Efficacy of a bivalent L1 virus-like particle vaccine in prevention of infection with human papillomavirus types 16 and 18 in young women: a randomised controlled trial. *The Lancet.* 2004; 364(9447): 1757-65.
13 Gok M, Coupe VM, Berkhof J et al. HPV16 and increased risk of recurrence after treatment for CIN. *Gynecologic Oncology.* 2007; 104(2): 273-5.
14 For example, Monsonego J, ed. *Emerging Issues on HPV Infections: From Science to Practice.* Basel: Karger; 2006.
15 See H. Krueger & Associates, Inc. *A Population Based HPV Immunization Program in British Columbia: Background Paper.* January 17, 2006. Prepared for the Cancer Prevention Program of the British Columbia Cancer Agency, available at www.krueger.ca. The table on page 77 of that document has been updated for Table 2.1. Additional details and references for Table 2.1 are available at www.krueger.ca.
16 Pantel K, Cote RJ, Fodstad O. Detection and clinical importance of micrometastatic disease. *Journal of the National Cancer Institute.* 1999; 91(13): 1113-24.
17 Mullin JM. Epithelial barriers, compartmentation, and cancer. *Science's STKE.* 2004; 2004(216): pe2.
18 zur Hausen H. *Infections Causing Human Cancer.* Heidelberg: Wiley-VCH; 2006.

19 Thus distinguishing them from the Polyomaviridae family, or the polyomaviruses. Previously, these two families were considered to be genera within the family Papovaviridae.
20 Derived from papilla, Latin for *nipple*.
21 zur Hausen H. *Infections Causing Human Cancer.* Heidelberg: Wiley-VCH; 2006.
22 Technically, demonstrating icosahedral symmetry.
23 Cheah PL, Looi LM. Biology and pathological associations of the human papillomaviruses: a review. *Malaysian Journal of Pathology.* 1998; 20(1): 1–10.
24 Bravo IG, Alonso A. Phylogeny and evolution of papillomaviruses based on the E1 and E2 proteins. *Virus Genes.* 2007; 34(3): 249–62.
25 Lin YY, Alphs H, Hung CF et al. Vaccines against human papillomavirus. *Frontiers in Bioscience.* 2007; 12: 246–64.
26 zur Hausen H. *Infections Causing Human Cancer.* Heidelberg: Wiley-VCH; 2006.
27 Bravo IG, Alonso A. Phylogeny and evolution of papillomaviruses based on the E1 and E2 proteins. *Virus Genes.* 2007; 34(3): 249–62.
28 Bernard HU. The clinical importance of the nomenclature, evolution and taxonomy of human papillomaviruses. *Journal of Clinical Virology.* 2005; 32(suppl 1): S1–6.
29 Calleja-Macias IE, Kalantari M, Allan B et al. Papillomavirus subtypes are natural and old taxa: phylogeny of human papillomavirus types 44 and 55 and 68a and -b. *Journal of Virology.* 2005; 79(10): 6565–9.
30 Calleja-Macias IE, Kalantari M, Huh J et al. Genomic diversity of human papillomavirus-16, 18, 31, and 35 isolates in a Mexican population and relationship to European, African, and Native American variants. *Virology.* 2004; 319(2): 315–23.
31 Tonon SA, Basiletti J, Badano I et al. Human papillomavirus type 16 molecular variants in Guarani Indian women from Misiones, Argentina. *International Journal of Infectious Diseases.* 2007; 11(1): 76–81.
32 Zheng ZM, Baker CC. Papillomavirus genome structure, expression, and post-transcriptional regulation. *Frontiers in Bioscience.* 2006; 11: 2286–302.
33 Bernard HU, Calleja-Macias IE, Dunn ST. Genome variation of human papillomavirus types: phylogenetic and medical implications. *International Journal of Cancer.* 2006; 118(5): 1071–6.
34 Sichero L, Villa LL. Epidemiological and functional implications of molecular variants of human papillomavirus. *Brazilian Journal of Medical and Biological Research.* 2006; 39(6): 707–17.
35 Munoz N, Bosch FX, Castellsague X et al. Against which human papillomavirus types shall we vaccinate and screen? The international perspective. *International Journal of Cancer.* 2004; 111(2): 278–85.
36 Padayachee A, Van Wyk CW. Human papillomavirus (HPV) in oral squamous cell papillomas. *Journal of Oral Pathology.* 1987; 16(7): 353–5.
37 Note that HPV-55 was subsequently found to be a subtype of HPV-44. Calleja-Macias IE, Kalantari M, Allan B et al. Papillomavirus subtypes are natural and old taxa: phylogeny of human papillomavirus types 44 and 55 and 68a and -b. *Journal of Virology.* 2005; 79(10): 6565–9.
38 Details are available at www.krueger.ca under the Projects tab.

39 Kremsdorf D, Jablonska S, Favre M et al. Human papillomaviruses associated with epidermodysplasia verruciformis. II. Molecular cloning and biochemical characterization of human papillomavirus 3a, 8, 10, and 12 genomes. *Journal of Virology.* 1983; 48(2): 340–51.
40 Calleja-Macias IE, Kalantari M, Allan B et al. Papillomavirus subtypes are natural and old taxa: phylogeny of human papillomavirus types 44 and 55 and 68a and -b. *Journal of Virology.* 2005; 79(10): 6565–9.
41 Hazard K, Eliasson L, Dillner J et al. Subtype HPV38b[FA125] demonstrates heterogeneity of human papillomavirus type 38. *International Journal of Cancer.* 2006; 119(5): 1073–7.
42 Taxonomy adapted from deVilliers E, Fauquet C, Broker TR et al. Classification of papillomaviruses. *Virology.* 2004; 324: 17–27.
43 Schiffman M, Kjaer SK. Natural history of anogenital human papillomavirus infection and neoplasia. *Journal of the National Cancer Institute Monograph.* Chapter 2, 2003; (31): 14–9.
44 Bekkers RL, Massuger LF, Bulten J et al. Epidemiological and clinical aspects of human papillomavirus detection in the prevention of cervical cancer. *Reviews in Medical Virology.* 2004; 14(2): 95–105.
45 Sellors JW, Karwalajtys TL, Kaczorowski J et al. Incidence, clearance and predictors of human papillomavirus infection in women. *Canadian Medical Association Journal.* 2003; 168(4): 421–5.
46 Kjaer SK, Chackerian B, van den Brule AJ et al. High-risk human papillomavirus is sexually transmitted: evidence from a follow-up study of virgins starting sexual activity (intercourse). *Cancer Epidemiology, Biomarkers and Prevention.* 2001; 10(2): 101–6.
47 Benevolo M, Mottolese M, Marandino F et al. HPV genotypes concordance between sex partners. *Journal of Experimental and Clinical Cancer Research.* 2007; 26(4): 609–12.
48 Rombaldi RL, Serafini EP, Villa LL et al. Infection with human papillomaviruses of sexual partners of women having cervical intraepithelial neoplasia. *Brazilian Journal of Medical and Biological Research.* 2006; 39(2): 177–87.
49 Bleeker MC, Snijders PF, Voorhorst FJ et al. Flat penile lesions: the infectious "invisible" link in the transmission of human papillomavirus. *International Journal of Cancer.* 2006; 119(11): 2505–12.
50 Gervaz P, Allal AS, Villiger P et al. Squamous cell carcinoma of the anus: another sexually transmitted disease. *Swiss Medical Weekly.* 2003; 133(25–26): 353–9.
51 Winer RL, Lee SK, Hughes JP et al. Genital human papillomavirus infection: incidence and risk factors in a cohort of female university students. *American Journal of Epidemiology.* 2003; 157(3): 218–26.
52 Marrazzo JM, Stine K, Koutsky LA. Genital human papillomavirus infection in women who have sex with women: a review. *American Journal of Obstetrics and Gynecology.* 2000; 183(3): 770–4.
53 Rintala M, Grenman S, Puranen M et al. Natural history of oral papillomavirus infections in spouses: a prospective Finnish HPV Family Study. *Journal of Clinical Virology.* 2006; 35(1): 89–94.
54 Scully C. Oral cancer; the evidence for sexual transmission. *British Dental Journal.* 2005; 199(4): 203–7.

55 Madsen BS, van den Brule AJ, Jensen HL et al. Risk factors for squamous cell carcinoma of the penis–population-based case-control study in Denmark. *Cancer Epidemiology Biomarkers and Prevention*. 2008; 17(10): 2683–91.
56 Haddad R, Crum C, Chen Z et al. HPV16 transmission between a couple with HPV-related head and neck cancer. *Oral Oncology*. 2008; 44(8): 812–5.
57 Rintala M, Grenman S, Puranen M et al. Natural history of oral papillomavirus infections in spouses: a prospective Finnish HPV Family Study. *Journal of Clinical Virology*. 2006; 35(1): 89–94.
58 Strauss S, Sastry P, Sonnex C et al. Contamination of environmental surfaces by genital human papillomaviruses. *Sexually Transmitted Infections*. 2002; 78(2): 135–8.
59 Ferenczy A, Bergeron C, Richart RM. Human papillomavirus DNA in fomites on objects used for the management of patients with genital human papillomavirus infections. *Obstetrics and Gynecology*. 1989; 74(6): 950–4.
60 Bruck LR, Zee S, Poulos B et al. Detection of cervical human papillomavirus infection by in situ hybridization in fetuses from women with squamous intra-epithelial lesions. *Journal of Lower Genital Tract Disease*. 2005; 9(2): 114–7.
61 Czegledy J. Sexual and non-sexual transmission of human papillomavirus. *Acta Microbiologica et Immunologica Hungarica*. 2001; 48(3–4): 511–7.
62 Tay SK. Genital oncogenic human papillomavirus infection: a short review on the mode of transmission. *Annals of the Academy of Medicine, Singapore*. 1995; 24(4): 598–601.
63 Rintala MA, Grenman SE, Jarvenkyla ME et al. High-risk types of human papillomavirus (HPV) DNA in oral and genital mucosa of infants during their first 3 years of life: experience from the Finnish HPV Family Study. *Clinical Infectious Diseases*. 2005; 41(12): 1728–33.
64 Dunne EF, Karem KL, Sternberg MR et al. Seroprevalence of human papillomavirus type 16 in children. *Journal of Infectious Diseases*. 2005; 191(11): 1817–9.
65 Cason J, Mant CA. High-risk mucosal human papillomavirus infections during infancy & childhood. *Journal of Clinical Virology*. 2005; 32(suppl 1): S52–8.
66 Rintala MA, Grenman SE, Puranen MH et al. Transmission of high-risk human papillomavirus (HPV) between parents and infant: a prospective study of HPV in families in Finland. *Journal of Clinical Microbiology*. 2005; 43(1): 376–81.
67 Syrjanen S, Puranen M. Human papillomavirus infections in children: the potential role of maternal transmission. *Critical Reviews in Oral Biology and Medicine*. 2000; 11(2): 259–74.
68 Arena S, Marconi M, Ubertosi M et al. HPV and pregnancy: diagnostic methods, transmission and evolution. *Minerva Ginecologica*. 2002; 54(3): 225–37.
69 Medeiros LR, Ethur AB, Hilgert JB et al. Vertical transmission of the human papillomavirus: a systematic quantitative review. *Cadernos de Saude Publica*. 2005; 21(4): 1006–15.
70 Smith EM, Ritchie JM, Yankowitz J et al. Human papillomavirus prevalence and types in newborns and parents: concordance and modes of transmission. *Sexually Transmitted Diseases*. 2004; 31(1): 57–62. See also Watts DH, Koutsky LA, Holmes KK et al. Low risk of perinatal transmission of human papillomavirus: results from a prospective cohort study. *American Journal of Obstetrics and Gynecology*. 1998; 178(2): 365–73.

71 Arena S, Marconi M, Ubertosi M et al. HPV and pregnancy: diagnostic methods, transmission and evolution. *Minerva Ginecologica*. 2002; 54(3): 225–37.
72 Bruck LR, Zee S, Poulos B et al. Detection of cervical human papillomavirus infection by in situ hybridization in fetuses from women with squamous intraepithelial lesions. *Journal of Lower Genital Tract Disease*. 2005; 9(2): 114–7.
73 Rombaldi RL, Serafini EP, Mandelli J et al. Transplacental transmission of human papillomavirus. *Virology Journal*. 2008; 5: 106–19.
74 Cason J, Mant CA. High-risk mucosal human papillomavirus infections during infancy & childhood. *Journal of Clinical Virology*. 2005; 32(suppl 1): S52–8.
75 Winer RL, Koutsky LA. Delivering reassurance to parents: perinatal human papillomavirus transmission is rare. *Sexually Transmitted Diseases*. 2004; 31(1): 63–4.
76 Bodaghi S, Wood LV, Roby G et al. Could human papillomaviruses be spread through blood? *Journal of Clinical Microbiology*. 2005; 43(11): 5428–34.
77 Tsai HJ, Peng YW, Lin LY et al. An association between human papillomavirus 16/18 deoxyribonucleic acid in peripheral blood with p16 protein expression in neoplastic cervical lesions. *Cancer Detection and Prevention*. 2005; 29(6): 537–43.
78 Schiffman M, Kjaer SK. Natural history of anogenital human papillomavirus infection and neoplasia. *Journal of the National Cancer Institute Monograph*. 2003; (31): 14–9.
79 Burchell AN, Richardson H, Mahmud SM et al. Modeling the sexual transmissibility of human papillomavirus infection using stochastic computer simulation and empirical data from a cohort study of young women in Montreal, Canada. *American Journal of Epidemiology*. 2006; 163(6): 534–43.
80 Weller SC, Stanberry LR. Estimating the population prevalence of HPV. *Journal of the American Medical Association*. 2007; 297(8): 876–8.
81 For example, Kjaer SK, Breugelmans G, Munk C et al. Population-based prevalence, type- and age-specific distribution of HPV in women before introduction of an HPV-vaccination program in Denmark. *International Journal of Cancer*. 2008; 123(8): 1864–70; Bhatla N, Lal N, Bao YP et al. A meta-analysis of human papillomavirus type-distribution in women from South Asia: implications for vaccination. *Vaccine*. 2008; 26(23): 2811–7; Asiimwe S, Whalen CC, Tisch DJ et al. Prevalence and predictors of high-risk human papillomavirus infection in a population-based sample of women in rural Uganda. *International Journal of STD and AIDS*. 2008; 19(9): 605–10; Lenselink CH, Melchers WJ, Quint WG et al. Sexual behaviour and HPV infections in 18 to 29 year old women in the pre-vaccine era in the Netherlands. *PLoS ONE*. 2008; 3(11): e3743.
82 Dunne EF, Unger ER, Sternberg M et al. Prevalence of HPV infection among females in the United States. *Journal of the American Medical Association*. 2007; 297(8): 813–9.
83 Manhart LE, Holmes KK, Koutsky LA et al. Human papillomavirus infection among sexually active young women in the United States: implications for developing a vaccination strategy. *Sexually Transmitted Diseases*. 2006; 33(8): 502–8.
84 Kahn JA, Lan D, Kahn RS. Sociodemographic factors associated with high-risk human papillomavirus infection. *Obstetrics and Gynecology*. 2007; 110(1): 87–95.

85 Goodman MT, Shvetsov YB, McDuffie K et al. Prevalence, acquisition, and clearance of cervical human papillomavirus infection among women with normal cytology: Hawaii Human Papillomavirus Cohort Study. *Cancer Research.* 2008; 68(21): 8813–24.
86 Clifford GM, Gallus S, Herrero R et al. Worldwide distribution of human papillomavirus types in cytologically normal women in the International Agency for Research on Cancer HPV prevalence surveys: a pooled analysis. *The Lancet.* 2005; 366(9490): 991–8. Note that, for reasons that are not clear, another study from a year later (involving some of the same researchers) that reviewed the same papers actually generated a somewhat different set of age-standardized values. Franceschi S, Herrero R, Clifford GM et al. Variations in the age-specific curves of human papillomavirus prevalence in women worldwide. *International Journal of Cancer.* 2006; 119(11): 2677–84.
87 Kjaer SK, Breugelmans G, Munk C et al. Population-based prevalence, type- and age-specific distribution of HPV in women before introduction of an HPV-vaccination program in Denmark. *International Journal of Cancer.* 2008; 123(8): 1864–70.
88 Bhatla N, Lal N, Bao YP et al. A meta-analysis of human papillomavirus type-distribution in women from South Asia: implications for vaccination. *Vaccine.* 2008; 26(23): 2811–7.
89 Dunne EF, Unger ER, Sternberg M et al. Prevalence of HPV infection among females in the United States. *Journal of the American Medical Association.* 2007; 297(8): 813–9.
90 Clifford GM, Gallus S, Herrero R et al. Worldwide distribution of human papillomavirus types in cytologically normal women in the International Agency for Research on Cancer HPV prevalence surveys: a pooled analysis. *The Lancet.* 2005; 366(9490): 991–8.
91 Verteramo R, Pierangeli A, Calzolari E et al. Direct sequencing of HPV DNA detected in gynaecologic outpatients in Rome, Italy. *Microbes and Infection.* 2006; 8(9–10): 2517–21.
92 Lehtinen M, Kaasila M, Pasanen K et al. Seroprevalence atlas of infections with oncogenic and non-oncogenic human papillomaviruses in Finland in the 1980s and 1990s. *International Journal of Cancer.* 2006; 119(11): 2612–9.
93 Thomas JO, Herrero R, Omigbodun AA et al. Prevalence of papillomavirus infection in women in Ibadan, Nigeria: a population-based study. *British Journal of Cancer.* 2004; 90(3): 638–45.
94 Jeng CJ, Phdl, Ko ML et al. Prevalence of cervical human papillomavirus in Taiwanese women. *Clinical and Investigative Medicine.* 2005; 28(5): 261–6.
95 Koutsky L. Epidemiology of genital human papillomavirus infection. *American Journal of Medicine.* 1997; 102(5A): 3–8.
96 Bhatla N, Lal N, Bao YP et al. A meta-analysis of human papillomavirus type-distribution in women from South Asia: implications for vaccination. *Vaccine.* 2008; 26(23): 2811–7.
97 Rodriguez AC, Schiffman M, Herroro R et al. Rapid clearance of human papillomavirus and implications for clinical focus on persistent infections. *Journal of the National Cancer Institute.* 2008; 100: 513–7.
98 Frazer IH, Cox JT, Mayeaux EJ et al. Advances in prevention of cervical cancer and other human papillomavirus-related diseases. *The Paediatric Infectious Disease Journal.* 2006; 25(2): S65–81.

99 Baseman JG, Koutsky LA. The epidemiology of human papillomavirus infections. *Journal of Clinical Virology.* 2005; 32(Suppl 1): S16–24.
100 Dillner J. Trends over time in the incidence of cervical neoplasia in comparison to trends over time in human papillomavirus infection. *Journal of Clinical Virology.* 2000; 19(1–2): 7–23.
101 Becker TM, Stone KM, Alexander ER. Genital human papillomavirus infection. A growing concern. *Obstetrics and Gynecology Clinics of North America.* 1987; 14(2): 389–96.
102 Kjaer SK, Lynge E. Incidence, prevalence and time trends of genital HPV infection determined by clinical examination and cytology. *IARC Scientific Publications.* 1989; (94): 113–24.
103 Armstrong BK, Allen OV, Brennan BA et al. Time trends in prevalence of cervical cytological abnormality in women attending a sexually transmitted diseases clinic and their relationship to trends in sexual activity and specific infections. *British Journal of Cancer.* 1986; 54(4): 669–75.
104 Vizcaino AP, Moreno V, Bosch FX et al. International trends in incidence of cervical cancer: II. Squamous-cell carcinoma. *International Journal of Cancer.* 2000; 86(3): 429–35.
105 Anttila A, Pukkala E, Soderman B et al. Effect of organised screening on cervical cancer incidence and mortality in Finland, 1963–1995: recent increase in cervical cancer incidence. *International Journal of Cancer.* 1999; 83(1): 59–65.
106 Hemminki K, Li X, Vaittinen P. Time trends in the incidence of cervical and other genital squamous cell carcinomas and adenocarcinomas in Sweden, 1958–1996. *European Journal of Obstetrics, Gynecology, and Reproductive Biology.* 2002; 101(1): 64–9.
107 Dillner J. Trends over time in the incidence of cervical neoplasia in comparison to trends over time in human papillomavirus infection. *Journal of Clinical Virology.* 2000; 19(1–2): 7–23.
108 Laukkanen P, Koskela P, Pukkala E et al. Time trends in incidence and prevalence of human papillomavirus type 6, 11 and 16 infections in Finland. *Journal of General Virology.* 2003; 84(Pt 8): 2105–9.
109 af Geijersstam V, Wang Z, Lewensohn-Fuchs I et al. Trends in seroprevalence of human papillomavirus type 16 among pregnant women in Stockholm, Sweden, during 1969–1989. *International Journal of Cancer.* 1998; 76(3): 341–4.
110 Rakoczy P, Sterrett G, Kulski J et al. Time trends in the prevalence of human papillomavirus infections in archival Papanicolaou smears: analysis by cytology, DNA hybridization, and polymerase chain reaction. *Journal of Medical Virology.* 1990; 32(1): 10–7.
111 Dunne EF, Unger ER, Sternberg M et al. Prevalence of HPV infection among females in the United States. *Journal of the American Medical Association.* 2007; 297(8): 813–9.
112 Leinonen M, Kotaniemi-Talonen L, Anttila A et al. Prevalence of oncogenic human papillomavirus infection in an organised screening population in Finland. *International Journal of Cancer.* 2008; 123(6): 1344–9.
113 Franceschi S, Herrero R, Clifford GM et al. Variations in the age-specific curves of human papillomavirus prevalence in women worldwide. *International Journal of Cancer.* 2006; 119(11): 2677–84.

114 Smith JS, Melendy A, Rana RK et al. Age-specific prevalence of infection with human papillomavirus in females: a global review. *Journal of Adolescent Health*. 2008; 43(4 suppl 1): S5–25, S e1–41.

115 Branca M, Ciotti M, Giorgi C et al. Predicting high-risk human papillomavirus infection, progression of cervical intraepithelial neoplasia, and prognosis of cervical cancer with a panel of 13 biomarkers tested in multivariate modeling. *International Journal of Gynecological Pathology*. 2008; 27(2): 265–73.

116 For example, Brown DR, Shew ML, Qadadri B et al. A longitudinal study of genital human papillomavirus infection in a cohort of closely followed adolescent women. *Journal of Infectious Diseases*. 2005; 191(2): 182–92.

117 For example, Sargent A, Bailey A, Almonte M et al. Prevalence of type-specific HPV infection by age and grade of cervical cytology: data from the ARTISTIC trial. *British Journal of Cancer*. 2008; 98(10): 1704–9.

118 Castle PE, Jeronimo J, Schiffman M et al. Age-related changes of the cervix influence human papillomavirus type distribution. *Cancer Research*. 2006; 66(2): 1218–24.

119 Lindau ST, Drum ML, Gaumer E et al. Prevalence of high-risk human papillomavirus among older women. *Obstetrics and Gynecology*. 2008; 112(5): 979–89.

120 Mammas IN, Sourvinos G, Michael C et al. Human papilloma virus in hyperplastic tonsillar and adenoid tissues in children. *Pediatric Infectious Disease Journal*. 2006; 25(12): 1158–62.

121 Stamataki S, Nikolopoulos TP, Korres S et al. Juvenile recurrent respiratory papillomatosis: still a mystery disease with difficult management. *Head and Neck*. 2007; 29(2): 155–62.

122 Maloney EM, Unger ER, Tucker RA et al. Longitudinal measures of human papillomavirus 6 and 11 viral loads and antibody response in children with recurrent respiratory papillomatosis. *Archives of Otolaryngology – Head and Neck Surgery*. 2006; 132(7): 711–5.

123 Freed GL, Derkay CS. Prevention of recurrent respiratory papillomatosis: role of HPV vaccination. *International Journal of Pediatric Otorhinolaryngology*. 2006; 70(10): 1799–803.

124 Draganov P, Todorov S, Todorov I et al. Identification of HPV DNA in patients with juvenile-onset recurrent respiratory papillomatosis using SYBR Green real-time PCR. *International Journal of Pediatric Otorhinolaryngology*. 2006; 70(3): 469–73.

125 Stamataki S, Nikolopoulos TP, Korres S et al. Juvenile recurrent respiratory papillomatosis: still a mystery disease with difficult management. *Head and Neck*. 2007; 29(2): 155–62.

126 Gerein V, Schmandt S, Babkina N et al. Human papilloma virus (HPV)-associated gynecological alteration in mothers of children with recurrent respiratory papillomatosis during long-term observation. *Cancer Detection and Prevention*. 2007; 31(4): 276–81.

127 Stamataki S, Nikolopoulos TP, Korres S et al. Juvenile recurrent respiratory papillomatosis: still a mystery disease with difficult management. *Head and Neck*. 2007; 29(2): 155–62.

128 Mount SL, Papillo JL. A study of 10,296 pediatric and adolescent Papanicolaou smear diagnoses in northern New England. *Pediatrics*. 1999; 103(3): 539–45.

129 Dunne EF, Unger ER, Sternberg M et al. Prevalence of HPV infection among females in the United States. *Journal of the American Medical Association.* 2007; 297(8): 813–9.
130 Antonsson A, Karanfilovska S, Lindqvist PG et al. General acquisition of human papillomavirus infections of skin occurs in early infancy. *Journal of Clinical Microbiology.* 2003; 41(6): 2509–14.
131 Mahe E, Bodemer C, Descamps V et al. High frequency of detection of human papillomaviruses associated with epidermodysplasia verruciformis in children with psoriasis. *British Journal of Dermatology.* 2003; 149(4): 819–25.
132 Sinal SH, Woods CR. Human papillomavirus infections of the genital and respiratory tracts in young children. *Seminars in Pediatric Infectious Diseases.* 2005; 16(4): 306–16.
133 Syrjanen S, Puranen M. Human papillomavirus infections in children: the potential role of maternal transmission. *Critical Reviews in Oral Biology and Medicine.* 2000; 11(2): 259–74.
134 Sinal SH, Woods CR. Human papillomavirus infections of the genital and respiratory tracts in young children. *Seminars in Pediatric Infectious Diseases.* 2005; 16(4): 306–16.
135 Syrjanen S, Puranen M. Human papillomavirus infections in children: the potential role of maternal transmission. *Critical Reviews in Oral Biology and Medicine.* 2000; 11(2): 259–74.
136 Rintala MA, Grenman SE, Jarvenkyla ME et al. High-risk types of human papillomavirus (HPV) DNA in oral and genital mucosa of infants during their first 3 years of life: experience from the Finnish HPV Family Study. *Clinical Infectious Diseases.* 2005; 41(12): 1728–33.
137 Rintala MA, Grenman SE, Puranen MH et al. Transmission of high-risk human papillomavirus (HPV) between parents and infant: a prospective study of HPV in families in Finland. *Journal of Clinical Microbiology.* 2005; 43(1): 376–81.
138 Puranen M, Yliskoski M, Saarikoski S et al. Vertical transmission of human papillomavirus from infected mothers to their newborn babies and persistence of the virus in childhood. *American Journal of Obstetrics and Gynecology.* 1996; 174(2): 694–9.
139 Koch A, Hansen SV, Nielsen NM et al. HPV detection in children prior to sexual debut. *International Journal of Cancer.* 1997; 73(5): 621–4.
140 Rice PS, Mant C, Cason J et al. High prevalence of human papillomavirus type 16 infection among children. *Journal of Medical Virology.* 2000; 61(1): 70–5.
141 Summersgill KF, Smith EM, Levy BT et al. Human papillomavirus in the oral cavities of children and adolescents. *Oral Surgery, Oral Medicine, Oral Pathology, Oral Radiology, and Endodontics.* 2001; 91(1): 62–9.
142 Kojima A, Maeda H, Kurahashi N et al. Human papillomaviruses in the normal oral cavity of children in Japan. *Oral Oncology.* 2003; 39(8): 821–8.
143 Rama CH, Roteli-Martins CM, Derchain SF et al. Serological detection of anti HPV 16/18 and its association with pap smear in adolescents and young women. *Revista da Associacao Medica Brasileira.* 2006; 52(1): 43–7.
144 Syrjanen S, Puranen M. Human papillomavirus infections in children: the potential role of maternal transmission. *Critical Reviews in Oral Biology and Medicine.* 2000; 11(2): 259–74.

145 Dunne EF, Karem KL, Sternberg MR et al. Seroprevalence of human papillomavirus type 16 in children. *Journal of Infectious Diseases*. 2005; 191(11): 1817–9.
146 Chen CJ, Viscidi RP, Chuang CH et al. Seroprevalence of human papillomavirus types 16 and 18 in the general population in Taiwan: implication for optimal age of human papillomavirus vaccination. *Journal of Clinical Virology*. 2007; 38(2): 126–30.
147 Powell J, Strauss S, Gray J et al. Genital carriage of human papilloma virus (HPV) DNA in prepubertal girls with and without vulval disease. *Pediatric Dermatology*. 2003; 20(3): 191–4.

3

HUMAN PAPILLOMAVIRUS: INFECTION, NATURAL HISTORY, AND CARCINOGENESIS

It is apparent that an intricate interplay of cellular and viral factors determines whether the outcome is active papillomavirus infection, viral latency, or ultimately, genital cancer.[1]

Over 150 different human papillomavirus (HPV) types are currently recognized; these are generally categorized in terms of their main target tissue, cutaneous or mucosal. The latter group is further divided into low-risk, intermediate-risk (sometimes called probable high-risk), and high-risk types, according to the strength of their association with malignant lesions at genital and extragenital mucosal sites. In this chapter, the tissues and sites where HPV "prefers" to cause cancer, the pathogenic processes connected to HPV (beginning with evading the immune system of the body), and the cofactors that play a role in HPV-related disease will all be described. Further details about the cancer-causing properties of HPV in specific body sites will be provided in subsequent chapters.

BODY SITES SUSCEPTIBLE TO HUMAN PAPILLOMAVIRUS INFECTION

While the connection between human papillomavirus (HPV) and many types of cancer is well known, health care professionals may be less familiar with the fact that the implicated tissues and body sites are highly specific. In short, the story of HPV carcinogenesis demands insight about the epithelial tissues of the human body. This is because papillomaviruses are essentially "epitheliotropic." Each member of the Papillomaviridae family appears to require the environment of differentiating squamous epithelium in a specific vertebrate in order to complete its life cycle.[2,3] Thus, HPV functions as a parasite, and more specifically as an obligate parasite.[4]

HPV infection seems to preferentially target keratinocytes within an epithelial lining. The virus does its most obvious damage in and through these types of cells, found in the upper (or suprabasal) layers of stratified squamous epithelia.[5] The name keratinocyte derives from the propensity of this type of cell to produce the substance known as keratin (or cytokeratin). Keratin refers to a class of tough, insoluble proteins that are the main component of body parts such as hair and fingernails. Keratin filaments are part of the cytoskeleton that creates cellular rigidity. Keratinization, also known as cornification, will be shown later to be an important aspect of HPV infection.

Why does HPV favor epithelial cells of skin and certain internal body sites? This is a fascinating question in its own right, and potentially relevant to understanding disease mechanisms and therefore preventive and therapeutic strategies. One possible explanation for the observed epitheliotropism is a reduced immunological response to HPV in those tissues. A tissue environment conducive to persistent infection by virtue of its compromised immune function may account for the evolution of the large number of papilloma types, each one ultimately adapting to epithelial cells in different animal species.[6]

There are different sites and kinds of epithelia, and all are not equally attractive to HPV. Proximity of the epithelium to the outside world appears to be important, reflecting the direct physical contact involved with most HPV transmission (as opposed to, e.g., transfer by blood or other bodily fluids). Skin clearly qualifies as a site susceptible to infection, but not the epithelial linings of internal body cavities. When ducts open to the outside surface of the body (e.g., in the digestive and reproductive systems), the epithelial layers at the exterior margins tend to have properties similar to skin epithelium. As is described below, the areas of transition from inside to outside the body often demonstrate an association with HPV-related disease. One epithelial tissue of great interest that does not fit easily into the preceding categories is the lining of lung spaces. In fact, the evidence for HPV involvement in lung carcinoma remains equivocal, which is consistent with limited physical access for the virus.[7]

For completeness, it may be noted that glandular tissues are also derived from epithelial cells during human development. This provides a biological context for the apparent association between malignancies of the breast and HPV infection.[8-11] Despite intensive investigation, it has not been possible to draw firm conclusions about HPV involvement with breast cancer.[12,13] The evidence for HPV connection with other glandular tissues (e.g., salivary, prostate) is absent or ambiguous.[14-18]

Target Tissues

Skin offers a paradigm for understanding the HPV connection to all epithelial tissues. The majority of epithelial cells in the skin are keratinocytes; these cells are known for progressively creating keratin (see below) as they gradually transform into the dead, denucleated cells found in the outermost layer of the skin. This surface layer of cells (sometimes referred to as corneocytes or squames) is integrated into a protective barrier called the stratum corneum; it offers a waterproof shield that is also resistant to noxious agents—whether chemical, biological, or mechanical.[19] Dead skin cells are continuously shed from the stratum corneum, a process known as exfoliation.[20] This phenomenon allows for the methods of HPV detection that depend on skin swabs.[21]

Skin epithelium may be characterized as a stratified lining, ranging from an innermost basal layer of cells that is the proposed primary target of HPV, through several layers of gradually differentiating keratinocytes, to the fully differentiated, squamous (=flattened) cells at the surface. Keratin can comprise up to 85% of the total cellular protein in the outermost cells.[22] In fact, they have sometimes been described as "sacs of keratin."

Keratin represents a family of 54 multifunctional proteins that provides structure and rigidity to epithelial cells. Specific types of keratin are found in various epithelial cells in the skin and other organs.[23] Keratinocyte is therefore an appropriate term for a cell from stratified squamous epithelia found anywhere in the body, even though the degree of progressive keratinization varies among different tissues.[24,25] In particular, keratinization in surface linings other than the skin may be markedly less than that found in the epidermis itself.[26] Not surprisingly, the skin tends to the be the physically toughest lining in the body; by comparison, the epithelium of more protected surfaces of the body have less keratin, even to the extent that they may be considered relatively nonkeratinized.

"Relatively nonkeratinized squamous linings" is a technical way of characterizing intermediate mucosal surfaces adjoining the surface of the body. As noted earlier, there is a key distinction between HPV types infecting skin or cutaneous keratinocytes and those preferring the keratinocytes on intermediate mucosal surfaces. There are other subcellular features that distinguish the latter tissues, some of which become important in disease processes. Notably, the lining of the vagina and oral cavity exhibit what is known as parakeratosis, where the cell nucleus is actually maintained in the outermost layer of the epithelium.

Having painted the histological background in some detail, it is useful to restate that HPV, particularly the cutaneous types, tends to target stratified squamous epithelium with a high degree of keratinization. Other HPV types prefer the less-keratinized mucosal epithelial cells found in a passageway near a body opening. Table 3.1 identifies the target tissues of the two main categories of HPV that preferentially infect humans.

The second category emphasizes the fact that the transitional areas between true mucosal epithelia and the exterior skin are of special clinical interest; these are regions where some physical abrasion or other insult may be expected, engendering therefore a higher degree of keratinization than will be found in mucosal surfaces fully internal to the body. Examples of these intermediate types of epithelia are found in the vagina and ectocervix and in parts of the mouth and anus. It is clear that there are regular epithelial insults at both ends of the digestive tract, deriving from mastication/swallowing and defecation, respectively. Penetrative sexual activity and oral-genital contact is also associated with potential abrasion and may plausibly be added to a full inventory of such risk areas.

Table 3.1. Categories of Stratified Squamous Epithelia

Feature	Site
More keratinized	Skin
	Tongue (dorsal)
	Hard palate
	Gums
	Anal margin
	Labia majora
Special susceptibility to mucosal HPV	Oral cavity
	Tonsil (crypt)
	Vocal folds
	Esophagus
	Anus (distal)
	Labia minora
	Vagina
	Ectocervix
	Glans penis (uncircumcized)
	Foreskin
	Cornea

It seems clear that transitional mucosal linings subject to microtrauma are of particular importance in terms of HPV transmission, infection, and sometimes cellular change. In two parts of the body, the cervix in females and the anal margin, this transitional lining has other distinctive histological features. For instance, one can clearly observe a gradual change from squamous cells near the surface of the body to the columnar epithelia of true mucosa; this accounts for the label given to this part of the cervix and anus, namely, the transformation zone. Significantly, the basal layer of cells in a transformation zone tends to be unusually close to the surface and thus more accessible to the virus. This phenomenon is often mentioned as a critical factor in the relatively high frequency of cancers of the cervix caused by HPV. Intriguingly, HPV infection may be found in various parts of the lower anogenital tract in women, but the incidence of cancer caused by HPV outside of the transformation zone of the cervix is very low—less than 0.003% for vulval and vaginal cancers combined.[27] The only other site where HPV-related cancer incidence matches that of the cervical transformation zone appears to be the similar zone found in the anal region, and then specifically in the context of men having sex with men.[28]

Potential Sites of HPV-Related Disease

The preceding categorical assessment of sites theoretically vulnerable to HPV-related disease is borne out by real world clinical experience. It is precisely those areas of the body marked by stratified squamous epithelium (with the potential for abnormal keratinization and other alterations) that have been most consistently associated with HPV-related cancer. The sites that are most susceptible to serious HPV-related disease (and especially to malignant transformation) are typically at or near body openings. They comprise the following: ectocervix, vagina, vulva (specifically the labia minora), the uncircumcised penis, distal anus, oral cavity, tonsillar crypts, vocal folds of the larynx, and esophagus. The changing anatomy of the cervix over the life span of women offers strong evidence for this anatomical characterization. As noted in Chapter 2, the transformation zone of the cervix shifts proximally over time; it is on the ectocervix in more than 90% of younger women but on the ectocervix in more than 90% of women 65 years of age and older. Dysplasia occurs twice as often when the transformation zone is on the ectocervix, partly explaining the higher rates of cervical cancer in younger women.[29]

The consistency of evidence concerning HPV tropism encourages hypothesizing about other locations where the virus should exert a disease impact. For example, one site noted in the inventory of relatively nonkeratinized epithelial tissues, namely, the cornea/conjunctiva, has attracted attention from investigators; however, the involvement of HPV in ocular malignancies has so far remained debatable.[30]

Similarly, one might be surprised at the absence of discussion about another area namely, the ear. Although evidence does exist of HPV involvement in ear diseases, the data are both modest and mixed. The epithelium in the auditory canal is basically an extension of the skin; given this fact, it is surprising that the key virus implicated in papilloma formation in the canal is a mucosal HPV type.[31]

The middle ear also presents a complex story, partly because of the histology allowed by the protection of the ear drum. However, while the epithelial tissue is dominated by low cuboidal cells, some squamous lining is also found in the middle ear. The cause of rare but serious cases of squamous cell carcinoma in this site appears to be twofold: (1) invasion of epithelial tissue via a cholesteatoma and (2) chronic inflammation. HPV involvement also appears to have two aspects. The virus has been implicated in cholesteatoma, a benign growth of skin that can penetrate the ear drum. As well, certain oncogenic types (notably HPV-16 and -18) appear to exploit the microenvironment associated with inner ear infections. As observed earlier, one ingredient in the "recipe" for HPV pathogenesis is physical access to the relevant target cells. In the case of ear infections, the virus may migrate from the oropharynx to the inner ear via the eustachian tube.[32]

The discussion to this point may be summarized before proceeding to the details of HPV-related disease processes. The HPV life cycle plays out in differentiating epithelial tissue, specifically the category known as stratified squamous epithelium. Particularly sensitive sites include the transitional areas at body openings, where distal squamous epithelium in effect is giving way to true, inner mucosal tissues (which in turn is typically composed of columnar epithelium). It is at these points of intermediate cellular keratinization that HPV infection, disordered cells, and cancerous transformation appear to occur relatively frequently.[33] Interestingly, the infected epithelial cells are marked by, among other features, changes in their normal keratin profile (see section "Processes of Disease").

In contrast with the list of susceptible sites, there is a relative absence of HPV infections in the linings found in various internal organs and gastrointestinal epithelia.[34] One intriguing exception to this "rule" has been the observed association between HPV and colorectal cancer.[35-37] Of course, the colorectum is also relatively near the surface of the body, so there may be macroscopic and microscopic explanations for HPV infection that are consistent with the general story developed in this chapter.

INFECTION AND IMMUNE EVASION

HPV infection requires access by the virus to the basal layer of stratified squamous epithelia. This appears to be facilitated by a natural entry point (e.g., via hair follicles or the deep ridges of plantar skin) or a break introduced in the epithelium, possibly a small cut or some other microtrauma.[38] While the specific character of the primary cellular target is still being investigated, some evidence points to epithelial stem cells.[39,40] Another possibility proposed in the case of the cervix is the mucosal columnar cells that merge into the stratified epithelium of the transformation zone.[41] As noted previously, the surface lining at this point is quite thin, perhaps increasing vulnerability to infection. While still an active area of research, many aspects of immune evasion, virus–host cell binding, internalization, and viral uncoating have begun to be clarified. A full description will ultimately explain how viral DNA is transported into the host nucleus and allowed to function there without effective opposition.[42]

The topic of immune evasion and HPV carcinogenesis is especially important because it is precisely the persistence of infection that is considered to be an essential component of cancer development.[43] As mentioned in Chapter 2, most HPV infections are cleared by the host within 2 years.[44,45] The rapid accumulation of infections after sexual debut is balanced in favor of viral clearance in women after age 25. This is why age-specific prevalence of HPV infection declines with age, at least until menopause. For reasons that are not well understood, some postmenopausal women do not clear the virus very well, leading to a second peak in HPV prevalence among older women in some populations in the world.[46]

When clearance does not occur, disease emerges. Technically, it is not incident HPV infection per se but rather a successfully evaded immune system that is the true risk factor for carcinogenesis.[47] This fact may help to explain the increased occurrence of HPV-related lesions in immunocompromised individuals.[48] Another intriguing finding is the fact that oncogenic HPV types tend to persist longer than low-risk types.[49] Full elucidation of the relationship between host immunity and HPV infection is ultimately vital to the development of immunotherapies and prophylactic vaccines.

The topic of immunity and cancer is complex. There are three categories of immune evasion required for viral carcinogenesis: mechanisms to allow the HPV infection to occur in the first place, mechanisms that prevent virally infected cells from being eliminated efficiently, and mechanisms "used" by tumor cells to evade the usual counterattacks mounted by the immune system.[50,51]

The first strategy employed by HPV to avoid detection and elimination has been described as "maintaining a low profile" or "operating by stealth." There are several features of HPV-related disease that support this characterization:

- The virus only infects epithelial cells
- Viral proteins are produced at low levels and are not secreted
- Viruses are produced in cells that are not lysed but are merely sloughed off at the end of their life span
- There is no viremia (i.e., viruses in the bloodstream), limiting antigen presentation and thus curtailing a systemic antibody response

This initial outline of the life cycle, focusing on the passive capacity of the virus to remain hidden, confirms that "HPV infection per se does not elicit any major damage likely to evoke the principal innate immunity danger signals."[52]

Immune evasion also involves more proactive measures. To fully appreciate the capabilities of HPV, it is important to acknowledge the defenses faced by the virus. The mucous membranes covering the urogenital and aerodigestive tracts (as well as the eye conjunctiva, the inner ear, and the ducts of all exocrine glands) have both mechanical and chemical cleansing mechanisms that manage to exclude most intruders. Furthermore, "a large and highly specialized innate and adaptive mucosal immune system protects these surfaces, and thereby also the body interior, against potential insults from the environment."[53] In an immunocompetent adult, the mucosal immune system, localized in various mucosa-associated lymphoid tissues, accounts for 80% of the body's immune cells.

Viral gene expression, in addition to driving viral production, helps HPV to evade the local immune system in its target tissue. In particular, E6 and E7 interrupt interferon pathways and regulate the production of certain chemokine factors involved with any inflammatory response. As well, by a variety of subtle means that are still being elucidated, HPV seems to directly disrupt the generation and delivery of cell-mediated adaptive immunity. This has been well documented in cervical cancer, but similar mechanisms have been found in viral skin lesions related to the genetic disorder known as epidermodysplasia verruciformis.[54]

One aspect of the immunity "battlefield" may be a reduced number of Langerhans cells (LCs) in cervical epithelium marked by dysplasia, though recent research has raised questions about the evidence for this phenomenon.[55,56] The LC is an essential component in adaptive immunity, functioning as an antigen-presenting cell during an adaptive immune response. A potentially important part of this story is the observation that LC distribution is affected by cervical cancer cofactors, such as HIV infection and smoking (see Chapter 4). A further consideration is the observation that the transformation zone itself has a lower density of LCs than found in the adjoining cervical epithelia.[57] The most significant mechanism may involve the role of E6 and E7 in decreasing the migration of LC and thereby compromising the immune response to infection. A 2009 study reported that experimentally silencing those two oncoproteins allowed LC migration to increase.[58]

Mutation of HPV types is another viral mechanism related to immune evasion. In particular, innate immunity that combats cervical cancer appears to be subverted by mutations in HPV capsid proteins.[59] This evolutionary process creates a continuing balance between host protection and viral persistence, so that both entities remain viable. This phenomenon is very common in the natural history of viruses; the ultimate "strategy" is to not kill the host nor impair its reproductive fitness.[60]

Host genetic makeup also appears to affect immune responses. The major histocompatibility complex (MHC) is pivotal in the functioning of the immune system. Genetic polymorphism in the host organism that may in turn influence the MHC is thought to predispose individuals toward cancer, especially when it is related to pathogenic infection.[61] This molecular variation in disease susceptibility has been examined in cervical cancer in particular.[62-64] The complexity of the story involves more than the host genome; certain viral genetic variations seem to exploit MHC polymorphisms to further increase the risk of cancer development.[65]

In sum, many HPV mechanisms (and host tissue conditions) appear to provide the foundation "for promoting viral persistence and avoiding innate immunity and the consequential activation of adaptive immunity."[66]

Finally, one intriguing observation is specific to unique immunological features of the cervix. In short, the phenomenon known as immune privilege could apply to this part of the female body; immune privilege refers to counter-regulating processes where destructive inflammation is attenuated and tissue function is preserved. The paradigm of such immunological exceptionalism is the eye. Researchers have postulated that the immune system could be similarly suppressed in the cervix, in part "to protect the integrity of the reproductive function."[67] A seemingly contrary result is the fact that certain mediators of immunity appear to be concentrated in the transformation zone between the ecto- and endocervix, a phenomenon that may increase susceptibility to HIV infection and ultimately immunosuppression.[68] Thus, although these proposed immunological features are heterogeneous, they actually lead to a similar result, that is, the cervix exhibiting a special propensity for cancer development.

PROCESSES OF DISEASE

Many aspects of the HPV carcinogenesis story have been worked out at a molecular level over the last two decades,[69–71] mostly based on cervical cancer as the prototypical malignancy.[72] Analysis of virus–host interactions has provided insight into the genes and pathways involved in the development of neoplasia. Viral proteins E6 and E7 are particularly key to such processes, though recently the role of E5 in disrupting cellular functions has also been elucidated.[73,74] Collateral benefits of this basic research on disease mechanisms include a growing understanding of normal cellular functions and the development of therapeutic and prophylactic vaccines that are designed to prevent or reverse the pathogenic disruption of those functions (see Chapter 7).[75,76]

As described earlier, all papillomaviruses have a parasitical relationship to their host. In each case of infection, they act as "obligatory intranuclear organisms" with tropism (i.e., affinity) for keratinocytes in the specific animal in question. Three possible courses of events can follow successful papillomavirus entry into target cells[77]:

1. Maintenance of viral DNA in an extrachromosomal form that replicates synchronously with the host cell; this basically constitutes a latent infection, where host epithelial cells (with their load of viral DNA) proliferate but new viruses are not produced
2. Conversion from latent into a productive infection that involves genome amplification and the assembly of complete virions, which ultimately may be transmitted to other hosts
3. Integration of viral DNA into host cellular genome, which is thought to be associated with malignant transformation

This section provides a brief synopsis of each of these expressions of HPV disease.

Proliferation Phase

The expression of viral gene products is closely regulated as the infected basal cell migrates toward the epithelial surface. The viral "strategy" at this point involves maintaining a molecular environment that is conducive for both viral genome replication and host cell proliferation.[78] Proliferation is marked by the expression of the initial "early" gene products that typify HPV. As noted earlier, these products are named after their controlling gene: E1, E2, etc. The E1 and E2 proteins appear to suppress viral replication when the infection is latent, so that only a low copy number of the virus genome is maintained in affected keratinocytes. Interestingly, this sort of controlled viral function is not restricted to human epithelia but can occur in other types of cells.[79] On the other hand, there is a so-called proliferation phase that is unique to disease in human keratinocytes; it is launched by E7, with E6 joining in. Both proteins have been implicated in mechanisms of cell immortalization, or the process of extending a cell's life, and increasing the number of its divisions, but without risk of developing into a tumor. Specifically, E7 has been associated with a reduction of retinoblastoma-associated protein (pRb), a substance that normally suppresses the cellular growth cycle. Similarly, E6 is involved with the interruption of p53, normally a mediator of growth suppression and cell death (=apoptosis).[80,81] A consistent interaction between E6 and the p53 pathway has been demonstrated across many oncogenic HPV types.[82] Another recent report described a reduced impact of E7 from HPV-26, 53, and 66, offering an elegant confirmation of the intermediate risk status of these viral types.[83] The immortalization role of E6 and/or E7 has also been demonstrated in skin neoplasia related to HPV types 8 and 38.[84,85]

Researchers have discovered several other molecular targets affected by E6 and E7, many having a direct role in malignant transformation (see below).[86-88] Interestingly, some dysregulation effects seem to differ across the range of HPV-16 E6 variants, suggesting the existence of viral phenotypes that are particularly "beneficial to carcinogenesis."[89] When viral functions are fully operational, the normal terminal differentiation of keratinocytes is disrupted, allowing them to continue proliferating in the affected epithelium. This microscopic feature of HPV disease accounts for the distinctive macroscopic feature, namely, the protuberances known as papilloma.

Evidence continues to emerge concerning the molecular mechanisms of HPV-related disease beyond the cervix. Recently, the proliferative capacity of oral keratinocytes (as driven by E6 and E7) was found to be enhanced when coinfected with HPV and HIV.[90] There is a suggestion of direct interaction between the two viruses; this phenomenon may become a more substantial concern given the growing understanding of oral-genital HIV transmission and the apparent ability of the virus to directly infect (and independently affect) oral mucosal cells.[91,92]

Keratinization as Mark and Marker

Adjustments of the keratin profile are an important part of the cellular change instigated by infection. Different types of keratin and various degrees of keratinization are exhibited in HPV-related disease states, including cancer.[93–96] The umbrella technical term for abnormal keratinization is dyskeratosis. The basic pattern of dyskeratosis involves an overall intensification of certain types of keratin in affected cells.[97] Such changes are distinct and generally observable when cells are examined for HPV-related disease, for example, in secondary prevention programs.

It is important to note that the conditions found in some normal tissues (e.g., parakeratosis, where the nucleus remains intact) can become hallmarks of disease in certain situations. A good example of this histological ambiguity is the presence of epithelial thickening. Hyperproliferative epidermis is perfectly natural where required for normal functioning (e.g., on the palms and soles). The same overproduction of keratinized cells, however, can become an expression of disease (technically designated as hyperkeratosis). Disorders of the epithelium involving this sort of condition include warts, corns, calluses, eczema, and psoriasis. It is notable that particular HPV types are strongly implicated in the hyperkeratosis associated with warts.

Warts are of course a clinically visible sign of HPV infection. But even preclinical, microscopic lesions can often be visually detected; low-level magnification provided by a colposcope, combined with the whitening effect produced by the application of acetic acid, routinely makes this possible in the case of the cervix. While the exact mechanism of the effect of acetic acid on epithelial cells is not clearly understood, the current consensus points to a process of cellular dehydration and the concomitant transformation of cellular proteins. This results in the reduction of surface transparency; the observed whitening is explained as a blockage of the underlying reddish color of vascular tissue.[98] In diagnostic terms, it is important to note that the proteins of abnormal cells are more dense, so an acetic acid wash yields more pronounced areas of white (often labeled as "acetowhite").[99,100] There are various opinions among researchers as to which cellular protein is most implicated in this telltale reaction of infected epithelium; some favor the role of nucleoproteins, whereas others look to cytokeratins.[101,102]

The fact that specific forms of keratin are generated during the proliferation of infected epithelial cells makes keratin typing a potentially useful diagnostic tool. In fact, "keratin filament proteins are regarded as the single invariable characteristic of epithelial cells, persisting even in metastatic tumors where all other identifying features are lost."[103]

Consequently, the role of keratin as a biomarker for tracking the presence and progression of epithelial disease has garnered increasing attention. This topic will be revisited in Chapter 6.

In sum, cellular proliferation and unique keratinization mark the first stage of the HPV infection life cycle. An important characteristic of this stage is the maintenance of the viral genome at a low copy number, which is mediated by the functioning of certain early viral proteins.[104]

Productive Infection and Virion Release

The daughter cells of dividing keratinocytes, each with a low copy number of replicated viral DNA, migrate "upward" and eventually reach the outer layers of the epithelium; at some point, the pattern of cellular regulation needs to change to allow the synthesis of new viruses. The basic molecular prerequisite of this phenomenon is amplification of the viral genome. All of the early viral proteins have been implicated in this process, though the precise roles of E4 and E5 are still being elucidated.[105,106]

As stated earlier, HPV encodes two structural proteins that are expressed once the process of genome amplification is completed. This occurs in the outermost layers of infected tissue. Multiple copies of the two late proteins, L1 and L2, combine into a viral capsid with icosahedral geometry.[107] Infected cells are not lysed; thus, to successfully complete its life cycle, the virus must reach the epithelial surface, be released within an exfoliated cell, and then survive until contact transmission and reinfection occurs.[108]

Malignant Transformation

The beginning of the development of cancerous cells constitutes in one sense a random accident; it may also be considered a "failure" for the virus as much as for the host. The viral life cycle, up to now closely linked to the epithelial differentiation process, is essentially disrupted during the development of malignancies. Sometimes this process is referred to as an abortive infection, that is, a manifest departure from a normal HPV life cycle. The sporadic nature of the initiating event accounts for the fact that the number of lesions leading to malignancies remains very low compared with the rate of HPV infection in the general population.

It has already been noted that proteins coded by the E6 and E7 genes are multifunctional; they interfere with a variety of important regulatory pathways in the cell cycle. In fact, E6 and E7 are also required for the initiation and maintenance of the malignant phenotype in HPV-positive cancers.[109] There is evidence, at least in the case of cervical cancer, that E5 may also play a critical role in the initiation of neoplasia, but a lesser role in cancer progression.[110]

Certain tissue sites seem to promote virus-induced malignancy. For instance, it is apparent that high-risk viral types such as HPV-16 "cannot reliably complete their life cycle" in the transformation zone of the cervix. In other words, rather than moving toward viral replication and release, the infection progresses in the direction of more profound cellular transformation and cancer.[111]

Expression of viral oncogenes such as E6 and E7 is normally tightly controlled in nondifferentiated keratinocytes. This is accomplished by at least two signaling pathways in the cell.[112] The initial factor that triggers carcinogenesis seems to be related to the viral genome itself. As a result of defects in HPV DNA, the expression of E6 or E7 is deregulated, leading to even greater cell proliferation. But this by itself would not be enough to generate malignancy. As one researcher has summarized: "While viral infection is a necessary prerequisite for the development of most cervical cancers, it is not by itself sufficient, indicating that secondary mutational events are also required."[113] Presumably, this is where cancer cofactors such as smoking may play a role. An important recent result showed that only one or two genetic changes are required in host cells after deregulation of HPV oncogenes for development of cervical cancer.[114]

This is not to say that the virus ever becomes a passive bystander. Abnormal viral protein expression helps to generate the susceptibility conditions related to cancer. In fact, the virus, especially one tuned to oncogenesis, promotes a triple threat: (1) increasing the incidence of host cell mutations, (2) interrupting DNA repair pathways in host cells, and (3) subverting intracellular safeguards "intended to eliminate cells that have acquired abnormalities that interfere with normal cell division."[115] In fact, one study described the impact on host cells of oncogenic HPV infections as "genomic chaos."[116] These manifest secondary changes in the host DNA, sometimes involving whole chromosomes, are critical contributors to cancer development.

In the normal HPV life cycle, the viral genome is maintained separately from that of the host. The final shift toward anogenital and oral carcinomas, especially those that become invasive, usually requires the integration of viral DNA into the host genome. Again, this phenomenon may be characterized as a form of molecular accident; it is essentially a terminal event interrupting the viral life cycle.[117] The uncontrolled expression of the E6 and E7 proteins that results from viral integration and the concomitant disruption of cell cycle regulators such as E2 is critical for progression toward a final carcinogenic state.[118,119]

This brief review of viral proteins in the development of malignancy underlines two potential cancer control levers at the molecular level: (1) the employment of biomarkers and (2) the development of therapies related to viral gene products.[120-122] Both areas have been the subject of intense investigation, as will be described in subsequent chapters. In addition, an understanding of disease mechanisms at a molecular level allows for better interpretation of emerging epidemiologic data, suggesting a causal role for HPV in malignancies beyond cervical cancer.[123]

NOTES

1. Turek LP, Smith EM. The genetic program of genital human papillomaviruses in infection and cancer. *Obstetrics and Gynecology Clinics of North America*. 1996; 23(4): 735–58.
2. Bodaghi S, Wood LV, Roby G et al. Could human papillomaviruses be spread through blood? *Journal of Clinical Microbiology*. 2005; 43(11): 5428–34.
3. Stanley MA, Pett MR, Coleman N. HPV: from infection to cancer. *Biochemical Society Transactions*. 2007; 35(Pt 6): 1456–60.
4. Huyse T, Poulin R, Theron A. Speciation in parasites: a population genetics approach. *Trends in Parasitology*. 2005; 21(10): 469–75.
5. Cason J, Mant CA. High-risk mucosal human papillomavirus infections during infancy & childhood. *Journal of Clinical Virology*. 2005; 32(suppl 1): S52–8.
6. zur Hausen H. Papillomaviruses causing cancer: evasion from host-cell control in early events in carcinogenesis. *Journal of the National Cancer Institute*. 2000; 92(9): 690–8.
7. Gillison ML, Shah KV. Role of mucosal human papillomavirus in nongenital cancers. *Journal of the National Cancer Institute*. Chapter 9, 2003; (31): 57–65.
8. Damin AP, Karam R, Zettler CG et al. Evidence for an association of human papillomavirus and breast carcinomas. *Breast Cancer Research and Treatment*. 2004; 84(2): 131–7.
9. Kan CY, Iacopetta BJ, Lawson JS et al. Identification of human papillomavirus DNA gene sequences in human breast cancer. *British Journal of Cancer*. 2005; 93(8): 946–8.
10. Kroupis C, Markou A, Vourlidis N et al. Presence of high-risk human papillomavirus sequences in breast cancer tissues and association with histopathological characteristics. *Clinical Biochemistry*. 2006; 39(7): 727–31.
11. Lindel K, Forster A, Altermatt HJ et al. Breast cancer and human papillomavirus (HPV) infection: no evidence of a viral etiology in a group of Swiss women. *Breast*. 2007; 16(2): 172–7.
12. Gillison ML, Shah KV. Role of mucosal human papillomavirus in nongenital cancers. *Journal of the National Cancer Institute*. Chapter 9, 2003; (31): 57–65.
13. Lindel K, Forster A, Altermatt HJ et al. Breast cancer and human papillomavirus (HPV) infection: no evidence of a viral etiology in a group of Swiss women. *Breast*. 2007; 16(2): 172–7.
14. Atula T, Grenman R, Klemi P et al. Human papillomavirus, Epstein-Barr virus, human herpesvirus 8 and human cytomegalovirus involvement in salivary gland tumours. *Oral Oncology*. 1998; 34(5): 391–5.

15 Shin KH, Park KH, Hong HJ et al. Prevalence of microsatellite instability, inactivation of mismatch repair genes, p53 mutation, and human papillomavirus infection in Korean oral cancer patients. *International Journal of Oncology.* 2002; 21(2): 297–302.
16 Sitas F, Urban M, Stein L et al. The relationship between anti-HPV-16 IgG seropositivity and cancer of the cervix, anogenital organs, oral cavity and pharynx, oesophagus and prostate in a black South African population. *Infectious Agents and Cancer.* 2007; 2: 6.
17 Korodi Z, Dillner J, Jellum E et al. Human papillomavirus 16, 18, and 33 infections and risk of prostate cancer: a Nordic nested case-control study. *Cancer Epidemiology, Biomarkers and Prevention.* 2005; 14(12): 2952–5.
18 Rosenblatt KA, Carter JJ, Iwasaki LM et al. Serologic evidence of human papillomavirus 16 and 18 infections and risk of prostate cancer. *Cancer Epidemiology, Biomarkers and Prevention.* 2003; 12(8): 763–8.
19 Nemes Z, Steinert PM. Bricks and mortar of the epidermal barrier. *Experimental and Molecular Medicine.* 1999; 31(1): 5–19.
20 Note that dandruff is essentially made up of dead skin keratinocytes.
21 Flores R, Abalos AT, Nielson CM et al. Reliability of sample collection and laboratory testing for HPV detection in men. *Journal of Virological Methods.* 2008; 149(1): 136–43.
22 Albers KM. Keratin biochemistry. *Clinics in Dermatology.* 1996; 14(4): 309–20.
23 Gu LH, Coulombe PA. Keratin function in skin epithelia: a broadening palette with surprising shades. *Current Opinion in Cell Biology.* 2007; 19(1): 13–23.
24 Maddox P, Szarewski A, Dyson J et al. Cytokeratin expression and acetowhite change in cervical epithelium. *Journal of Clinical Pathology.* 1994; 47(1): 15–7.
25 Smedts F, Ramaekers FC, Vooijs PG. The dynamics of keratin expression in malignant transformation of cervical epithelium: a review. *Obstetrics and Gynecology.* 1993; 82(3): 465.
26 Presland RB, Jurevic RJ. Making sense of the epithelial barrier: what molecular biology and genetics tell us about the functions of oral mucosal and epidermal tissues. *Journal of Dental Education.* 2002; 66(4): 564–74.
27 Incidence data taken from Duarte-Franco E, Franco EL. Other gynecologic cancers: endometrial, ovarian, vulvar and vaginal cancers. *BMC Women's Health.* 2004; 4(suppl 1): S14. Combined with HPV causality data in Chapter 2 (Figure 2.1). Cervical cancer incidence is 3 to 5 times higher, depending on the region of the world.
28 Doorbar J. Molecular biology of human papillomavirus infection and cervical cancer. *Clinical Science.* 2006; 110(5): 525–41.
29 Autier P, Coibion M, Huet F et al. Transformation zone location and intraepithelial neoplasia of the cervix uteri. *British Journal of Cancer.* 1996; 74(3): 488–90.
30 Tornesello ML, Duraturo ML, Waddell KM et al. Evaluating the role of human papillomaviruses in conjunctival neoplasia. *British Journal of Cancer.* 2006; 94(3): 446–9.
31 Xia MY, Zhu WY, Lu JY et al. Ultrastructure and human papillomavirus DNA in papillomatosis of external auditory canal. *International Journal of Dermatology.* 1996; 35(5): 337–9.

32 Jin YT, Tsai ST, Li C et al. Prevalence of human papillomavirus in middle ear carcinoma associated with chronic otitis media. *American Journal of Pathology*. 1997; 150(4): 1327–33.
33 Crum CP. Contemporary theories of cervical carcinogenesis: the virus, the host, and the stem cell. *Modern Pathology*. 2000; 13(3): 243–51.
34 zur Hausen H. Papillomaviruses causing cancer: evasion from host-cell control in early events in carcinogenesis. *Journal of the National Cancer Institute*. 2000; 92(9): 690–8.
35 Damin DC, Caetano MB, Rosito MA et al. Evidence for an association of human papillomavirus infection and colorectal cancer. *European Journal of Surgical Oncology*. 2007; 33(5): 569–74.
36 Bodaghi S, Yamanegi K, Xiao SY et al. Colorectal papillomavirus infection in patients with colorectal cancer. *Clinical Cancer Research*. 2005; 11(8): 2862–7.
37 Perez LO, Abba MC, Laguens RM et al. Analysis of adenocarcinoma of the colon and rectum: detection of human papillomavirus (HPV) DNA by polymerase chain reaction. *Colorectal Disease*. 2005; 7(5): 492–5.
38 Jimenez-Flores R, Mendez-Cruz R, Ojeda-Ortiz J et al. High-risk human papilloma virus infection decreases the frequency of dendritic Langerhans' cells in the human female genital tract. *Immunology*. 2006; 117(2): 220–8.
39 Egawa K. Do human papillomaviruses target epidermal stem cells? *Dermatology*. 2003; 207(3): 251–4.
40 Martens JE, Arends J, Van der Linden PJ et al. Cytokeratin 17 and p63 are markers of the HPV target cell, the cervical stem cell. *Anticancer Research*. 2004; 24(2B): 771–5.
41 Doorbar J. The papillomavirus life cycle. *Journal of Clinical Virology*. 2005; 32(suppl 1): S7–15.
42 Kanodia S, Fahey LM, Kast WM. Mechanisms used by human papillomaviruses to escape the host immune response. *Current Cancer Drug Targets*. 2007; 7(1): 79–89.
43 Brummer O, Hollwitz B, Bohmer G et al. Human papillomavirus-type persistence patterns predict the clinical outcome of cervical intraepithelial neoplasia. *Gynecologic Oncology*. 2006; 102(3): 517–22.
44 Plummer M, Schiffman M, Castle PE et al. A 2-year prospective study of human papillomavirus persistence among women with a cytological diagnosis of atypical squamous cells of undetermined significance or low-grade squamous intraepithelial lesion. *Journal of Infectious Diseases*. 2007; 195(11): 1582–9.
45 Lai CH, Chao A, Chang CJ et al. Host and viral factors in relation to clearance of human papillomavirus infection: a cohort study in Taiwan. *International Journal of Cancer*. 2008; 123(7): 1685–92.
46 Syrjanen K. Mechanisms and predictors of high-risk human papillomavirus (HPV) clearance in the uterine cervix. *European Journal of Gynaecological Oncology*. 2007; 28(5): 337–51.
47 Rodriguez AC, Schiffman M, Herrero R et al. Rapid clearance of human papillomavirus and implications for clinical focus on persistent infections. *Journal of the National Cancer Institute*. 2008; 100(7): 513–7.
48 Tyring SK. Human papillomavirus infections: epidemiology, pathogenesis, and host immune response. *Journal of the American Academy of Dermatology*. 2000; 43(1 Pt 2): S18–26.

49 Trottier H, Mahmud S, Prado JC et al. Type-specific duration of human papillomavirus infection: implications for human papillomavirus screening and vaccination. *Journal of Infectious Diseases.* 2008; 197(10): 1436–47.
50 Kanodia S, Fahey LM, Kast WM. Mechanisms used by human papillomaviruses to escape the host immune response. *Current Cancer Drug Targets.* 2007; 7(1): 79–89.
51 Sheu BC, Chang WC, Lin HH et al. Immune concept of human papillomaviruses and related antigens in local cancer milieu of human cervical neoplasia. *Journal of Obstetrics and Gynaecology Research.* 2007; 33(2): 103–13.
52 Stern PL. Immune control of human papillomavirus (HPV) associated anogenital disease and potential for vaccination. *Journal of Clinical Virology.* 2005; 32(suppl 1): S72–81.
53 Holmgren J, Czerkinsky C. Mucosal immunity and vaccines. *Nature Medicine.* 2005; 11(4 suppl): S45–53.
54 Orth G. Genetics of epidermodysplasia verruciformis: insights into host defense against papillomaviruses. *Seminar in Immunology.* 2006; 18: 362–74.
55 Connor JP, Ferrer K, Kane JP et al. Evaluation of Langerhans' cells in the cervical epithelium of women with cervical intraepithelial neoplasia. *Gynecologic Oncology.* 1999; 75(1): 130–5.
56 Campaner AB, Nadais RF, Galvao MA et al. Evaluation of density of Langerhans cells in human cervical intraepithelial neoplasia. *Acta Obstetricia et Gynecologica Scandinavica.* 2007; 86(3): 361–6.
57 Giannini SL, Hubert P, Doyen J et al. Influence of the mucosal epithelium microenvironment on Langerhans cells: implications for the development of squamous intraepithelial lesions of the cervix. *International Journal of Cancer.* 2002; 97(5): 654–9.
58 Caberg JH, Hubert P, Herman L et al. Increased migration of Langerhans cells in response to HPV16 E6 and E7 oncogene silencing: role of CCL20. *Cancer Immunology, Immunotherapy.* 2009; 58(1): 39–47.
59 Yang R, Wheeler CM, Chen X et al. Papillomavirus capsid mutation to escape dendritic cell-dependent innate immunity in cervical cancer. *Journal of Virology.* 2005; 79(11): 6741–50.
60 Frazer IH. Interaction of human papillomaviruses with the host immune system: a well evolved relationship. *Virology.* 2009; 384(2): 410–4.
61 Little AM, Stern PL. Does HLA type predispose some individuals to cancer? *Molecular Medicine Today.* 1999; 5(8): 337–42.
62 Hildesheim A, Wang SS. Host and viral genetics and risk of cervical cancer: a review. *Virus Research.* 2002; 89(2): 229–40.
63 Madeleine MM, Brumback B, Cushing-Haugen KL et al. Human leukocyte antigen class II and cervical cancer risk: a population-based study. *Journal of Infectious Diseases.* 2002; 186(11): 1565–74.
64 Beskow AH, Moberg M, Gyllensten UB. HLA class II allele control of HPV load in carcinoma in situ of the cervix uteri. *International Journal of Cancer.* 2005; 117(3): 510–4.
65 Wu Y, Liu B, Lin W et al. HPV16 E6 variants and HLA class II polymorphism among Chinese women with cervical cancer. *Journal of Medical Virology.* 2007; 79(4): 439–46.

66 Stern PL. Immune control of human papillomavirus (HPV) associated anogenital disease and potential for vaccination. *Journal of Clinical Virology.* 2005; 32(suppl 1): S72–81.
67 Hoglund P, Karre K, Klein G. The uterine cervix—a new member of the family of immunologically exceptional sites? *Cancer Immunity.* 2003; 3: 6.
68 Pudney J, Quayle AJ, Anderson DJ. Immunological microenvironments in the human vagina and cervix: mediators of cellular immunity are concentrated in the cervical transformation zone. *Biology of Reproduction.* 2005; 73(6): 1253–63.
69 Munger K, Phelps WC, Bubb V et al. The E6 and E7 genes of the human papillomavirus type 16 together are necessary and sufficient for transformation of primary human keratinocytes. *Journal of Virology.* 1989; 63(10): 4417–21.
70 Stubenrauch F, Laimins LA. Human papillomavirus life cycle: active and latent phases. *Seminars in Cancer Biology.* 1999; 9(6): 379–86.
71 Whiteside MA, Siegel EM, Unger ER. Human papillomavirus and molecular considerations for cancer risk. *Cancer.* 2008; 113(suppl 10): 2981–94.
72 DiMaio D, Liao JB. Human papillomaviruses and cervical cancer. *Advances in Virus Research.* 2006; 66: 125–59.
73 Kivi N, Greco D, Auvinen P et al. Genes involved in cell adhesion, cell motility and mitogenic signaling are altered due to HPV 16 E5 protein expression. *Oncogene.* 2008; 27(18): 2532–41.
74 Krawczyk E, Suprynowicz FA, Liu X et al. Koilocytosis: a cooperative interaction between the human papillomavirus E5 and E6 oncoproteins. *American Journal of Pathology.* 2008; 173(3): 682–8.
75 Ghim SJ, Sundberg J, Delgado G et al. The pathogenesis of advanced cervical cancer provides the basis for an empirical therapeutic vaccine. *Experimental and Molecular Pathology.* 2001; 71(3): 181–5.
76 Dell G, Gaston K. Human papillomaviruses and their role in cervical cancer. *Cellular and Molecular Life Sciences.* 2001; 58(12–13): 1923–42.
77 Cheah PL, Looi LM. Biology and pathological associations of the human papillomaviruses: a review. *Malaysian Journal of Pathology.* 1998; 20(1): 1–10.
78 Doorbar J. The papillomavirus life cycle. *Journal of Clinical Virology.* 2005; 32 (suppl 1): S7–15.
79 Desaintes C, Demeret C. Control of papillomavirus DNA replication and transcription. *Seminars in Cancer Biology.* 1996; 7(6): 339–47.
80 Jones EE, Wells SI. Cervical cancer and human papillomaviruses: inactivation of retinoblastoma and other tumor suppressor pathways. *Current Molecular Medicine.* 2006; 6(7): 795–808.
81 Narisawa-Saito M, Kiyono T. Basic mechanisms of high-risk human papillomavirus-induced carcinogenesis: roles of E6 and E7 proteins. *Cancer Science.* 2007; 98(10): 1505–11.
82 Hiller T, Poppelreuther S, Stubenrauch F et al. Comparative analysis of 19 genital human papillomavirus types with regard to p53 degradation, immortalization, phylogeny, and epidemiologic risk classification. *Cancer Epidemiology, Biomarkers and Prevention.* 2006; 15(7): 1262–7.
83 Mansour M, Touka M, Hasan U et al. E7 properties of mucosal human papillomavirus types 26, 53 and 66 correlate with their intermediate risk for cervical cancer development. *Virology.* 2007; 367(1): 1–9.

84 Akgul B, Ghali L, Davies D et al. HPV8 early genes modulate differentiation and cell cycle of primary human adult keratinocytes. *Experimental Dermatology.* 2007; 16(7): 590–9.
85 Gabet AS, Accardi R, Bellopede A et al. Impairment of the telomere/telomerase system and genomic instability are associated with keratinocyte immortalization induced by the skin human papillomavirus type 38. *FASEB Journal.* 2008; 22(2): 622–32.
86 Scheurer ME, Tortolero-Luna G, Adler-Storthz K. Human papillomavirus infection: biology, epidemiology, and prevention. *International Journal of Gynecological Cancer.* 2005; 15(5): 727–46.
87 Mammas IN, Sourvinos G, Giannoudis A et al. Human papilloma virus (HPV) and host cellular interactions. *Pathology Oncology Research.* 2008; 14(4): 345–54.
88 Liu X, Roberts J, Dakic A et al. HPV E7 contributes to the telomerase activity of immortalized and tumorigenic cells and augments E6-induced hTERT promoter function. *Virology.* 2008; 375(2): 611–23.
89 Zehbe I, Richard C, DeCarlo CA et al. Human papillomavirus 16 E6 variants differ in their dysregulation of human keratinocyte differentiation and apoptosis. *Virology.* 2009; 383(1): 69–77.
90 Kim RH, Yochim JM, Kang MK et al. HIV-1 Tat enhances replicative potential of human oral keratinocytes harboring HPV-16 genome. *International Journal of Oncology.* 2008; 33(4): 777–82.
91 Liu X, Zha J, Chen H et al. Human immunodeficiency virus type 1 infection and replication in normal human oral keratinocytes. *Journal of Virology.* 2003; 77(6): 3470–6.
92 Acheampong EA, Parveen Z, Muthoga LW et al. Molecular interactions of human immunodeficiency virus type 1 with primary human oral keratinocytes. *Journal of Virology.* 2005; 79(13): 8440–53.
93 Lam KY, Loke SL, Shen XC et al. Cytokeratin expression in non-neoplastic oesophageal epithelium and squamous cell carcinoma of the oesophagus. *Virchows Archiv.* 1995; 426(4): 345–9.
94 Maddox P, Sasieni P, Szarewski A et al. Differential expression of keratins 10, 17, and 19 in normal cervical epithelium, cervical intraepithelial neoplasia, and cervical carcinoma. *Journal of Clinical Pathology.* 1999; 52(1): 41–6.
95 Chu PG, Weiss LM. Keratin expression in human tissues and neoplasms. *Histopathology.* 2002; 40(5): 403–39.
96 Akgul B, Ghali L, Davies D et al. HPV8 early genes modulate differentiation and cell cycle of primary human adult keratinocytes. *Experimental Dermatology.* 2007; 16(7): 590–9.
97 Smedts F, Ramaekers F, Leube RE et al. Expression of keratins 1, 6, 15, 16, and 20 in normal cervical epithelium, squamous metaplasia, cervical intraepithelial neoplasia, and cervical carcinoma. *American Journal of Pathology.* 1993; 142(2): 403–12.
98 Sankaranarayanan R, Wesley R, Somanathan T et al. Visual inspection of the uterine cervix after the application of acetic acid in the detection of cervical carcinoma and its precursors. *Cancer.* 1998; 83(10): 2150–6.
99 Maddox P, Szarewski A, Dyson J et al. Cytokeratin expression and acetowhite change in cervical epithelium. *Journal of Clinical Pathology.* 1994; 47(1): 15–7.

100 Jonsson M, Karlsson R, Evander M et al. Acetowhitening of the cervix and vulva as a predictor of subclinical human papillomavirus infection: sensitivity and specificity in a population-based study. *Obstetrics and Gynecology.* 1997; 90(5): 744–7.
101 MacLean AB. Acetowhite epithelium. *Gynecologic Oncology.* 2004; 95(3): 691–4.
102 Lambert R, Rey JF, Sankaranarayanan R. Magnification and chromoscopy with the acetic acid test. *Endoscopy.* 2003; 35(5): 437–45.
103 Maddox P, Szarewski A, Dyson J et al. Cytokeratin expression and acetowhite change in cervical epithelium. *Journal of Clinical Pathology.* 1994; 47(1): 15–7.
104 Doorbar J. The papillomavirus life cycle. *Journal of Clinical Virology.* 2005; 32(suppl 1): S7–15.
105 Genther SM, Sterling S, Duensing S et al. Quantitative role of the human papillomavirus type 16 E5 gene during the productive stage of the viral life cycle. *Journal of Virology.* 2003; 77(5): 2832–42.
106 Doorbar J. The papillomavirus life cycle. *Journal of Clinical Virology.* 2005; 32(suppl 1): S7–15.
107 Hebner CM, Laimins LA. Human papillomaviruses: basic mechanisms of pathogenesis and oncogenicity. *Reviews in Medical Virology.* 2006; 16: 83–97.
108 Doorbar J. The papillomavirus life cycle. *Journal of Clinical Virology.* 2005; 32(suppl 1): S7–15.
109 zur Hausen H. Papillomaviruses in human cancers. *Proceedings of the Association of American Physicians.* 1999; 111(6): 581–7.
110 Kim SW, Yang JS. Human papillomavirus type 16 E5 protein as a therapeutic target. *Yonsei Medical Journal.* 2006; 47(1):1–14.
111 Doorbar J. The papillomavirus life cycle. *Journal of Clinical Virology.* 2005; 32(suppl 1): S7–15.
112 zur Hausen H. Papillomaviruses in human cancers. *Proceedings of the Association of American Physicians.* 1999; 111(6): 581–7.
113 Laimins L. Human papillomaviruses target differentiating epithelia for virion production and malignant conversion. *Seminars in Virology.* 1996; 7(5): 305–13.
114 Narisawa-Saito M, Yoshimatsu Y, Ohno S et al. An in vitro multistep carcinogenesis model for human cervical cancer. *Cancer Research.* 2008; 68(14): 5699–705.
115 Munger K, Hayakawa H, Nguyen CL. Viral carcinogenesis and genomic instability. *EXS.* 2006; 96: 179–99.
116 von Knebel Doeberitz M. New markers for cervical dysplasia to visualise the genomic chaos created by aberrant oncogenic papillomavirus infections. *European Journal of Cancer.* 2002; 38(17): 2229–42.
117 Munger K. The role of human papillomaviruses in human cancers. *Frontiers in Bioscience.* 2002; 7: d641–9.
118 Turek LP, Smith EM. The genetic program of genital human papillomaviruses in infection and cancer. *Obstetrics and Gynecology Clinics of North America.* 1996; 23(4): 735–58.
119 Furumoto H, Irahara M. Human papilloma virus (HPV) and cervical cancer. *Journal of Medical Investigation.* 2002; 49(3–4): 124–33.

120 Middleton K, Peh W, Southern S et al. Organization of human papillomavirus productive cycle during neoplastic progression provides a basis for selection of diagnostic markers. *Journal of Virology.* 2003; 77(19): 10186–201.

121 Govan VA. Strategies for human papillomavirus therapeutic vaccines and other therapies based on the E6 and E7 oncogenes. *Annals of the New York Academy of Sciences.* 2005; 1056: 328–43.

122 Kim SW, Yang JS. Human papillomavirus type 16 E5 protein as a therapeutic target. *Yonsei Medical Journal.* 2006; 47(1):1–14.

123 Whiteside MA, Siegel EM, Unger ER. Human papillomavirus and molecular considerations for cancer risk. *Cancer.* 2008; 113(suppl 10): 2981–94.

4

HUMAN PAPILLOMAVIRUS: ASSOCIATIONS WITH CERVICAL CANCER

Beyond any doubt, oncogenic HPV types are the single most important etiological agents of cervical cancer and CIN lesions.[1]

The investigation of infections associated with cancer has been strongly influenced by the story of human papillomavirus (HPV), dating from even before the virus was isolated and characterized. Indirect evidence of possible cancer causation was accumulated over many decades at a macro- rather than a microscopic level. Early insights were based on the connection between cervical cancer and sexual behavior.[2–4] As early as 1842, it was noticed that cervical cancers occurred only in married women[5]; in a similar vein, the low cervical cancer rates among nuns pointed to a connection with coitus. In general, cervical cancer was found to share "many characteristics with communicable diseases that follow a venereal mode of transmission."[6] The suspected sexually transmitted agent was eventually identified as HPV. As introduced in Chapter 2, the pool of cancers associated with HPV has greatly expanded since the discoveries about cervical cancer, although cancer of the cervix continues to occupy the majority of research attention.

Globally, cervical cancer is the second most common female cancer. Thus, it is of particular importance that vital information is available concerning its etiology. HPV in fact occupies a unique position in this regard. As Walboomers and colleagues famously concluded in 1999, "the presence of HPV in virtually all cervical cancers implies the highest worldwide attributable fraction so far reported for a specific cause of any major human cancer."[7] In short, HPV has been proposed as the first necessary cause of a human cancer ever identified, accounting for its dominant status in biological and clinical studies of infection and cancer, and its high profile in the present book.[8]

Adding to the important etiologic role of the virus, public health and clinical concerns about cervical cancer have also helped to propel HPV to the forefront of research agendas related to infection and cancer. In fact, only one or two other infectious agents compete with HPV in terms of the intensity of investigation. One by-product of the substantial research focus on HPV has been the growing understanding of the role of the virus in many other diseases, both malignant and benign.

HPV INFECTION AND CANCER

While it is clear that cervical cancer dominates the story, it is important to understand from the start the full range of cancers associated with the virus. These malignancies notably include other genital carcinomas, such as those affecting the vulva or penis. The fraction of these cancers attributable to HPV infection is quite substantial, as high as 50%.[9] The HPV-related cancers also comprise various mucosal neoplasms of the head and neck and certain skin tumors.[10-12] A particularly serious cancer connected to HPV, especially in high-risk male subpopulations, is squamous cell carcinoma of the anus.[13]

Other HPV–cancer associations are being actively investigated, including lung tumors.[14] The main benign disorders associated with HPV are different types of genital and cutaneous warts and recurrent respiratory papillomatosis.

For the balance of the present chapter, the focus will be on the connection between HPV and cervical cancer. The growing information in this area has offered a basic paradigm for understanding the other HPV-related cancers, which will be the topic of Chapter 5. The main agenda in each case will be to describe and, as much as possible, quantify the connection between these cancers and HPV infection.

For cervical cancer, an overview of disease burden in the United States and Canada will be provided, with the information being situated within a global context. Tracking cervical cancer statistics is a particularly appropriate exercise for understanding the impact of HPV, given the close association between viral infection and malignancy. In this situation, combining this comprehensive insight about disease burden and viral etiology may directly shape prevention priorities and strategies.

BURDEN OF CERVICAL CANCER

As noted above, cervical cancer represents the second most common malignant neoplasm in women worldwide; the annual number of incident cases approaches half a million. It is second only to breast cancer in terms of the global incidence of female cancers.

Global Variation

The burden of cervical cancer relative to all female malignancies is generally higher in the developing world. Indeed, in certain developing countries, such as Mexico and India, it is the most common female cancer.[15,16] The distribution of cervical cancer impact according to a crude stratification by level of national development is summarized in Table 4.1; the information was compiled by the International Agency for Research on Cancer (IARC) from numerous national and regional cancer registries.[17] The mortality due to cervical cancer, which continues to rise in global terms, is particularly high in South Asia, sub-Saharan Africa, and parts of Latin America.

On the basis of the aggregate data, a strong case can certainly be made for prevention initiatives in the developing world. A number of other statistics may be marshaled to further motivate such an effort, including the fact that cervical cancer is the largest contributor to years of life lost due to cancer in two highly populous regions, sub-Saharan Africa and south-central Asia; even more, it is the most important cause of years of life lost due to any cause in Latin America and the Caribbean.[18]

It is clear that most developed countries are at an advantage in terms of cervical cancer burden. As an illustration of this, the rates of cervical cancer in the United States and Canada are compared against incidence data from selected countries in Figure 4.1.[19]

United States and Canada

The United States and Canada boast cervical cancer rates that are among the lowest in the world. In contrast with the sizeable global burden, the

Table 4.1. Cervical Cancer in the World (2002)

	Cases	Deaths	5-Year Prevalence
World	492,800	273,200	1,409,200
More developed countries	83,400	39,500	309,900
Less developed countries	409,400	233,700	1,099,300

Source: Sankaranarayanan, *International Journal of Gynecology & Obstetrics*, 2006. Used by permission.

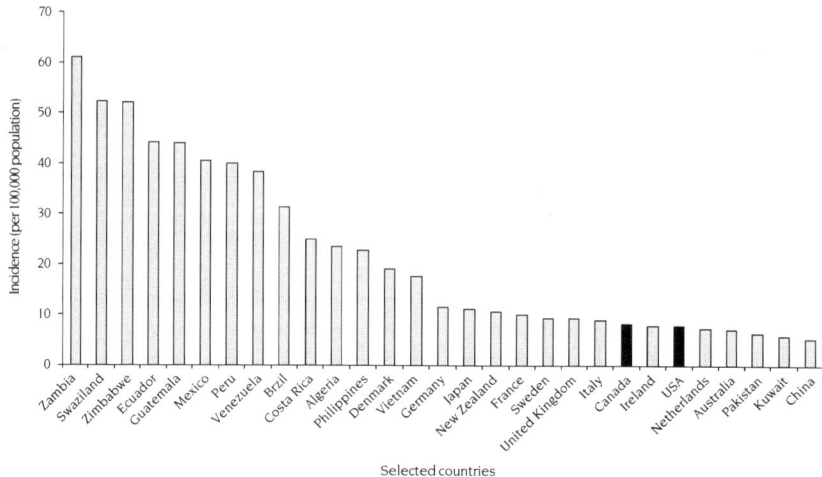

Figure 4.1. Cervical cancer incidence, by country, 2003. *Source:* Steckley et al., *Biomedicine & Pharmacotherapy*, 2003.

number of new cases in the United States was estimated at only 12,000 in 2004, whereas 3,850 deaths were attributed to the disease. An even more modest 1,350 new cases of cervical cancer occurred in Canada in 2007 (making it the 11th most common cancer diagnosed among Canadian women); there were an estimated 390 deaths due to cancer of the cervix in the country that year.[20] While small on a global scale, the figures in the United States and Canada still demonstrate that cervical cancer is an important prevention target. Even more urgent is the need to learn from the successes in controlling incidence and mortality in developed countries, and to enhance prevention efforts in other parts of the world. This perspective is strengthened by the existence of relatively simple prevention strategies that were proven and in use long before the advent of HPV vaccines.

Although the relatively modest disease burden is enjoyed across both countries, important regional variations do exist in terms of incidence and mortality. In the United States, incidence and mortality rates for cervical cancer tend to be higher in the South, Appalachia, and areas bordering Mexico.[21–23] Intraregional variation also exists, for example, among the five Appalachian states.[24]

A pattern of variability may be seen across the provinces of Canada, as detailed in Figure 4.2.[25] For example, in 2003, incidence rates per 100,000 population ranged from a low of 6.0 in British Columbia to a high of 11.2 in Nova Scotia, and mortality rates from 1.3 in Quebec to 3.9 in New Brunswick. The favorable situation in British Columbia may

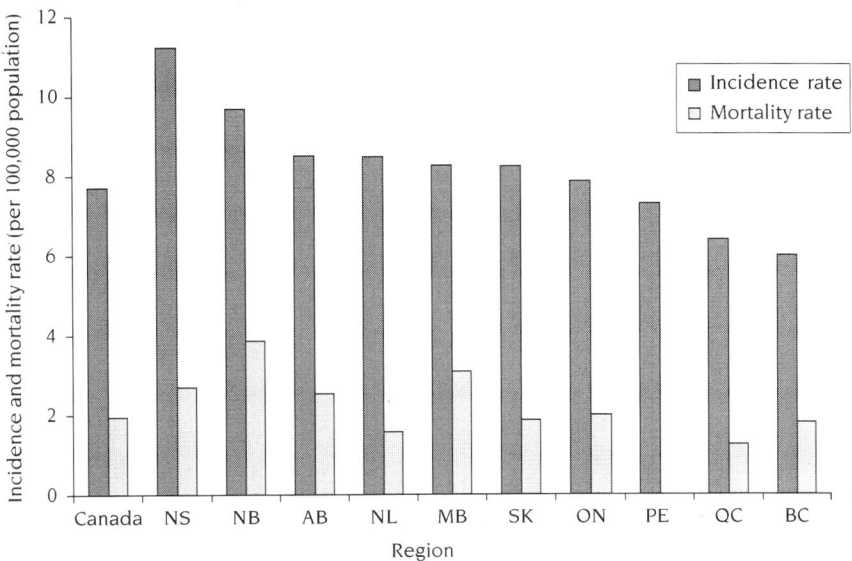

Figure 4.2. Age-standardized incidence and mortality rates for cervical cancer, Canada and the provinces, 2003. Source: *Canadian Cancer Statistics, 2007*.

Table 4.2. Female Cancers in the United States, by Time Period Average Age-adjusted Incidence Rates (per 100,000)

	1974–1978	1979–1983	1989–1993	1999–2003
Breast	104.1	105.7	130.6	134.1
Cervix	13.9	11.4	10.2	7.6

Source: SEER Cancer Registry as cited by Hayat et al., *The Oncologist*, 2007.

reflect the fact that, in 1949, the province became the first jurisdiction in the world to implement an organized, population-based program to screen for cervical cancer.[26]

Trends and Target Groups

Not only are the incidence and mortality rates for cervical cancer in the United States and Canada low by global standards, the current status is the result of a positive trend over several decades. Table 4.2 provides average age-adjusted incidence rates for two important female cancers in the United States for selected 5-year time periods; it is clear that there has been opposing developments with respect to cervical cancer and breast cancer at the population health level since the 1970s.[27] Breast cancer incidence has steadily risen, whereas cervical cancer occurrence has declined.

A similar situation for cervical cancer occurs in Canada. As seen in Figure 4.3, between 1978 and 2007 the age-standardized incidence rate for cervical cancers decreased from 14.8 cases per 100,000 to 7.3. The age-standardized mortality rate also declined, shifting from 4.7 to 1.8 per 100,000.[28] This pattern is repeated in the provinces. For instance, a 2008 analysis in Manitoba revealed that cervical cancer had shifted from being the 5th most frequent cancer diagnosis for women in 1970 to the 11th by 1999.[29]

The already low and, up to now, steadily declining rate of cervical cancer in the United States and Canada needs to be taken into consideration when planning new prevention investments to combat HPV-related disease. This is not to say that public health efforts should not be maintained or even increased, especially to guard against any exceptions or reversal in the positive general pattern and to make equitable progress among groups not well served in terms of cervical cancer prevention. There are examples of the latter concern in many developed countries, including Aboriginal peoples in Canada (see section "Canadian Aboriginal Groups and Cervical Cancer") and ethnic and low-income groups in the United States. Results from one recent study in the U.S. context are summarized in Table 4.3.[30] While different methods of collecting data seem to generate deviations from the

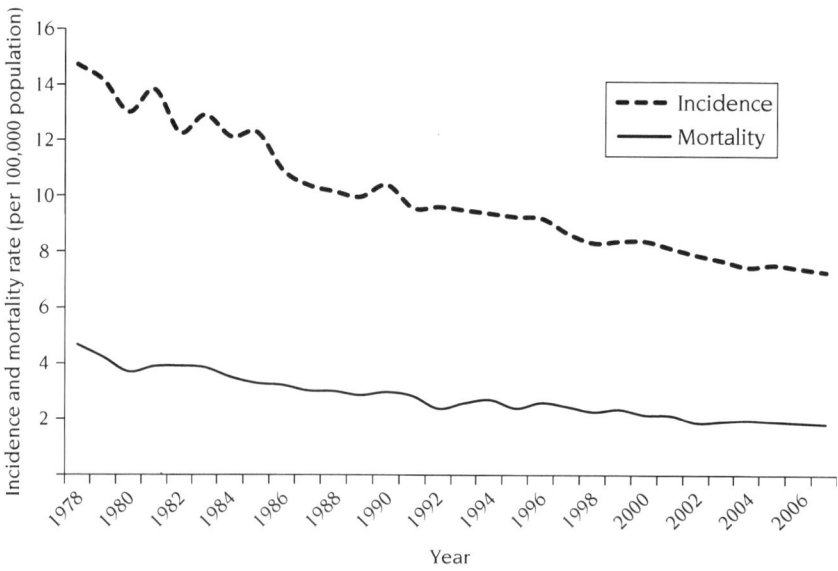

Figure 4.3. Age-standardized incidence and mortality rates for cervical cancer, Canada 1978–2007. *Source: Canadian Cancer Statistics*, 2007.

overall population totals presented in Table 4.2, the basic phenomenon of ethnic and socioeconomic variation is still evident. Indeed, the results immediately point to some important demographic targets for enhanced prevention initiatives among, for instance, Hispanic and African American populations; this conclusion is consistent with results from other recent studies.[31–35]

Other statistical reports indicate that the picture for Asian-Americans is complex.[36] Vietnamese and Korean groups demonstrate notably high incidence, a phenomenon that seems to be driving the cervical cancer rate for all Asian and Pacific Islanders higher than that of non-Hispanic whites.[37] This trend, which is contrary to that seen in Table 4.3, may reflect recent shifts in Asian immigration patterns, variations in cervical cancer susceptibility, and low rates of cervical cancer screening and precursor control among certain ethnic populations. On the other hand, some Asian groups, such as Chinese- and Japanese-Americans, appear to continue to enjoy a lower cervical cancer incidence rate compared with non-Hispanic white women. Older research from British Columbia, Canada, suggests a different picture, with incidence (and mortality) of cervical cancer elevated among the Chinese population.[38] This is similar to the pattern seen for Chinese Americans in Los Angeles reported in the same era (the early 1990s).[39] Interestingly, this was part of a period where Asian and Pacific Islander groups as a whole did not enjoy an advantage compared with U.S. Caucasians in terms of cervical cancer rates.[40]

In sum, it appears that three cautions should be observed when drawing conclusions about specific ethnic populations and cervical cancer, at least in North America: the information sometimes is quite limited, it is

Table 4.3. Average Age-adjusted Incidence Rates for Cervical Cancer, by Social Category (United States), 1998–2001

	Rate (per 100,000)	95% C.I.
Overall	12.0	(11.9–12.2)
Non-Hispanic white	11.6	(11.5–11.7)
Hispanic	16.6	(16.2–17.1)
African American	17.1	(16.7–17.6)
Asian or Pacific Islander	9.9	(9.3–10.5)
American Indian or Alaskan Native	7.2	(6.2–8.4)
<20% below poverty line	11.6	(11.5–11.7)
≥20% below poverty line	16.7	(16.2–17.1)

Source: United States Cancer Statistics: 2001 Incidence and Mortality as cited by Benard et al., Obstetrics & Gynecology, 2007.

often dated, and apparently the data are subject to fluctuations over a relatively short period of time.

While remaining cognizant of the challenges regarding the underlying data, at least some information indicates that the cervical cancer picture for Aboriginal groups in the United States may be the reverse of that found in Canada. For example, the recent study summarized in Table 4.3 found an incident rate of approximately 7 per 100,000 American Aboriginal women compared with 12 per 100,000 in the general population; indeed, some ethnic groups demonstrated a rate more than double that of American Indians.[41] By contrast, cervical cancer incidence (and mortality) is known to be higher among Aboriginal women of Canada.[42] This important topic will be explored in some detail in the next section, including a review of alternate information concerning Aboriginal groups in the United States. The ultimate aim is to provide a comparison for other countries assessing and responding to cancer among indigenous populations.

Canadian Aboriginal Groups and Cervical Cancer

The various Aboriginal groups of Canada, referred to collectively as First Nations, Inuit, or Métis, appear to be an exception to the generally favorable national statistics concerning cervical cancer. The most extensive research on cervical cancer among Aboriginal women in Canada has been conducted in Ontario, Manitoba, Saskatchewan, British Columbia, and northern regions. The inclusion of Manitoba and Saskatchewan in this list is not surprising, as Aboriginal women (at 14%) represent the largest share of the overall female provincial population compared with other jurisdictions in the country. The proportions in the northern territories are even more dramatic; for example, 87% of women in Nunavut are Aboriginal. Shifting to absolute terms, the largest numbers of Aboriginal women live in Ontario, 20% of the national complement; not far behind, 17% of Canadian Aboriginal women live in British Columbia.[43]

The available research, which is somewhat dated, indicates that Aboriginal women tend to have higher rates of cervical cancer than the general female population in Canada. For instance, the age-standardized incidence rate of invasive cervical cancer from 1984 to 1997 among Aboriginals in Manitoba was 3.6 times that for non-Aboriginal women.[44] The elevated rate of cervical cancer was consistent with an earlier report examining Manitoba First Nations reserves.[45] Citing a 1991 Canadian cancer statistics report, Franco et al. noted that 29% of all malignancies among Saskatchewan Aboriginal women were cancers of the cervix, reflecting an age-standardized incidence rate six times the national average.[46]

A study of 437 women with cervical cancer in British Columbia (detected from 1985 to 1988) indicated that 10% of invasive cervical cancers were found in Aboriginals, even though they only constitute 4% of the women in the province.[47] An oft-cited report from the same period demonstrated substantially higher cervical cancer mortality among Aboriginals in the province. While this introduces the possibility of elevated occurrence, it is only one among many potential explanations (such as poor access to detection services and follow-up care).[48]

Women from the Inuit and possibly other Aboriginal groups in the Northwest Territories also demonstrate higher cervical cancer rates than the general Canadian population—up to three times higher.[49,50] According to 1991–1996 statistics, cervical cancer was the most common female malignancy in the region.[51] A parallel result seems to apply among the Inuit women of northern Quebec (the so-called Nunavik region), where cervical cancer was second only to lung cancer as the leading cause of cancer-related deaths from 1984 to 1993.[52] It should be acknowledged that, especially in the northern territories, the absolute number of Aboriginal patients underlying most cancer statistics is very small.

The general picture of cancer among Aboriginal peoples that has been described so far in this section was confirmed in a meta-analysis of data up to 1991 in North Americaas a whole. It showed that, in the case of most cancers, incidence rates among Aboriginals actually tend to be *lower* than the general population (although this varies geographically).[53] Cancer of the cervix was one of the notable exceptions. The meta-analysis of data from the United States and Canada suggested that cervical cancer rates are elevated among Aboriginal females.[54] More recent research seems to support this conclusion in the U.S. context, contrary to the picture described earlier based on Table 4.3. In short, the balance of evidence indicates higher cervical cancer incidence rates among Aboriginal groups compared with non-Hispanic whites and the U.S. general population.[55,56] Interestingly, among Indian Health Service regions in the United States, the highest rates for cervical cancer are found in the Northern and Southern plains, a result that may relate in part to HPV prevalence.[57]

Whereas most data indicate a consistent cervical cancer situation in Canada and the United States, suggesting the need for increased prevention efforts directed toward Aboriginal females, there are also some positive trends. First, recent secondary prevention efforts targeted at Aboriginal communities appear to be gaining traction. In fact, cervical cancer screening utilization rates among some Aboriginal groups now exceed those in the general Canadian population,[58,59] although this is not likely to be typical for Aboriginal women who live off-reserve.

Table 4.4. Cervical Cancer and First Nations, by Time Period Ages 15–74, Ontario, Canada

Year of Diagnosis	Incidence (per 100,000)		Incidence Rate Ratio
	First Nations Population	General Population	First Nations vs. General Population
1968–1975	33.6 (22.9–47.6)	24.5	1.37 (0.93–1.94)
1976–1983	23.6 (15.9–33.9)	16.4	1.43 (0.96–2.05)
1984–1991	22.8 (17.6–29.1)	13.4	1.69 (1.30–2.15)
1992–2001	14.2 (8.5–22.4)	11.2	1.26 (0.75–1.98)

Source: Cancer Care Ontario, Dr. L. Marrett, personal communication.

Note: 95% confidence interval in brackets.

Second, and likely a reflection of the first point, cervical cancer rates in Canadian Aboriginal women are decreasing. For instance, incidence declined sharply between 1992 and 1998 in what is now the Nunavut territory.[60] In Ontario, the incidence of cervical cancers in Aboriginal women has declined from an average annual 33.6 cases per 100,000 population between 1968 and 1975 to 14.2 cases per 100,000 between 1992 and 2001 (Table 4.4). While this decrease is substantial and important, it should be noted that the most recent incidence rates are still higher than in the general population.[61]

Care must be taken in attributing recent changes in cervical cancer rates among Aboriginals to targeted secondary prevention efforts rather than changes in underlying primary causes such as HPV infection and smoking, or increases in the prevalence of hysterectomy.[62] Nonetheless, the fact that there appear to have been improvements in cervical cancer incidence is certainly positive and worthy of further investigation as to underlying factors.

HPV AS A NECESSARY CAUSE OF CERVICAL CANCER

For all practical purposes, a one-to-one connection exists between cervical cancer and the presence of HPV DNA in disease tissue. This discovery has generated a great deal of excitement, especially related to the implied promise that "the prevention of HPV infection would virtually eliminate cervical cancer."[63]

There is a strong evidence base specifically implicating so-called high-risk (i.e., oncogenic) HPV types as the main risk factor for the development of cervical cancer. Extensive epidemiologic data on the association between the virus and cervical cancer has been confirmed by molecular biological research. For example, a recent study suggested that the presence of integrated HPV-18 genome in tumor-free mucosal tissue is a strong marker of adjacent tumor development.[64]

The gradually increasing disclosure of the natural history of HPV infections within cervical tissues has been an important part of the scientific evidence uncovered to date. The present conclusion is unequivocal: high-grade cervical intraepithelial neoplasia (CIN) develops as a result of persistent oncogenic HPV infections.[65] The same type of infections put women at a significantly increased risk of invasive cervical cancer.[66]

It is important to recognize that cervical cancer occurs in three main histological categories: squamous cell carcinoma, adenocarcinoma, and adenosquamous carcinoma. Squamous cell carcinoma clearly dominates. For example, of nearly 8,500 cases of invasive cervical cancer recorded in the Michigan cancer registry from 1985 to 2003, 72% were squamous cell carcinoma, 17% were adenocarcinoma, and 4% were adenosquamous carcinoma.[67]

Sometimes multiple histologies present at the same time.[68] While evidence has suggested that squamous lesions coexisting with glandular lesions have a different etiology than squamous lesions appearing on their own,[69,70] the most critical observation is that HPV has been clearly implicated in all three forms of cancer of the cervix. For example, a 2006 study revealed a connection between HPV infection in the underlying squamous epithelium and the development of cervical adenocarcinoma.[71] Only a few rare histological variants of cervical adenocarcinoma seem unrelated to HPV infection.[72] For the rest of cervical cancer cases, HPV is the clear culprit. Intriguingly, there appears to be a differential pattern of HPV-type involvement with the various forms of cervical cancer, as will be described below. It is useful to note that the histological specificity related to cervical cancer parallels the broader patterns of tissue tropism seen with HPV types. As seen in Chapter 2, various viral types beyond HPV-16 and 18 preferentially cause different forms of malignant and nonmalignant disease in the human body. A notable example is the essential connection between genital warts and HPV-6 and 11.

High-Risk Viral Types

A clear pattern has emerged in terms of HPV types and the propensity for cancer occurrence. The "high-risk" label has traditionally been defined in terms of the probability of development of cervical cancer, as that malignancy stands out in the inventory of HPV-related cancers. For the most part, however, the key HPV types implicated in cervical cancer reappear for the other HPV-related malignancies; the main exception is skin cancer, which involves an additional set of HPV types.

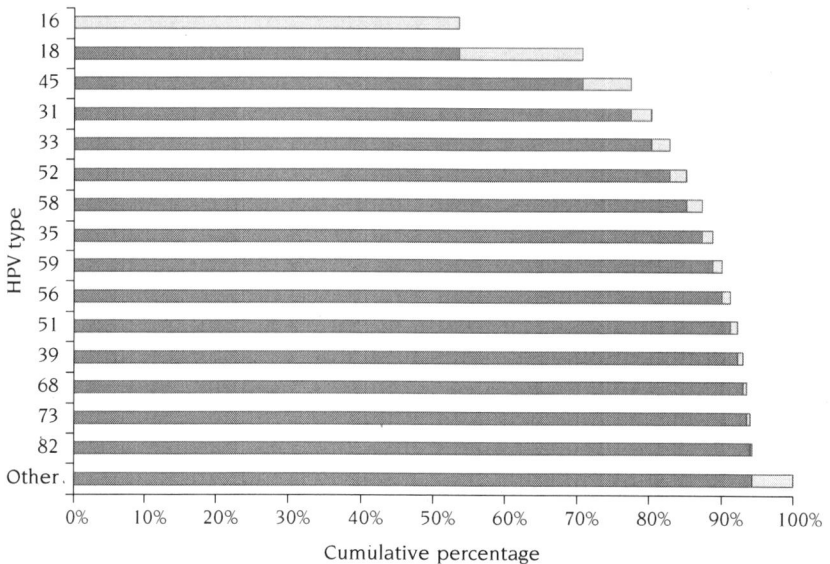

Figure 4.4. Cumulative proportion of cervical cancers by HPV type. *Source*: Bosch et al., *International Journal of Gynecology and Obstetrics*, 2006. Used by permission.

Of the more than 40 HPV types transmitted through sexual contact and infecting the anogenital region, a handful is found most frequently within malignant cells. According to pooled data from 1,700 HPV-positive cervical cancer patients in nine countries from different parts of the world, HPV-16 dominated the spectrum, being detected in more than half the cases; types 18, 45, and 31 together accounted for another 27% of cervical cancer incidence (Figure 4.4).[73-75] Other high-risk HPV types implicated in cervical cancer were (in descending order) 33, 52, 58, 35, 59, plus several other proven or candidate forms.[76]

A meta-analysis published in the same year yielded very similar results, with HPV-16 and 18 observed at the highest rate in 8,500 cervical cancer patients (at 54.3% and 12.6%, respectively). The next five types were comparable to the pattern observed in the other study, though in a different order: HPV-33, 45, 31, 58 and, finally, 52.[77]

A further project examined 55 reports (dated 1996–2004) from across the world, with a specific focus on HPV typology associated with low-grade squamous intraepithelial lesions (LSIL) of the cervix. In addition to demonstrating geographical variation in HPV type-specific distribution, the research showed that infection rates for high-risk types were lower in patients with low-grade dysplasia compared with the known occurrence in individuals with full cancer; in other words, there

Table 4.5. Risk Factors Over 2 Year Follow-up for Cervical Cancer Progression, by HPV Type

Viral Type	% of ASC-US Cases Leading to CIN3	% of LSIL Cases Leading to CIN3	Odds Ratio of Progressing to CIN3 (Compared to HPV-Negative Cases)
HPV-16	32.5 (28.4–36.8)	39.1 (33.8–44.7)	38 (22–68)
All other HPV types	8.4 (6.9–10.4)	9.9 (8.0–12.0)	7.2 (4.2–13)

Source: Castle et al., *Journal of the National Cancer Institute*, 2005. Used by permission.

Note: 95% confidence interval in brackets.

is a disproportionate involvement of these viral types in malignancy, confirming their status as high-risk types. This was especially notable for HPV-16 and 18, "highlighting the importance of HPV genotype in the risk of progression from LSIL to malignancy."[78]

Other papers have also reported variations in HPV association with cervical cancer and its precursors. For example, in a 2005 study, 5,060 women with equivocal cytology (i.e., atypical squamous cells of undetermined significance, or ASCUS) or mildly abnormal results (i.e., LSIL) were tested for HPV DNA. The prevalence of HPV-16 among these cases was much lower than observed in high-grade lesions or full cervical cancer.[79] The conclusion was that there was a marked difference between HPV-16 and all other viral types in terms of their propensity to move tissue from mildly dysplastic to the most serious grade of precursor (Table 4.5).

In sum, HPV-16 is the most common type found in cervical neoplasia and cancer, a finding that holds across all parts of the world.[80,81] Putting it in different terms, HPV-16 demonstrates the highest risk for disease progression,[82] and equivalently the lowest propensity for spontaneous tumor regression.[83] Additional research has shown that patients with cervical HPV-16 have a higher risk for recurrent or residual CIN3 after treatment for neoplasia.[84] Such results reinforce the conclusion that HPV-16 is the most critical focus of any preventive, therapeutic, or surveillance initiative.

Tumor Histology and HPV Types

The preceding conclusions apply in particular to squamous cell carcinomas and precursors; a different story emerges when other tissues are considered.[85–87] For example, in certain jurisdictions, HPV-18 appears to be equally or even more prevalent than HPV-16 in cervical adenocarcinomas.[88–90] This was recently demonstrated in a dramatic way among cervical adenocarcinoma patients in Indonesia.[91] Likewise, HPV-18 appears to predominate in the presentation of adenosquamous carcinoma of the cervix.[92] Such results have serious implications for prevention efforts. Adenocarcinoma and adenosquamous carcinoma precursors are not as easily detected by Pap smears. This may be part of the reason for a worldwide increase in the prevalence of cervical adenocarcinoma; currently, it may represent a quarter of all cervical cancers.[93] As a consequence, the benefit of molecular screening or a vaccine targeting HPV-18 becomes elevated as a way to compensate for the limitations of the Pap smear.[94–96] Research has been conducted on the etiology of very rare malignancies of the cervix. In some cases these appear to be associated with HPV, although there is a "greater tendency toward more unusual HPV types."[97] Because of low prevalence and the resulting challenges of epidemiologic studies, the etiology of many of the more unusual cervical tumors has not been elucidated.[98]

As noted earlier, declining cervical cancer incidence rates ought not to lead to complacency in public health initiatives in developed countries. Reinforcing this perspective, it seems that while the incidence of squamous cell carcinoma of the cervix has been declining in recent decades, adenocarcinoma has been on the rise.[99] For example, the incidence rate of adenocarcinoma in Canada has increased since 1970.[100] The upward trend-line related to adenocarcinoma is true both in absolute terms, presumably driven by factors such as high-risk HPV infections, and relative to squamous cell carcinoma rates; the explanation for the latter pattern usually involves the lower sensitivity of screening tests with respect to adenocarcinoma precursors (see Chapter 6). Regions within Canada offer evidence of these phenomena. For example, according to a 2008 study, the proportion of cervical cancer cases in the province of Manitoba that were adenocarcinomas rose from 7% to 22% between 1970 and 1999.[101] On the other hand, improved screening techniques in the province of Ontario during the late 1990s seem to have reversed the rising incidence of cervical adenocarcinoma.[102]

Multiple Viral Types

Several studies have demonstrated a high frequency of multiple HPV infections in cervical carcinomas.[103–105] For the most part, coinfections seem to reflect random combinations of HPV types.[106] There has been some evidence that multiple infections are found more often in adenosquamous carcinomas of the cervix.[107,108]

Details about the pattern of multiple infections have begun to emerge. While detecting different HPV types may ultimately be traced back to more than one lesion on the cervix, multiple types have also been clearly isolated from a single lesion.[109] Some research has even suggested that single tumor cells can contain multiple HPV genomes.[110] The physical status of the multiple types of HPV DNA may vary from tumor to tumor. In a recent study of three cervical cancers demonstrating HPV-16 and -18, integration of only one genome was seen in two cases (HPV-16 in one, and HPV-18 in the other), whereas in the remaining case both genomes remained in an episomal state.[111]

There is mixed evidence concerning the pathological implications of simultaneous HPV infections. Some authorities have suggested that "each genotype of HPV acts as an independent infection, with differing carcinogenic risks linked to evolutionary species."[112] However, coinfections with two or more viral types have also been associated with a higher risk of CIN or cervical cancer. For example, a 2006 study of a Brazilian cohort concluded that "infections with multiple HPV types seem to act synergistically in cervical carcinogenesis."[113] Other research has suggested that there is no increased risk with multiple types compared with situations with single HPV infections.[114] One recent study even suggested that the frequency of single infections increased with the severity of the cervical lesion.[115]

The complex interactions between HPV types in carcinogenesis remain an important topic of research, with potential implication for prevention measures such as prophylactic vaccination. For example, there may be lower prevalence of HPV-16 integration in the presence of HPV-18 coinfection, possibly indicating lower oncogenicity.[116] Such intratypic modulation in tissues with multiple infections may partially account for the difference between vaccine efficacy under experimental conditions and more recent effectiveness data related to real-world reductions in high-grade cervical lesions.[117]

Geographical Variation

The HPV-type distribution associated with cervical cancer varies geographically. The disease-related patterns of infection appear to parallel the differences in HPV prevalence in the general female population (see Chapter 2).[118] IARC and other agencies have analyzed the many studies that establish the distribution of HPV types in cytologically abnormal cervixes. Substantial meta-analyses were published in 2003 and 2005, in each case covering a decade worth of reports.[119-121] A 2007 update by Smith et al. of data gathered from different parts of the world yielded a further summary of oncogenic types most frequently observed in cervical cancer patients (Figure 4.5).[122]

The various meta-analyses confirm that HPV-16/18 dominate the inventory of viral types detected in cervical cancer in all parts of the

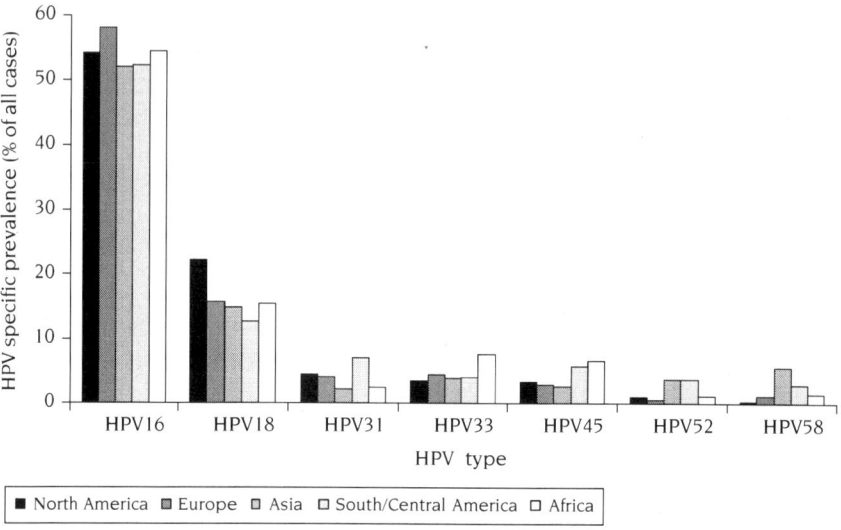

Figure 4.5. Proportion of selected HPV types in cervical cancer, by region. *Source*: Smith et al., *International Journal of Cancer*, 2007.

world. One notable regional difference is the lower proportion of HPV-18-related cases in the developing world as compared with North America, and the higher prevalence of cervical cancer cases featuring HPV-52 and 58 in Asia and South/Central America. This type profile for cancer in such regions may impact the effectiveness of any vaccine targeting only two oncogenic types, that is, HPV-16/18. On the other hand, the absolute numbers of cervical cancer cases in developing countries is much higher; thus, a vaccine against HPV-16/18, whatever the variation in its impact in different regions of the world, will arguably prevent a large number of cervical cancers wherever it is deployed.

Meta-analyses suffer from a standard set of limitations, including variable detection methods and different sample sizes (e.g., the number of patients from sub-Saharan Africa available to Smith et al. was less than 25% of the combined sample used to generate European information). As a counterpoint, the comparison of recent data from four representative countries provided in Table 4.6 was designed to reflect similar sample sizes.

The information in Table 4.6 confirms previously discussed points about the preferential involvement of HPV-16 in higher grade lesions, and about geographical variation of disease specific types. Certain HPV types appear to have a proportionately higher impact on carcinogenesis outside of the West. This is especially true of the family of viral types related to HPV-16, known collectively as genus α, species 9 (or $\alpha 9$). For

Table 4.6. Geographic Variation in Oncogenic HPV Genotypes, by Cytological Grade

HPV Types Categorized by Species	Italy (2006) N = 231		Taiwan (2006) N = 552		Costa Rica (2006) N = 6		Senegal (2003) N = 172	
	LSIL (%)	HSIL/CIS/ICC (%)	LSIL (%)	HSIL/CIS/ICC (%)	LSIL (%)	HSIL/CIS/ICC (%)	LSIL (%)	HSIL/CIS/ICC (%)
	n = 101	n = 130	n = 241	n = 311	n = 391	n = 291	n = 86	n = 86
α9								
HPV 16	37	52	8	32	7	32	8	23
HPV 31	3	4	1	2	5	9	1	6
HPV 33	2	5	2	12	1	1	2	8
HPV 35	0	1	2	1	1	1	3	1
HPV 52	1	0	18	19	4	2	3	8
HPV 58	1	2	7	20	6	8	9	13
α7								
HPV 18	0	6	5	2	2	2	5	5
HPV 39	0	0	6	1	5	1	0	1
HPV 45	1	0	2	1	0	0	0	0
HPV 59	–	–	4	2	1	1	2	0
HPV 68	1	0	3	0	1	1	0	1
HPV 70	0	1	0	0	8	0	–	–

(Continued)

Table 4.6. (Continued)

HPV Types Categorized by Species	Italy (2006) N = 231		Taiwan (2006) N = 552		Costa Rica (2006) N = 682		Senegal (2003) N = 172	
	LSIL (%) n = 101	HSIL/CIS/ICC (%) n = 130	LSIL (%) n = 241	HSIL/CIS/ICC (%) n = 311	LSIL (%) n = 391	HSIL/CIS/ICC (%) n = 291	LSIL (%) n = 86	HSIL/CIS/ICC (%) n = 86
α5								
HPV 51	1	0	10	3	5	4	1	3
HPV 82	0	1	–	–	0	0	0	2
α6								
HPV 53	2	2	11	2	5	5	3	2
HPV 56	0	1	2	0	6	0	1	1
HPV 66	2	0	7	0	3	0	1	2
% of n cases	50	74	89	97	60	68	42	78

Sources: Italy: Tornsello et al., *Journal of Medical Virology*, 2006. Taiwan: Chen et al., *International Journal of Gynecological Cancer*, 2006. Costa Rica: Kovacic et al., *Cancer Research*, 2006. Senegal: Xi et al., *International Journal of Cancer*, 2003.

example, the high prevalence of HPV-52 and 58 stands out in cervical cancers among the Chinese population in Taiwan, a phenomenon also identified in several other studies.[123–128] The importance of these two types has also recently been noted in Singapore and Hong Kong.[129]

Given the national and regional variations in HPV distribution related to cervical disease, there may be concerns related to immigration and potential health care costs. For instance, certain West African immigrants in south Italy have been shown to have very high HPV prevalence, with the most common types being those other than HPV-16 and 18. In other words, apart from the effect of any cross-protection, the viral types involved may not be prevented by the vaccines currently on the market.[130] A recent Canadian study further underlined this concern; HPV-31 was found to contribute more significantly to cervical cancer in the province of Saskatchewan than type 18, the significance of which "will depend on the level of cross protection offered by the new vaccines."[131] In sum, many authorities have suggested that the knowledge of unique HPV genotype distribution patterns in CIN or cervical cancer should inform effectiveness and cost-effectiveness analyses and national guidelines for both screening and vaccine deployment.[132,133] When there is substantial involvement of nonvaccine HPV types in cancer development within a particular population, it can raise doubts about the degree of protection afforded by vaccination.[134]

Whatever the final conclusion concerning HPV-type distribution in cervical lesions in a particular jurisdiction, it is important to also incorporate the effect of HPV-type variation in the general female population (as described in Chapter 2). As an IARC-led study group acknowledged in 2003, the "heterogeneity in HPV-type distribution among women from different populations should be taken into account when developing screening tests for the virus and predicting the effect of vaccines on the incidence of infection."[135]

Subtypes and Variants

Complexity is multiplied when HPV types are further divided into subtypes or variants based on diversity in one or more viral genes.[136] Several reports have been recently published on the variations within HPV-16/18 and other types from the same HPV species.[137–142] Some researchers are attempting to map the fascinating story of human migrations over the last four centuries by tracking the mutation and geographic spread of specific HPV genotypes. As part of this work, investigators have identified European, Asian, American-Asian, and African forms of HPV-16.

Most pertinent to the prevention theme is the implication of HPV-type variation on vaccine efficacy. Questions have been raised, but few conclusions advanced, about this topic for over a decade.[143] Even the most recent studies continue in a speculative vein, suggesting that further research will be required to fully elucidate the impact of genetic variation within HPV types on both prophylactic and therapeutic strategies.[144–151] Only two informative reports were found in the review for this book; both were related to genetic variations in the L1 capsid gene of HPV-16, and both were reassuring. The suggestion from a 2006 study was that there was little impact from a known variant on the antigenicity of the virus-like particle (VLP) that is the foundation of current prophylactic vaccines.[152] An earlier paper went further, concluding that, from vaccination perspective, HPV-16 variants belong to one serotype; this creates the potential for VLP-generated antibodies that "confer a similar degree of protection against all known branches of HPV 16."[153]

Also potentially relevant to prevention, researchers have investigated variations in viral genomes that may account for higher cervical cancer rates in specific populations.[154] For example, the prevalence of highly carcinogenic variants of HPV-16 and related types may explain the elevated cervical cancer burden in Mexico.[155] The research examining the relative carcinogenicity of HPV-16 variants has yielded mixed results. One older study showed that non-European viral types are more persistent in the human body.[156]

Clinical Utility of HPV Genotyping

Implications of the data concerning type-specific disease development extend beyond vaccine effectiveness to the potential utility of HPV DNA testing.[157] While comprehensive screening applications are still being evaluated, there is already compelling evidence for the cost-effectiveness of HPV testing following equivocal Pap smears or detection and treatment for CIN.[158–162]

Consideration of future HPV testing programs raises three important areas of practical discussion. First, a "double negative" result, that is, a normal Pap smear combined with no detected HPV, may allow for "the safe extension of the interval between cervical screenings."[163]

More pertinent to genotyping, the detection of high-risk HPV as a result of primary screening using HPV DNA testing could be used to guide more intensive follow-up.[164]

Finally, the detection of specific genotypes, in turn allowing predictions concerning progression to cancer or prognosis after cancer, could further clarify management approaches.[165] For instance, infection with HPV-31 has been associated with better survival, and HPV-18 with worse survival, in cervical cancer patients,[166,167] although this finding has been questioned in a more recent study.[168] On the other hand, there is little doubt about the connection between HPV-18 and the development of adenocarcinoma; thus, testing for this particular viral type, followed by targeted management, could reduce the incidence of cervical adenocarcinoma worldwide.[169]

A more complete coverage of the topics of HPV vaccination and testing will be offered in subsequent chapters.

AGE, OTHER RISK CORRELATES, AND TARGETED PREVENTION

Cervical cancer is extremely rare in women under the age of 20; for example, there were no cases diagnosed in this age group in the United States between 1998 and 2002.[170] This phenomenon is presumably attributable to the timing of high-risk HPV acquisition and the typical latency period involved with cancer development. Similar mechanisms are at work in creating a peak in cervical cancer incidence around age 40. Interestingly, a second peak in the number of cases is observed among older women in some populations, including the United Kingdom.[171] The bimodal pattern may reflect the distribution of HPV infection in the population ; this in turn may be related to endogenous host factors or increasingly liberal sexual activity in older adults. It was noted in Chapter 2 that some countries demonstrate a second peak in HPV prevalence in women over age 55. Indeed, relatively high acquisition and persistence of HPV infection in postmenopausal women have been reported in various studies,[172,173] as well as a tendency to progress toward single-type infections and select for an integrated viral clone that can aggressively move toward malignancy.[174] Compounding the impact of current high-risk infection, older women, especially after menopause, sometimes participate less frequently in cervical cancer screening and, even when they do, the test proves to be less sensitive.[175]

A general correlation between sexual activity and cervical cancer incidence would be expected given the involvement of a sexually transmitted infection (STI) such as HPV. Important factors in this regard include the number of sexual partners (lifetime and recent), young age at first sexual intercourse, and risky sexual behavior in a woman's male partners.[176-178] A recent pooled analysis of studies covering more than 11,000 women confirmed that certain factors related to risky sexual behavior are associated with HPV positivity.[179]

Sexual debut is particularly critical; research has shown that the earlier HPV infection occurs in young women, the higher the risk of developing cervical malignancies.[180] This phenomenon persists even when the latency period is controlled for, indicating that there is some independent effect of sexual activity at a young age; this may involve the continuous metaplastic changes that happen at the junction between the endocervix and ectocervix, a process that is more active at puberty (and in pregnancy), thus producing increased susceptibility to HPV infection.[181–183]

Past or current STIs with a microbe other than HPV provide another obvious correlation with cervical cancer occurrence. Consistent with the earlier suggestions about sexual behavior in seniors, there are indications that the rate of STIs in older cohorts has been increasing.[184]

The associations under consideration in this section raise the promise of identifying high-risk cohorts, such as commercial sex workers, and targeting prevention activities accordingly.[185] Unfortunately, effective strategies related to lifestyle interventions (including sexual health promotion and counseling) that might reduce the risk of cervical cancer development have been slow to emerge and be disseminated.[186,187]

On a related (and controversial) front, a recent U.S. study did not demonstrate increased oncogenic HPV infection in women of low socioeconomic status, once the researchers had controlled for age, number of sexual partners, and smoking history.[188] The implication is that poverty does not offer a consistent marker of HPV prevalence and related disease risk. This topic continues to be studied in other jurisdictions, sometimes with different results.[189]

Incidence and mortality need to be distinguished when assessing cervical cancer burden and its correlation with risk factors, including socioeconomic status. Thus, income-related disparities in cervical cancer mortality rates have been observed in Canada, though these have declined markedly since 1971. While more equitable cervical cancer screening probably accounts for most of the narrowing gap, favorable changes in disease cofactors (see section "Disease Cofactors") may also be involved; candidate influences in this regard include declines in parity and improved diets.[190]

DISEASE COFACTORS

While HPV has been identified as a necessary cause of cervical cancer, the fact that a large percentage of women infected with high-risk HPV types do not progress to cancerous states demonstrates that the presence of the virus is not a sufficient cause of disease.[191] This conclusion is reinforced on an epidemiologic level; while varying cervical cancer rates sometimes can be traced to varying HPV prevalence[192]; the relationship does not seem to hold for every country.[193] The implication is that other risk factors, possibly causal ones, are at work in such situations. In fact, several cofactors have been posited to interact with the natural history of HPV infection and related carcinogenesis.[194-196] Some of the suggestions continue to be controversial, including smoking and oral contraceptive use.[197]

The mechanisms related to increased susceptibility may be classified as follows:

1. Creation of the conditions for persistent HPV infection
2. Reactivation of a latent infection
3. Enhancement of the carcinogenic potency of HPV molecular products
4. Promotion of malignancy in the target tissue in some other way

The most robust form of the first three mechanisms would be the existence of another necessary cause of cervical cancer, that is, a full and formal instance of cocarcinogenesis. Such a factor has not yet been identified in cervical cancer. On the other hand, the most substantial expression of the fourth category would be a factor that could cause cervical cancer independently of HPV infection. Again, no such factor has been identified. Smoking offers an example of limitations affecting candidate risk factors. While apparently increasing the risk of cervical cancer (see below), use of tobacco products is neither required for carcinogenesis nor able to cause cervical tumors apart from HPV infection.

Unless otherwise noted, the brief overview that follows will focus on factors involved with squamous cell carcinoma in particular. One exception will involve pointing out where the etiologic impact of a risk factor varies with respect to adenocarcinoma and adenosquamous carcinoma. In fact, the main forms of cervical cancer share most risk factors, with the exception of smoking.[198,199]

Genetic Factors

Endogenous factors, notably the genetic susceptibility of the host, have been an area of intense research interest. It is part of the ongoing quest to explain why only a subset of women infected with HPV develop cervical cancer.[200,201] In particular, polymorphisms of the p53 gene in the host have been investigated, although with somewhat divergent results.[202,203] Various genes have also been studied with reference to possible gene–gene interactions.[204] The fact that some of the host genetic variation may have a link to ethnic or geographic differences only adds to the complexity.[205,206]

Reflecting the important role of immunologic responses in controlling HPV infection, research has also focused on differences in the major histocompatability complex. This is a region of the host genome responsible for generating immune system proteins known as human leukocyte antigens.[207-209]

The story becomes even more complicated when the subtle variants within HPV types are factored into the equation. For example, polymorphisms of the p53 gene in the host seem to interact most intensely with certain variants of HPV-16 in the modulation of disease progression.[210,211] Likewise, polymorphisms of the human leukocyte antigen have been shown to interact with HPV-16 variants and thereby modify cervical cancer risk.[212] Even as such information continues to accumulate, it must be acknowledged that the relationship between host polymorphisms and HPV variants remains "poorly understood."[213] Nonetheless, the promise is held out of one day routinely screening for genetic predisposing factors that may help to predict the persistence of HPV infection and the probability of tumor development.[214]

Smoking

Of all the non-HPV candidates introduced into multifactorial explanations of cervical cancer, smoking stands out. Over two decades of epidemiologic studies, including several multicenter projects, have established that smoking increases the risk of cervical cancer.[215-217] Sometimes such results have been interpreted as an artifact of the association between smoking and risky sexual activity. As recently as 2008, Syrjanen reported that elevated cervical cancer rates among smokers could be attributed to increased HPV acquisition that is ultimately traceable to sexual behavior patterns.[218] It should be noted that this author and colleagues have posited similar mechanisms for the connection between drug addiction and cervical cancer.[219] However, several studies on smoking and cervical cancer have specifically controlled for such confounding effects.[220] A recent reanalysis of results involving 13,541 cervical squamous carcinoma cases confirmed that there was a significant and substantial relative risk (1.95, 95% C.I. 1.43–2.65) of cervical cancer incidence in current smokers compared with never smokers; control data included age, age at first intercourse, duration of oral contraceptive use, number of full-term pregnancies, and lifetime number of sexual partners.[221] Interestingly, an association with smoking was not found for adenocarcinoma in this and other studies,[222] reinforcing the suggestion of direct mechanisms rather than an artifact of risky sexual behavior.

Recent studies have confirmed a true synergistic effect between smoking and infection, which may be particularly strong for HPV-16.

The potential etiologic mechanisms related to tobacco smoke are still under investigation. The suggested interactions include localized immunosuppression, a direct influence on malignant transformation of HPV-infected cells, and the creation of genotoxic DNA adducts in the cervical epithelium.[223,224] The immune effects of smoking related to HPV have been shown to apply mostly to women under 30 years of age, suggesting that preventing smoking initiation and promoting cessation in younger women may be particularly important.[225] In regard to genotoxicity, it is known that certain smoking-related carcinogens do accumulate in cervical tissues.[226] Indeed, researchers have suggested that some cancers arise specifically due to an interaction between oncogenic viruses and tar exposure in the cervix. Smoking is not the only culprit in such cases. In addition to tobacco use, tar exposure can result from application of certain vaginal douches and using fossil-fuel burning stoves in poorly ventilated dwellings.[227]

This area continues to be an intensive focus of study. As with many other cancers, researchers are interested in genetic polymorphisms that may increase cervical cancer susceptibility in the presence of smoking.[228–230] Another growing area of research involves second-hand or environmental smoke. Several recent studies have demonstrated a link between CIN and passive or involuntary exposure to cigarette smoke.[231–233] Furthermore, an association between passive smoking and certain genetic polymorphisms in the causation of cervical cancer has been reported by a research team in India.[234,235]

Oral Contraceptives and Parity

Sex hormones have received a great deal of attention as potential cofactors in cervical carcinogenesis. Suggested mechanisms of action include the induction of metaplasia in the cervical transformation zone, direct interaction with HPV gene expression, and modulation of the local immune microenvironment.[236,237] The classic influences on sex hormone levels have not always been implicated in cervical cancer risk. For example, it seems that age at menarche is not an independent risk factor for high-risk HPV infections or cervical lesions.[238] On the other hand, there have long been suggestions that extended hormonal contraceptive use, a high number of pregnancies, and an early age at first pregnancy increase the risk of cervical cancer development. Many studies on these relationships have been published, allowing for a meta-analysis across large datasets.

Oral contraception continues to be a controversial topic. The current conclusion, based on research from 14 regions in the world, is that long-term use of oral contraceptives is not associated with HPV prevalence, although it might be implicated in the "transition from HPV infection to neoplastic lesions."[239] While this result is consistent with earlier systematic reviews,[240,241] the latest studies have generated further questions about oral contraceptive use, HPV infection, and related disease.[242,243] Recent research has landed on either side of the debate concerning disease progression. For example, a 2005 study in the United States found no association between oral contraceptive use and CIN3 incidence.[244] In contrast, research published in 2007 implicated longer term use in cervical cancer risk.[245] Similar to active and passive smoking, attention has been focused on genetic polymorphisms that may increase cervical cancer susceptibility with oral contraception.[246,247]

The potential mechanisms of a causal connection between oral contraceptive use and cervical neoplasia are still being investigated. Explanations involving a particular hormonal profile and the acceleration of carcinogenesis are similar to those sometimes advanced in the context of parity. A recent hypothesis suggested that oral contraceptives might affect the structure of the mucous barrier in the female reproductive tract, accounting for differential responses to HPV infection.[248]

The findings from research on reproductive history have perhaps been more consistent. A 2006 reanalysis of studies covering a total of 16,563 cases of cervical cancer and 33,542 controls showed an increased risk of cervical carcinoma in women with seven or more full-term deliveries (compared with one or two). A similar result was found when the first birth occurred at age less than 17 years, compared with 25 years or more. Such conclusions have been traditionally challenged in the face of the notorious "difficulty of disentangling the effect of reproductive variables from sexual behavior and HPV infection."[249] However, research where these confounding variables have been controlled has confirmed the associations between pregnancy and cervical cancer.[250] It is disconcerting from a public health standpoint that the biological forces at work in breast cancer may move in the opposite direction; thus, multiparous women or those giving birth at a young age appear to have a reduced risk of breast cancer.[251]

Again, the increased risk related to a woman's reproductive history seems to focus on cancer development per se rather than high-risk HPV positivity.[252] In other words, an explanation for elevated risk due to early or many pregnancies cannot necessarily be attributed to increased susceptibility to HPV infection but rather to factors that come into play after infection has occurred. Adding complexity to the discussion, past IARC research across multiple study centers suggested that increased risk of disease pertains to squamous cell cancers, not adenocarcinoma or adenosquamous carcinoma.[253] A recent pooled analysis of eight papers arrived at a contrary conclusion.[254] At the other extreme, one 2005 study questioned whether number of pregnancies or age of first pregnancy are actually associated with an increased risk of CIN3 at all, demonstrating again that this area of research remains very fluid.[255]

Coinfection

Coinfections with two or more types of agents is a complex topic in epidemiology, and one that has a particular relevance to understanding the infectious mechanism of cancer. Several forms of infection beyond HPV have been implicated in cervical cancer development. While modest attention has been paid to human T-cell lymphotropic virus type 1 and other agents that are endemic to specific regions,[256] the dominant focus has been on more universal STIs, such as herpes simplex virus (HSV), *Chlamydia trachomatis*, and human immunodeficiency virus (HIV). A recent comprehensive review identified three other viruses that may also influence cervical cancer development: cytomegalovirus, Epstein-Barr virus, and adeno-associated virus.[257]

Before HPV was established as the key pathogen involved with cervical cancer, HSV was actively examined as a causative agent.[258,259] Although some recent research supports the notion of HSV type 1 or 2 infection acting in concert with HPV to increase the risk of cervical malignancy,[260,261] the balance of evidence raises doubts about such an association.[262–266]

There also has been extensive research with respect to *C. trachomatis* and cervical cancer. A pooled analysis of studies up to 2004 suggested that there was an association between *C. trachomatis* and squamous cell carcinoma, but not adenocarcinoma or adenosquamous carcinoma.[267] Increased risk of cancer in women infected with Chlamydia may be mediated by chronic inflammation.[268] This is consistent with established and investigational models emphasizing the carcinogenic role of inflammation in tissue microenvironments affected by infection.[269–271] Despite the plausibility of the underlying biological mechanism, it is important to note that recent studies have been more equivocal about a causal connection between *C. trachomatis* and cervical cancer.[272–275] An intriguing result from one study suggested that multiple HPV infections may operate antagonistically in the presence of *C. trachomatis*, actually reducing the incidence of cervical cancer.[276]

The topic of HIV and HPV coinfection is a large and complex one in its own right. While the mechanisms are certainly not fully understood,[277] the prevailing understanding is that HIV is not a direct causal factor in cervical cancer but that it does interact somehow with HPV infection to increase the risk of dysplasia.[278,279] For example, in a recent South African study, women infected with both HIV and high-risk HPV had a 40-fold higher risk of developing intraepithelial lesions compared with women infected with neither virus.[280]

Having accounted for the confounding impact of exposure to common lifestyle factors such as smoking and unsafe sexual activity, the remaining potential mechanisms related to HIV fall into two categories. The first and most obvious involves immunodeficiency, the signature effect of HIV that allows other infections to take hold and/or carcinogenic processes to continue uncontained. Of the sequelae related to HIV, the persistence of HPV infection in the face of HIV infection, while certainly observed,[281] appears not to be a dominant outcome; this may partly explain why cervical cancer rates have not reached more epidemic proportions in HIV-positive women. Incident HPV rates, however, do appear to be elevated with HIV coinfection, some of which "may reflect HPV reactivation."[282] Other phenomena related to immunodeficiency remain unexplained. For instance, HPV-16 has been found to be underrepresented in HIV-positive women, whereas higher levels of other HPV types, single and multiple, are detected.[283] Whatever the impact on infection per se, the main immunity impact of HIV seems to be the suppression of tumor surveillance and control. In short, HIV infection facilitates a hospitable environment for both the initiation and progression of certain forms of cancer, leading in particular to so-called AIDS-defining malignancies.

The second category of possible disease-increasing interactions is driven by an even more complex epidemiologic relationship between HIV, HPV, and cancer. The circumstantial evidence for the existence of an alternate type of impact is the fact that acquired immunodeficiency caused by HIV has a cancer risk profile that differs from other immunosuppressed conditions (such as created by transplantation).[284] Various models have been put forward to explain a higher risk for cancer that is not related to a compromised immune system per se. The proposals include direct effects of HIV on different stages of tumor development, and direct effects of HIV on other carcinogenic viruses.[285] Evidence for such pathways is beginning to emerge in the context of HPV, including the cytokine-mediated impact of HIV-infected cells circulating below the basement membrane of the epithelium, and the modulation of HPV gene expression via the HIV-encoded Tat protein.[286]

A final intriguing aspect of coinfection is offered by the adeno-associated virus (AAV), which in fact is negatively associated with cervical cancer.[287] The protective effect seems to be mediated by complex, bidirectional interactions between AAV and HPV.[288]

Micronutrients, Diet, and Obesity

The effect of plasma micronutrients on cervical cancer has been an intensive area of investigation.[289] Perhaps not surprisingly, the evidence to date has been mixed. A key focus has been the impact on HPV clearance. In one 2007 study from Hawaii, *cis*-lycopene, β-carotene, and several other micronutrients were associated with a "significant decrease in the clearance time of type-specific HPV infection, particularly during the early stages of infection."[290] The Ludwig-McGill study, which is following a Brazilian cohort, also found results suggestive of potential prevention, but for a more modest range of micronutrients.[291] Sometimes the data for a particular vitamin, such as B12, may diverge when the target outcome is shifted from persistent HPV infection to cervical dysplasia.[292,293] Folate supplementation, on the other hand, has been associated with reductions in the development of CIN.[294]

Data related to nutrient intake and energy balance is much sparser. One recent study suggested that total fruit and vegetable intake may protect against cervical cancer; this was consistent with the evidence of a preventive effect for various plant-based micronutrients.[295] The few studies related to obesity may point to an impact on cervical adenocarcinoma incidence.[296] The evidence for an unfavorable influence on cervical cancer mortality is stronger; while a mediated effect by way of risky sexual behavior seems to have been ruled out,[297] there is a definite possibility that higher mortality is related mostly to poor screening rates among obese women.[298,299]

Public Health Implications

While the vital role of HPV in cervical carcinogenesis will inevitably dominate both research agendas and preventive interventions, the evidence for a multifactorial etiology for most if not all cases of cervical cancer continues to generate other options to potentially reduce the risk of tumor development. Based on a review of the literature, the strongest candidates for such efforts are smoking cessation (or avoiding tobacco use in the first place) and preventing or treating other STIs. Targeted screening and management programs for HIV-positive women would appear to be particularly relevant. The challenge that remains for even such well-established categories is the large number of at-risk women that would need to be the target of prevention programs and the relatively modest reduction in cervical cancer risk that is achievable.

The evidence base for other potential intervention categories is equivocal. For instance, initiatives to curtail the use of hormonal contraception "depend largely on the extent to which the observed associations remain long after use [is ended], and this cannot be evaluated properly from published data."[300] Other intriguing associations remain investigational, including the apparent increase in HPV infection and detected cervical dysplasia in summer months in the northern hemisphere, with different indirect effects of light on HPV infection and cancer development being suggested as an explanation; an argument has been advanced that screening and follow-up should occur mostly in seasons other than summer in order to minimize false-positive PAP smear rates.[301]

NOTES

1. Syrjanen K. PL8 The causal role of genital human papillomavirus (hpv) infections in cervical carcinogenesis. *Oral Diseases*. 2006; 12(suppl 1): 2.
2. Rent CS, Rent GS, Northcutt TJ, Jr. Behavioral factors related to the onset of cervical cancer. *Journal of Health and Social Behavior*. 1972; 13(4): 437–45.
3. Moscicki AB, Palefsky J, Gonzales J et al. Human papillomavirus infection in sexually active adolescent females: Prevalence and risk factors. *Pediatric Research*. 1990; 28(5): 507–13.
4. Vaccarella S, Franceschi S, Herrero R et al. Sexual behavior, condom use, and human papillomavirus: Pooled analysis of the IARC human papillomavirus prevalence surveys. *Cancer Epidemiology, Biomarkers and Prevention*. 2006; 15(2): 326–33.
5. Al-Daraji WI, Smith JH. Infection and cervical neoplasia: facts and fiction. *International Journal of Clinical and Experimental Pathology*. 2009; 2(1): 48–64.
6. Menczer J. The low incidence of cervical cancer in Jewish women: Has the puzzle finally been solved? *Israel Medical Association Journal*. 2003; 5(2): 120–3.
7. Walboomers JM, Jacobs MV, Manos MM et al. Human papillomavirus is a necessary cause of invasive cervical cancer worldwide. *Journal of Pathology*. 1999; 189(1): 12–9.
8. Bosch FX, Lorincz A, Munoz N et al. The causal relation between human papillomavirus and cervical cancer. *Journal of Clinical Pathology*. 2002; 55(4): 244–65.
9. Dillner J, Meijer CJ, von Krogh G et al. Epidemiology of human papillomavirus infection. *Scandinavian Journal of Urology and Nephrology. Supplementum*. 2000; (205): 194–200.
10. Mork J, Lie AK, Glattre E et al. Human papillomavirus infection as a risk factor for squamous-cell carcinoma of the head and neck. *New England Journal of Medicine*. 2001; 344(15): 1125–31.
11. Gillison ML, Koch WM, Capone RB et al. Evidence for a causal association between human papillomavirus and a subset of head and neck cancers. *Journal of the National Cancer Institute*. 2000; 92(9): 709–20.
12. Masini C, Fuchs PG, Gabrielli F et al. Evidence for the association of human papillomavirus infection and cutaneous squamous cell carcinoma in immunocompetent individuals. *Archives of Dermatology*. 2003; 139(7): 890–4.

13 Xi LF, Critchlow CW, Wheeler CM et al. Risk of anal carcinoma in situ in relation to human papillomavirus type 16 variants. *Cancer Research.* 1998; 58(17): 3839–44.
14 Cheng YW, Chiou HL, Sheu GT et al. The association of human papillomavirus 16/18 infection with lung cancer among nonsmoking Taiwanese women. *Cancer Research.* 2001; 61(7): 2799–803.
15 Lizano M, De la Cruz-Hernandez E, Carrillo-Garcia A et al. Distribution of HPV16 and 18 intratypic variants in normal cytology, intraepithelial lesions, and cervical cancer in a Mexican population. *Gynecologic Oncology.* 2006; 102(2): 230–5.
16 Gheit T, Vaccarella S, Schmitt M et al. Prevalence of human papillomavirus types in cervical and oral cancers in central India. *Vaccine.* 2009; 27(5): 636–9.
17 Sankaranarayanan R. Overview of cervical cancer in the developing world. FIGO 6th Annual Report on the Results of Treatment in Gynecological Cancer. *International Journal of Gynaecology and Obstetrics.* 2006; 95(suppl 1): S205–10.
18 Yang BH, Bray FI, Parkin DM et al. Cervical cancer as a priority for prevention in different world regions: An evaluation using years of life lost. *International Journal of Cancer.* 2004; 109(3): 418–24.
19 The chart is adapted from Steckley SL, Pickworth WB, Haverkos HW. Cigarette smoking and cervical cancer: PART II: a geographic variability study. *Biomedicine and Pharmacotherapy.* 2003; 57(2): 78–83.
20 *Canadian Cancer Statistics 2007.* 2007. Available at www.cancer.ca. Accessed August 2007.
21 Saraiya M, Ahmed F, Krishnan S et al. Cervical cancer incidence in a prevaccine era in the United States, 1998–2002. *Obstetrics and Gynecology.* 2007; 109(2 Pt 1): 360–70.
22 Yabroff KR, Lawrence WF, King JC et al. Geographic disparities in cervical cancer mortality: what are the roles of risk factor prevalence, screening, and use of recommended treatment? *Journal of Rural Health.* 2005; 21(2): 149–57.
23 Coughlin SS, Richards TB, Nasseri K et al. Cervical cancer incidence in the United States in the US-Mexico border region, 1998–2003. *Cancer.* 2008; 113(suppl 10): 2964–73.
24 Hopenhayn C, King JB, Christian A et al. Variability of cervical cancer rates across 5 Appalachian states, 1998–2003. *Cancer.* 2008; 113(suppl 10): 2974–80.
25 The chart is adapted from *Canadian Cancer Statistics 2007.* 2007. Available at www.cancer.ca. Accessed August 2007.
26 See http://www.bccancer.bc.ca/PPI/Screening/Cervical/default.htm. Accessed August 2007.
27 Hayat MJ, Howlader N, Reichman ME et al. Cancer statistics, trends, and multiple primary cancer analyses from the Surveillance, Epidemiology, and End Results (SEER) Program. *Oncologist.* 2007; 12(1): 20–37.
28 *Canadian Cancer Statistics 2007.* 2007. Available at www.cancer.ca. Accessed August 2007.
29 Gari A, Lotocki R, Krepart G et al. Cervical cancer in the province of Manitoba: a 30-year experience. *Journal of Obstetrics and Gynaecology Canada.* 2008; 30(9): 788–95.

30 Benard VB, Coughlin SS, Thompson T et al. Cervical cancer incidence in the United States by area of residence, 1998–2001. *Obstetrics and Gynecology.* 2007; 110(3): 681–6.
31 Watson M, Saraiya M, Benard V et al. Burden of cervical cancer in the United States, 1998–2003. *Cancer.* 2008; 113(suppl 10): 2855–64.
32 Downs LS, Smith JS, Scarinci I et al. The disparity of cervical cancer in diverse populations. *Gynecologic Oncology.* 2008; 109(suppl 2): S22–30.
33 Smith JS. Ethnic disparities in cervical cancer illness burden and subsequent care: a prospective view in managed care. *American Journal of Managed Care.* 2008; 14(6 suppl 1): S193–9.
34 McDougall JA, Madeleine MM, Daling JR et al. Racial and ethnic disparities in cervical cancer incidence rates in the United States, 1992–2003. *Cancer Causes and Control.* 2007; 18(10): 1175–86.
35 Merrill RM. Impact of hysterectomy and bilateral oophorectomy on race-specific rates of corpus, cervical, and ovarian cancers in the United States. *Annals of Epidemiology.* 2006; 16(12): 880–7.
36 For example, Bates JH, Hofer BM, Parikh-Patel A. Cervical cancer incidence, mortality, and survival among Asian subgroups in California, 1990–2004. *Cancer.* 2008; 113(suppl 10): 2955–63.
37 McCracken M, Olsen M, Chen MS, Jr. et al. Cancer incidence, mortality, and associated risk factors among Asian Americans of Chinese, Filipino, Vietnamese, Korean, and Japanese ethnicities. *CA: A Cancer Journal for Clinicians.* 2007; 57(4): 190–205.
38 Archibald CP, Coldman AJ, Wong FL et al. The incidence of cervical cancer among Chinese and Caucasians in British Columbia. *Canadian Journal of Public Health.* 1993; 84(4): 283–5.
39 Ralston JD, Taylor VM, Yasui Y et al. Knowledge of cervical cancer risk factors among Chinese immigrants in Seattle. *Journal of Community Health.* 2003; 28(1): 41–57.
40 Akers AY, Newmann SJ, Smith JS. Factors underlying disparities in cervical cancer incidence, screening, and treatment in the United States. *Current Problems in Cancer.* 2007; 31(3): 157–81.
41 Benard VB, Coughlin SS, Thompson T et al. Cervical cancer incidence in the United States by area of residence, 1998–2001. *Obstetrics and Gynecology.* 2007; 110(3): 681–6.
42 Marrett LD, Chaudhry M. Cancer incidence and mortality in Ontario First Nations, 1968–1991 (Canada). *Cancer Causes and Control.* 2003; 14(3): 259–68.
43 *Women in Canada: A Gender-based Statistical Report.* 2006. Statistics Canada. Available at www.statcan.ca/english/freepub/89–503-XIE/0010589-503-XIE.pdf. Accessed July 2007.
44 Young TK, Kliewer E, Blanchard J et al. Monitoring disease burden and preventive behavior with data linkage: cervical cancer among aboriginal people in Manitoba, Canada. *Amercian Journal of Public Health.* 2000; 90(9): 1466–8.
45 Rosenberg T, Martel S. Cancer trends from 1972–1991 for Registered Indians living on Manitoba Reserves. *International Journal of Circumpolar Health.* 1998; 57(suppl 1): 391–8.
46 Franco EL, Duarte-Franco E, Ferenczy A. Cervical cancer: epidemiology, prevention and the role of human papillomavirus infection. *Canadian Medical Association Journal.* 2001; 164(7): 1017–25.

47   Anderson GH, Benedet JL, Le Riche JC et al. Invasive cancer of the cervix in British Columbia: a review of the demography and screening histories of 437 cases seen from 1985–1988. *Obstetrics and Gynecology.* 1992; 80(1): 1–4.
48   Band PR, Gallagher RP, Threlfall WJ et al. Rate of death from cervical cancer among native Indian women in British Columbia. *Canadian Medical Association Journal.* 1992; 147(12): 1802–4.
49   Gaudette LA, Gao RN, Freitag S et al. Cancer incidence by ethnic group in the Northwest Territories (NWT) 1969–1988. *Health reports/Statistics Canada, Canadian Centre for Health Information.* 1993; 5(1): 23–32.
50   Kjaer SK, Nielsen NH. Cancer of the female genital tract in Circumpolar Inuit. *Acta Oncologica.* 1996; 35(5): 581–7.
51   *EpiNorth: The Northwest Territories Epidemiology Newsletter.* 1997. Northwest Territories Health and Social Services. Available at http://www.hlthss.gov.nt.ca/pdf/newsletters/Epinorth/1997/1997_March.pdf. Accessed August 2007.
52   Hodgins S. *Health and what affects it in Nunavik: How is the situation changing?* 1997. Nunavik Regional Board of Health and Social Services. Available at http://www.rrsss17.gouv.qc.ca/en/doc/publications/default.aspx. Accessed July 2007.
53   Wiggins CL, Espey DK, Wingo PA et al. Cancer among American Indians and Alaska Natives in the United States, 1999–2004. *Cancer.* 2008; 113(suppl 5): 1142–52.
54   Mahoney MC, Michalek AM. A meta-analysis of cancer incidence in United States and Canadian native populations. *International Journal of Epidemiology.* 1991; 20(2): 323–7.
55   Becker TM, Espey DK, Lawson HW et al. Regional differences in cervical cancer incidence among American Indians and Alaska Natives, 1999–2004. *Cancer.* 2008; 113(suppl 5): 1234–43.
56   Leman RF, Espey D, Cobb N. Invasive cervical cancer among American Indian women in the Northern Plains, 1994–1998: incidence, mortality, and missed opportunities. *Public Health Reports.* 2005; 120(3): 283–7.
57   Bell MC, Schmidt-Grimminger D, Patrick S et al. There is a high prevalence of human papillomavirus infection in American Indian women of the Northern Plains. *Gynecologic Oncology.* 2007; 107(2): 236–41.
58   *Cancer in the Northwest Territories 1990–2000.* 2003. Northwest Territories Health and Social Services. Available at http://www.hlthss.gov.nt.ca/pdf/reports/diseases_and_conditions/2003/english/cancer_in_the_nwt.pdf. Accessed August 2007.
59   *The NWT Health Status Report 2005.* 2005. Northwest Territories Health and Social Services. Available at http://www.hlthss.gov.nt.ca/pdf/reports/health_care_system/2005/english/nwt_health_status_report_2005.pdf. Accessed August 2007.
60   Healey S, Plaza D, Osborne G. *A Ten-Year Profile of Cancer in Nunavut: 1992–2001.* 2003. Nunavut Department of Health and Social Services. Available at http://www.gov.nu.ca/hsssite/Cancer_NunavutEng.pdf. Accessed August 2007.
61   Dr. L.D. Marrett, personal communication with Dr. H. Krueger, August 19 and 23, 2007. The cervical cancer numbers in the table are standardized to the 1991 Canadian population and are restricted to ages 15–74. A cautionary note from Dr. Marrett indicates that the 1992–2001 data "are of poorer quality than earlier data. The reason is that updates to the Status Indian Register, which

was used in part to produce these estimates, are not available after 1991. As a result, the cervical cancer incidence rate estimated for Ontario First Nations women in 1992–2001 is likely too low."

62 *Cervical Cancer Screening in Canada: 1998 Surveillance Report.* 2002. Health Canada. Available at http://www.phac-aspc.gc.ca/publicat/ccsic-dccuac/pdf/cervical-e3.pdf. Accessed August 2007. Denominators for cervical cancer incidence should include only women who still have a cervix, that is have not had a hysterectomy. This information is often not known. Changing hysterectomy prevalence over time in Aboriginal women could therefore affect the trend in incidence. Historical differences between Aboriginal and women in the general population in the prevalence of hysterectomy could affect rates.

63 Gillison ML, Shah KV. Role of mucosal human papillomavirus in nongenital cancers. *Journal of the National Cancer Institute Monographs.* Chapter 9, 2003; (31): 57–65.

64 Badaracco G, Venuti A. Physical status of HPV types 16 and 18 in topographically different areas of genital tumours and in paired tumour-free mucosa. *International Journal of Oncology.* 2005; 27(1): 161–7.

65 Koshiol J, Lindsay L, Pimenta JM et al. Persistent human papillomavirus infection and cervical neoplasia: a systematic review and meta-analysis. *American Journal of Epidemiology.* 2008; 168(2): 123–37.

66 Syrjanen K. PL8 The causal role of genital human papillomavirus (hpv) infections in cervical carcinogenesis. *Oral Diseases.* 2006; 12(suppl 1): 2.

67 Copeland G, Datta SD, Spivak G et al. Total burden and incidence of in situ and invasive cervical carcinoma in Michigan, 1985–2003. *Cancer.* 2008; 113(suppl 10): 2946–54.

68 Tase T, Okagaki T, Clark BA et al. Human papillomavirus DNA in adenocarcinoma in situ, microinvasive adenocarcinoma of the uterine cervix, and coexisting cervical squamous intraepithelial neoplasia. *International Journal of Gynecological Pathology.* 1989; 8(1): 8–17.

69 Bekkers RL, Bulten J, Wiersma-van Tilburg A et al. Coexisting high-grade glandular and squamous cervical lesions and human papillomavirus infections. *British Journal of Cancer.* 2003; 89(5): 886–90.

70 Ueda Y, Miyatake T, Okazawa M et al. Clonality and HPV infection analysis of concurrent glandular and squamous lesions and adenosquamous carcinomas of the uterine cervix. *American Journal of Clinical Pathology.* 2008; 130(3): 389–400.

71 Ogura K, Ishi K, Matsumoto T et al. Human papillomavirus localization in cervical adenocarcinoma and adenosquamous carcinoma using in situ polymerase chain reaction: review of the literature of human papillomavirus detection in these carcinomas. *Pathology International.* 2006; 56(6): 301–8.

72 Pirog EC, Kleter B, Olgac S et al. Prevalence of human papillomavirus DNA in different histological subtypes of cervical adenocarcinoma. *American Journal of Pathology.* 2000; 157(4): 1055–62.

73 Burd EM. Human papillomavirus and cervical cancer. *Clinical Microbiology Reviews.* 2003; 16(1): 1–17.

74 Munoz N, Bosch FX, de Sanjose S et al. Epidemiologic classification of human papillomavirus types associated with cervical cancer. *New England Journal of Medicine.* 2003; 348(6): 518–27.

75 Bosch FX, Qiao Y, Castellsague X. The epidemiology of human papillomavirus infection and its association with cervical cancer. *International Journal of Gynecology and Obstetrics*. 2006; 94(suppl 1): S8–21.
76 Andersson S, Mints M, Sallstrom J et al. The relative distribution of oncogenic types of human papillomavirus in benign, pre-malignant and malignant cervical biopsies. A study with human papillomavirus deoxyribonucleic acid sequence analysis. *Cancer Detection and Prevention*. 2005; 29(1): 37–41.
77 Clifford GM, Smith JS, Aguado T et al. Comparison of HPV type distribution in high-grade cervical lesions and cervical cancer: a meta-analysis. *British Journal of Cancer*. 2003; 89(1): 101–5.
78 Clifford GM, Rana RK, Franceschi S et al. Human papillomavirus genotype distribution in low-grade cervical lesions: comparison by geographic region and with cervical cancer. *Cancer Epidemiology, Biomarkers and Prevention*. 2005; 14(5): 1157–64.
79 Castle PE, Solomon D, Schiffman M et al. Human papillomavirus type 16 infections and 2-year absolute risk of cervical precancer in women with equivocal or mild cytologic abnormalities. *Journal of the National Cancer Institute*. 2005; 97(14): 1066–71.
80 See, for example, Herrero R, Castle PE, Schiffman M et al. Epidemiologic profile of type-specific human papillomavirus infection and cervical neoplasia in Guanacaste, Costa Rica. *Journal of Infectious Diseases*. 2005; 191(11): 1796–807; Del Mistro A, Salamanca HF, Trevisan R et al. Human papillomavirus typing of invasive cervical cancers in Italy. *Infectious Agents and Cancer*. 2006; 1: 9; Roberts CC, Tadesse AS, Sands J et al. Detection of HPV in Norwegian cervical biopsy specimens with type-specific PCR and reverse line blot assays. *Journal of Clinical Virology*. 2006; 36(4): 277–82; Medeiros R, Prazeres H, Pinto D et al. Characterization of HPV genotype profile in squamous cervical lesions in Portugal, a southern European population at high risk of cervical cancer. *European Journal of Cancer Prevention*. 2005; 14(5): 467–71; Amrani M, Lalaoui K, El Mzibri M et al. Molecular detection of human papillomavirus in 594 uterine cervix samples from Moroccan women (147 biopsies and 447 swabs). *Journal of Clinical Virology*. 2003; 27(3): 286–95; Wall SR, Scherf CF, Morison L et al. Cervical human papillomavirus infection and squamous intraepithelial lesions in rural Gambia, West Africa: viral sequence analysis and epidemiology. *British Journal of Cancer*. 2005; 93(9): 1068–76; Peedicayil A, Abraham P, Sathish N et al. Human papillomavirus genotypes associated with cervical neoplasia in India. *International Journal of Gynecological Cancer*. 2006; 16(4): 1591–5; Maehama T. Epidemiological study in Okinawa, Japan, of human papillomavirus infection of the uterine cervix. *Infectious Diseases in Obstetrics and Gynecology*. 2005; 13(2): 77–80; Kim CJ, Jeong JK, Park M et al. HPV oligonucleotide microarray-based detection of HPV genotypes in cervical neoplastic lesions. *Gynecologic Oncology*. 2003; 89(2): 210–7; Wu Y, Chen Y, Li L et al. Associations of high-risk HPV types and viral load with cervical cancer in China. *Journal of Clinical Virology*. 2006; 35(3): 264–9.
81 Bosch FX, Burchell AN, Schiffman M et al. Epidemiology and natural history of human papillomavirus infections and type-specific implications in cervical neoplasia. *Vaccine*. 2008; 26(suppl 10): K1–16.
82 Evans MF, Adamson CS, Papillo JL et al. Distribution of human papillomavirus types in ThinPrep Papanicolaou tests classified according to the Bethesda

2001 terminology and correlations with patient age and biopsy outcomes. *Cancer.* 2006; 106(5): 1054–64.
83 Trimble CL, Piantadosi S, Gravitt P et al. Spontaneous regression of high-grade cervical dysplasia: effects of human papillomavirus type and HLA phenotype. *Clinical Cancer Research.* 2005; 11(13): 4717–23.
84 Gok M, Coupe VM, Berkhof J et al. HPV16 and increased risk of recurrence after treatment for CIN. *Gynecologic Oncology.* 2007; 104(2): 273–5.
85 Wilczynski SP, Bergen S, Walker J et al. Human papillomaviruses and cervical cancer: analysis of histopathologic features associated with different viral types. *Human Pathology.* 1988; 19(6): 697–704.
86 Zehbe I, Wilander E. Human papillomavirus infection and invasive cervical neoplasia: a study of prevalence and morphology. *Journal of Pathology.* 1997; 181(3): 270–5.
87 Shyu JS, Chen CJ, Chiu CC et al. Correlation of human papillomavirus 16 and 18 with cervical neoplasia in histological typing and clinical stage in Taiwan: an in-situ polymerase chain reaction approach. *Journal of Surgical Oncology.* 2001; 78(2): 101–9.
88 Clifford GM, Smith JS, Plummer M et al. Human papillomavirus types in invasive cervical cancer worldwide: a meta-analysis. *British Journal of Cancer.* 2003; 88(1): 63–73.
89 Andersson S, Rylander E, Larsson B et al. The role of human papillomavirus in cervical adenocarcinoma carcinogenesis. *European Journal of Cancer.* 2001; 37(2): 246–50.
90 Andersson S, Rylander E, Larson B et al. Types of human papillomavirus revealed in cervical adenocarcinomas after DNA sequencing. *Oncology Reports.* 2003; 10(1): 175–9.
91 De Boer MA, Peters LA, Aziz MF et al. Human papillomavirus type 18 variants: histopathology and E6/E7 polymorphisms in three countries. *International Journal of Cancer.* 2005; 114(3): 422–5.
92 Huang LW, Chao SL, Chen PH et al. Multiple HPV genotypes in cervical carcinomas: improved DNA detection and typing in archival tissues. *Journal of Clinical Virology.* 2004; 29(4): 271–6.
93 Baalbergen A, Ewing-Graham PC, Eijkemans MJ et al. Prognosis of adenocarcinoma of the uterine cervix: p53 expression correlates with higher incidence of mortality. *International Journal of Cancer.* 2007; 121(1): 106–10.
94 Wright VC. Cervical squamous and glandular intraepithelial neoplasia: identification and current management approaches. *Salud Publica de Mexico.* 2003; 45(suppl 3): S417–29.
95 Moreira MA, Longato-Filho A, Taromaru E et al. Investigation of human papillomavirus by hybrid capture II in cervical carcinomas including 113 adenocarcinomas and related lesions. *International Journal of Gynecological Cancer.* 2006; 16(2): 586–90.
96 Kovacic MB, Castle PE, Herrero R et al. Relationships of human papillomavirus type, qualitative viral load, and age with cytologic abnormality. *Cancer Research.* 2006; 66(20): 10112–9.
97 Matthews-Greer J, Dominguez-Malagon H, Herrera GA et al. Human papillomavirus typing of rare cervical carcinomas. *Archives of Pathology and Laboratory Medicine.* 2004; 128(5): 553–6.

98 Chauhan SC, Kumar D, Bell MC et al. Molecular markers of miscellaneous primary and metastatic tumors of the uterine cervix. *European Journal of Gynaecological Oncology.* 2007; 28(1): 5–14.
99 International Collaboration of Epidemiological Studies of Cervical Cancer. Comparison of risk factors for invasive squamous cell carcinoma and adenocarcinoma of the cervix: collaborative reanalysis of individual data on 8,097 women with squamous cell carcinoma and 1,374 women with adenocarcinoma from 12 epidemiological studies. *International Journal of Cancer.* 2007; 120(4): 885–91.
100 Liu S, Semenciw R, Mao Y. Cervical cancer: the increasing incidence of adenocarcinoma and adenosquamous carcinoma in younger women. *Canadian Medical Association Journal.* 2001; 164(8): 1151–2.
101 Gari A, Lotocki R, Krepart G et al. Cervical cancer in the province of Manitoba: a 30-year experience. *Journal of Obstetrics and Gynaecology Canada.* 2008; 30(9): 788–95.
102 Howlett RI, Marrett LD, Innes MK et al. Decreasing incidence of cervical adenocarcinoma in Ontario: is this related to improved endocervical Pap test sampling? *International Journal of Cancer.* 2007; 120(2): 362–7.
103 Bekkers RL, Melchers WJ, Bulten J et al. Localized distribution of human papillomavirus genotypes in the uterine cervix. *European Journal of Gynaecological Oncology.* 2002; 23(3): 203–6.
104 Huang LW, Chao SL, Chen PH et al. Multiple HPV genotypes in cervical carcinomas: improved DNA detection and typing in archival tissues. *Journal of Clinical Virology.* 2004; 29(4): 271–6.
105 Trottier H, Mahmud S, Costa MC et al. Human papillomavirus infections with multiple types and risk of cervical neoplasia. *Cancer Epidemiology, Biomarkers and Prevention.* 2006; 15(7): 1274–80.
106 Chaturvedi AK, Myers L, Hammons AF et al. Prevalence and clustering patterns of human papillomavirus genotypes in multiple infections. *Cancer Epidemiology, Biomarkers and Prevention.* 2005; 14(10): 2439–45.
107 Schellekens MC, Dijkman A, Aziz MF et al. Prevalence of single and multiple HPV types in cervical carcinomas in Jakarta, Indonesia. *Gynecologic Oncology.* 2004; 93(1): 49–53.
108 Hadzisejdc I, Krasevic M, Haller H et al. Distribution of human papillomavirus types in different histological subtypes of cervical adenocarcinoma. *Collegium Antropologicum.* 2007; 31(suppl 2): 97–102.
109 Bekkers RL, Melchers WJ, Bulten J et al. Localized distribution of human papillomavirus genotypes in the uterine cervix. *European Journal of Gynaecological Oncology.* 2002; 23(3): 203–6.
110 Ciotti M, Paba P, Bonifacio D et al. Single or multiple HPV types in cervical cancer and associated metastases. *Oncology Reports.* 2006; 15(1): 143–8.
111 Vermeulen CF, Jordanova ES, Szuhai K et al. Physical status of multiple human papillomavirus genotypes in flow-sorted cervical cancer cells. *Cancer Genetics and Cytogenetics.* 2007; 175(2): 132–7.
112 Schiffman M, Castle PE, Jeronimo J et al. Human papillomavirus and cervical cancer. *The Lancet.* 2007; 370(9590): 890–907.
113 Trottier H, Mahmud S, Costa MC et al. Human papillomavirus infections with multiple types and risk of cervical neoplasia. *Cancer Epidemiology, Biomarkers and Prevention.* 2006; 15(7): 1274–80.

114 Gargiulo F, De Francesco MA, Schreiber C et al. Prevalence and distribution of single and multiple HPV infections in cytologically abnormal cervical samples from Italian women. *Virus Research.* 2007; 125(2): 176–82.
115 Briolat J, Dalstein V, Saunier M et al. HPV prevalence, viral load and physical state of HPV-16 in cervical smears of patients with different grades of CIN. *International Journal of Cancer.* 2007; 121(10): 2198–204.
116 Badaracco G, Venuti A, Sedati A et al. HPV16 and HPV18 in genital tumors: significantly different levels of viral integration and correlation to tumor invasiveness. *Journal of Medical Virology.* 2002; 67(4): 574–82.
117 FUTURE II Study Group. Quadrivalent vaccine against human papillomavirus to prevent high-grade cervical lesions. *New England Journal of Medicine.* 2007; 356: 1915–27.
118 de Boer MA, Vet JN, Aziz MF et al. Human papillomavirus type 18 and other risk factors for cervical cancer in Jakarta, Indonesia. *International Journal of Gynecological Cancer.* 2006; 16(5): 1809–14.
119 Clifford GM, Smith JS, Plummer M et al. Human papillomavirus types in invasive cervical cancer worldwide: a meta-analysis. *British Journal of Cancer.* 2003; 88(1): 63–73.
120 Clifford GM, Smith JS, Aguado T et al. Comparison of HPV type distribution in high-grade cervical lesions and cervical cancer: a meta-analysis. *British Journal of Cancer.* 2003; 89(1): 101–5.
121 Clifford GM, Rana RK, Franceschi S et al. Human papillomavirus genotype distribution in low-grade cervical lesions: comparison by geographic region and with cervical cancer. *Cancer Epidemiology, Biomarkers and Prevention.* 2005; 14(5): 1157–64.
122 Smith JS, Lindsay L, Hoots B et al. Human papillomavirus type distribution in invasive cervical cancer and high-grade cervical lesions: a meta-analysis update. *International Journal of Cancer.* 2007; 121(3): 621–32.
123 Ding DC, Hsu HC, Huang RL et al. Type-specific distribution of HPV along the full spectrum of cervical carcinogenesis in Taiwan: an indication of viral oncogenic potential. *European Journal of Obstetrics, Gynecology, and Reproductive Biology.* 2008; 140(2): 245–51.
124 Lai CH, Huang HJ, Hsueh S et al. Human papillomavirus genotype in cervical cancer: a population-based study. *International Journal of Cancer.* 2007; 120(9): 1999–2006.
125 Ho CM, Chien TY, Huang SH et al. Integrated human papillomavirus types 52 and 58 are infrequently found in cervical cancer, and high viral loads predict risk of cervical cancer. *Gynecologic Oncology.* 2006; 102(1): 54–60.
126 Ho CM, Yang SS, Chien TY et al. Detection and quantitation of human papillomavirus type 16, 18 and 52 DNA in the peripheral blood of cervical cancer patients. *Gynecologic Oncology.* 2005; 99(3): 615–21.
127 Huang S, Afonina I, Miller BA et al. Human papillomavirus types 52 and 58 are prevalent in cervical cancers from Chinese women. *International Journal of Cancer.* 1997; 70(4): 408–11.
128 Liaw KL, Hsing AW, Chen CJ et al. Human papillomavirus and cervical neoplasia: a case-control study in Taiwan. *International Journal of Cancer.* 1995; 62(5): 565–71.
129 Tay SK, Ngan HY, Chu TY et al. Epidemiology of human papillomavirus infection and cervical cancer and future perspectives in Hong Kong, Singapore and Taiwan. *Vaccine.* 2008; 26(suppl 12): M60–70.

130 Tornesello ML, Duraturo ML, Buonaguro L et al. Prevalence of human papillomavirus genotypes and their variants in high risk West Africa women immigrants in South Italy. *Infectious Agents and Cancer.* 2007; 2: 1.
131 Antonishyn NA, Horsman GB, Kelln RA et al. The impact of the distribution of human papillomavirus types and associated high-risk lesions in a colposcopy population for monitoring vaccine efficacy. *Archives of Pathology and Laboratory Medicine.* 2008; 132(1): 54–60.
132 Lai CH, Huang HJ, Hsueh S et al. Human papillomavirus genotype in cervical cancer: a population-based study. *International Journal of Cancer.* 2007; 120(9): 1999–2006.
133 Blossom DB, Beigi RH, Farrell JJ et al. Human papillomavirus genotypes associated with cervical cytologic abnormalities and HIV infection in Ugandan women. *Journal of Medical Virology.* 2007; 79(6): 758–65.
134 Gonzalez-Bosquet E, Esteva C, Munoz-Almagro C et al. Identification of vaccine human papillomavirus genotypes in squamous intraepithelial lesions (CIN2-3). *Gynecologic Oncology.* 2008; 111(1): 9–12.
135 Clifford GM, Gallus S, Herrero R et al. Worldwide distribution of human papillomavirus types in cytologically normal women in the International Agency for Research on Cancer HPV prevalence surveys: A pooled analysis. *The Lancet.* 2005; 366(9490): 991–8.
136 Prado JC, Calleja-Macias IE, Bernard HU et al. Worldwide genomic diversity of the human papillomaviruses-53, 56, and 66, a group of high-risk HPVs unrelated to HPV-16 and HPV-18. *Virology.* 2005; 340(1): 95–104.
137 Xi LF, Kiviat NB, Hildesheim A et al. Human papillomavirus type 16 and 18 variants: race-related distribution and persistence. *Journal of the National Cancer Institute.* 2006; 98(15): 1045–52.
138 Ortiz M, Torres M, Munoz L et al. Oncogenic human papillomavirus (HPV) type distribution and HPV type 16 E6 variants in two Spanish population groups with different levels of HPV infection risk. *Journal of Clinical Microbiology.* 2006; 44(4): 1428–34.
139 Arias-Pulido H, Peyton CL, Torrez-Martinez N et al. Human papillomavirus type 18 variant lineages in United States populations characterized by sequence analysis of LCR-E6, E2, and L1 regions. *Virology.* 2005; 338(1): 22–34.
140 De Boer MA, Peters LA, Aziz MF et al. Human papillomavirus type 18 variants: histopathology and E6/E7 polymorphisms in three countries. *International Journal of Cancer.* 2005; 114(3): 422–5.
141 Calleja-Macias IE, Villa LL, Prado JC et al. Worldwide genomic diversity of the high-risk human papillomavirus types 31, 35, 52, and 58, four close relatives of human papillomavirus type 16. *Journal of Virology.* 2005; 79(21): 13630–40.
142 Calleja-Macias IE, Kalantari M, Allan B et al. Papillomavirus subtypes are natural and old taxa: phylogeny of human papillomavirus types 44 and 55 and 68a and -b. *Journal of Virology.* 2005; 79(10): 6565–9; Calleja-Macias IE, Kalantari M, Huh J et al. Genomic diversity of human papillomavirus-16, 18, 31, and 35 isolates in a Mexican population and relationship to European, African, and Native American variants. *Virology.* 2004; 319(2): 315–23.
143 Yamada T, Manos MM, Peto J et al. Human papillomavirus type 16 sequence variation in cervical cancers: a worldwide perspective. *Journal of Virology.* 1997; 71(3): 2463–72.

144 Sichero L, Ferreira S, Trottier H et al. High grade cervical lesions are caused preferentially by non-European variants of HPVs 16 and 18. *International Journal of Cancer.* 2007; 120(8): 1763–8.
145 Tornesello ML, Duraturo ML, Salatiello I et al. Analysis of human papillomavirus type-16 variants in Italian women with cervical intraepithelial neoplasia and cervical cancer. *Journal of Medical Virology.* 2004; 74(1): 117–26.
146 Lizano M, De la Cruz-Hernandez E, Carrillo-Garcia A et al. Distribution of HPV16 and 18 intratypic variants in normal cytology, intraepithelial lesions, and cervical cancer in a Mexican population. *Gynecologic Oncology.* 2006; 102(2): 230–5.
147 Tu JJ, Kuhn L, Denny L et al. Molecular variants of human papillomavirus type 16 and risk for cervical neoplasia in South Africa. *International Journal of Gynecological Cancer.* 2006; 16(2): 736–42.
148 Schlecht NF, Burk RD, Palefsky JM et al. Variants of human papillomaviruses 16 and 18 and their natural history in human immunodeficiency virus-positive women. *Journal of General Virology.* 2005; 86(Pt 10): 2709–20.
149 Sichero L, Villa LL. Epidemiological and functional implications of molecular variants of human papillomavirus. *Brazilian Journal of Medical and Biological Research.* 2006; 39(6): 707–17.
150 Garbuglia AR, Carletti F, Minosse C et al. Genetic variability in E6 and E7 genes of human papillomavirus -16, -18, -31 and -33 from HIV-1-positive women in Italy. *New Microbiologica.* 2007; 30(4): 377–82.
151 Chen Z, DeSalle R, Schiffman M et al. Evolutionary dynamics of variant genomes of human papillomavirus types 18, 45, and 97. *Journal of Virology.* 2009; 83(3): 1443–55.
152 Varsani A, Williamson AL, Jaffer MA et al. A deletion and point mutation study of the human papillomavirus type 16 major capsid gene. *Virus Research.* 2006; 122(1–2): 154–63.
153 Pastrana DV, Vass WC, Lowy DR et al. NHPV16 VLP vaccine induces human antibodies that neutralize divergent variants of HPV16. *Virology.* 2001; 279(1): 361–9.
154 Junes-Gill K, Sichero L, Maciag PC et al. Human papillomavirus type 16 variants in cervical cancer from an admixtured population in Brazil. *Journal of Medical Virology.* 2008; 80(9): 1639–45.
155 Calleja-Macias IE, Kalantari M, Huh J et al. Genomic diversity of human papillomavirus-16, 18, 31, and 35 isolates in a Mexican population and relationship to European, African, and Native American variants. *Virology.* 2004; 319(2): 315–23.
156 Villa LL, Sichero L, Rahal P et al. Molecular variants of human papillomavirus types 16 and 18 preferentially associated with cervical neoplasia. *Journal of General Virology.* 2000; 81(Pt 12): 2959–68.
157 Meijer CJ, Snijders PJ, Castle PE. Clinical utility of HPV genotyping. *Gynecologic Oncology.* 2006; 103(1): 12–7.
158 Verguts J, Bronselaer B, Donders G et al. Prediction of recurrence after treatment for high-grade cervical intraepithelial neoplasia: the role of human papillomavirus testing and age at conisation. *British Journal of Obstetrics and Gynaecology.* 2006; 113(11): 1303–7.
159 Allan BR, Marais DJ, Denny L et al. The agreement between cervical abnormalities identified by cytology and detection of high-risk types of human papillomavirus. *South African Medical Journal.* 2006; 96(11): 1186–90.

160 Arbyn M, Buntinx F, Van Ranst M et al. Virologic versus cytologic triage of women with equivocal Pap smears: a meta-analysis of the accuracy to detect high-grade intraepithelial neoplasia. *Journal of the National Cancer Institute.* 2004; 96(4): 280–93.
161 Srodon M, Parry Dilworth H, Ronnett BM. Atypical squamous cells, cannot exclude high-grade squamous intraepithelial lesion: diagnostic performance, human papillomavirus testing, and follow-up results. *Cancer.* 2006; 108(1): 32–8.
162 Wheeler CM, Hunt WC, Schiffman M et al. Human papillomavirus genotypes and the cumulative 2-year risk of cervical precancer. *Journal of Infectious Diseases.* 2006; 194(9): 1291–9.
163 Cox JT. Human papillomavirus testing in primary cervical screening and abnormal Papanicolaou management. *Obstetrical and Gynecological Survey.* 2006; 61(6 suppl 1): S15–25.
164 Berkhof J, Bulkmans NW, Bleeker MC et al. Human papillomavirus type-specific 18-month risk of high-grade cervical intraepithelial neoplasia in women with a normal or borderline/mildly dyskaryotic smear. *Cancer Epidemiology, Biomarkers and Prevention.* 2006; 15(7): 1268–73.
165 Zuna RE, Allen RA, Moore WE et al. Distribution of HPV genotypes in 282 women with cervical lesions: evidence for three categories of intraepithelial lesions based on morphology and HPV type. *Modern Pathology.* 2007; 20(2): 167–74.
166 Huang LW, Chao SL, Hwang JL. Human papillomavirus-31-related types predict better survival in cervical carcinoma. *Cancer.* 2004; 100(2): 327–34.
167 Burger RA, Monk BJ, Kurosaki T et al. Human papillomavirus type 18: association with poor prognosis in early stage cervical cancer. *Journal of the National Cancer Institute.* 1996; 88(19): 1361–8.
168 Tong SY, Lee YS, Park JS et al. Human papillomavirus genotype as a prognostic factor in carcinoma of the uterine cervix. *International Journal of Gynecological Cancer.* 2007; 17(6): 1307–13.
169 Castellsague X, Diaz M, de Sanjose S et al. Worldwide human papillomavirus etiology of cervical adenocarcinoma and its cofactors: implications for screening and prevention. *Journal of the National Cancer Institute.* 2006; 98(5): 303–15.
170 *SEER Cancer Statistics Review,* 2005. Available at seer.cancer.gov/csr/1975_2005/index.html.
171 *Cancer Research UK statistics,* 2005. Available at info.cancerresearchuk.org/cancerstats/types/cervix/.
172 Smith EM, Johnson SR, Ritchie JM et al. Persistent HPV infection in postmenopausal age women. *International Journal of Gynaecology and Obstetrics.* 2004; 87(2): 131–7.
173 Grainge MJ, Seth R, Guo L et al. Cervical human papillomavirus screening among older women. *Emerging Infectious Diseases.* 2005; 11(11): 1680–5.
174 Syrjanen K. New concepts on risk factors of HPV and novel screening strategies for cervical cancer precursors. *European Journal of Gynaecological Oncology.* 2008; 29(3): 205–21.
175 Bosch FX, de Sanjose S. Human papillomavirus and cervical cancer—burden and assessment of causality. *Journal of the National Cancer Institute Monographs.* Chapter 1, 2003; (31): 3–13.
176 International Collaboration of Epidemiological Studies of Cervical Cancer. Comparison of risk factors for invasive squamous cell carcinoma and

adenocarcinoma of the cervix: collaborative reanalysis of individual data on 8,097 women with squamous cell carcinoma and 1,374 women with adenocarcinoma from 12 epidemiological studies. *International Journal of Cancer.* 2007; 120(4): 885–91.
177 Franco EL, Duarte-Franco E, Ferenczy A. Cervical cancer: epidemiology, prevention and the role of human papillomavirus infection. *Canadian Medical Association Journal.* 2001; 164(7): 1017–25.
178 Ho GY, Bierman R, Beardsley L et al. Natural history of cervicovaginal papillomavirus infection in young women. *New England Journal of Medicine.* 1998; 338(7): 423–8.
179 Vaccarella S, Franceschi S, Herrero R et al. Sexual behavior, condom use, and human papillomavirus: pooled analysis of the IARC human papillomavirus prevalence surveys. *Cancer Epidemiology, Biomarkers and Prevention.* 2006; 15(2): 326–33.
180 Biswas LN, Manna B, Maiti PK et al. Sexual risk factors for cervical cancer among rural Indian women: a case-control study. *International Journal of Epidemiology.* 1997; 26(3): 491–5.
181 Burd EM. Human papillomavirus and cervical cancer. *Clinical Microbiology Reviews.* 2003; 16(1): 1–17.
182 Ng WK, Cheung LK, Li AS et al. Transitional cell metaplasia of the uterine cervix is related to human papillomavirus: molecular analysis in seven patients with cytohistologic correlation. *Cancer Cytopathology.* 2002; 96(4): 250–8.
183 Castle PE, Jeronimo J, Schiffman M et al. Age-related changes of the cervix influence human papillomavirus type distribution. *Cancer Research.* 2006; 66(2): 1218–24.
184 Bodley-Tickell AT, Olowokure B, Bhaduri S et al. Trends in sexually transmitted infections (other than HIV) in older people: analysis of data from an enhanced surveillance system. *Sexually Transmitted Infections.* 2008; 84(4): 312–7.
185 Mak R, Van Renterghem L, Cuvelier C. Cervical smears and human papillomavirus typing in sex workers. *Sexually Transmitted Infections.* 2004; 80(2): 118–20.
186 Benedet JL, Cabero-Roura L. Strategies for the modification of risk factors in gynecological cancers. *European Journal of Gynaecological Oncology.* 2002; 23(1): 5–10.
187 Fernandez-Esquer ME, Ross MW, Torres I. The importance of psychosocial factors in the prevention of HPV infection and cervical cancer. *International Journal of STD and AIDS.* 2000; 11(11): 701–13.
188 Khan MJ, Partridge EE, Wang SS et al. Socioeconomic status and the risk of cervical intraepithelial neoplasia grade 3 among oncogenic human papillomavirus DNA-positive women with equivocal or mildly abnormal cytology. *Cancer.* 2005; 104(1): 61–70.
189 Flores YN, Bishai DM, Shah KV et al. Risk factors for cervical cancer among HPV positive women in Mexico. *Salud Publica de Mexico.* 2008; 50(1): 49–58.
190 Ng E, Wilkins R, Fung MF et al. Cervical cancer mortality by neighbourhood income in urban Canada from 1971 to 1996. *Canadian Medical Association Journal.* 2004; 170(10): 1545–9.
191 Castle PE. Beyond human papillomavirus: the cervix, exogenous secondary factors, and the development of cervical precancer and cancer. *Journal of Lower Genital Tract Disease.* 2004; 8(3): 224–30.

192 Dillner J. Trends over time in the incidence of cervical neoplasia in comparison to trends over time in human papillomavirus infection. *Journal of Clinical Virology.* 2000; 19(1–2): 7–23.
193 Maucort-Boulch D, Franceschi S, Plummer M. International correlation between human papillomavirus prevalence and cervical cancer incidence. *Cancer Epidemiology, Biomarkers and Prevention.* 2008; 17(3): 717–20.
194 Castellsague X, Munoz N. Cofactors in human papillomavirus carcinogenesis—role of parity, oral contraceptives, and tobacco smoking. *Journal of the National Cancer Institute Monographs.* Chapter 3, 2003; 31: 20–8.
195 Tjalma WA, Van Waes TR, Van den Eeden LE et al. Role of human papillomavirus in the carcinogenesis of squamous cell carcinoma and adenocarcinoma of the cervix. Best Practice and Research. *Clinical Obstetrics and Gynaecology.* 2005; 19(4): 469–83.
196 Munoz N, Bosch FX. Cervical cancer and human papillomavirus: epidemiological evidence and perspectives for prevention. *Salud Publica de Mexico.* 1997; 39(4): 274–82.
197 Syrjanen K. New concepts on risk factors of HPV and novel screening strategies for cervical cancer precursors. *European Journal of Gynaecological Oncology.* 2008; 29(3): 205–21.
198 International Collaboration of Epidemiological Studies of Cervical Cancer. Comparison of risk factors for invasive squamous cell carcinoma and adenocarcinoma of the cervix: collaborative reanalysis of individual data on 8,097 women with squamous cell carcinoma and 1,374 women with adenocarcinoma from 12 epidemiological studies. *International Journal of Cancer.* 2007; 120(4): 885–91.
199 Berrington de Gonzalez A, Sweetland S, Green J. Comparison of risk factors for squamous cell and adenocarcinomas of the cervix: a meta-analysis. *British Journal of Cancer.* 2004; 90(9): 1787–91.
200 Hildesheim A, Wang SS. Host and viral genetics and risk of cervical cancer: a review. *Virus Research.* 2002; 89(2): 229–40.
201 Horng JT, Hu KC, Wu LC et al. Identifying the combination of genetic factors that determine susceptibility to cervical cancer. *IEEE Transactions on Information Technology in Biomedicine.* 2004; 8(1): 59–66.
202 Andersson S, Rylander E, Strand A et al. The significance of p53 codon 72 polymorphism for the development of cervical adenocarcinomas. *British Journal of Cancer.* 2001; 85(8): 1153–6.
203 de Araujo Souza PS, Villa LL. Genetic susceptibility to infection with human papillomavirus and development of cervical cancer in women in Brazil. *Mutation Research.* 2003; 544(2–3): 375–83.
204 Lee SA, Kim JW, Roh JW et al. Genetic polymorphisms of GSTM1, p21, p53 and HPV infection with cervical cancer in Korean women. *Gynecologic Oncology.* 2004; 93(1): 14–8.
205 Govan VA, Loubser S, Saleh D et al. No relationship observed between human p53 codon-72 genotype and HPV-associated cervical cancer in a population group with a low arginine-72 allele frequency. *International Journal of Immunogenetics.* 2007; 34(3): 213–7.
206 Au WW. Life style, environmental and genetic susceptibility to cervical cancer. *Toxicology.* 2004; 198(1–3): 117–20.
207 Zoodsma M, Nolte IM, Schipper M et al. Analysis of the entire HLA region in susceptibility for cervical cancer: a comprehensive study. *Journal of Medical Genetics.* 2005; 42(8): e49.

208 Maciag PC, Schlecht NF, Souza PS et al. Major histocompatibility complex class II polymorphisms and risk of cervical cancer and human papillomavirus infection in Brazilian women. *Cancer Epidemiology, Biomarkers and Prevention.* 2000; 9(11): 1183–91.

209 Munoz N, Bosch FX. Cervical cancer and human papillomavirus: epidemiological evidence and perspectives for prevention. *Salud Publica de Mexico.* 1997; 39(4): 274–82.

210 Zehbe I, Voglino G, Wilander E et al. p53 codon 72 polymorphism and various human papillomavirus 16 E6 genotypes are risk factors for cervical cancer development. *Cancer Research.* 2001; 61(2): 608–11.

211 van Duin M, Snijders PJ, Vossen MT et al. Analysis of human papillomavirus type 16 E6 variants in relation to p53 codon 72 polymorphism genotypes in cervical carcinogenesis. *Journal of General Virology.* 2000; 81(Pt 2): 317–25.

212 de Araujo Souza PS, Maciag PC, Ribeiro KB et al. Interaction between polymorphisms of the human leukocyte antigen and HPV-16 variants on the risk of invasive cervical cancer. *BMC Cancer.* 2008; 8: 246.

213 Heilmann V, Kreienberg R. Molecular biology of cervical cancer and its precursors. *Current Women's Health Reports.* 2002; 2(1): 27–33.

214 Magnusson PK, Lichtenstein P, Gyllensten UB. Heritability of cervical tumours. *International Journal of Cancer.* 2000; 88(5): 698–701.

215 Gunnell AS, Tran TN, Torrang A et al. Synergy between cigarette smoking and human papillomavirus type 16 in cervical cancer in situ development. *Cancer Epidemiology, Biomarkers and Prevention.* 2006; 15(11): 2141–7.

216 Hellberg D, Stendahl U. The biological role of smoking, oral contraceptive use and endogenous sexual steroid hormones in invasive squamous epithelial cervical cancer. *Anticancer Research.* 2005; 25(4): 3041–6.

217 Plummer M, Herrero R, Franceschi S et al. Smoking and cervical cancer: pooled analysis of the IARC multi-centric case–control study. *Cancer Causes and Control.* 2003; 14(9): 805–14.

218 Syrjanen K. New concepts on risk factors of HPV and novel screening strategies for cervical cancer precursors. *European Journal of Gynaecological Oncology.* 2008; 29(3): 205–21.

219 Syrjanen K, Naud P, Derchain S et al. Drug addiction is not an independent risk factor for oncogenic human papillomavirus infections or high-grade cervical intraepithelial neoplasia: case-control study nested within the Latin American Screening study cohort. *International Journal of STD and AIDS.* 2008; 19(4): 251–8.

220 Haverkos H, Rohrer M, Pickworth W. The cause of invasive cervical cancer could be multifactorial. *Biomedicine and Pharmacotherapy.* 2000; 54(1): 54–9.

221 International Collaboration of Epidemiological Studies of Cervical Cancer. Carcinoma of the cervix and tobacco smoking: collaborative reanalysis of individual data on 13,541 women with carcinoma of the cervix and 23,017 women without carcinoma of the cervix from 23 epidemiological studies. *International Journal of Cancer.* 2006; 118: 1481–95.

222 International Collaboration of Epidemiological Studies of Cervical Cancer. Comparison of risk factors for invasive squamous cell carcinoma and adenocarcinoma of the cervix: collaborative reanalysis of individual data on 8,097 women with squamous cell carcinoma and 1,374 women with adenocarcinoma from 12 epidemiological studies. *International Journal of Cancer.* 2007; 120(4): 885–91.

223 Gunnell AS, Tran TN, Torrang A et al. Synergy between cigarette smoking and human papillomavirus type 16 in cervical cancer in situ development. *Cancer Epidemiology, Biomarkers and Prevention.* 2006; 15(11): 2141–7.
224 Wiley DJ, Wiesmeier E, Masongsong E et al. Smokers at higher risk for undetected antibody for oncogenic human papillomavirus type 16 infection. *Cancer Epidemiology, Biomarkers and Prevention.* 2006; 15(5): 915–20.
225 Simen-Kapeu A, Kataja V, Yliskoski M et al. Smoking impairs human papillomavirus (HPV) type 16 and 18 capsids antibody response following natural HPV infection. *Scandinavian Journal of Infectious Diseases.* 2008: 1–7.
226 Prokopczyk B, Cox JE, Hoffmann D et al. Identification of tobacco-specific carcinogen in the cervical mucus of smokers and nonsmokers. *Journal of the National Cancer Institute.* 1997; 89(12): 868–73.
227 Haverkos HW. Multifactorial etiology of cervical cancer: a hypothesis. *Medscape General Medicine.* 2005; 7(4): 57.
228 Nishino K, Sekine M, Kodama S et al. Cigarette smoking and glutathione S-transferase M1 polymorphism associated with risk for uterine cervical cancer. *Journal of Obstetrics and Gynaecology Research.* 2008; 34(6): 994–1001.
229 Singh H, Jain M, Mittal B. MMP-7 (-181A>G) promoter polymorphisms and risk for cervical cancer. *Gynecologic Oncology.* 2008; 110(1): 71–5.
230 Juarez-Cedillo T, Vallejo M, Fragoso JM et al. The risk of developing cervical cancer in Mexican women is associated to CYP1A1 MspI polymorphism. *European Journal of Cancer.* 2007; 43(10): 1590–5.
231 Tsai HT, Tsai YM, Yang SF et al. Lifetime cigarette smoke and second-hand smoke and cervical intraepithelial neoplasm—a community-based case-control study. *Gynecologic Oncology.* 2007; 105(1): 181–8.
232 Trimble CL, Genkinger JM, Burke AE et al. Active and passive cigarette smoking and the risk of cervical neoplasia. *Obstetrics and Gynecology.* 2005; 105(1): 174–81.
233 Wu MT, Lee LH, Ho CK et al. Lifetime exposure to environmental tobacco smoke and cervical intraepithelial neoplasms among nonsmoking Taiwanese women. *Archives of Environmental Health.* 2003; 58(6): 353–9.
234 Sobti RC, Shekari M, Tamandani DM et al. Association of interleukin-18 gene promoter polymorphism on the risk of cervix carcinogenesis in north Indian population. *Oncology Research.* 2008; 17(4): 159–66.
235 Sobti RC, Kaur S, Kaur P et al. Interaction of passive smoking with GST (GSTM1, GSTT1, and GSTP1) genotypes in the risk of cervical cancer in India. *Cancer Genetics and Cytogenetics.* 2006; 166(2): 117–23.
236 Delvenne P, Herman L, Kholod N et al. Role of hormone cofactors in the human papillomavirus-induced carcinogenesis of the uterine cervix. *Molecular and Cellular Endocrinology.* 2007; 264(1–2): 1–5.
237 Remoue F, Jacobs N, Miot V et al. High intraepithelial expression of estrogen and progesterone receptors in the transformation zone of the uterine cervix. *American Journal of Obstetrics and Gynecology.* 2003; 189(6): 1660–5.
238 Syrjanen K, Shabalova I, Petrovichev N et al. Age at menarche is not an independent risk factor for high-risk human papillomavirus infections and cervical intraepithelial neoplasia. *International Journal of STD and AIDS.* 2008; 19(1): 16–25.
239 Vaccarella S, Herrero R, Dai M et al. Reproductive factors, oral contraceptive use, and human papillomavirus infection: pooled analysis of the IARC

HPV prevalence surveys. *Cancer Epidemiology, Biomarkers and Prevention.* 2006; 15(11): 2148–53.
240 Green J, Berrington de Gonzalez A, Smith JS et al. Human papillomavirus infection and use of oral contraceptives. *British Journal of Cancer.* 2003; 88(11): 1713–20.
241 Smith JS, Green J, Berrington de Gonzalez A et al. Cervical cancer and use of hormonal contraceptives: A systematic review. *The Lancet.* 2003; 361(9364): 1159–67.
242 Syrjanen K, Shabalova I, Petrovichev N et al. Oral contraceptives are not an independent risk factor for cervical intraepithelial neoplasia or high-risk human papillomavirus infections. *Anticancer Research.* 2006; 26(6C): 4729–40.
243 Cotton SC, Sharp L, Seth R et al. Lifestyle and socio-demographic factors associated with high-risk HPV infection in UK women. *British Journal of Cancer.* 2007; 97(1): 133–9.
244 Castle PE, Walker JL, Schiffman M et al. Hormonal contraceptive use, pregnancy and parity, and the risk of cervical intraepithelial neoplasia 3 among oncogenic HPV DNA-positive women with equivocal or mildly abnormal cytology. *International Journal of Cancer.* 2005; 117(6): 1007–12.
245 International Collaboration of Epidemiological Studies of Cervical Cancer. Comparison of risk factors for invasive squamous cell carcinoma and adenocarcinoma of the cervix: collaborative reanalysis of individual data on 8,097 women with squamous cell carcinoma and 1,374 women with adenocarcinoma from 12 epidemiological studies. *International Journal of Cancer.* 2007; 120(4): 885–91.
246 Sobti RC, Shekari M, Kordi Tamandani DM et al. Effect of NBS1 gene polymorphism on the risk of cervix carcinoma in a northern Indian population. *International Journal of Biological Markers.* 2008; 23(3): 133–9.
247 Shekari M, Sobti RC, Tamandani DM et al. Association of genetic polymorphism of the DNA base excision repair gene (APE-1 Asp/148 Glu) and HPV type (16/18) with the risk of cervix cancer in north Indian population. *Cancer Biomarkers.* 2008; 4(2): 63–71.
248 Guven S, Kart C, Guvendag Guven ES et al. The underlying cause of cervical cancer in oral contraceptive users may be related to cervical mucus changes. *Medical Hypotheses.* 2007; 69(3): 550–2.
249 International Collaboration of Epidemiological Studies of Cervical Cancer. Cervical carcinoma and reproductive factors: collaborative reanalysis of individual data on 16,563 women with cervical carcinoma and 33,542 women without cervical carcinoma from 25 epidemiological studies. *International Journal of Cancer.* 2006; 119: 1108–24.
250 Brinton LA, Reeves WC, Brenes MM et al. Parity as a risk factor for cervical cancer. *American Journal of Epidemiology.* 1989; 130: 486–96.
251 Britt K, Ashworth A, Smalley M. Pregnancy and the risk of breast cancer. *Endocrine-Related Cancer.* 2007; 14(4): 907–33.
252 Vaccarella S, Herrero R, Dai M et al. Reproductive factors, oral contraceptive use, and human papillomavirus infection: pooled analysis of the IARC HPV prevalence surveys. *Cancer Epidemiology, Biomarkers and Prevention.* 2006; 15(11): 2148–53.
253 Munoz N, Franceschi S, Bosetti C et al. Role of parity and human papillomavirus in cervical cancer: the IARC multicentric case-control study. *The Lancet.* 2002; 359(9312): 1093–101.

254 Castellsague X, Diaz M, de Sanjose S et al. Worldwide human papillomavirus etiology of cervical adenocarcinoma and its cofactors: implications for screening and prevention. *Journal of the National Cancer Institute*. 2006; 98(5): 303–15.
255 Castle PE, Walker JL, Schiffman M et al. Hormonal contraceptive use, pregnancy and parity, and the risk of cervical intraepithelial neoplasia 3 among oncogenic HPV DNA-positive women with equivocal or mildly abnormal cytology. *International Journal of Cancer*. 2005; 117(6): 1007–12.
256 Castle PE, Escoffery C, Schachter J et al. Chlamydia trachomatis, herpes simplex virus 2, and human T-cell lymphotrophic virus type 1 are not associated with grade of cervical neoplasia in Jamaican colposcopy patients. *Sexually Transmitted Diseases*. 2003; 30(7): 575–80.
257 Al-Daraji WI, Smith JH. Infection and cervical neoplasia: facts and fiction. *International Journal of Clinical and Experimental Pathology*. 2009; 2(1): 48–64.
258 Haverkos H, Rohrer M, Pickworth W. The cause of invasive cervical cancer could be multifactorial. *Biomedicine and Pharmacotherapy*. 2000; 54(1): 54–9.
259 zur Hausen H. Human genital cancer: synergism between two virus infections or synergism between a virus infection and initiating events? *The Lancet*. 1982; 2(8312): 1370–2.
260 Smith JS, Herrero R, Bosetti C et al. Herpes simplex virus-2 as a human papillomavirus cofactor in the etiology of invasive cervical cancer. *Journal of the National Cancer Institute*. 2002; 94(21): 1604–13.
261 Finan RR, Musharrafieh U, Almawi WY. Detection of Chlamydia trachomatis and herpes simplex virus type 1 or 2 in cervical samples in human papilloma virus (HPV)-positive and HPV-negative women. *Clinical Microbiology and Infection*. 2006; 12(9): 927–30.
262 Zereu M, Zettler CG, Cambruzzi E et al. Herpes simplex virus type 2 and Chlamydia trachomatis in adenocarcinoma of the uterine cervix. *Gynecologic Oncology*. 2007; 105(1): 172–5.
263 Perez LO, Barbisan G, Abba MC et al. Herpes simplex virus and human papillomavirus infection in cervical disease in Argentine women. *International Journal of Gynecological Pathology*. 2006; 25(1): 42–7.
264 Kwasniewska A, Korobowicz E, Visconti J et al. Chlamydia trachomatis and herpes simplex virus 2 infection in vulvar intraepithelial neoplasia associated with human papillomavirus. *European Journal of Gynaecological Oncology*. 2006; 27(4): 405–8.
265 Tran-Thanh D, Provencher D, Koushik A et al. Herpes simplex virus type II is not a cofactor to human papillomavirus in cancer of the uterine cervix. *American Journal of Obstetrics and Gynecology*. 2003; 188(1): 129–34.
266 Lehtinen M, Koskela P, Jellum E et al. Herpes simplex virus and risk of cervical cancer: a longitudinal, nested case-control study in the nordic countries. *American Journal of Epidemiology*. 2002; 156(8): 687–92.
267 Smith JS, Bosetti C, Munoz N et al. Chlamydia trachomatis and invasive cervical cancer: a pooled analysis of the IARC multicentric case-control study. *International Journal of Cancer*. 2004; 111(3): 431–9.
268 Smith JS, Munoz N, Herrero R et al. Evidence for Chlamydia trachomatis as a human papillomavirus cofactor in the etiology of invasive cervical cancer in Brazil and the Philippines. *Journal of Infectious Diseases*. 2002; 185(3): 324–31.

269 Mumm JB, Oft M. Cytokine-based transformation of immune surveillance into tumor-promoting inflammation. *Oncogene.* 2008; 27(45): 5913–9.
270 Farinati F, Cardin R, Cassaro M et al. Helicobacter pylori, inflammation, oxidative damage and gastric cancer: a morphological, biological and molecular pathway. *European Journal of Cancer Prevention.* 2008; 17(3): 195–200.
271 Klein EA, Silverman R. Inflammation, infection, and prostate cancer. *Current Opinion in Urology.* 2008; 18(3): 315–9.
272 de Paula FD, Fernandes AP, Carmo BB et al. Molecular detection of Chlamydia trachomatis and HPV infections in cervical samples with normal and abnormal cytopathological findings. *Diagnostic Cytopathology.* 2007; 35(4): 198–202.
273 Zereu M, Zettler CG, Cambruzzi E et al. Herpes simplex virus type 2 and Chlamydia trachomatis in adenocarcinoma of the uterine cervix. *Gynecologic Oncology.* 2007; 105(1): 172–5.
274 Kwasniewska A, Korobowicz E, Visconti J et al. Chlamydia trachomatis and herpes simplex virus 2 infection in vulvar intraepithelial neoplasia associated with human papillomavirus. *European Journal of Gynaecological Oncology.* 2006; 27(4): 405–8.
275 Feher E, Szalmas A. Prevalence of Chlamydia trachomatis and oncogenic human papillomavirus types in cytologic atypia of the uterine cervix. *Acta Microbiologica et Immunologica Hungarica.* 2006; 53(4): 479–87.
276 Luostarinen T, Lehtinen M, Bjorge T et al. Joint effects of different human papillomaviruses and Chlamydia trachomatis infections on risk of squamous cell carcinoma of the cervix uteri. *European Journal of Cancer.* 2004; 40(7): 1058–65.
277 Cameron JE, Hagensee ME. Human papillomavirus infection and disease in the HIV+ individual. *Cancer Treatment and Research.* 2007; 133: 185–213.
278 Lehtovirta P, Finne P, Nieminen P et al. Prevalence and risk factors of squamous intraepithelial lesions of the cervix among HIV-infected women - a long-term follow-up study in a low-prevalence population. *International Journal of STD and AIDS.* 2006; 17(12): 831–4.
279 De Vuyst H, Lillo F, Broutet N et al. HIV, human papillomavirus, and cervical neoplasia and cancer in the era of highly active antiretroviral therapy. *European Journal of Cancer Prevention.* 2008; 17(6): 545–54.
280 Moodley JR, Hoffman M, Carrara H et al. HIV and pre-neoplastic and neoplastic lesions of the cervix in South Africa: a case-control study. *BioMed Central Cancer.* 2006; 6: 135.
281 Hawes SE, Critchlow CW, Sow PS et al. Incident high-grade squamous intraepithelial lesions in Senegalese women with and without human immunodeficiency virus type 1 (HIV-1) and HIV-2. *Journal of the National Cancer Institute.* 2006; 98(2): 100–9.
282 Strickler HD, Burk RD, Fazzari M et al. Natural history and possible reactivation of human papillomavirus in human immunodeficiency virus-positive women. *Journal of the National Cancer Institute.* 2005; 97(8): 577–86.
283 Clifford GM, Goncalves MA, Franceschi S. Human papillomavirus types among women infected with HIV: a meta-analysis. *AIDS.* 2006; 20(18): 2337–44.
284 Busnach G, Piselli P, Arbustini E et al. Immunosuppression and cancer: a comparison of risks in recipients of organ transplants and in HIV-positive individuals. *Transplantation Proceedings.* 2006; 38(10): 3533–5.

285 Branca M, Costa S, Mariani L et al. Assessment of risk factors and human papillomavirus (HPV) related pathogenetic mechanisms of CIN in HIV-positive and HIV-negative women. Study design and baseline data of the HPV-PathogenISS study. *European Journal of Gynaecological Oncology.* 2004; 25(6): 689–98.

286 Theodore C, Androulakis N, Spatz A et al. An explosive course of squamous cell penile cancer in an AIDS patient. *Annals of Oncology.* 2002; 13(3): 475–9.

287 Agorastos T, Chrisafi S, Lambropoulos AF et al. Adeno-associated virus infection and cervical neoplasia: is there a protective role against human papillomavirus-related carcinogenesis? *European Journal of Cancer Prevention.* 2008; 17(4): 364–8.

288 Hermonat PL, You H, Chiriva-Internati CM et al. Analysis of adeno-associated virus and HPV interaction. *Methods in Molecular Medicine.* 2005; 119: 397–409.

289 Piyathilake CJ. Update on micronutrients and cervical dysplasia. *Ethnicity and Disease.* 2007; 17(2 suppl 2): S2-14-7.

290 Goodman MT, Shvetsov YB, McDuffie K et al. Hawaii cohort study of serum micronutrient concentrations and clearance of incident oncogenic human papillomavirus infection of the cervix. *Cancer Research.* 2007; 67(12): 5987–96.

291 Siegel EM, Craft NE, Duarte-Franco E et al. Associations between serum carotenoids and tocopherols and type-specific HPV persistence: the Ludwig-McGill cohort study. *International Journal of Cancer.* 2007; 120(3): 672–80.

292 Sedjo RL, Inserra P, Abrahamsen M et al. Human papillomavirus persistence and nutrients involved in the methylation pathway among a cohort of young women. *Cancer Epidemiology, Biomarkers and Prevention.* 2002; 11(4): 353–9.

293 Goodman MT, McDuffie K, Hernandez B et al. Case-control study of plasma folate, homocysteine, vitamin B(12), and cysteine as markers of cervical dysplasia. *Cancer.* 2000; 89(2): 376–82.

294 Piyathilake CJ. Update on micronutrients and cervical dysplasia. *Ethnicity and Disease.* 2007; 17(2 suppl 2): S2-14-7.

295 Ghosh C, Baker JA, Moysich KB et al. Dietary intakes of selected nutrients and food groups and risk of cervical cancer. *Nutrition and Cancer.* 2008; 60(3): 331–41.

296 Lane G. Obesity and gynaecological cancer. *Menopause International.* 2008; 14(1): 33–7.

297 Wee CC, Huang A, Huskey KW et al. Obesity and the likelihood of sexual behavioral risk factors for HPV and cervical cancer. *Obesity.* 2008; 16(11): 2552–5.

298 Maruthur NM, Bolen SD, Brancati FL et al. The association of obesity and cervical cancer screening: a systematic review and meta-analysis. *Obesity (Silver Spring).* 2009; 17(2): 375–81.

299 Mitchell RS, Padwal RS, Chuck AW et al. Cancer screening among the overweight and obese in Canada. *American Journal of Preventive Medicine.* 2008; 35(2): 127–32.

300 Smith JS, Green J, Berrington de Gonzalez A et al. Cervical cancer and use of hormonal contraceptives: a systematic review. *The Lancet.* 2003; 361(9364): 1159–67.

301 Hrushesky WJ, Sothern RB, Rietveld WJ et al. Season, sun, sex, and cervical cancer. *Cancer Epidemiology, Biomarkers and Prevention.* 2005; 14(8): 1940–7.

5

HUMAN PAPILLOMAVIRUS: ASSOCIATIONS WITH NONCERVICAL CANCER

Papillomaviruses have attracted increasing scientific attention, as they are quantitatively the most important group of viruses associated with benign and malignant neoplasia in humans.[1]

Although the evidence for a human papillomavirus (HPV) connection to cervical cancer is the most extensive and compelling, there are clear indications that the virus is involved in malignancies at many other sites. Indeed, the annual incidence of HPV-associated noncervical cancers approximates the number of cervical cancers in the United States, with similar numbers of noncervical cases for men and women.[2] In contrast with cervical cancer, the incidence of anal and oropharyngeal cancers, some of which are traceable to HPV infection and for which there are no effective or widely used screening programs, has actually been increasing. This has focused greater attention on the possible utility of new HPV vaccines in reducing this burden, including the associated economic costs to society.[3,4]

As detailed in Chapter 2, HPV demonstrates a remarkable tropism for cutaneous and mucosal epithelia. Oncogenic HPV types appear to target the basal cells of squamous linings at or near the surface of the body; these epithelia demonstrate limited "natural" keratinization combined with the potential for keratinization to increase as part of certain disease processes. Precise knowledge of HPV tropism allows for the logical characterization of an inventory of tissues and body sites with susceptibility to both infection and carcinoma development. The clear evidence of tropism also may explain the apparent skepticism in the literature about finding a direct role for HPV in tumor formation beyond the world of squamous epithelia, for instance, in breast cancer or cancer of the urinary bladder.

Lesions at the predictable sites of susceptibility are typically broken into two major categories: anogenital cancers (which include cervical cancer) and head and neck cancers. In addition to these two groups, the known link between HPV and skin cancer will be considered; as well, a brief review will be offered concerning other locations and cancers where the HPV association is under investigation. The main agenda in each section is to describe the HPV involvement with the various cancers. An important finding that emerges over and over in the following commentary is the dominance of HPV-16 in malignant phenotypes, "regardless of the organ of origin."[5]

ANOGENITAL CANCERS

The best known category of HPV-related malignancy after cervical cancer comprises the other susceptible sites in the anogenital region, including the vulva and vagina. These cancers are generally much rarer than cervical cancer. As suggested above, however, there are indications in some populations that the burden may be expanding. For example, a 2008 report indicated that the incidence of anal cancer in women and of vulvar cancer had increased in the province of Quebec; survival rates for penile cancer and male anal cancer have also shown a recent decline.[6]

The relevant noncervical gynecological cancers will be the first focus of this section, followed by penile cancer; the latter will offer a good opportunity to revisit the topic of HPV infection in males. Finally, cancer of the anus, a malignancy of increasing concern, will be considered. A key fact emerging from the following overview is that there is substantial overlap between the role of HPV in the cervix and its impact in other anogenital sites. Indeed, the close relationship between these malignancies has been traced to the molecular level, specifically to the genetic perturbations involved with carcinogenesis.[7]

Cancer of the Vulva

Vulvar[8] and vaginal cancers are rare, together accounting for only 7% of cancers of the female genital tract in the United States[9] Consequently, the research attention paid to these diseases has been quite limited, especially compared with the flood of literature on cervical cancer.[10] This situation may change, as there are indications of increased incidence in the United States for in situ vulvar carcinoma and, to a lesser extent, for invasive cancer.[11] Similar trends have recently been reported for vulvar cancer in Germany.[12]

HPV has been implicated in a variety of lesions in the vulva, including genital warts, vulvar intraepithelial neoplasia (VIN), and malignancies.[13] About 75–90% of vulvar cancers are squamous cell carcinomas, with the balance including melanoma, adenocarcinoma, and other rarer forms.[14–16] In recent years, researchers have discovered that vulvar carcinomas and related VIN represent two distinct disease pathways.[17,18] One form involves differentiated, keratinizing squamous cell tumors, likely developing from VIN that are sometimes related to other epithelial disorders (e.g., lichen sclerosus).[19] Such tumors usually occur in patients of advanced age, and are characterized by poor prognosis.[20,21] Significantly, HPV is rarely detected in these lesions.

In contrast, the other type of vulvar cancer (and associated VIN) does appear to involve HPV infection. These lesions, sometimes referred to as the "classic type," tend to be nonkeratinizing carcinomas, characterized as basaloid or warty.[22,23] Biomarkers, especially p16 expression, are being investigated to help distinguish the two types of vulvar cancer at an early stage so that so that the appropriate therapies can be applied.[24–29]

As already suggested, age is associated with the HPV status of vulvar cancer; patients with HPV-positive cancers tend to be younger.[30,31] This pattern was confirmed in a 1999 study of about 300 women with VIN or stage I vulvar carcinoma; 61.5% of the younger women (under age 45 years) demonstrated an HPV infection, compared with only 17.5% of the older subset.[32]

There are variable estimates of the breakdown between HPV-related and other forms of vulvar cancer. Older clinical studies detected HPV DNA in 20–80% of tumors (with a median figure of around 40%).[33] Variation is also evident in more recent data. Thus, the figure reported by Ngan et al. (1999) was 48%, by Menczer et al. (2000) 64% (for HPV-16 and -18 only), by Koyamatsu et al. (2003) only 13%, and by Huang et al. (2005) 75%.[34–37] At least two factors may be influencing the wide range of results: small sample sizes and changes in the detection technology applied in each study.

A final example from research published in 2006 demonstrated HPV positivity in vulvar cancer of about 60%. A summary of the study results is provided in Table 5.1, demonstrating the different data according to lesion progression, including average patient age at diagnosis.[38] Note that, at 92%, HPV-positivity was substantially higher in VIN than in vulvar cancer. This suggests that the propensity to progress to cancer is actually lower in cases involving HPV infection compared with women with HPV-negative vulvar lesions.

Table 5.1. HPV Infections in Women with Vulvar Intraepithelial Neoplasia and Carcinoma

	VIN 2/3	*Vulvar Carcinoma*
Subjects	168	48
Samples	183	48
Mean age at diagnosis	47 years	55 years
HPV-positive samples	169 (92.3%)	29 (60.4%)
Mean age at diagnosis	46 years	51 years
HPV-negative samples	14 (7.6%)	19 (39.6%)
Mean age at diagnosis	55 years	61 years

Source: Hampl et al., Obstetrics and Gynecology, 2006.

High-risk HPV is the viral category most often found in vulvar cancer or high-grade precursor lesions. In other words, the pattern for vulvar neoplasia matches that seen in cervical tumors. For example, a recent study of 30 VIN patients found that 80% demonstrated high-risk viral types, with HPV-16 clearly in the lead.[39] Other research among VIN patients has found even higher prevalence rates for HPV-16—up to 90%.[40,41] A 2006 study drew a clear distinction between low-grade and high-grade lesions, with low-risk HPV being more prevalent in the former and HPV-16 dominating in the latter.[42]

Turning to cancer proper, the 1999 study by Ngan et al. (noted earlier) suggested that HPV-16 and -18 accounted for 96% of the cases involving viral infection. This result is comparable to an earlier study that focused on one viral type, ultimately detecting HPV-16 in 83% of the total vulvar cancer patients infected with the virus.[43] Overall, these data suggest that the first proposed HPV vaccination programs (which in fact target HPV-16 and -18) could have a substantial impact on vulvar cancer.[44] While promise is also held out for therapies that target infection,[45] it is the prevention potential that truly excites health care planners. Indeed, one study has suggested that a prophylactic vaccine could prevent about half of the vulvar cancers that occur in younger women.[46] The final impact may depend on the true distribution of viral types in HPV-related cancer.[47] A recent systematic review suggested that HPV-33 rather than -18 is the second most frequent cause (after HPV-16) of virally related vulvar cancer.[48]

HPV is important not only in the origin, prevention, and early treatment of certain vulvar cancers but also in long-term follow-up. Patients who are HPV positive are more likely to experience recurrent VIN, a factor that should be considered when establishing a surveillance plan.[49]

It should be acknowledged that "the presence and role of various oncogenic types of HPV in vulvar intraepithelial neoplasia and in the promotion and development of vulvar carcinoma is still under discussion."[50] The growing evidence base admittedly is drawn from quite variable data that may in part reflect ongoing challenges in classifying different types of vulvar lesions.[51] The International Society for the Study of Vulvar Disease has formulated new terminology that may help to distinguish forms of cancer related to HPV, but the proposals are still being evaluated.[52,53]

The research obstacles notwithstanding, the involvement of HPV in the etiology of vulvar malignancy is now quite well established. The known etiologic pattern both differs from and parallels cervical cancer. Since HPV is only implicated in 40–60% of vulvar cancers, the virus cannot be construed as a necessary carcinogen.[54] It is not a sufficient agent either. Thus, it is clear that, like cervical cancer, vulvar tumors have a multifactorial origin. The implicated correlates and cofactors are now also familiar, including multiple sexual partners, early sexual debut, and smoking.[55-57] There are definitely other factors involved; a notable proportion of older women with vulvar cancer are neither infected with HPV nor are they smokers.[58]

Local spread of gynecological cancers complicates the epidemiological picture; such extensions must be distinguished from truly new cancers. There is a high risk of current cervical cancer spreading to the vulvar area. Cervical tumors tend to spread locally before metastasizing; this phenomenon probably has even more relevance for the development of vaginal cancer (see section "Cancer of the Vagina").[59,60] An intriguing pathway potentially explaining local advancement of cancer involves HPV-infected, transformed cells in one site disseminating throughout the genital mucosa.[61,62] Multiple locations of cancer, even in adjacent sites, are not always considered to be a local extension. In fact, when tumors in different sites occur more than 2 months apart, the new occurrence is usually defined as a second primary cancer (SPC). Different mechanism may be at work to generate an SPC related to HPV, from the simple reality of an underlying infection in multiple sites to shared exposure to risk factors that promote reinfection. For example, a primary cancer in the vulva following cervical cancer may be explicable in terms of ongoing exposure to a number of social or lifestyle factors that are known to increase persistent HPV infection.[63,64]

Whatever the final explanation for multiple cancers in the female lower genital tract, it is important to recognize that a history of cervical intraepithelial neoplasia (CIN) or cervical cancer elevates the risk of second primary vulvar cancers.[65] Having a history of VIN operates in a similar way; lesions in the vulva demonstrate an association with recurrent and/or multifocal HPV infection elsewhere in the female lower genital tract, which can lead to SPC.[66] The topic of second primary malignancies related to HPV will be revisited in a later section.

Coinfection with other microbes appears to elevate the risk of vulvar cancer. In particular, there is limited evidence that HIV increases the risk of persistent HPV infection and, as a result, vulvar disease progression.[67,68] The recent increase in high-grade VIN and vulvar cancer among young women is still not well understood; it has been attributed to rising HPV infection rates, as well as to the impact of HIV coinfection.[69-71] Finally, recent research has found no correlation between herpes simplex virus type 2 (HSV-2) or *Chlamydia trachomatis* and HPV infection in the vulva.[72] Interestingly, some earlier studies did support the idea of HSV-2 as an independent risk factor for vulvar cancer development.[73]

Other common risk factors for carcinomas may not increase the occurrence of the subset of vulvar lesions related to HPV. In fact, there is evidence that exposure to solar radiation, in particular ultraviolet-B (UVB), protects against vulvar cancers. The mechanism of effect must be systemic, as the vulva is not typically exposed directly to sunlight; the most likely candidate is vitamin D production.[74] Although not likely to be related to HPV infection, there is evidence of a different pattern of melanoma occurrence in the vulva, one that is also traceable to levels of solar exposure; purported mechanisms include the protective effect of some form of sun-induced melanoma-inhibitory factor and melanin interference with carcinogenesis.[75] Discussion has arisen on whether the increase in sunbathing and nude artificial tanning will influence the incidence of vulvar melanomas.[76] Again, HPV is not thought to be connected to the occurrence of melanoma, and so is not implicated in this changing picture.

Cancer of the Vagina

Partly because of the rarity of vaginal lesions (both absolute and relative to other sites in the female lower genital tract),[77] the evidence of HPV association has been only gradually emerging. A study in 1997 found an 83% HPV positivity rate across 71 cases of vaginal intraepithelial neoplasia (VaIN). Over 20 types of HPV were detected.[78] A more recent and larger study showed similar results for malignancies, with 82% positivity for in situ cancers and 64% for invasive cancers. Although a variety of HPV types were again detected, HPV-16 was dominant, showing up in over half the cases.[79] This result may be compared with a report published in 2003 that detected HPV-16 or 18 DNA in 44% of a small series of vaginal tumors.[80] Finally, a 2006 study found HPV in 76% of VaIN 1 and 94% of VaIN 3 cases, with 15 different types ultimately detected.[81] A spectrum of HPV types has also been found in vaginal specimens from women without lesions; the affinity of HPV for vaginal and cervical epithelium appears to be similar, though non-oncogenic viral types may be found more frequently in vaginal samples from a general population.[82]

The other risk factors connected to HPV-related lesions are similar to those seen in the vulva and the cervix. A population-based study found that lifetime number of sexual partners, early age at first intercourse, and smoking were all associated with an increased risk of in situ and invasive vaginal cancer.[83] The role of smoking in high-grade VaIN was recently confirmed in a U.S. study.[84] Beyond personal lifestyle factors, there is also some evidence for an effect of host genetic susceptibility, and possibly chemical carcinogens, especially in early life.[85] The best known example of the latter is prenatal exposure to the medication diethylstibestrol, or DES, which was once used as a treatment during pregnancy.[86,87] It is unlikely that this (now discontinued) iatrogenic source of a very rare vaginal cancer has any connection to HPV infection. Finally, HIV infection appears to increase the incidence of vaginal lesions, though the specific relationship to HPV coinfection has not been clarified.[88]

The general conclusion is that vaginal neoplasia, as with other genital tract tumors, shares many risk factors and cytological markers with lesions of the cervix.[89,90] In particular, a common susceptibility to HPV infection may help to explain the elevated risk for vaginal cancer in women previously treated for CIN or for cancer of the cervix.[91,92] This phenomenon alone should motivate intensified detection of HPV infection and surveillance for new primary lesions in survivors of cervical cancer.[93] High-risk HPV has also been associated with vaginal cancer recurrence, again underlining the potential value of HPV DNA tests in focusing a surveillance program.[94]

As HPV-16 and -18 seem to be the dominant types found in VaIN and vaginal carcinomas,[95,96] currently available prophylactic vaccines will likely decrease vaginal cancers, though the rarity of these tumors means the impact on total cancer incidence will be small. Important reductions may be seen in the subset of cases comprising second primary vaginal cancers following other anogenital tumors. In fact, emerging evidence suggests that high-grade tumors in the female lower genital tract, including those in the vagina, are mostly "monoclonal lesions from a transformed cell population derived from the uterine cervix," which in turn may be traced to high-risk HPV infection.[97] This and other aspects of vaginal neoplasia continue to be investigated, including the evidence for variations in the natural history of disease depending on the specific subsite of HPV-related VaIN.[98]

Cancer of the Penis

Penile cancer is an "aggressive and mutilating disease that deeply affects the patient's self-esteem."[99] The malignancy is much more common in emerging economies such as Brazil and India compared with the developed world. While there is variability across ethnic groups, the incidence of penile cancer in the United States is generally very low, and perhaps even on the decline.[100–102] This may explain why the impact of HPV in males has not been as intensively investigated by researchers as the involvement of the virus with female genital cancer.[103] Nonetheless, in the studies that have been conducted, researchers consistently detect HPV DNA in lesions of the male genitals.[104,105] Although the evidence is accumulating in this way, an etiological connection between HPV and penile cancer is not yet fully established.[106–108] Indeed, alternate causal factors continue to be proposed that are independent of HPV infection.[109]

Earlier reports suggested that HPV DNA is present in 75–100% of penile intraepithelial neoplasia (PIN).[110,111] This result, which has been confirmed in recent studies, would be more compelling were it not for the fact that PIN does not seem to be a precursor for all penile cancer, but only for a subset of carcinomas characterized as basaloid or warty.[112] Consistent with this observation is the fact that, among all forms of penile cancer, these tumors typically demonstrate the highest prevalence for HPV infection (47–80% for basaloid and 75–100% for warty).[113,114] By contrast, while HPV has in fact been detected in the most common type of penile cancer (i.e., keratinizing or verrucous carcinoma), it is consistently found in much lower proportions than seen either in PIN or in the other two forms of penile cancer just noted.[115]

The variation in HPV association with different types of penile lesions suggests the existence of more than one causal pathway. This is similar to the situation for vulvar cancer described earlier, as is the fact that cases of penile cancer related to HPV tend to occur in younger patients and to demonstrate better prognosis.[116–118] Proposals have been offered to explain the better survival in HPV-positive penile cancers; these include the "lower degree of gross genetic alterations" in such cancers (a phenomenon also seen in head and neck carcinomas), as well as increased immune surveillance prompted by the presence of infection.[119]

Taking penile cancers together (i.e., regardless of etiologic pathway) and excluding PIN, the HPV prevalence in carcinomas has been reported as anywhere from 15% to 82%.[120–127] The variation may reflect the sensitivity of detection methods, different definitions of penile cancer, or geographical diversity in the prevalence of HPV infection.[128,129] Despite the research challenges, a consistent picture has begun to emerge. According to various older reviews, HPV prevalence in penile cancer falls between 40% and 50%.[130–132] This aligns well with the weighted average of 44% for HPV positivity across penile cancer patient series from 1993 to 2001, all of which were studied using the same detection method (i.e., polymerase chain reaction).[133] Finally, a 2008 systematic review of 30 studies yielded an unadjusted overall HPV rate of 47.9%, which is likely the best assessment of the matter at the current time.[134]

As with other anogenital cancers, a variety of HPV types have been detected in penile lesions.[135] However, HPV-16 once again dominates the spectrum in both premalignant and malignant lesions, a finding that is consistent across the spectrum of patient ages and histological categories.[136,137] HPV-18 is usually a distant second in terms of prevalence (but see the exception discussed below). The precise distribution has varied considerably, as seen in the summary of larger patient series in Table 5.2. The percentages in the table were derived by using the total number of cancer cases as the denominator. If the analysis were restricted to HPV-positive cases, then the percentage of type 16 would range higher, between 52% and 95%. The results shown by Senba et al. in Thailand (where incidence of penile cancer is much higher than in North America) indicate that type 18 was the most prevalent, followed by HPV-6. This population also showed the incidence of high-risk HPV increasing significantly with age. This unusual pattern further underlines the need to carefully consider geographical variation when shaping public health policy in reference to HPV infection.[138]

Summarizing the epidemiological evidence to date, a conservative estimate would be that HPV infection is involved with just under 50% of penile cancer cases, with well over half of HPV-positive cases demonstrating the presence of viral type 16 specifically. This certainly positions the malignancy as another appropriate target for emerging HPV vaccine technologies.

It should be noted that multiple HPV types are commonly found in penile tumors. For instance, in the study by Rubin and others noted in Table 5.2, only 30% of the cases presented with a single HPV type.[139] Surprisingly, the mixed infections sometimes involved low-risk types 6 and 11, usually associated with benign genital warts.[140] Highly specific cancer associations have been reported in the literature. For example, coinfection with HPV-8 has been strongly linked to erythroplasia of Queyrat (or Bowen disease of the glans penis), a form of squamous cell carcinoma that almost exclusively affects uncircumcised males.[141] There is also emerging evidence of an association between low-risk HPV types, such as 6 and 11, and penile cancer in South America.[142]

Table 5.2. Prevalence of HPV Types in Penile Cancer

Study	Cancer Cases	HPV-16 (%)	HPV-18 (%)	HPV-16 and -18 (%)	Other High-Risk Types and/or HPV-6 and 11 (%)
McCance et al. (1986) *International Journal of Cancer*	53	51			
Iwasawa et al. (1993) *Journal of Urology*	123	57	2		
Cupp et al. (1995) *Journal of Urology*	42	40	5		12
Levi et al. (1998) *International Journal of Cancer*	50	32	6		24
Bezerra et al. (2001) *Cancer*	82	16	5	1	9
Carter et al. (2001) *Cancer Research*	33	70	3		21
Rubin et al. (2001) *American Journal of Pathology*	142	25	1		11
Daling et al. (2005) *International Journal of Cancer*	94	69			8
Senba et al. (2006) *Journal of Medical Virology*	65		55		43 (HPV-6)
Lont et al. (2006) *International Journal of Cancer*	171	22	2	>1	5
Pascual et al. (2007) *Histology and Histopathology*	49	65	8		
Scheiner et al. (2008) *International Braz J Urol*	45	27	2		
Tornesello et al. (2008) *International Journal of Cancer*	41	44			

Finally, there appear to be variants of HPV-16 that show a higher risk of progression to penile cancer, which parallels the pattern seen in cervical cancer etiology.[143,144]

Other risk factors for penile cancer include number of sexual partners, penile trauma, phimosis (i.e., an unretractable foreskin), poor penile hygiene, and smoking.[145-149] There is an increased risk of penile squamous carcinoma in men with a history of anogenital warts, which seems plausible.[150] Some posited risk factors remain equivocal, including race, herpes simplex virus infection, a family history of penile cancer, and cervical cancer in sexual partners.[151,152] Coinfections of other microbes and HPV, as well as UV radiation (used in the treatment of psoriasis), may play a role in carcinogenesis.[153,154] Surveillance to allow early detection of lesions has been recommended by some authors in the case of HIV infection,[155] even though it seems that only a handful of penile carcinoma cases have been observed in HIV-positive males.[156] While PIN is frequent in HIV-positive men with anal dysplasia, penile carcinoma may only be modestly elevated in such patients.[157]

Circumcision. Lack of neonatal circumcision is consistently revealed to be the strongest risk factor for cancer of the penis, though the practice and its implications have a long history of controversy.[158-164] Although penile cancer does occur infrequently among circumcised males, a review by Moses et al. concluded that neonatal circumcision reduced the risk by at least 10-fold.[165] Squamous cell carcinomas of the penis are particularly rare among males circumcised as neonates, though recent instances have been reported.[166,167] Despite (rare) counterexamples and an understandable reluctance to support an invasive (and painful) procedure in neonates, the most recent studies continue to indicate a protective effect for circumcision against all categories of HPV infection, at all subsites on the penis.[168-171]

It is fair to say that, regardless of the evidence, many authorities are reluctant to classify or promote circumcision as a preventive measure, especially later in life. In fact, there are questions about whether adult circumcision is protective.[172] But the reluctance to advocate circumcision cuts across all client ages. Instead, prevention planners have been focusing on less invasive strategies related to sexual health and hygiene, with their obvious benefits in terms of avoiding sexually transmitted infections (STIs) such as HPV. In keeping with this conservative bent, there are contemporary movements to limit prepuce (foreskin) removal to cases of phimosis, that is, an abnormal constriction or tightness preventing its retraction over the glans.[173,174] As noted above, phimosis is in fact another risk factor for penile cancer development, which has focused attention on the idea "that factors within the inner preputial environment promote carcinogenesis."[175] Intense debate will no doubt continue concerning the rationale for circumcision, in part fuelled by the contrary evidence from countries such as Denmark. The Danes, though they demonstrate a very low circumcision rate (of about 1.6%), also enjoy a declining incidence of penile cancer.[176] Furthermore, a recent study has raised questions about the value of circumcision in protecting against HIV, HPV, and other STIs in men who have sex with men (MSM).[177]

Potentially fruitful insight on this complicated topic may found by studying the impact of circumcision on histological mechanisms that have a connection with HPV. The starting point is to recognize that the penile cancer that does occur in circumcised males tends to be the type not associated with HPV. In fact, such tumors often emerge in conjunction with the mild form of dysplasia known as lichen sclerosus, which matches the pattern seen with vulvar cancers that are also unrelated to HPV infection.[178-180] This fact raises the following question: Is it possible that the preventive effect of circumcision in penile cancer is mostly tied to HPV-driven disease, which might be expected to show a tropism for mucosal sites such as the prepuce and glans penis? If this were true, then the preventive mechanism of circumcision might simply relate to removal of HPV-susceptible tissue, specifically the inner layer of the prepuce, which is histologically continuous with the mucosal epithelium of the glans penis.[181,182]

Nothing is straightforward when the topic is circumcision. The very localization of HPV infection on the penis is a matter of some controversy.[183,184] Studies in 2006 and 2007 concluded that the penile shaft was the subsite most likely to be HPV positive.[185,186] But other recent research has suggested that there are few instances where HPV is found on the penile shaft alone, that is, apart from concurrent infection on the glans/coronal sulcus.[187] Likewise, while there is a known association between HPV and urethral lesions,[188] there have been no examples of infection detected at this subsite but not on the glans.[189]

In sum, the glans, combined with the foreskin mucosa, appears to be a key zone for primary HPV infection; these tissues also reflect a high degree of HPV-related disease susceptibility. This is not surprising, given that the inner surface of the foreskin is "lined by variably keratinized squamous epithelium similar to frictional mucosa of the mouth, vagina, and esophagus."[190] As such, it is plausible that simply reducing the availability of such tissue could limit penile cancers, whatever the indirect effects due to lower infection rates may be. Not coincidentally, one practical by-product of circumcision involves the harvesting of foreskin keratinocytes, which have offered the best in vitro system for the "production and amplification of the large quantities of infectious HPV that are required for reinfection and passage studies."[191]

Also of relevance to HPV infection and disease are any protective changes in the surface tissues of the penis after circumcision. As with all aspects of this topic, the concept of such changes is surrounded by controversy. Some authorities maintain that the epithelium of the glans and distal shaft of the penis is not keratinized in uncircumcised males but becomes keratinized (and thus less susceptible to HPV infection) after circumcision, while others offer contrary evidence.[192,193] Circumstantial evidence supporting the idea of histological changes may be found in the fact that circumcision does not alter the risk of HPV infection in the urethral mucosa; however, this is exactly as one might expect, since foreskin removal does not generate additional physical exposure and subsequent keratinization in the urethral opening.[194]

Despite the preceding analysis, the main conclusion probably should be that more research is required. As if to confirm this situation, two recent reviews of the same body of literature drew diametrically opposite conclusions, one questioning and one supporting the premise that circumcision reduces the risk for genital HPV infection in men.[195,196]

Finally, it is important to note that the protective effect of circumcision on HIV infection has also been traced in part to histological features in the foreskin.[197-200] Not surprisingly, the role of circumcision in HIV prevention has engendered similar lively debate, combined with intensive ongoing investigation.[201,202] If the preventive effects with regards to HIV and other STIs are ultimately confirmed, then there could be additional positive implications for penile cancer in light of the synergies between coinfections and HPV that were noted above.

HPV Infection in Males

This is an opportune point to review the topic of HPV infection in males. The prevalence of the virus in asymptomatic men has not been as intensively studied; females have been the main focus of HPV researchers, presumably due to higher rates of associated disease.[203] Indeed, most of the studies taking males into account have been concerned with HPV transmission to women from men with genital infections.[204,205] Although the evidence is not uniform,[206] several recent studies have suggested that HPV infection and penile lesions are frequent in the male sexual partners of women with CIN and VIN.[207-210] There is evidence that male partners may constitute a reservoir for high-risk HPV, possibly localized in flat penile lesions that are sometimes difficult to detect.[211] One 2002 study generated much comment (and even some controversy) when it concluded that circumcision in men, even those with a history of multiple sexual partners, led to a reduced risk of cervical cancer in current female partners.[212] The fact first described in Chapter 2 should be repeated here, namely, that there is little evidence for oral sex leading to oral HPV infection in men or women.

Research on HPV infection in general male populations has mainly focused on the anogenital region, and especially on the penis. Two systematic reviews of HPV infection in asymptomatic males were completed in 2006. There has been very little publishing relevant to the topic since that time. In seven of the relatively recent reports, the rate of detection of any HPV type varied from 33% to 70%. Although two studies reported only a single-digit detection rate, the general consensus remains that "HPV infection is highly prevalent in sexually active men."[213] This has been confirmed in the few very recent studies not covered in the 2006 reviews; this research, which has covered several different parts of the world, yielded HPV prevalence data of 50–65%.[214–216] One recent study focusing on anal HPV infection suggested that rates might be lower in this site, at least in a cohort restricted to men who had not had sex with men (see section "Cancer of the Anus").[217]

HPV-16 seems to be the most common type detected. One study looked at viral loads for HPV-16; there was a correlation in data from proximal sites (e.g., perianal and anal, scrotum, and penile shaft), suggesting a role for autoinoculation.[218] There is some evidence that rarer or undetermined HPV types, as well as multiple types, may be found more often in men than in women. Detection of more than one HPV type has also been associated with the important etiologic variable of viral persistence.[219,220]

The factors that increase the risk of HPV infection in males generally appear to parallel the experience in females. The categories include number of sexual partners, history of STIs, and smoking. However, it should be noted that the data related to increasing risk of infection are highly variable; the influence of each posited risk factor has been questioned by recent studies.[221] The research varies in quality, with only a subset of studies controlling for confounding by using multivariate analysis.[222] An intriguing recent result from Jamaica demonstrated that a decrease in poverty was correlated with a decrease in penile (and vulvar) cancer; since the type of screening program used for cervical cancer does not exist for these cancers, the decline in cases suggests an actual improvement in underlying causes, such as HPV rates.[223]

One of the most consistent risk factors for HPV acquisition in men appears to be HIV coinfection. There is a high prevalence of HPV in HIV-positive men; this is especially true of high-risk HPV in the anal region of MSM.[224–227] Generally, HIV appears to be more strongly associated with viral persistence or reactivation of latent infection rather than acquisition of new HPV infections.[228] MSM who are HIV-negative also demonstrate high prevalence of anal HPV infection across all age groups.[229] This fact likely accounts for the high frequency of anal intraepithelial neoplasia (AIN) among the HIV-negative cohort.[230] The topic of anal lesions will be considered more fully in section "Cancer of the Anus."

It is clear that further investigation of HPV infection in males is required, preferably based on comprehensive sampling across all anogenital sites and sensitive detection of a wide range of HPV types.[231,232] The topic of HPV detection in men will be touched on again in Chapter 6. There seems to be a growing understanding of the importance of this subset of the HPV topic. Expanding the information on male infections may ultimately have implications for "modeling the potential impact of a prophylactic HPV vaccine."[233] Certainly, the calls to consider HPV vaccination in males have only intensified as the campaign to vaccinate females has been launched in different jurisdictions.[234,235]

Cancer of the Anus

Anal cancer occurs at a higher rate than found in vulvar, vaginal, or penile tumors. This is especially true in certain well-defined subpopulations. Whereas vulvar, vaginal, and penile cancers must be classified as rare malignancies, and even anal cancer is relatively uncommon in a general population,[236] the incidence of anal cancer among high-risk male groups approaches the rate of cervical cancer in the developing world and eclipses the current rate in developed countries.[237,238] Furthermore, anal cancer incidence continues to rise in some developed countries, especially among men. For example, between 1973 and 2004, the rate of anal cancer increased in the United States from 0.5 to 1.3 per 100,000.[239] This trend was initially paralleled by the growing impact of HIV infection and related acquired immunodeficiency.[240–242] Most alarmingly, the pattern has not been reversed by the introduction of medical treatments for HIV. In fact, antiretroviral therapies may be worsening the situation, as the survival of HIV-positive patients now makes subsequent anal cancers a potential problem.[243–246] Such data highlight the urgency of learning as much as possible about cancers of the anus, especially insights about prevention; it also explains the fact that the volume of publishing on the topic of anal HPV infection is second only to that seen for HPV and the cervix.[247]

Particularly salient to the prevention theme is the conclusion that anal malignancies are etiologically more related to cancers of the genital region than to those of the digestive tract.[248] Consequently, theories about the cause of anal cancer have steadily shifted away from chronic irritation (due to hemorrhoids, inflammatory bowel disease, etc.) toward a carcinogenic, sexually transmitted agent, namely, HPV.[249,250]

The true prevalence of anal HPV infection in the general population is not well characterized, but it seems to range between 5% and 15% in women; data for men have been heterogeneous, sometimes appearing to be less than the rate for women, but with one study generating a figure close to 25%.[251,252] Research has shown that the rate of HPV infection can range much higher in HIV-positive women, as well as in those who are HIV-negative but engage in high-risk lifestyles.[253] As introduced in section "HPV Infection in Males," the same pattern holds for HIV-positive men and MSM, where the prevalence of HPV can exceed 50%.[254]

Research on the detection rate of HPV in anal cancers has also been modest. The data varied widely in older studies (from 0 to 85%).[255] As seen in Table 5.3, more recent research has consistently pegged the rate at 80–90%. In turn, the HPV-16 proportion of cases positive for HPV runs between 73% and 93%, which translates into 50–60% of all cancer cases. This strong involvement of HPV-16 has been confirmed in molecular analyses of gene expression.[256]

In sum, the very high proportion of neoplasia with detectable virus suggests that infection with high-risk HPV is likely to be a necessary cause of anal cancer.[257] In short, there appears to be epidemiological

Table 5.3. Prevalence of HPV Types in Anal Cancer

Study	Cancer Cases	HPV Positive (%)	HPV-16	HPV-18	Other Types
			Percent of Positive Cases		
Holm et al. (1994) *Modern Pathology*	99	81	93		
Frisch et al. (1997) *New England Journal of Medicine*	388	88	73	6	11
Daling et al. (2004) *Cancer*	306	88	73	7	
Varnai et al. (2006) *International Journal of Colorectal Disease*	47	81	87	3	10
Tachezy et al. (2007) *Acta Pathologica, Microbiologica, et Immunologica Scandinavica*	22	81	82		

parallels between cervical and anal cancer. One explanation for this is the presence of a transitional area between different types of epithelium in both the cervix and the anus; as noted earlier, this type of tissue "is suggested to be more susceptible to HPV-mediated transformation."[258] The so-called transformation zone is precisely where the majority of AIN and anal cancers develop.[259] A more generalized form of HPV tropism may pertain to this phenomenon; studies have revealed a higher rate of HPV infection in cancers of the mucosal epithelium in the anal canal proper as opposed to cutaneous tumors at the anal margin (which may be better defined as skin cancers). Distinguishing these two areas of the anal region becomes an important part of accurately gauging the true role of HPV in anal cancer.[260]

Another similarity with the cervix is the fact that anal HPV infection commonly clears, or remains latent with no disease development. There is also the observation that AIN often regresses; this once again indicates that necessary is not the same as sufficient for causation.[261,262] In short, factors beyond HPV infection are likely involved with the emergence of both AIN and the progression to malignancy. The impact of HIV-positivity on persistent, active HPV infection of the anal region was already noted in the previous section. Being HIV-positive also increases the likelihood of having infections involving multiple HPV types and of developing precursor lesions, high-grade AIN, and full cancer.[263-268] In fact, studies have shown that HIV-positive MSM develop AIN about six times more often than MSM who are HIV-negative. A plausible related finding is the fact that the risk of AIN is inversely correlated with CD4 counts, which is a measure of immune competence.[269] The probability of developing anal cancer per se has been reported as 2–14 times higher in HIV-positive MSM compared with those who are HIV-negative.[270] Comparisons with the general population are even more dramatic, yielding a relative risk for anal cancer as high as 37 among HIV-positive men.[271] Anal tumors also arise at an earlier age than in HIV-negative individuals.[272] Given these sorts of data, it is not surprising that there have been calls to "upgrade" anal cancer from an AIDS-associated malignancy to the AIDS-defining category. It also explains why screening for HPV-related anal dysplasia among HIV-positive individuals (or those at risk of being infected with HIV) is being increasingly investigated and promoted.[273,274]

Some research has shown that being immunocompromised by any cause (including transplantation regimens) may be as important in mediating higher risks for infection and disease progression as any specific behaviors, including anal sex.[275-280] Nonetheless, engaging in receptive anal intercourse continues to stand out as a strong independent risk factor for progression to anal cancer, especially in men.[281] The idea that microtraumas caused by anal intercourse contribute to both HPV infection and disease development remains a distinct possibility.[282]

The evidence related to specific sexual practices in women has been more mixed. For example, recent research noted a lack of association between anal intercourse and anal HPV infection in adolescent females.[283] In contrast, a 2005 study of a large sample of women concluded that HPV infection in the anal region was common among sexually active females, and that concurrent infection of the cervix often involved the same viral subtype. This genotype concordance suggests a common transmission pathway, such as engaging in vaginal and anal intercourse with the same infected partner(s).[284] In another recent study, the odds ratio of anal cancer in women practicing receptive anal intercourse was 2.2 (95% C.I. 1.4–3.3).[285] This is consistent with the results of earlier research that focused on anal sex in women and the prevalence of AIN.[286]

Several other risk factors may be correlates or even play a direct role in HPV infection and related disease in the anal region. These include various measures of sexual activity, history of anal warts, history or presence of other anogenital lesions, sexually transmitted coinfections (other than HIV), and smoking.[287-292]

Second Primary Cancers

A recent case report described two patients with HPV-related anal carcinoma who subsequently developed oral squamous cell carcinoma.[293] The latter represents an SPC. These are malignancies occurring in a person with a history of cancer, but originating in a site different than that of the first primary. The phenomenon is of both clinical and preventive interest when the risk of the second primary is greater than what one would expect for that type of cancer in a general population. Explanations for the increased risk fall into three categories: (1) a common genetic pathway for the first and second primary, (2) an iatrogenic effect of treatment (e.g., radiation) for the first primary, and (3) a common environmental factor (such as exposure to a viral infection).[294] For the purposes of this book, two potentially HPV-related cancers developing in the same person would be of interest. One implication is the potential for primary prevention efforts and/or intensive surveillance following the first primary.[295]

Given the fact that data from large cohorts of patients are required to detect elevated SPC risk, and that cervical cancer is the first primary with an HPV link that occurs in sizeable numbers, most of the relevant information has been gathered on that malignancy. As well, because

HPV tends to be a localized rather than a systemic infection, one might hypothesize that the HPV-related SPCs following cervical cancer would also be localized. This turns out to be the case. At least six studies of SPC following cervical cancer have been published in the last decade. The results consistently showed that the sites of greatest excess cancer risk following cervical cancer were found in the anogenital region.[296] One of the most recent (and largest) studies examined over 100,000 women with cervical cancer, analyzing rates of SPC. There was an almost five times higher risk of a cervical cancer survivor being diagnosed with a cancer of the female genitals (i.e., vulva, vagina) compared with the general population.[297] This coincides well with the elevated rates of vaginal lesions found in series of patients who underwent hysterectomy for cervical cancer.[298,299] It seems highly likely that susceptibility to a latent or incident HPV infection is driving at least part of this phenomenon, though clonal propagation of transformed cervical cells is another mechanism that is suspected.[300] The risk of anal cancer is also elevated following cervical cancer, as much as six times.[301,302] This result is consistent with the higher prevalence of anal HPV found in women with cervical HPV infections and lesions.[303,304] While far less researched, there have been indications that HPV (and especially HPV-16) can drive the development of multiple lesions in the anogenital region of men as well.[305]

Although a history of cervical cancer has generally been associated with a protective effect against breast cancer, HPV DNA has actually been detected in breast cancers in cervical cancer survivors[306,307]; this opens up the controversial topic of possible HPV involvement in breast malignancies, which will be addressed below. As will become clear in the next section, the observed excess of SPCs found in head and neck sites following cervical cancer could be deemed a more expected result.[308] Common HPV infection is again the proposed explanation, notwithstanding the ongoing uncertainties about HPV transmission involving the cervix and the oral cavity, oropharynx, etc. One of the most dramatic indications of a potential common etiology between anogenital and head and neck cancers emerged in a recent case report of a woman with synchronous cervical, vaginal, and laryngeal carcinomas, who was found to be seropositive for HPV-16.[309] Similar to the discussion of HPV detected in breast cancer (see below), the possibility must be acknowledged that the virus is only a benign "passenger" in such cases.[310,311] In other words, rather than being an etiologic agent, HPV in certain tissues may be a sign of reduced immune function in the host, with poor cancer control in turn being the true explanation for emergence of tumors in multiple sites.

The preceding qualification is not meant to take away from the growing evidence that HPV does in fact play a causative role specifically in cancers of the larynx and many other head and neck sites. The next section will provide an overview of HPV involvement in head and neck cancers.

CANCERS OF THE HEAD AND NECK

HPV has been detected in a wide variety of nongenital human cancers. In particular, there is a growing appreciation of the role of HPV as an explanation for a subset of head and neck cancers that lack the classic risk factors of tobacco and alcohol use.[312] While smoking perhaps dominates in the larynx and alcohol use in the oral cavity, even in "never smokers" and light drinkers there may be up to a 30-fold increased risk of oropharyngeal cancer in people who are seropositive for HPV-16.[313] Indeed, epidemiologic data supporting a connection between HPV and oropharyngeal (especially tonsillar) cancers are compelling.[314-316]

Despite the available evidence, a decisive conclusion remains to be reached about the etiologic link between HPV and such cancers.[317,318]

The HPV types associated with head and neck cancers are similar to those implicated in cervical cancer; HPV-16 dominates, with HPV-18 a distant second.[319,320] These facts immediately suggest the potential impact for current prophylactic HPV vaccines, which target HPV-16 and -18. It will be important to monitor the effect that HPV vaccines have on the incidence rates of such cancers in coming years.[321,322] Other viral types appear to be involved in some head and neck cancers. This includes HPV-6, best known for causing benign genital warts; one study showed that HPV-6, operating independently of HPV-16, doubled the risk of oropharyngeal cancer.[323]

Among the main categories of human malignancy, the survival rate for head and neck cancers is one of the worst. Mortality results from early signs of cellular transformation being missed, so that the malignancy presents in an advanced stage that is not very amenable to treatment. Further, the recurrence rate even for lesions with adequate treatment is very high. On the other hand, HPV involvement with cancers in head and neck sites has been linked to better prognosis.[324] This pattern, which matches the survival profile in some anogenital cancers associated with the virus, may be mostly driven by clinical experience in the oropharyngeal subregion.[325,326] One explanation may be that the irritation associated with infection is prompting detection of lesions at an earlier stage. However, researchers have found that even patients with metastases, specifically involving HPV-positive lymph nodes, enjoy better survival than those with advanced head and neck cancers not caused by the virus.[327]

The differential etiology and disease course and prognosis makes it very important to detect HPV directly or indirectly in head and neck cancer patients.[328] Confirming oncogenic viral types such as HPV-16 offers increased possibilities for secondary prevention among at least a portion of head and neck cancers.[329,330] There are also decisions related to managing a frank malignancy; the concern is to apply the appropriate therapeutic responses, and especially to avoid overtreatment in the case of less aggressive HPV-related tumors.[331] The topic of HPV detection is discussed in Chapter 6.

A few studies have begun the task of unraveling the viral genetic and host immunologic profiles of head and neck cancers related to HPV, which may in turn guide targeted management strategies.[332,333] The emerging understanding of cellular disease processes in the presence of the virus has confirmed that the cancers operate differently at the molecular level compared with HPV-negative head and neck tumors (see section "Aspects of Transformation").[334,335] As a result, molecular interventions may need to be calibrated accordingly. It is important to note that not all HPV-positive tumors express the products of viral oncogenes, suggesting that a smaller proportion of head and neck cancers are caused by HPV than sometimes thought.[336]

The primary prevention strategies begin by acknowledging that there are essentially two types of cancer at work in the head and neck. Risk for the HPV-positive category does not respond to reductions in smoking or alcohol use, but has been recently associated with practices such as oral sex and marijuana use.[337] Furthermore, human herpes virus type 8 has been found to potentiate the cellular effects of HPV-16, increasing the risk of head and neck cancer.[338] The importance of this viral cofactor may be elevated by its multiple transmission routes, including vertical, sexual, blood/transplant, and especially horizontal by means of saliva.[339] Other clues about prevention emerge from an understanding of HPV transmission that precedes head and neck cancers caused by the virus.

Aspects of Transmission

While the natural history of oral HPV infection generally appears to mimic that found in the anogenital region, there are differences. For instance, oral HPV prevalence increases with age, compared to the decline with age that is seen in infections of the cervix.[340] As the cause of head and neck cancers continues to be investigated, researchers are being careful to ensure that viral associations "fit coherently within our current framework of knowledge of the epidemiology and biology of HPV infection."[341] Consequently, the known patterns of high-risk HPV infection and disease development have been tested against expressions seen in the head and neck region, and especially in oral and oropharyngeal cancers. One study indicated that high-risk HPV prevalence in the oral cavity and oropharynx is elevated in people "whose sexual practices are typically associated with sexual transmission of the virus."[342] HPV-16 prevalence in particular has been linked to sexual history.[343] As well, women with genital HPV infections have demonstrated a higher risk of HPV infection in their oral mucosa.[344] As noted in Chapter 2, what is not clear is how genital HPV makes it to the mouth. Adding to the mystery, the precise HPV types in the two regions of the body are routinely discordant.[345,346] This is consistent with the fact that research has not supported the otherwise plausible idea that oral-genital contact itself is associated with oral HPV infection.[347,348]

Other potential transmission routes (e.g., sharing saliva through kissing, normal intrafamilial contact) demonstrate little or no support in the literature. The plausible pathway of vertical transmission is known to mostly lead to transient infections.[349,350] One qualification of the perinatal route was recently posited, namely, the potential for infection to remain latent in a child and be reactivated later, even in adulthood.[351] Recent studies have suggested nonsexual horizontal transmission as an explanation for anogenital and head and neck infections in pediatric cases where sexual abuse is not suspected.[352,353] However, oral high-risk HPV infection and related disease in adolescents and adults are still mainly attributed to sexual activity. Unfortunately, the actual transmission mechanisms remain obscure.

Autoinnoculation via hand warts has been offered as an explanation of HPV-related benign lesions in the oral cavity, as well as some anogenital warts in children.[354,355] This pathway may explain the apparent spread of oncogenic HPV types in the reverse direction, from the anogenital region to the hands.[356] It has been hypothesized that such transfer could conceivably lead all the way to infections of the oral cavity and even deeper into the aerodigestive tract, though recent evidence has contradicted this theory.[357] The only real conclusion on this topic for now seems to be that "the mechanism of transmission of HPV to the oral cavity warrants further investigation."[358]

Aspects of Transformation

There is some evidence that one or more distinct molecular pathways are involved in many of the head and neck tumors that are HPV-positive, similar to certain genital cancers that develop in different ways depending on whether the virus is implicated.[359–364] HPV-related tumors are characterized as nonkeratinizing.[365,366] The distinctive keratin profile is sometimes traceable even in the metastases of laryngeal, nasopharyngeal, and oral cancers.[367] The inference is that HPV DNA may be implicated in the entire process of head and neck cancers, from tumor initiation through to lymph node involvement.[368,369] Smoking and alcohol consumption are known to increase the risk of HPV-negative head and neck cancers. By contrast, there is an *inverse* relationship between smoking (with or without alcohol consumption) and HPV-positive tumors in the head and neck.[370–372]

Established or investigational sites in the head and neck region of the body that have been linked to HPV infection will now be examined. Specific head and neck sites of interest include the oral cavity, the tonsils, the larynx, and the sinonasal area.[373] For convenience, ocular, aural and esophageal cancers will be included under this category, though they are often classified separately. Note that there is a strong overlap between the head and neck region and the sites sometimes known collectively as the aerodigestive tract, though the latter category can include structures below the neck per se (e.g., the bronchus and lung).[374]

Oral Cavity Cancers

The fact that "oral cavity" is a nonspecific anatomical term presents some challenges. Usually a distinction is made between two important subregions in the head and neck: oral and oropharyngeal. Distinguishing the various oral cancers from oropharyngeal malignancies may be clinically important (see below). Subsites typically identified within the oral cavity include the alveolus, the gingiva (gums), the tongue (usually specified as the oral or mobile tongue), and sometimes the floor of the mouth.[375] There are terminological overlaps that create confusion; for example, the base of the tongue is often considered alongside the tonsils as an intrinsic part of the oropharynx (see below).[376] A further complexity in the literature is the fact that oral and oropharyngeal cancers are sometimes conflated as one category for statistical purposes.[377–380]

When the head and neck subsites are clearly distinguished, there appears to be a stronger association between HPV and oropharyngeal cancers compared with tumors in the oral cavity. The evidence in this regard remains mixed for certain subsites; for example, there have been reports of high HPV prevalence in carcinomas of the oral (or mobile) tongue, but also indications that HPV is more common in the cancers of the base of the tongue.[381–385]

A review of research from 1985 to 2003 found HPV positivity ranging anywhere from 0 to 100% in oral squamous cell carcinoma.[386] In one larger study, HPV DNA was detected in 3.9% of 766 oral cavity cancers; by contrast, the prevalence among 142 tumors in the oropharynx (including the tonsils) was 18.3%.[387] Another review from 2005 indicated that 22% of oral cancers were found to be positive for HPV.[388] Finally, several recent studies have reinforced the evidence of HPV involvement in a subset of oral squamous cell carcinomas.[389–392] The specific detection method used in the different studies found in the literature may account for most of the variation in prevalence results.[393–395] As noted earlier, investigations of HPV involvement in the oral cavity have sometimes been localized to subsites such as the floor of the mouth and especially the tongue.[396,397]

HPV-16 and -18 appear to be the most prevalent types involved with oral squamous cell carcinomas, though other types (and sometimes multiple types) are certainly detected.[398–400] Some evidence suggests that HPV-16 is not as common in oral cancers compared with oropharyngeal tumors.[401–403] When HPV-16 is detected, it has actually been associated with improved survival compared with HPV-negative oral cancers; this is consistent with the pattern suggested for head and neck cancers in general (see above).[404]

It should be acknowledged that a definite viral connection has not yet been confirmed for the oral cavity (or even, according to some authorities, for the oropharynx).[405–408] According to current evidence, the most that can be said with complete confidence is that HPV is one of several risk factors in oral squamous cell carcinomas, with differing degrees of importance in various populations.[409–412]

Notwithstanding the ongoing questions about etiology, the proportion of oral carcinoma cases attributable to HPV infection appears to be increasing in the United States[413] There is a concern that disease caused by HPV may be on the rise in the HIV-positive population in the United States, specifically HPV-32-associated oral warts and HPV-16-associated carcinomas.[414]

At the same time that an enlarged benefit of vaccination is being promoted, the rationale for a population program to screen for oral cancer is under examination. One challenge involves the identification of at-risk cohorts that might benefit from more intensive testing. Even if potential triage methods could be validated, such as detecting oncogenic HPV in exfoliated oral epithelial cells, their value may be limited, since factors other than HPV are involved in malignant transformation. Even detecting HPV in the anogenital regions does not automatically drive a screening program for the oral mucosa as studies have shown that mucosal compartments in the human body tend to operate independently of one another in terms of HPV infection (see Chapter 3 on transmission).[415]

So far, the search for factors to allow for risk stratification has not yielded conclusive results.[416] Whether there is influence from tobacco, alcohol, or coinfection with other viruses on HPV-related oral cancer remains obscure.[417] Notably, there appears to be little increase in the incidence of HPV-related oral cancer among HIV-positive individuals.[418] This means that targeting the HIV-positive or MSM cohort of a population, which offers a cornerstone in anal cancer screening, is simply not a useful option in the case of oral cancer.

In sum, evidence continues to accumulate that HPV plays a role in oral carcinogenesis, with the precise mechanisms still to be elucidated.[419] Studies remain divided on the extent of the HPV role in cancers of the oral cavity proper.[420,421]

Oropharyngeal Cancers

Most of the evidence concerning HPV involvement in head and neck cancers actually relates to the oropharynx, which accounts for about 25% of all malignancies in the head and neck region.[422] This means that most of the results noted earlier about head and neck cancers were actually driven by data derived from oropharyngeal malignancies. This applies, for instance, to the evidence that HPV involvement in an oropharyngeal cancer appears to confer a better prognosis and survival rate,[423] which in turn may generate concern about overtreatment of HPV-related oropharyngeal carcinomas.[424] Notwithstanding the favorable mortality implications, the incidence trends are still alarming. Cancers in the oropharynx appears to be on the increase in the United States and in other jurisdictions.[425,426] The suggestion is that the trend is being driven by rising attribution of tumors related to HPV.[427]

As recently reinforced by a Canadian study, the localization of HPV carcinogenicity may be further refined, ultimately focusing on two subsites: the tonsils (see below) and the base of the tongue.[428] HPV is strongly associated with any cancers in these subsites that are not related to smoking or drinking. It appears that HPV-related cancer susceptibility may be increased by certain host polymorphisms related to tumor suppression.[429,430]

HPV-16 appears to be the dominant type detected in malignancies in the oropharynx[431]; this is especially true for cancer of the tonsils.[432] In fact, the greatest potential impact for vaccination against HPV-16 outside the anogenital region is assumed to be with respect to the tonsils.[433] Similar to oral cancers, the drive toward vaccine solutions is complemented by occasional calls for increased surveillance for HPV in the oropharynx, especially in nonsmokers and nondrinkers.[434] Any suggestion of a screening program must be moderated by the reality that the cancers involved are relatively rare.

Cancer of the tonsils. As suggested above, the most compelling evidence concerning HPV involvement in head and neck cancer involves the oropharynx, and especially the tonsils.[435,436] Circumstantial evidence for the role of HPV is derived from the fact that the risk of tonsillar cancer is elevated in people with anogenital carcinomas.[437] In addition, one study has shown that husbands of women with cervical cancer had an increased risk of tonsillar cancer.[438]

Molecular evidence has also been steadily accumulating. HPV DNA was first detected in tonsillar squamous cell carcinoma in 1989. Based on many patient series since that time, it is now accepted that HPV occurs in about half of all tonsillar cancers—one of the highest rates of association outside of the anogenital region.[439,440] This has confirmed the tonsils as a "hot spot" for viral transformation.[441,442] In fact, consistent with the thesis developed in this book, the viral initiation of carcinogenesis is localized specifically in the tonsillar crypts, precisely where one finds the stratified squamous epithelium targeted by HPV infection.[443,444]

The role that HPV plays in tonsillar cancer appears to vary geographically. For example, the proportion of cancers attributable to the virus is lower in Hong Kong than in Australia.[445] Generally, Asian populations seem to demonstrate a lower prevalence of HPV-related tonsillar cancer.[446]

Epidemiology and molecular analysis have been combined in order to understand the rising incidence of tonsillar cancer in the United States and other developed countries.[447-449] The increase cannot be explained by smoking and alcohol consumption rates, as these have generally been declining in the affected jurisdictions. HPV infection appears to be the likely culprit, as the proportion of tonsillar cancers positive for the virus has increased; in turn, it has been suggested that this reflects changing patterns of sexual activity in recent decades.[450]

There is a growing understanding that HPV-related cancers in the tonsils are a distinct clinicopathologic entity compared with HPV-negative tumors.[451-453] In fact, the latter variety of cancer is influenced mostly by smoking and alcohol consumption,[454] a pattern that was first noted within the general category of head and neck tumors, and then again in the subcategory of oropharyngeal cancers. The tumors in which HPV is found demonstrate nonkeratinizing cellular characteristics.[455] Clinically, patients with HPV-positive cancers demonstrate better survival[456-461]; this effect appears to be enhanced with higher viral load.[462] On the other hand, there is mixed evidence concerning the rate of recurrence and of SPCs following HPV-related primary tonsillar cancer.[463,464] Overall, there are indications that tonsillar malignancy involving HPV can be managed with more moderate interventions, making the detection of virus a priority in such patients.[465]

On the prevention front, the lack of influence from "classic" head and neck cancer risk factors, that is, smoking and excessive alcohol drinking,[466,467] has steered researchers of HPV-positive tonsillar malignancy toward other risk topics. This has included the protective effect of certain genetic polymorphisms.[468,469]

HPV-16 is the viral type that appears to be detected most frequently in normal tonsillar tissue,[470] though the profile in tumor-free individuals or in cases of benign disease is still being elucidated.[471,472] The picture with respect to cancer of the tonsils is clearer. The complete breakdown for HPV types analyzed in a 2004 review is found in Table 5.4 (note that cases with multiple HPV types are reported redundantly, resulting in a total percentage higher than 100).[473]

Recent research supports the conclusion that HPV-16 dominates in tonsillar carcinogenesis.[474] In a 2006 study, HPV was detected in 49% of cases of tonsillar cancer; type 16 was found in 87% of those cases.[475] The weight of evidence allowed a 2005 review to conclude that "therapeutic and preventive HPV-16 antiviral immune vaccination trials may be worthwhile not only in cervical cancer but also in tonsillar cancer."[476] The trend of increasing incidence of cancers of the tonsils, which is likely related for the most part to HPV-16 infection, only serves to underline the potential value of a prophylactic vaccine targeting this viral type.[477]

Cancer of the Larynx

With respect to infection and cancer of the larynx, a 2002 review offered a succinct cautious conclusion: the "role of HPV in laryngeal carcinogenesis remains unclear."[478] Past evidence indicated that up to 20% of laryngeal carcinomas contain HPV; more recent studies have measured 25–37% HPV-positivity in laryngeal carcinoma samples.[479–481]

A possible reason for some variability in the rate of HPV involvement in laryngeal cancer is that most studies do not distinguish between

Table 5.4. HPV Involvement in Tonsillar Cancer

HPV Type	Proportion of HPV-Positive Cases
16	84%
16/18	3
6/11	3
16/33	1
31	3
33	5
Unknown	6

Source: Syrjanen, *Journal of Clinical Pathology*, 2004.

the glottic and supraglottic larynx; one subsite or the other tends to dominate in terms of cancer risk in different parts of the world.[482,483] It is also possible that the different study results reflect variations in detection methods.[484]

In contrast with the relatively modest involvement of HPV in laryngeal carcinomas, it is well established that virtually 100% of laryngeal papillomas contain HPV-6 or 11.[485,486] Interestingly, malignant transformation of these benign lesions appears to be a rare occurrence.[487] Such developments are more common in patients with a history of smoking or radiation therapy. The fact that progression sometimes occur in the absence of these known risk factors has suggested a possible carcinogenic role for HPV in a patient with laryngeal papillomas; however, this proposal continues to be debated.[488,489]

The carcinomas of the larynx that are (rarely) found in laryngeal papilloma patients generally harbor the same type of HPV DNA seen in benign tumors, namely, types 6 and 11.[490] In some benign and malignant tumors, HPV-16 and -18 and other high-risk types have also been detected.[491,492,493] On the whole, the association between HPV-16 and laryngeal cancer is not as strong as found in many other types of head and neck cancers,[494] even though in vitro studies have demonstrated the carcinogenic effect of HPV-16 oncoproteins in laryngeal cells.[495]

In sum, present research suggests that HPV is implicated in some cases of laryngeal carcinoma, though involving carcinogenetic mechanisms that differ from those seen in anogenital tumors.[496] There are also some parallels with anogenital disease. The larynx demonstrates transformation zones between squamous and columnar epithelia that are similar to the well-known subsite in the cervix that is susceptible to HPV. There is some suggestion that the susceptible zones in the larynx may be affected by smoking habits, as opposed to HPV-positive oral cancers, which generally seem to be independent of tobacco use.[497] Although smoking cessation may play some role in preventing a subset of laryngeal cancers, there has been even greater interest in the impact of prophylactic HPV vaccines.[498]

Sinonasal Cancers

Many characteristics of cancer in the sinonasal area are similar to those seen with HPV-related lesions at other mucosal sites.[499] For example, high-risk HPV types exhibit tropism for the nonkeratinizing forms of sinonasal squamous cell carcinoma, the same pattern seen in other head and neck subsites, such as the tonsils.[500]

A synthesis of the literature up to 2001 reported that HPV was detected in 70 of 322 sinonasal carcinomas (i.e., 22%). Types 16 or 18 (or both) were present in 80% of the HPV-positive cases.[501] A 2005 study confirmed a 20% rate of HPV (exclusively type 16) among sinonasal squamous cell carcinomas. By contrast, HPV DNA was not detected in clinically intact mucosa or in benign nasal papilloma.[502] The most recent research continues to produce very consistent results, albeit based on small patient series; for example, one 2006 study reported HPV-16/18 in 17% of invasive tumors.[503] One pathway toward malignancy that has been intensively investigated involves the transformation of sinonasal inverted papilloma; HPV has been clearly implicated in this process.[504–506]

Cancer of the Esophagus

An association between HPV and esophageal cancer was first proposed in 1982, but the evidence developed since that time has been mixed. Studies using a variety of detection methods have identified HPV prevalence rates ranging from 0 to 67% in cancers of the esophagus or precursor lesions such as Barrett's esophagus; there is also some evidence of geographical variation in the prevalence pattern.[507–512] Rates of HPV-positive esophageal cancer generally appear to be higher in Asian and southern European populations, as well as among Alaska natives.[513–515] On the other hand, a 2008 study suggested that HPV is not associated with esophageal carcinogenesis in Korea.[516]

An example of the conflicting results seen in the literature is offered by two studies from Germany. Research published in 2003 found no association between HPV and esophageal cancer, but did identify Epstein-Barr virus (EBV) in about one-third of samples; in contrast, HPV-16 and -18 were detected in esophageal tumor samples in a 2007 study.[517,518] International interest in this topic continues to be strong. For example, Iranian researchers recently reported HPV prevalence of 24% in esophageal cancers.[519]

HPV-16 is the most frequently identified viral type connected to esophageal cancers, similar to head and neck cancers as a whole. One 2007 study also suggested a role for HPV-11.[520] However, unlike other HPV-related tumors in this part of the body, the involvement of the virus in esophageal cancer is not associated with better survival outcomes compared with HPV-negative forms.[521,522] Furthermore, there is evidence that HPV infection and tobacco or alcohol abuse may act synergistically to increase the risk of esophageal cancer[523]; such susceptibility has also been related to genetic polymorphisms in the host.[524]

In sum, though current evidence could not be characterized as conclusive, the available data justify further research on the involvement of HPV in the etiology of esophageal cancer.[525]

Cancer of the Ocular Surface

HPV has been detected in a majority of benign and malignant ocular lesions in some patient series; the virus is also prevalent in healthy eye tissues.[526–528] Nonetheless, the evidence for an etiological link between HPV and squamous cell carcinoma of the surface of the eye remains mixed.[529–534] A recent summary noted that "the association between HPV and conjunctival neoplasias is variable in different geographical areas and also depends on the methods of detection used."[535]

Indication of the dramatic differences in the literature is offered by two small studies of precursor lesions; one found HPV-16 or -18 in *all* cases of conjunctival intraepithelial neoplasia, whereas HPV was not detected in the tumors of the other patient series.[536,537]

The dominance of HPV-16 and -18 in squamous cell carcinogenesis at the ocular surface was suggested in older studies.[538] Other types of HPV, especially those related to the disease known as epidermodysplasia verruciformis (EV), have also been implicated in more recent research.[539] HPV-6 and 11 are common in benign conjunctival papilloma.[540]

The role of HPV in the development of other rare cancers of the eye, including retinoblastoma, is also being investigated; most research suggests that retinoblastoma is not caused by HPV, as there is no evidence that it infects the retina or other neural tissue.[541,542]

Other Head and Neck Tumors and Lung Cancer

Tracing the complex anatomy of the head and neck identifies additional cancer sites with possible connections to HPV. These include the hypopharynx, nasopharynx, and even tracheal and bronchial neoplasia (though the latter two are often considered cancers of the upper aerodigestive tract rather than of the head and neck proper).[543,544]

Limited evidence has been found for HPV involvement in nasopharyngeal carcinomas, a type of cancer that is also known to be strongly associated with EBV infection.[545–547] The facts and implications of this phenomenon are still being elucidated, including whether HPV infection acts as a cofactor alongside EBV, with smoking offering additional risk modification.[548,549] An intriguing finding in one study was the preponderance of HPV-31 in nasopharyngeal carcinoma.[550]

A 2002 review noted that HPV DNA had been detected in a cumulative 2,468 cases of bronchial carcinoma reported in the literature.[551] One of the intriguing lines of investigation considers the whole extent of the aerodigestive tract, from the oral cavity to different lung tissues. The suggestion is that oncogenic HPV originating in the anogenital region may somehow be transferred to the mouth and then "migrate" from one susceptible site to the next. In fact, versions of the squamous-columnar junction (i.e., transformation zone) that has been strongly connected to HPV-related cancer in the cervix have also been identified in the pharynx, larynx, and bronchi.[552]

The theory of viral migration notwithstanding, there has been great variability in HPV detection in lung tumors, with the observed rates ranging from 0 to 79%.[553] There are indications of both gender and geographic variations.[554,555] However, recent teams as far apart as Latin America and Iran have actually found very consistent results, pegging HPV prevalence in lung cancer around 26–28%.[556,557] This is very close to the global total of 24.5% derived from a 2008 meta-analysis of 4,508 cases over 53 studies.[558]

The conclusion of the meta-analysis, namely, that HPV is the second most important cause of lung cancer (after smoking), may be premature. However, there certainly is sufficient evidence to inspire further research on the potential role of the virus in pulmonary tumors.[559] One line of inquiry will involve determining the differential impact of infection in various lung tissues.[560–562] Another question revolves around the HPV types that are implicated in lung or upper aerodigestive tract cancers; as might be expected, HPV-16 and -18 dominate, but other types have been detected in lung cancer at varying rates depending on the geographic region.[563–567] Finally, potential host risk factors and viral disease mechanisms are being worked out at a molecular level.[568] A Taiwanese research team is leading the investigation of the role of HPV oncoproteins in lung tissues.[569–571]

The investigations of HPV involvement in aural cancers have not been very extensive, with the available information mostly drawn from decade-old studies. Most research has been related to ear infections and cholesteatoma (i.e., scar tissue from infections); evidence exists of primary transformation of mucosal tissues that have undergone this sort of insult. There is also indication of high-risk HPV involvement in benign and malignant tumors of the middle ear, but research results are still very mixed.[572–574] One unique aspect of this topic is the physical barrier of the tympanum (i.e., ear drum) protecting any mucosal tissue of the ear from ready exposure to infection. An interesting possibility is that HPV infection and disease may access the middle ear from the pharynx by way of the eustachian tube, thus creating connection with the broader discussion of head and neck cancers.[575,576] This situation parallels the modest evidence for HPV involvement in lacrimal sac epithelial lesions that may, in rare cases, spread via the nasolacrimal duct to the nasal cavity itself.[577,578]

The accumulating data related to these and other investigational sites may play a part, albeit a modest one, in the developing HPV vaccination story. If a substantial role for HPV were confirmed in a prevalent malignancy such as lung cancer, then the prevention implications would multiply dramatically. In this regard, the evidence for HPV involvement in other cancers will be briefly reviewed, including the remainder of the "big four" category that generates the greatest public health impact; besides lung cancer, this category comprises malignancies of the prostate, colorectum, and female breast. Then, in the final section of the chapter, the state of the science will be reviewed concerning HPV and the most common malignancy in humans, skin cancer.

CANCER AT OTHER SITES

Given the extensive range of sites in which HPV has been detected, it is reasonable to wonder if there are any tissues, and especially epithelial ones, where the virus has not been implicated in cancer development. Indeed, the arena of HPV-associated cancer seems to only be getting larger, increasing the potential efficacy of any vaccination program. The list of investigational interests includes gender-specific sites such as the ovary and the prostate gland. While there has been evidence offered for HPV (especially type 16) involvement in ovarian carcinomas,[579-581] the preponderance of recent research has pointed to explanations other than primary infection/disease for any weak HPV DNA signal.[582-585] Results for endometrial tissues, though limited, have been more compelling, with evidence of HPV involvement being particularly strong for adenosquamous carcinomas.[586,587] On the male side, results for prostate cancer have also been consistent, though in the opposite direction; there has been essentially no research evidence supporting a role for HPV in tumors at this site.[588-590] This conclusion was recently confirmed in a brief review of the latest research.[591]

As noted earlier, a key approach to understanding HPV and disease development involves tracing the physical access of the virus to susceptible tissues. For this reason, much of the focus has been on body sites that are adjacent to the surface, or that otherwise communicate with the outside world relatively easily. This is also why microabrasions and other forms of trauma are sometimes regarded as plausible mechanisms in HPV exposure and infection.[592] Access to susceptible tissues is the theme that links these ideas together. In this way, a perspective may be offered on HPV involvement in malignancies such as renal carcinoma and colorectal cancer. The balance of evidence suggests no HPV involvement in cancers of the kidney, but a potential role in the case of the colorectum.[593-595] The kidney is simply less accessible physically, whereas the colorectal area offers both a direct route to the surface of the body and the type of epithelial tissue that may be more susceptible to HPV infection and carcinogenesis.

Such considerations also may inform the understanding of the role of HPV in cancers of the urinary bladder and the female breast. As is often the case, the evidence is controversial. Routine involvement of HPV in the (unique) transitional epithelium of the (relatively inaccessible) urinary bladder does not seem likely. In fact, the available evidence in this regard has proven to be insufficient and/or conflicting, notwithstanding the suggested interaction with another infection-based risk factor for bladder cancer, namely, schistosomiasis.[596–600] In sum, the evidence is inadequate to confirm or contradict ideas about the role of HPV infection, but both the location of the bladder and its tissue type points toward a negative conclusion.

A number of studies have supported the involvement of HPV in at least the progression of breast carcinoma,[601,602] though the most recent analyses have been more equivocal.[603–605] Research in this area is plagued by a familiar problem: the detection of virus in a tissue is not proof of etiology.[606] If primary carcinomas are found to be caused by HPV, then the following mechanisms may be important: (1) viral transmission from the anogenital region to the mamillae and ductal tissue by hand (i.e., autoinoculation)[607,608] or possibly by the bloodstream[609,610]; and (2) mammary epithelial cells that "partly lose control in proliferation" and thus are more susceptible to persistent HPV infection.[611] Recently, the involvement of HPV in breast cancer has been explored in terms of plausible molecular mechanisms, including viral oncoproteins, host genetic polymorphisms, and estrogen function.[612–614] Intriguingly, the basal-like and similar aggressive breast carcinomas that have recently been characterized demonstrate a microscopic histology and a molecular phenotype that resembles HPV-related carcinomas.[615]

Whatever the eventual fate of these hypothesized linkages, there is no doubt that clarification of the role of HPV in female breast tumors could have a substantial bearing on both the primary and secondary prevention of cancer. As such, it is not surprising that investigations of HPV involvement in breast cancer continue at a high pace, with the evidence trending away from a likely role for the virus in carcinogenesis.[616–619]

SKIN CANCER

Cutaneous malignancies have also received substantial attention among researchers of HPV, though it is not the only infectious agent investigated in connection with skin cancer.[620] Viral skin infections are especially found in immunosuppressed individuals, including organ transplant patients.[621,622] For example, all eight of the known human herpes viruses have been studied in the context of transplantation.[623] Human herpes virus 8, the causative agent in Kaposi sarcoma, is notable because of its connection to the immunodeficiency condition associated with HIV. As well, human T-cell lymphotropic virus type 1 has also been known to cause skin eruptions that share some features with cutaneous T-cell lymphoma.[624] Recently, a melanoma-associated retrovirus has been identified in mice and humans.[625] These examples notwithstanding, it is fair to say that most of the research on infections and skin cancer has focused on HPV.

As the final part of the long account of HPV-related carcinogenesis, the key information on skin cancers will be reviewed, focusing on the epidermis that lies outside of the anogenital region. The latter distinction is important, as consideration of the anogenital epithelia on or near the surface of the body clearly overlaps with the topic of the skin. An example of this overlap is the recent report of HPV involvement with VIN that in turn demonstrated a connection with the skin disease known as lichen sclerosus.[626]

Research Complexity

There are two immediate challenges encountered when investigating skin cancer and infections:

- Dealing with the wide range of lesions (both benign and malignant) found on skin surfaces—though the ultimate interest is squamous cell carcinomas
- Distinguishing the viruses and other agents that may be accidentally present in or near a lesion from those that are a causative factor

The first category of complexity is generated by both histological and terminological confusion. Thus, in addition to the difficulty involved with placing a skin lesion accurately within the multistep sequence of neoplastic progression, the many labels for skin lesions have been inconsistently applied.[627] This is true of a term such as actinic keratosis (also known as solar keratosis), which is sometimes defined so that it essentially overlaps with Bowen's disease. Clinical classification of keratoses depends almost on a philosophical decision: either a keratosis is a late stage of cancer precursor that has not yet spread to the dermis, and therefore (by analogy with cervical lesions) a type of keratinocytic intraepithelial neoplasia or it is an early form of cancer (usually referred to as squamous cell carcinoma in situ). If any distinction is made between actinic keratoses and Bowen's disease, it is usually along these very lines—the first lesion is nonmalignant (perhaps stabilizing as a benign tumor, or even regressing) and the second is a premalignant form that may progress to a true cancer. Thus, it may be difficult to apply the proper label to a particular lesion because of uncertainty about how it will progress.

Adding to the confusion of definitions, sometimes the term Bowen's disease is simply reserved for that subset of actinic keratoses not exposed to sunlight. As noted in the earlier section "Cancer of the Penis", such lesions have a special label when found on the glans penis, namely, erythroplasia of Queyrat. Keratoses at different sites have been traced to arsenic exposure; this cause is actually suspected when the lesion is on a cutaneous surface not normally exposed to UV radiation. All of these distinctions become important when ascertaining whether HPV is involved with the malignant transformation of skin cells. As a final consideration, all malignant or potentially malignant lesions of the keratotic sort need to be distinguished from the (usually) benign Bowenoid papules[628] that also appear to have an HPV connection. Interestingly, when Bowenoid papulosis does progress to squamous cell carcinoma, the HPV types detected are often the high-risk mucosal types.[629]

The second category of research challenge, that is, interpreting the detection of HPV, is no less complex. Most HPV types may be found on the skin of both healthy and (especially) immunocompromised individuals.[630] They seem to be part of the "normal flora," sometimes existing as infections within hair follicles.[631] However, there is increasing evidence that conditions such as impaired immunity and sun exposure may move HPV beyond a routine life on the surface of the body toward various disease involvements, from proliferative lesions to premalignancies and, ultimately, nonmelanoma skin cancer (NMSC).[632,633] Given its very high incidence, NMSC is a serious public health concern. In fact, NMSC is the most frequent cancer in Caucasian populations (100–150 annual cases per 100,000).[634] Viral involvement turns out to be a mitigating factor in skin cancer. HPV-related squamous cell carcinomas appear to be less aggressive than other forms of skin cancer.[635,636]

HPV Types and Skin Diseases

Although HPV types that populate the skin were the first to be identified, knowledge of how they function has not kept pace with the investigation of mucosal HPV types (HPV-6, -16, etc.).[637] Of just over 100 HPV types that have been fully characterized to date, almost half seem to have a specific tropism for the skin. While fully 34 types come from the beta (β) and gamma (γ) genera alone, even a few well-known alphapapillomaviruses also exhibit cutaneous disease involvement (e.g., types 2, 7, and 10). Figure 5.1 indicates the distribution of types with known skin tropism. HPV-101 and -103 have been recently classified as gammapapillomaviruses, and therefore are destined to join this skin-related inventory.[638] In whatever way HPV typology evolves, it is clear that for now the beta (β) genus dominates in skin cancer.

The beta and gamma categories of HPV are characterized as low risk from the point of view of mucosal oncogenesis; this follows by definition since the HPV types in question tend to infect the skin rather than mucosal surfaces anyway. Aligning with that pattern, a recent study reported that 133 putative beta and gamma types (defined as having a genome >10% different than any other type) have been detected on human skin.[639] This means that the number of skin-related HPV types is triple that found on mucosal surfaces, which suggests that this area of research will expand in the near future.

There are also nonmalignant skin lesions related to a subset of the αgenus, and to certain HPV types from the other genera. Some of the

Genus	Species	Prototype	Other types ⟶									
α papillomavirus	1											
	2	HPV-10	HPV-3	HPV-28	HPV-29	HPV-78	HPV-94					
	3											
	4	HPV-2	HPV-27	HPV-57								
	5											
	6											
	7											
	8	HPV-7	HPV-40									
	9											
	10											
	11											
	13											
	14											
	15											
β papillomavirus	1	**HPV-5**	HPV-8	HPV-12	HPV-14	HPV-19	HPV-20	HPV-21	HPV-24	HPV-25	HPV-36	HPV-47	HPV-93
	2	**HPV-9**	HPV-15	HPV-17	HPV-22	HPV-23	HPV-37	HPV-38	HPV-80				
	3	HPV-49	HPV-75	HPV-76									
	4	HPV-92											
	5	**HPV-96**											
γ papillomavirus	1	HPV-4	HPV-65	HPV-95									
	2	HPV-48											
	3	**HPV-50**											
	4	HPV-60											
	5	HPV-88											
μ-papillomavirus	1	HPV-1											
	2	HPV-63											
υ papillomavirus	1	HPV-41											

Legend
Skin cancer or precursor: **HPV type**
Other skin lesions: HPV type

Figure 5.1. Skin disease characteristics of HPV genera and species. *Source*: de Villiers et al., *Virology*, 2004. Used by permission.

best-characterized cutaneous associations of this sort (essentially involving various types of skin wart) are summarized in Table 5.5.[640]

In addition to these conditions, a wide range of HPV types has been detected in the skin of patients with NMSC.[641,642] The first evidence of an HPV connection was reported in patients with epidermodysplasia verruciformis (EV), a rare autosomal recessive disorder that demonstrates distinctive skin lesions. Infection with more than 20 types of HPV from the betapapillomavirus genus (specifically species 1 and 2) is associated with EV.[643] These so-called HPV-EV types include HPV-5, -8, -9, -14, -23, -24, and -25, among others. They appear to have a tropism for sun-exposed skin, a pattern revealed in both healthy and diseased surfaces.[644,645] Investigation of the HPV-EV linkage with disease is still at an early stage of development. Emerging research has connected certain HPV-EV types to psoriasis and other similar nonmalignant skin conditions, though possibly not as causal factors.[646-649] Most important, the EV condition appears to lead to squamous cell carcinoma, most likely under the influence of HPV infection.[650,651]

Of the EV types, HPV-5 and -8 have been especially related to the development of carcinomas in EV exposed to UV radiation, though the activating effect of UV is not consistent across the HPV-EV spectrum.[652,653] A recent study suggested that these and other species 1 types of the betapapillomavirus genus tend to cause squamous cell rather than basal cell carcinomas.[654] Other research has indicated that species 1 types such as HPV-5 and -8 may be mostly restricted to benign presentations, with species 2 actually predominating in skin cancer.[655] Other 2008 studies seemed to confirm the important role of species 2 betapapillomaviruses (as well as the gamma genus) in the etiology of skin cancer.[656-658] This continues to be an active area of research, which is being pursued on multiple fronts. For instance, biopsy assays and in vitro research have suggested that types from both species 1 and 2 demonstrate transforming potential.[659,660]

Table 5.5. HPV Types and "Benign" Skin Lesions

HPV Type	Skin Lesion
HPV-1, -2, -3, -4, -27, -29, -57	Common wart
HPV-1 (especially)	Deep palmoplantar wart
HPV-3, -10, -28	Flat wart
HPV-7	Butcher's wart
HPV-60	Cystic wart

On a final note, EV is a model of a group of genetic syndromes with skin manifestations that are linked in some way with HPV. A summary of several other genetic conditions that have been implicated in HPV-related skin lesions (from dysplasia to full carcinomas) is found in Table 5.6.[661]

Complex Disease Processes

As with investigations of other infectious diseases, the mechanism of transmission involved with HPV-related skin disease is of paramount interest. Family members tend to display a similar spectrum of HPV types, a phenomenon that is first observed in infants. On the basis of this observation, it seems clear that cutaneous transmission results from close domestic contact of a routine nature. However, regular exposure to any one viral type does not automatically lead to persistent infection. This implies a role for certain "type-specific susceptibilities of different individuals."[662]

Even when an infection does persist, it is not carcinogenic by itself. UV radiation, sometimes interacting with genetic promoters, is an important causative risk factor in cutaneous cancers. Although the mechanism has not been completely elucidated, the best understanding may be that HPV is a co-carcinogen with UV in the development of some cases of NMSC.[663–666] One pathway that may be involved is UV-induced immunosuppression, as it may permit HPV infection to persist. HPV may then complete the pathogenetic cycle by interfering with normal DNA repair responses to any UV-induced mutations.[667] Evidence related to the immunosuppression theory is mixed. Individuals who have experienced sunburn do seem to exhibit a higher prevalence of infection with HPV-EV types, whereas those with increased lifetime sun exposure are associated with a lower risk of HPV infection.[668] This reinforces the reality that a full understanding of the relationship among UV, HPV, and skin cancer remains elusive.

The connection with EV also continues to be elucidated at the molecular level.[669–673] Intriguingly, EV-specific HPV types are defective for an important growth-promoting function (normally encoded by an E5/E8 gene present in other HPV types); moreover, the inactivation of so-called EVER proteins (a distinctive aspect of the EV disorder) precisely compensates for the missing viral function.[674] While the entire relationship continues to be worked out, this appears to be part of the synergy between EV and HPV that creates susceptibility to skin cancer formation.[675]

It is important to reiterate that the HPV types involved with skin neoplasia are not restricted to the HPV-EV types, or even to the classic cutaneous genera. In short, mucosal HPV types have also been implicated in skin pathogenesis.[676,677] One of the clearest associations identified exists between HPV-16 and Bowen's disease.[678–680] Acknowledging

Table 5.6. Genetic Syndromes with Skin Involvement and Possible HPV Association

Syndrome	Inheritance	Features	Skin Manifestation	HPV Association	Lead Author
Xeroderma pigmentosum	Autosomal recessive	Rare; predisposes children to skin cancers; causes DNA repair deficiency	Hypersensitivity to ultraviolet irradiation	Half of 40 squamous cell carcinomas from patients tested positive for HPV	Luron (2007)
Cowden syndrome (CS)	Autosomal dominant	Rare (1 in 200,000 affected); associated with cancer; symptoms typically appear by late 20s	Hamartomas (benign tumours); facial trichilemmomas (benign hair follicle tumours); other lesions	Majority of cutaneous lesions in CS contain HPV DNA	Schaller (2003)
Netherton syndrome	Autosomal recessive	Rare, causes complex immunological dysfunction	Ichthyosis, eczema, and alopecia with abnormal hair shafts	Immunodeficiency leads to HPV infection; 7 of 22 biopsies positive for HPV DNA	Weber (2001)
Hailey-Hailey disease	Autosomal dominant	Manifestation in late teenage years or in adulthood	Uncomfortable skin plaques, which may smell unpleasant	HPV-16 and -39 found in squamous cell carcinoma adjacent to Hailey-Hailey lesions	Ochiai (1999)
Fanconi anemia	Autosomal recessive	Rare bone marrow failure syndrome	Development of squamous cell carcinomas observed	HPV DNA detected in 84% of squamous cell carcinoma specimens from case subjects	Kutler (2003)

the previous discussion of somewhat fluid terms such as Bowen's disease, a lesion positive for HPV-16 usually is assumed to be on the malignancy spectrum, rather than being classified as a benign manifestation. That said, such characterizations are not straightforward; molecular evidence concerning HPV-16 involvement in skin disease continues to be an emerging area of science.[681] In fact, some research has pointed to mechanisms involving HPV-16 that may work against the development or maintenance of skin dysplasia. Thus, in suspected precancerous tumors, the so-called transient stage[682] may contain keratinocytes immortalized by HPV-16 that are actually susceptible to UV-induced apoptosis (i.e., cellular death).[683] This counteracts the general tendency for UV-affected tissues to resist apoptosis of damaged cells, which in turn increases the risk of skin cancers.[684] Other research has suggested that the effects on apoptosis may vary according to other molecular factors.[685] Thus, some evidence points to an antiapoptotic impact of infection, including (at least under certain conditions) infection with HPV-16.[686] A similar effect has been recently seen with species 1 betapapillomavirus types.[687] The increased keratinocyte survival that is a consequence of reduced apoptosis in turn allows HPV infection to persist, which is a prerequisite for the now familiar carcinogenic pathway induced by the virus. Summing up these apparently countervailing molecular forces, it seems that an individual may get skin cancer due to UV radiation, HPV-16 infection, or some complex interaction between these two factors.

Future Research

Beyond the general research challenges already described, there are several technical obstacles involved with establishing a clear association between skin cancer and HPV. For instance, it can be difficult to determine where best to obtain a control sample, especially to overcome the low copy number normally associated with HPV infection of the skin.[688] The current significance of detected virus is also unclear. A recent study demonstrated that HPV is not only present on healthy skin but can persist there for several years.[689] Another complication is the suggestion that some HPV types are inversely associated with lesions of the skin induced by UV, apparently offering a kind of protective effect.[690,691] As well, there is some limited evidence of HPV involvement in melanomas of the skin; given the high mortality rate of this cancer, the public health implications of any new information on causation would be far-reaching.[692] In sum, the full role of HPV in skin cancers is clearly not yet determined. It will continue to be a subject of serious investigation, possibly leading to improved understanding of the full benefits of prophylactic vaccine applications.[693]

NOTES

1. Chan SY, Delius H, Halpern AL et al. Analysis of genomic sequences of 95 papillomavirus types: uniting typing, phylogeny, and taxonomy. *Journal of Virology.* 1995; 69(5): 3074–83.
2. Gillison ML, Chaturvedi AK, Lowy DR. HPV prophylactic vaccines and the potential prevention of noncervical cancers in both men and women. *Cancer.* 2008; 113(suppl 10): 3036–46.
3. Myers ER. The economic impact of HPV vaccines: not just cervical cancer. *American Journal of Obstetrics and Gynecology.* 2008; 198(5): 487–8.
4. Hu D, Goldie S. The economic burden of noncervical human papillomavirus disease in the United States. *American Journal of Obstetrics and Gynecology.* 2008; 198(5): 500 e1–7.
5. Monk BJ, Tewari KS. The spectrum and clinical sequelae of human papillomavirus infection. *Gynecologic Oncology.* 2007; 107(2 suppl 1): S6–13.
6. Louchini R, Goggin P, Steben M. The evolution of HPV-related anogenital cancers reported in Quebec—Incidence rates and survival probabilities. *Chronic Diseases in Canada.* 2008; 28(3): 99–106.
7. Huang FY, Kwok YK, Lau ET et al. Genetic abnormalities and HPV status in cervical and vulvar squamous cell carcinomas. *Cancer Genetics and Cytogenetics.* 2005; 157(1): 42–8.
8. Also known as vulval.
9. Duong TH, Flowers LC. Vulvo-vaginal cancers: risks, evaluation, prevention and early detection. *Obstetrics and Gynecology Clinics of North America.* 2007; 34(4): 783–802.
10. Madsen BS, Jensen HL, van den Brule AJ et al. Risk factors for invasive squamous cell carcinoma of the vulva and vagina–population-based case-control study in Denmark. *International Journal of Cancer.* 2008; 122(12): 2827–34.
11. Judson PL, Habermann EB, Baxter NN et al. Trends in the incidence of invasive and in situ vulvar carcinoma. *Obstetrics and Gynecology.* 2006; 107(5): 1018–22.
12. Hampl M, Deckers-Figiel S, Hampl JA et al. New aspects of vulvar cancer: changes in localization and age of onset. *Gynecologic Oncology.* 2008; 109(3): 340–5.
13. Kennedy CM, Boardman LA. New approaches to external genital warts and vulvar intraepithelial neoplasia. *Clinical Obstetrics and Gynecology.* 2008; 51(3): 518–26.
14. Giles GG, Kneale BL. Vulvar cancer: the Cinderella of gynaecological oncology. *Australian and New Zealand Journal of Obstetrics and Gynaecology.* 1995; 35(1): 71–5.
15. Saraiya M, Watson M, Wu X et al. Incidence of in situ and invasive vulvar cancer in the US, 1998–2003. *Cancer.* 2008; 113(suppl 10): 2865–72.
16. Giuliano AR, Tortolero-Luna G, Ferrer E et al. Epidemiology of human papillomavirus infection in men, cancers other than cervical and benign conditions. *Vaccine.* 2008; 26(suppl 10): K17–28.
17. Crum CP. Carcinoma of the vulva: epidemiology and pathogenesis. *Obstetrics and Gynecology.* 1992; 79(3): 448–54.

18 Bonvicini F, Venturoli S, Ambretti S et al. Presence and type of oncogenic human papillomavirus in classic and in differentiated vulvar intraepithelial neoplasia and keratinizing vulvar squamous cell carcinoma. *Journal of Medical Virology.* 2005; 77(1): 102–6.
19 van der Avoort IA, Shirango H, Hoevenaars BM et al. Vulvar squamous cell carcinoma is a multifactorial disease following two separate and independent pathways. *International Journal of Gynecological Pathology.* 2006; 25(1): 22–9.
20 Fox H, Wells M. Recent advances in the pathology of the vulva. *Histopathology.* 2003; 42(3): 209–16.
21 Monk BJ, Burger RA, Lin F et al. Prognostic significance of human papillomavirus DNA in vulvar carcinoma. *Obstetrics and Gynecology.* 1995; 85(5 Pt 1): 709–15.
22 Santos M, Landolfi S, Olivella A et al. p16 overexpression identifies HPV-positive vulvar squamous cell carcinomas. *American Journal of Surgical Pathology.* 2006; 30(11): 1347–56.
23 Srodon M, Stoler MH, Baber GB et al. The distribution of low and high-risk HPV types in vulvar and vaginal intraepithelial neoplasia (VIN and VaIN). *American Journal of Surgical Pathology.* 2006; 30(12): 1513–8.
24 Santos M, Landolfi S, Olivella A et al. p16 overexpression identifies HPV-positive vulvar squamous cell carcinomas. *American Journal of Surgical Pathology.* 2006; 30(11): 1347–56.
25 Rufforny I, Wilkinson EJ, Liu C et al. Human papillomavirus infection and p16(INK4a) protein expression in vulvar intraepithelial neoplasia and invasive squamous cell carcinoma. *Journal of Lower Genital Tract Disease.* 2005; 9(2): 108–13.
26 Riethdorf S, Neffen EF, Cviko A et al. p16INK4A expression as biomarker for HPV 16-related vulvar neoplasias. *Human Pathology.* 2004; 35(12): 1477–83.
27 Hampl M, Wentzensen N, Vinokurova S et al. Comprehensive analysis of 130 multicentric intraepithelial female lower genital tract lesions by HPV typing and p16 expression profile. *Journal of Cancer Research and Clinical Oncology.* 2007; 133(4): 235–45.
28 de Koning MN, Quint WG, Pirog EC. Prevalence of mucosal and cutaneous human papillomaviruses in different histologic subtypes of vulvar carcinoma. *Modern Pathology.* 2008; 21(3): 334–44.
29 McCluggage WG. Recent developments in vulvovaginal pathology. *Histopathology.* 2009; 54(2): 156–73.
30 Kagie MJ, Kenter GG, Zomerdijk-Nooijen Y et al. Human papillomavirus infection in squamous cell carcinoma of the vulva, in various synchronous epithelial changes and in normal vulvar skin. *Gynecologic Oncology.* 1997; 67(2): 178–83.
31 Goffin F, Mayrand MH, Gauthier P et al. High-risk human papillomavirus infection of the genital tract of women with a previous history or current high-grade vulvar intraepithelial neoplasia. *Journal of Medical Virology.* 2006; 78(6): 814–9.
32 Basta A, Adamek K, Pitynski K. Intraepithelial neoplasia and early stage vulvar cancer. Epidemiological, clinical and virological observations. *European Journal of Gynaecological Oncology.* 1999; 20(2): 111–4.
33 Hildesheim A, Han CL, Brinton LA et al. Human papillomavirus type 16 and risk of preinvasive and invasive vulvar cancer: results from a seroepidemiological case-control study. *Obstetrics and Gynecology.* 1997; 90(5): 748–54.

34 Ngan HY, Cheung AN, Liu SS et al. Abnormal expression or mutation of TP53 and HPV in vulvar cancer. *European Journal of Cancer.* 1999; 35(3): 481–4.
35 Menczer J, Fintsi Y, Arbel-Alon S et al. The presence of HPV 16, 18 and p53 immunohistochemical staining in tumor tissue of Israeli Jewish women with cervical and vulvar neoplasia. *European Journal of Gynaecological Oncology.* 2000; 21(1): 30–4.
36 Koyamatsu Y, Yokoyama M, Nakao Y et al. A comparative analysis of human papillomavirus types 16 and 18 and expression of p53 gene and Ki-67 in cervical, vaginal, and vulvar carcinomas. *Gynecologic Oncology.* 2003; 90(3): 547–51.
37 Huang FY, Kwok YK, Lau ET et al. Genetic abnormalities and HPV status in cervical and vulvar squamous cell carcinomas. *Cancer Genetics and Cytogenetics.* 2005; 157(1): 42–8.
38 Hampl M, Sarajuuri H, Wentzensen N et al. Effect of human papillomavirus vaccines on vulvar, vaginal, and anal intraepithelial lesions and vulvar cancer. *Obstetrics and Gynecology.* 2006; 108(6): 1361–8.
39 Hillemanns P, Wang X. Integration of HPV-16 and HPV-18 DNA in vulvar intraepithelial neoplasia. *Gynecologic Oncology.* 2006; 100(2): 276–82.
40 Almeida G, do Val I, Gondim C et al. Human papillomavirus, Epstein-Barr virus and p53 mutation in vulvar intraepithelial neoplasia. *Journal of Reproductive Medicine.* 2004; 49(10): 796–9.
41 Bonvicini F, Venturoli S, Ambretti S et al. Presence and type of oncogenic human papillomavirus in classic and in differentiated vulvar intraepithelial neoplasia and keratinizing vulvar squamous cell carcinoma. *Journal of Medical Virology.* 2005; 77(1): 102–6.
42 Srodon M, Stoler MH, Baber GB et al. The distribution of low and high-risk HPV types in vulvar and vaginal intraepithelial neoplasia (VIN and VaIN). *American Journal of Surgical Pathology.* 2006; 30(12): 1513–8.
43 Kagie MJ, Kenter GG, Tollenaar RA et al. p53 protein overexpression is common and independent of human papillomavirus infection in squamous cell carcinoma of the vulva. *Cancer.* 1997; 80(7): 1228–33.
44 Maclean AB. Vulval cancer: prevention and screening. Best Practice and Research. *Clinical Obstetrics and Gynaecology.* 2006; 20(2): 379–95.
45 van Poelgeest MI, van Seters M, van Beurden M et al. Detection of human papillomavirus (HPV) 16-specific CD4+ T-cell immunity in patients with persistent HPV16-induced vulvar intraepithelial neoplasia in relation to clinical impact of imiquimod treatment. *Clinical Cancer Research.* 2005; 11(14): 5273–80.
46 Hampl M, Sarajuuri H, Wentzensen N et al. Effect of human papillomavirus vaccines on vulvar, vaginal, and anal intraepithelial lesions and vulvar cancer. *Obstetrics and Gynecology.* 2006; 108(6): 1361–8.
47 Skapa P, Zamecnik J, Hamsikova E et al. Human papillomavirus (HPV) profiles of vulvar lesions: possible implications for the classification of vulvar squamous cell carcinoma precursors and for the efficacy of prophylactic HPV vaccination. *American Journal of Surgical Pathology.* 2007; 31(12): 1834–43.
48 Insinga RP, Liaw KL, Johnson LG et al. A systematic review of the prevalence and attribution of human papillomavirus types among cervical, vaginal, and vulvar precancers and cancers in the United States. *Cancer Epidemiology, Biomarkers and Prevention.* 2008; 17(7): 1611–22.
49 Ahr A, Rody A, Kissler S et al. [Risk factors for recurrence of vulvar intraepithelial neoplasia III (VIN III)]. *Zentralblatt fur Gynakologie.* 2006; 128(6): 347–51.

50 Bonvicini F, Venturoli S, Ambretti S et al. Presence and type of oncogenic human papillomavirus in classic and in differentiated vulvar intraepithelial neoplasia and keratinizing vulvar squamous cell carcinoma. *Journal of Medical Virology.* 2005; 77(1): 102–6.
51 Medeiros F, Nascimento AF, Crum CP. Early vulvar squamous neoplasia: advances in classification, diagnosis, and differential diagnosis. *Advances in Anatomic Pathology.* 2005; 12(1): 20–6.
52 Scurry J, Wilkinson EJ. Review of terminology of precursors of vulvar squamous cell carcinoma. *Journal of Lower Genital Tract Disease.* 2006; 10(3): 161–9.
53 Sideri M, Jones RW, Wilkinson EJ et al. Squamous vulvar intraepithelial neoplasia: 2004 modified terminology, ISSVD Vulvar Oncology Subcommittee. *Journal of Reproductive Medicine.* 2005; 50(11): 807–10.
54 Goffin F, Mayrand MH, Gauthier P et al. High-risk human papillomavirus infection of the genital tract of women with a previous history or current high-grade vulvar intraepithelial neoplasia. *Journal of Medical Virology.* 2006; 78(6): 814–9.
55 Basta A, Adamek K, Pitynski K. Intraepithelial neoplasia and early stage vulvar cancer. Epidemiological, clinical and virological observations. *European Journal of Gynaecological Oncology.* 1999; 20(2): 111–4.
56 Madeleine MM, Daling JR, Carter JJ et al. Cofactors with human papillomavirus in a population-based study of vulvar cancer. *Journal of the National Cancer Institute.* 1997; 89(20): 1516–23.
57 Hussain SK, Madeleine MM, Johnson LG et al. Cervical and vulvar cancer risk in relation to the joint effects of cigarette smoking and genetic variation in interleukin 2. *Cancer Epidemiology Biomarkers and Prevention.* 2008; 17(7): 1790–9.
58 Giles GG, Kneale BL. Vulvar cancer: the Cinderella of gynaecological oncology. *Australian and New Zealand Journal of Obstetrics and Gynaecology.* 1995; 35(1): 71–5.
59 Denny L, Ngan HYS. Section B: malignant manifestations of HPV infection: carcinoma of the cervix, vulva, vagina, anus, and penis. *International Journal of Gynecology and Obstetrics.* 2006; 94(suppl 1): S50–5.
60 Monk BJ, Tewari KS, Koh WJ. Multimodality therapy for locally advanced cervical carcinoma: state of the art and future directions. *Journal of Clinical Oncology.* 2007; 25(20): 2952–65.
61 Vinokurova S, Wentzensen N, Einenkel J et al. Clonal history of papillomavirus-induced dysplasia in the female lower genital tract. *Journal of the National Cancer Institute.* 2005; 97(24): 1816–21.
62 Hampl M, Wentzensen N, Vinokurova S et al. Comprehensive analysis of 130 multicentric intraepithelial female lower genital tract lesions by HPV typing and p16 expression profile. *Journal of Cancer Research and Clinical Oncology.* 2007; 133(4): 235–45.
63 Edgren G, Sparen P. Risk of anogenital cancer after diagnosis of cervical intraepithelial neoplasia: a prospective population-based study. *Lancet Oncology.* 2007; 8(4): 311–6.
64 Mourton SM, Sonoda Y, Abu-Rustum NR et al. Resection of recurrent cervical cancer after total pelvic exenteration. *International Journal of Gynecological Cancer.* 2007; 17(1): 137–40.

65 Evans HS, Newnham A, Hodgson SV et al. Second primary cancers after cervical intraepithelial neoplasia III and invasive cervical cancer in Southeast England. *Gynecologic Oncology.* 2003; 90(1): 131–6.
66 Goffin F, Mayrand MH, Gauthier P et al. High-risk human papillomavirus infection of the genital tract of women with a previous history or current high-grade vulvar intraepithelial neoplasia. *Journal of Medical Virology.* 2006; 78(6): 814–9.
67 Jamieson DJ, Paramsothy P, Cu-Uvin S et al. Vulvar, vaginal, and perianal intraepithelial neoplasia in women with or at risk for human immunodeficiency virus. *Obstetrics and Gynecology.* 2006; 107(5): 1023–8.
68 Conley LJ, Ellerbrock TV, Bush TJ et al. HIV-1 infection and risk of vulvovaginal and perianal condylomata acuminata and intraepithelial neoplasia: a prospective cohort study. *The Lancet.* 2002; 359(9301): 108–13.
69 Santegoets LA, Seters M, Helmerhorst TJ et al. HPV related VIN: highly proliferative and diminished responsiveness to extracellular signals. *International Journal of Cancer.* 2007; 121(4): 759–66.
70 Casolati E, Agarossi A, Valieri M et al. Vulvar neoplasia in HIV positive women: a review. *Medycyna Wieku Rozwojowego.* 2003; 7(4 Pt 1): 487–93.
71 Duarte-Franco E, Franco EL. Other gynecologic cancers: endometrial, ovarian, vulvar and vaginal cancers. *BMC Womens Health.* 2004; 4(suppl 1): S14.
72 Kwasniewska A, Korobowicz E, Visconti J et al. Chlamydia trachomatis and herpes simplex virus 2 infection in vulvar intraepithelial neoplasia associated with human papillomavirus. *European Journal of Gynaecological Oncology.* 2006; 27(4): 405–8.
73 Hildesheim A, Han CL, Brinton LA et al. Human papillomavirus type 16 and risk of preinvasive and invasive vulvar cancer: results from a seroepidemiological case-control study. *Obstetrics and Gynecology.* 1997; 90(5): 748–54.
74 Boscoe FP, Schymura MJ. Solar ultraviolet-B exposure and cancer incidence and mortality in the United States, 1993–2002. *BMC Cancer.* 2006; 6: 264.
75 Weinstock MA. Malignant melanoma of the vulva and vagina in the United States: patterns of incidence and population-based estimates of survival. *American Journal of Obstetrics and Gynecology.* 1994; 171(5): 1225–30.
76 Isenberg A, Paul Shackelford D. The value of tan lines: vulvar melanoma and ultraviolet rays. *Obstetrical and Gynecological Survey.* 2001; 56(6): 377–80.
77 Wu X, Matanoski G, Chen VW et al. Descriptive epidemiology of vaginal cancer incidence and survival by race, ethnicity, and age in the United States. *Cancer.* 2008; 113(suppl 10): 2873–82.
78 Sugase M, Matsukura T. Distinct manifestations of human papillomaviruses in the vagina. *International Journal of Cancer.* 1997; 72(3): 412–5.
79 Daling JR, Madeleine MM, Schwartz SM et al. A population-based study of squamous cell vaginal cancer: HPV and cofactors. *Gynecologic Oncology.* 2002; 84(2): 263–70.
80 Koyamatsu Y, Yokoyama M, Nakao Y et al. A comparative analysis of human papillomavirus types 16 and 18 and expression of p53 gene and Ki-67 in cervical, vaginal, and vulvar carcinomas. *Gynecologic Oncology.* 2003; 90(3): 547–51.
81 Srodon M, Stoler MH, Baber GB et al. The distribution of low and high-risk HPV types in vulvar and vaginal intraepithelial neoplasia (VIN and VaIN). *American Journal of Surgical Pathology.* 2006; 30(12): 1513–8.

82 Castle PE, Rodriguez AC, Porras C et al. A comparison of cervical and vaginal human papillomavirus. *Sexually Transmitted Diseases.* 2007; 34(11): 849–55.
83 Daling JR, Madeleine MM, Schwartz SM et al. A population-based study of squamous cell vaginal cancer: HPV and cofactors. *Gynecologic Oncology.* 2002; 84(2): 263–70.
84 Sherman JF, Mount SL, Evans MF et al. Smoking increases the risk of high-grade vaginal intraepithelial neoplasia in women with oncogenic human papillomavirus. *Gynecologic Oncology.* 2008; 110(3): 396–401.
85 Barton HA, Cogliano VJ, Flowers L et al. Assessing susceptibility from early-life exposure to carcinogens. *Environmental Health Perspectives.* 2005; 113(9): 1125–33.
86 Swan SH. Intrauterine exposure to diethylstilbestrol: long-term effects in humans. *Acta Pathologica, Microbiologica et Immunologica Scandinavica.* 2000; 108(12): 793–804.
87 Veurink M, Koster M, Berg LT. The history of DES, lessons to be learned. *Pharmacy World and Science.* 2005; 27(3): 139–43.
88 Jamieson DJ, Paramsothy P, Cu-Uvin S et al. Vulvar, vaginal, and perianal intraepithelial neoplasia in women with or at risk for human immunodeficiency virus. *Obstetrics and Gynecology.* 2006; 107(5): 1023–8.
89 Daling JR, Madeleine MM, Schwartz SM et al. A population-based study of squamous cell vaginal cancer: HPV and cofactors. *Gynecologic Oncology.* 2002; 84(2): 263–70.
90 Indraccolo U, Chiocci L, Baldoni A. Does vaginal intraepithelial neoplasia have the same evolution as cervical intraepithelial neoplasia? *European Journal of Gynaecological Oncology.* 2008; 29(4): 371–3.
91 Edgren G, Sparen P. Risk of anogenital cancer after diagnosis of cervical intraepithelial neoplasia: a prospective population-based study. *Lancet Oncology.* 2007; 8(4): 311–6.
92 Daling JR, Madeleine MM, Schwartz SM et al. A population-based study of squamous cell vaginal cancer: HPV and cofactors. *Gynecologic Oncology.* 2002; 84(2): 263–70.
93 Barzon L, Pizzighella S, Corti L et al. Vaginal dysplastic lesions in women with hysterectomy and receiving radiotherapy are linked to high-risk human papillomavirus. *Journal of Medical Virology.* 2002; 67(3): 401–5.
94 Frega A, French D, Piazze J et al. Prediction of persistent vaginal intraepithelial neoplasia in previously hysterectomized women by high-risk HPV DNA detection. *Cancer Letters.* 2007; 249(2): 235–41.
95 Insinga RP, Liaw KL, Johnson LG et al. A systematic review of the prevalence and attribution of human papillomavirus types among cervical, vaginal, and vulvar precancers and cancers in the United States. *Cancer Epidemiology, Biomarkers and Prevention.* 2008; 17(7): 1611–22.
96 Ferreira M, Crespo M, Martins L et al. HPV DNA detection and genotyping in 21 cases of primary invasive squamous cell carcinoma of the vagina. *Modern Pathology.* 2008; 21(8): 968–72.
97 Vinokurova S, Wentzensen N, Einenkel J et al. Clonal history of papillomavirus-induced dysplasia in the female lower genital tract. *Journal of the National Cancer Institute.* 2005; 97(24): 1816–21.
98 Indraccolo U, Del Frate E, Cenci S et al. Vaginal intraepithelial neoplasia and human papillomavirus infection: a report of 75 cases. *Minerva Ginecologica.* 2006; 58(2): 101–8.

99 Favorito LA, Nardi AC, Ronalsa M et al. Epidemiologic study on penile cancer in Brazil. *Official Journal of the Brazilian Society of Urology.* 2008; 34(5): 587–93.
100 Hernandez BY, Barnholtz-Sloan J, German RR et al. Burden of invasive squamous cell carcinoma of the penis in the United States, 1998–2003. *Cancer.* 2008; 113(suppl 10): 2883–91.
101 Goodman MT, Hernandez BY, Shvetsov YB. Demographic and pathologic differences in the incidence of invasive penile cancer in the United States, 1995–2003. *Cancer Epidemiology, Biomarkers and Prevention.* 2007; 16(9): 1833–9.
102 Barnholtz-Sloan JS, Maldonado JL, Pow-sang J et al. Incidence trends in primary malignant penile cancer. *Urologic Oncology.* 2007; 25(5): 361–7.
103 Giuliano AR, Tortolero-Luna G, Ferrer E et al. Epidemiology of human papillomavirus infection in men, cancers other than cervical and benign conditions. *Vaccine.* 2008; 26(suppl 10): K17–28.
104 Dianzani C, Calvieri S, Pierangeli A et al. Identification of human papilloma viruses in male dysplastic genital lesions. *New Microbiologica.* 2004; 27(1): 65–9.
105 Daling JR, Madeleine MM, Johnson LG et al. Penile cancer: importance of circumcision, human papillomavirus and smoking in in situ and invasive disease. *International Journal of Cancer.* 2005; 116(4): 606–16.
106 Mosconi AM, Roila F, Gatta G et al. Cancer of the penis. *Critical Reviews in Oncology/Hematology.* 2005; 53(2): 165–77.
107 Culkin DJ, Beer TM. Advanced penile carcinoma. *Journal of Urology.* 2003; 170(2 Pt 1): 359–65.
108 Salazar EL, Mercado E, Calzada L. Human papillomavirus hpv-16 DNA as an epitheliotropic virus that induces hyperproliferation in squamous penile tissue. *Archives of Andrology.* 2005; 51(4): 327–34.
109 Kayes O, Ahmed HU, Arya M et al. Molecular and genetic pathways in penile cancer. *Lancet Oncology.* 2007; 8(5): 420–9.
110 Aynaud O, Ionesco M, Barrasso R. Penile intraepithelial neoplasia. Specific clinical features correlate with histologic and virologic findings. *Cancer.* 1994; 74(6): 1762–7.
111 Dillner J, von Krogh G, Horenblas S et al. Etiology of squamous cell carcinoma of the penis. *Scandinavian Journal of Urology and Nephrology.* 2000; (205): 189–93.
112 Gross G, Pfister H. Role of human papillomavirus in penile cancer, penile intraepithelial squamous cell neoplasias and in genital warts. *Medical Microbiology and Immunology.* 2004; 193(1): 35–44.
113 Rubin MA, Kleter B, Zhou M et al. Detection and typing of human papillomavirus DNA in penile carcinoma: evidence for multiple independent pathways of penile carcinogenesis. *American Journal of Pathology.* 2001; 159(4): 1211–8.
114 Gregoirc L, Cubilla AL, Reuter VF et al. Preferential association of human papillomavirus with high-grade histologic variants of penile-invasive squamous cell carcinoma. *Journal of the National Cancer Institute.* 1995; 87(22): 1705–9. A 2001 result for warty carcinoma was somewhat lower, but still in excess of the HPV prevalence in squamous cell carcinoma. Bezerra AL, Lopes A, Landman G et al. Clinicopathologic features and human papillomavirus DNA prevalence of warty and squamous cell carcinoma of the penis. *American Journal of Surgical Pathology.* 2001; 25(5): 673–8.

115 Across different older studies, the variation in HPV prevalence for squamous cell carcinoma has been wide, from 5 to 48%. Melbye M, Frisch M. The role of human papillomaviruses in anogenital cancers. *Seminars in Cancer Biology*. 1998; 8(4): 307–13. A more recent result in a small sample was 67%. Humbey O, Cairey-Remonnay S, Guerrini JS et al. Detection of the human papillomavirus and analysis of the TP53 polymorphism of exon 4 at codon 72 in penile squamous cell carcinomas. *European Journal of Cancer*. 2003; 39(5): 684–90.

116 Rubin MA, Kleter B, Zhou M et al. Detection and typing of human papillomavirus DNA in penile carcinoma: evidence for multiple independent pathways of penile carcinogenesis. *American Journal of Pathology*. 2001; 159(4): 1211–8.

117 Micali G, Nasca MR, Innocenzi D et al. Penile cancer. *Journal of the American Academy of Dermatology*. 2006; 54(3): 369–91.

118 Nehal KS, Levine VJ, Ashinoff R. Basal cell carcinoma of the genitalia. *Dermatologic Surgery*. 1998; 24(12): 1361–3.

119 Lont AP, Kroon BK, Horenblas S et al. Presence of high-risk human papillomavirus DNA in penile carcinoma predicts favorable outcome in survival. *International Journal of Cancer*. 2006; 119(5): 1078–81.

120 Daling JR, Madeleine MM, Johnson LG et al. Penile cancer: importance of circumcision, human papillomavirus and smoking in in situ and invasive disease. *International Journal of Cancer*. 2005; 116(4): 606–16.

121 Perceau G, Derancourt C, Clavel C et al. Lichen sclerosus is frequently present in penile squamous cell carcinomas but is not always associated with oncogenic human papillomavirus. *British Journal of Dermatology*. 2003; 148(5): 934–8.

122 Rubin MA, Kleter B, Zhou M et al. Detection and typing of human papillomavirus DNA in penile carcinoma: evidence for multiple independent pathways of penile carcinogenesis. *American Journal of Pathology*. 2001; 159(4): 1211–8.

123 Bezerra AL, Lopes A, Santiago GH et al. Human papillomavirus as a prognostic factor in carcinoma of the penis: analysis of 82 patients treated with amputation and bilateral lymphadenectomy. *Cancer*. 2001; 91(12): 2315–21.

124 Bunker CB. Topics in penile dermatology. *Clinical and Experimental Dermatology*. 2001; 26(6): 469–79.

125 Carter JJ, Madeleine MM, Shera K et al. Human papillomavirus 16 and 18 L1 serology compared across anogenital cancer sites. *Cancer Research*. 2001; 61(5): 1934–40.

126 Scheiner MA, Campos MM, Ornellas AA et al. Human papillomavirus and penile cancers in Rio de Janeiro, Brazil: HPV typing and clinical features. *Official Journal of the Brazilian Society of Urology*. 2008; 34(4): 467–76.

127 Tornesello ML, Duraturo ML, Losito S et al. Human papillomavirus genotypes and HPV16 variants in penile carcinoma. *International Journal of Cancer*. 2008; 122(1): 132–7.

128 Pascual A, Pariente M, Godinez JM et al. High prevalence of human papillomavirus 16 in penile carcinoma. *Histology and Histopathology*. 2007; 22(2): 177–83.

129 Giovannelli L, Migliore MC, Capra G et al. Penile, urethral, and seminal sampling for diagnosis of human papillomavirus infection in men. *Journal of Clinical Microbiology*. 2007; 45(1): 248–51.

130 Cupp MR, Malek RS, Goellner JR et al. The detection of human papillomavirus deoxyribonucleic acid in intraepithelial, in situ, verrucous and invasive carcinoma of the penis. *Journal of Urology.* 1995; 154(3): 1024–9.
131 Melbye M, Frisch M. The role of human papillomaviruses in anogenital cancers. *Seminars in Cancer Biology.* 1998; 8(4): 307–13.
132 Dillner J, von Krogh G, Horenblas S et al. Etiology of squamous cell carcinoma of the penis. *Scandinavian Journal of Urology and Nephrology.* 2000; (205): 189–93.
133 Calculated from data summarized by Rubin MA, Kleter B, Zhou M et al. Detection and typing of human papillomavirus DNA in penile carcinoma: evidence for multiple independent pathways of penile carcinogenesis. *American Journal of Pathology.* 2001; 159(4): 1211–8.
134 Backes DM, Kurman RJ, Pimenta JM et al. Systematic review of human papillomavirus prevalence in invasive penile cancer. *Cancer Causes and Control.* 2009; 20(4): 449–57.
135 Meyer T, Arndt R, Christophers E et al. Association of rare human papillomavirus types with genital premalignant and malignant lesions. *Journal of Infectious Diseases.* 1998; 178(1): 252–5.
136 Salazar EL, Mercado E, Calzada L. Human papillomavirus hpv-16 DNA as an epitheliotropic virus that induces hyperproliferation in squamous penile tissue. *Archives of Andrology.* 2005; 51(4): 327–34.
137 Heideman DA, Waterboer T, Pawlita M et al. Human papillomavirus-16 is the predominant type etiologically involved in penile squamous cell carcinoma. *Journal of Clinical Oncology.* 2007; 25(29): 4550–6.
138 Senba M, Kumatori A, Fujita S et al. The prevalence of human papillomavirus genotypes in penile cancers from northern Thailand. *Journal of Medical Virology.* 2006; 78(10): 1341–6.
139 Rubin MA, Kleter B, Zhou M et al. Detection and typing of human papillomavirus DNA in penile carcinoma: evidence for multiple independent pathways of penile carcinogenesis. *American Journal of Pathology.* 2001; 159(4): 1211–8.
140 Turazza E, Lapena A, Sprovieri O et al. Low-risk human papillomavirus types 6 and 11 associated with carcinomas of the genital and upper aerodigestive tract. *Acta Obstetricia et Gynecologica Scandinavica.* 1997; 76(3): 271–6.
141 Wieland U, Jurk S, Weissenborn S et al. Erythroplasia of queyrat: coinfection with cutaneous carcinogenic human papillomavirus type 8 and genital papillomaviruses in a carcinoma in situ. *Journal of Investigative Dermatology.* 2000; 115(3): 396–401.
142 Dorfman S, Cavazza M, Cardozo J. Penile cancer associated with so-called low-risk human papilloma virus. Report of five cases from rural Venezuela. *Tropical Doctor.* 2006; 36(4): 232–3.
143 Kalantari M, Villa LL, Calleja-Macias IE et al. Human papillomavirus-16 and -18 in penile carcinomas: DNA methylation, chromosomal recombination and genomic variation. *International Journal of Cancer.* 2008; 123(8): 1832–40.
144 Tornesello ML, Duraturo ML, Losito S et al. Human papillomavirus genotypes and HPV16 variants in penile carcinoma. *International Journal of Cancer.* 2008; 122(1): 132–7.

145 Maden C, Sherman KJ, Beckmann AM et al. History of circumcision, medical conditions, and sexual activity and risk of penile cancer. *Journal of the National Cancer Institite.* 1993; 85(1): 19–24.
146 Dillner J, von Krogh G, Horenblas S et al. Etiology of squamous cell carcinoma of the penis. *Scandinavian Journal of Urology and Nephrology.* 2000; (205): 189–93.
147 Daling JR, Madeleine MM, Johnson LG et al. Penile cancer: importance of circumcision, human papillomavirus and smoking in in situ and invasive disease. *International Journal of Cancer.* 2005; 116(4): 606–16.
148 Bleeker MC, Heideman DA, Snijders PJ et al. Penile cancer: epidemiology, pathogenesis and prevention. *World Journal of Urology.* 2009; 27(2): 141–50.
149 Madsen BS, van den Brule AJ, Jensen HL et al. Risk factors for squamous cell carcinoma of the penis—population-based case-control study in Denmark. *Cancer Epidemiology Biomarkers and Prevention.* 2008; 17(10): 2683–91.
150 Denny L, Ngan HYS. Section B: malignant manifestations of HPV infection: carcinoma of the cervix, vulva, vagina, anus, and penis. *International Journal of Gynecology and Obstetrics.* 2006; 94(suppl 1): S50–5.
151 Micali G, Nasca MR, Innocenzi D et al. Penile cancer. *Journal of the American Academy of Dermatology.* 2006; 54(3): 369–91.
152 Mosconi AM, Roila F, Gatta G et al. Cancer of the penis. *Critical Reviews in Oncology/Hematology.* 2005; 53(2): 165–77.
153 Tsen HF, Morgenstern H, Mack T et al. Risk factors for penile cancer: results of a population-based case-control study in Los Angeles County (United States). *Cancer Causes and Control.* 2001; 12(3): 267–77.
154 Aubin F, Puzenat E, Arveux P et al. Genital squamous cell carcinoma in men treated by photochemotherapy. A cancer registry-based study from 1978 to 1998. *British Journal of Dermatology.* 2001; 144(6): 1204–6.
155 Cubilla AL, Velazquez EF, Young RH. Epithelial lesions associated with invasive penile squamous cell carcinoma: a pathologic study of 288 cases. *International Journal of Surgical Pathology.* 2004; 12(4): 351–64.
156 Aboulafia DM, Gibbons R. Penile cancer and human papilloma virus (HPV) in a human immunodeficiency virus (HIV)-infected patient. *Cancer Investigation.* 2001; 19(3): 266–72.
157 Kreuter A, Brockmeyer NH, Weissenborn SJ et al. Penile intraepithelial neoplasia is frequent in HIV-positive men with anal dysplasia. *Journal of Investigative Dermatology.* 2008; 128(9): 2316–24.
158 Ozsahin M, Jichlinski P, Weber DC et al. Treatment of penile carcinoma: to cut or not to cut? *International Journal of Radiation Oncology, Biology, Physics.* 2006; 66(3): 674–9.
159 Siow WY, Cheng C. Penile cancer: current challenges. *Canadian Journal of Urology.* 2005; 12(suppl 1): 18–23.
160 Castellsague X, Bosch FX, Munoz N et al. Male circumcision, penile human papillomavirus infection, and cervical cancer in female partners. *New England Journal of Medicine.* 2002; 346(15): 1105–12.
161 Schoen EJ, Wiswell TE, Moses S. New policy on circumcision—cause for concern. *Pediatrics.* 2000; 105(3 Pt 1): 620–3.
162 Bunker CB. Topics in penile dermatology. *Clinical and Experimental Dermatology.* 2001; 26(6): 469–79.

163 Micali G, Innocenzi D, Nasca MR et al. Squamous cell carcinoma of the penis. *Journal of the American Academy of Dermatology*. 1996; 35(3 Pt 1): 432–51.
164 Maden C, Sherman KJ, Beckmann AM et al. History of circumcision, medical conditions, and sexual activity and risk of penile cancer. *Journal of the National Cancer Institute*. 1993; 85(1): 19–24.
165 Moses S, Bailey RC, Ronald AR. Male circumcision: assessment of health benefits and risks. *Sexually Transmitted Infections*. 1998; 74(5): 368–73.
166 Ross BS, Levine VJ, Dixon C et al. Squamous cell carcinoma of the penis in a circumcised man: a case for dermatology and urology, and review of the literature. *Cutis*. 1998; 61(1): 41–3.
167 Saibishkumar EP, Crook J, Sweet J. Neonatal circumcision and invasive squamous cell carcinoma of the penis: a report of 3 cases and a review of the literature. *Canadian Urological Association Journal*. 2008; 2(1): 39–42.
168 Nielson CM, Schiaffino MK, Dunne EF et al. Associations between Male Anogenital Human Papillomavirus Infection and Circumcision by Anatomic Site Sampled and Lifetime Number of Female Sex Partners. *Journal of Infectious Diseases*. 2009; 199(1): 7–13.
169 Giuliano AR, Lazcano E, Villa LL et al. Circumcision and sexual behavior: factors independently associated with human papillomavirus detection among men in the HIM study. *International Journal of Cancer*. 2009; 124(6): 1251–7.
170 Hernandez BY, Wilkens LR, Zhu X et al. Circumcision and human papillomavirus infection in men: a site-specific comparison. *Journal of Infectious Diseases*. 2008; 197(6): 787–94.
171 Auvert B, Sobngwi-Tambekou J, Cutler E et al. Effect of male circumcision on the prevalence of high-risk human papillomavirus in young men: results of a randomized controlled trial conducted in orange farm, South Africa. *Journal of Infectious Diseases*. 2009; 199(1): 14–9.
172 Thami GP, Kaur S. Genital lichen sclerosus, squamous cell carcinoma and circumcision. *British Journal of Dermatology*. 2003; 148(5): 1083–4.
173 Busby JE, Pettaway CA. What's new in the management of penile cancer? *Current Opinion in Urology*. 2005; 15(5): 350–7.
174 Kroon BK, Horenblas S, Nieweg OE. Contemporary management of penile squamous cell carcinoma. *Journal of Surgical Oncology*. 2005; 89(1): 43–50.
175 Kayes O, Ahmed HU, Arya M et al. Molecular and genetic pathways in penile cancer. *Lancet Oncology*. 2007; 8(5): 420–9.
176 Frisch M, Friis S, Kjaer SK et al. Falling incidence of penis cancer in an uncircumcised population (Denmark 1943–90). *British Medical Journal*. 1995; 311(7018): 1471.
177 Millett GA, Flores SA, Marks G et al. Circumcision status and risk of HIV and sexually transmitted infections among men who have sex with men: a meta-analysis. *Journal of the American Medical Association*. 2008; 300(14): 1674–84.
178 Thami GP, Kaur S. Genital lichen sclerosus, squamous cell carcinoma and circumcision. *British Journal of Dermatology*. 2003; 148(5): 1083–4.
179 Velazquez EF, Cubilla AL. Lichen sclerosus in 68 patients with squamous cell carcinoma of the penis: frequent atypias and correlation with special carcinoma variants suggests a precancerous role. *American Journal of Surgical Pathology*. 2003; 27(11): 1448–53.

180 Recently, some connection was also drawn between lichen sclerosus and high-risk HPV infection, which only serves to show that the topic of penile lesions and HPV remains a fluid area of investigation. Nasca MR, Innocenzi D, Micali G. Association of penile lichen sclerosus and oncogenic human papillomavirus infection. *International Journal of Dermatology.* 2006; 45(6): 681-3.

181 Cold CJ, Taylor JR. The prepuce. *British Journal of Urology International.* 1999; 83(suppl 1): 34-44.

182 Velazquez EF, Soskin A, Bock A et al. Epithelial abnormalities and precancerous lesions of anterior urethra in patients with penile carcinoma: a report of 89 cases. *Modern Pathology.* 2005; 18(7): 917-23.

183 Weaver BA, Feng Q, Holmes KK et al. Evaluation of genital sites and sampling techniques for detection of human papillomavirus DNA in men. *Journal of Infectious Diseases.* 2004; 189(4): 677-85.

184 Van Howe RS. Reply to "HPV and circumcision: a biased, inaccurate and misleading meta-analysis". *British Infection Society.* 2007; 55(1): 93-6.

185 Hernandez BY, McDuffie K, Goodman MT et al. Comparison of physician- and self-collected genital specimens for detection of human papillomavirus in men. *Journal of Clinical Microbiology.* 2006; 44(2): 513-7.

186 Nielson CM, Flores R, Harris RB et al. Human papillomavirus prevalence and type distribution in male anogenital sites and semen. *Cancer Epidemiology, Biomarkers and Prevention.* 2007; 16(6): 1107-14.

187 Smith JS, Moses S, Hudgens MG et al. Human papillomavirus detection by penile site in young men from Kenya. *Sexually Transmitted Diseases.* 2007; 34(11): 928-34.

188 Aynaud O, Ionesco M, Barrasso R. Cytologic detection of human papillomavirus DNA in normal male urethral samples. *Urology.* 2003; 61(6): 1098-101.

189 Aguilar LV, Lazcano-Ponce E, Vaccarella S et al. Human papillomavirus in men: comparison of different genital sites. *Sexually Transmitted Infections.* 2006; 82(1): 31-3.

190 Taylor JR, Lockwood AP, Taylor AJ. The prepuce: specialized mucosa of the penis and its loss to circumcision. *British Journal of Urology.* 1996; 77(2): 291-5.

191 Christensen ND, Koltun WA, Cladel NM et al. Coinfection of human foreskin fragments with multiple human papillomavirus types (HPV-11, -40, and -LVX82/MM7) produces regionally separate HPV infections within the same athymic mouse xenograft. *Journal of Virology.* 1997; 71(10): 7337-44.

192 Allen DC, Cameron RI, eds. *Histological Specimens: Clinical, Pathological and Laboratory Aspects.* London: Springer, 2004.

193 Szabo R, Short RV. How does male circumcision protect against HIV infection? *British Medical Journal.* 2000; 320(7249): 1592-4.

194 Aynaud O, Piron D, Bijaoui G et al. Developmental factors of urethral human papillomavirus lesions: correlation with circumcision. *British Journal of Urology International.* 1999; 84(1): 57-60.

195 Van Howe RS. Human papillomavirus and circumcision: a meta-analysis. *Journal of Infection.* 2007; 54(5): 490-6.

196 Castellsague X, Albero G, Cleries R et al. HPV and circumcision: a biased, inaccurate and misleading meta-analysis. *Journal of Infection.* 2007; 55(1): 91-3.

197 Szabo R, Short RV. How does male circumcision protect against HIV infection? *British Medical Journal.* 2000; 320(7249): 1592–4.
198 Patterson BK, Landay A, Siegel JN et al. Susceptibility to human immunodeficiency virus-1 infection of human foreskin and cervical tissue grown in explant culture. *American Journal of Pathology.* 2002; 161(3): 867–73.
199 Donoval BA, Landay AL, Moses S et al. HIV-1 target cells in foreskins of African men with varying histories of sexually transmitted infections. *American Journal of Clinical Pathology.* 2006; 125(3): 386–91.
200 McCoombe SG, Short RV. Potential HIV-1 target cells in the human penis. *AIDS.* 2006; 20(11): 1491–5.
201 Van Howe RS. Does circumcision influence sexually transmitted diseases?: a literature review. *British Journal of Urology International.* 1999; 83(suppl 1): 52–62.
202 Weiss HA. Male circumcision as a preventive measure against HIV and other sexually transmitted diseases. *Current Opinion in Infectious Diseases.* 2007; 20(1): 66–72.
203 Partridge JM, Koutsky LA. Genital human papillomavirus infection in men. *Lancet Infectious Diseases.* 2006; 6(1): 21–31.
204 Castellsague X, Bosch FX, Munoz N. The male role in cervical cancer. *Salud Publica de Mexico.* 2003; 45(suppl 3): S345–53.
205 Giuliano AR, Tortolero-Luna G, Ferrer E et al. Epidemiology of human papillomavirus infection in men, cancers other than cervical and benign conditions. *Vaccine.* 2008; 26(suppl 10): K17–28.
206 Rosenblatt C, Lucon AM, Pereyra EA et al. HPV prevalence among partners of women with cervical intraepithelial neoplasia. *International Journal of Gynaecology and Obstetrics.* 2004; 84(2): 156–61.
207 Rombaldi RL, Serafini EP, Villa LL et al. Infection with human papillomaviruses of sexual partners of women having cervical intraepithelial neoplasia. *Brazilian Journal of Medical and Biological Research.* 2006; 39(2): 177–87.
208 Nicolau SM, Camargo CG, Stavale JN et al. Human papillomavirus DNA detection in male sexual partners of women with genital human papillomavirus infection. *Urology.* 2005; 65(2): 251–5.
209 Bleeker MC, Hogewoning CJ, Van Den Brule AJ et al. Penile lesions and human papillomavirus in male sexual partners of women with cervical intraepithelial neoplasia. *Journal of the American Academy of Dermatology.* 2002; 47(3): 351–7.
210 Taner MZ, Taskiran C, Onan MA et al. Genital human papillomavirus infection in the male sexual partners of women with isolated vulvar lesions. *International Journal of Gynecological Cancer.* 2006; 16(2): 791–4.
211 Bleeker MC, Snijders PF, Voorhorst FJ et al. Flat penile lesions: the infectious "invisible" link in the transmission of human papillomavirus. *International Journal of Cancer.* 2006; 119(11): 2505–12.
212 Castellsague X, Bosch FX, Munoz N et al. Male circumcision, penile human papillomavirus infection, and cervical cancer in female partners. *New England Journal of Medicine.* 2002; 346(15): 1105–12.
213 Dunne EF, Nielson CM, Stone KM et al. Prevalence of HPV infection among men: a systematic review of the literature. *Journal of Infectious Diseases.* 2006; 194(8): 1044–57.

214 Smith JS, Moses S, Hudgens MG et al. Human papillomavirus detection by penile site in young men from Kenya. *Sexually Transmitted Diseases*. 2007; 34(11): 928–34.
215 Giuliano AR, Lazcano-Ponce E, Villa LL et al. The human papillomavirus infection in men study: human papillomavirus prevalence and type distribution among men residing in Brazil, Mexico, and the United States. *Cancer Epidemiology, Biomarkers and Prevention*. 2008; 17(8): 2036–43.
216 Giuliano AR, Lu B, Nielson CM et al. Age-specific prevalence, incidence, and duration of human papillomavirus infections in a cohort of 290 US men. *Journal of Infectious Diseases*. 2008; 198(6): 827–35.
217 Nyitray A, Nielson CM, Harris RB et al. Prevalence of and risk factors for anal human papillomavirus infection in heterosexual men. *Journal of Infectious Diseases*. 2008; 197(12): 1676–84.
218 Flores R, Beibei L, Nielson C et al. Correlates of human papillomavirus viral load with infection site in asymptomatic men. *Cancer Epidemiology, Biomarkers and Prevention*. 2008; 17(12): 3573–6.
219 Kjaer SK, Munk C, Winther JF et al. Acquisition and persistence of human papillomavirus infection in younger men: a prospective follow-up study among Danish soldiers. *Cancer Epidemiology, Biomarkers and Prevention*. 2005; 14(6): 1528–33.
220 Lajous M, Mueller N, Cruz-Valdez A et al. Determinants of prevalence, acquisition, and persistence of human papillomavirus in healthy Mexican military men. *Cancer Epidemiology, Biomarkers and Prevention*. 2005; 14(7): 1710–6.
221 Partridge JM, Koutsky LA. Genital human papillomavirus infection in men. *Lancet Infectious Diseases*. 2006; 6(1): 21–31.
222 Dunne EF, Nielson CM, Stone KM et al. Prevalence of HPV infection among men: a systematic review of the literature. *Journal of Infectious Diseases*. 2006; 194(8): 1044–57.
223 Fletcher HM, Hanchard B. Poverty eradication and decreased human papilloma virus related cancer of the penis and vulva in Jamaica. *Journal of Obstetrics and Gynaecology*. 2008; 28(3): 333–5.
224 Sirera G, Videla S, Pinol M et al. High prevalence of human papillomavirus infection in the anus, penis and mouth in HIV-positive men. *AIDS*. 2006; 20(8): 1201–4.
225 Smits PH, Bakker R, Jong E et al. High prevalence of human papillomavirus infections in urine samples from human immunodeficiency virus-infected men. *Journal of Clinical Microbiology*. 2005; 43(12): 5936–9.
226 Kreuter A, Brockmeyer NH, Hochdorfer B et al. Clinical spectrum and virologic characteristics of anal intraepithelial neoplasia in HIV infection. *Journal of the American Academy of Dermatology*. 2005; 52(4): 603–8.
227 van der Snoek EM, Niesters HG, Mulder PG et al. Human papillomavirus infection in men who have sex with men participating in a Dutch gay-cohort study. *Sexually Transmitted Diseases*. 2003; 30(8): 639–44.
228 Partridge JM, Koutsky LA. Genital human papillomavirus infection in men. *Lancet Infectious Diseases*. 2006; 6(1): 21–31.
229 Chin-Hong PV, Vittinghoff E, Cranston RD et al. Age-Specific prevalence of anal human papillomavirus infection in HIV-negative sexually active men who have sex with men: the EXPLORE study. *Journal of Infectious Diseases*. 2004; 190(12): 2070–6.

230 Chin-Hong PV, Vittinghoff E, Cranston RD et al. Age-related prevalence of anal cancer precursors in homosexual men: the EXPLORE study. *Journal of the National Cancer Institute*. 2005; 97(12): 896–905.

231 Nielson CM, Flores R, Harris RB et al. Human papillomavirus prevalence and type distribution in male anogenital sites and semen. *Cancer Epidemiology, Biomarkers and Prevention*. 2007; 16(6): 1107–14.

232 Giuliano AR, Nielson CM, Flores R et al. The optimal anatomic sites for sampling heterosexual men for human papillomavirus (HPV) detection: the HPV detection in men study. *Journal of Infectious Diseases*. 2007; 196(8): 1146–52.

233 Dunne EF, Nielson CM, Stone KM et al. Prevalence of HPV infection among men: a systematic review of the literature. *Journal of Infectious Diseases*. 2006; 194(8): 1044–57.

234 Kubba T. Human papillomavirus vaccination in the United Kingdom: what about boys? *Reproductive Health Matters*. 2008; 16(32): 97–103.

235 Giuliano AR. Human papillomavirus vaccination in males. *Gynecologic Oncology*. 2007; 107(2 suppl 1): S24–6.

236 Joseph DA, Miller JW, Wu X et al. Understanding the burden of human papillomavirus-associated anal cancers in the US. *Cancer*. 2008; 113(suppl 10): 2892–900.

237 Steenbergen RD, de Wilde J, Wilting SM et al. HPV-mediated transformation of the anogenital tract. *Journal of Clinical Virology*. 2005; 32(suppl 1): S25–33.

238 Palefsky J. Human papillomavirus and anal neoplasia. *Current HIV/AIDS Reports*. 2008; 5(2): 78–85.

239 Nyitray A, Nielson CM, Harris RB et al. Prevalence of and risk factors for anal human papillomavirus infection in heterosexual men. *Journal of Infectious Diseases*. 2008; 197(12): 1676–84.

240 Johnson LG, Madeleine MM, Newcomer LM et al. Anal cancer incidence and survival: the surveillance, epidemiology, and end results experience, 1973–2000. *Cancer*. 2004; 101(2): 281–8.

241 Zbar AP, Fenger C, Efron J et al. The pathology and molecular biology of anal intraepithelial neoplasia: comparisons with cervical and vulvar intraepithelial carcinoma. *International Journal of Colorectal Disease*. 2002; 17(4): 203–15.

242 Herat A, Whitfeld M, Hillman R. Anal intraepithelial neoplasia and anal cancer in dermatological practice. *Australasian Journal of Dermatology*. 2007; 48(3): 143–55.

243 Palefsky JM. Anal squamous intraepithelial lesions: relation to HIV and human papillomavirus infection. *Journal of Acquired Immune Deficiency Syndromes*. 1999; 21(suppl 1): S42–8.

244 Piketty C, Darragh TM, Heard I et al. High prevalence of anal squamous intraepithelial lesions in HIV-positive men despite the use of highly active antiretroviral therapy. *Sexually Transmitted Diseases*. 2004; 31(2): 96–9.

245 D'Souza G, Wiley DJ, Li X et al. Incidence and epidemiology of anal cancer in the multicenter AIDS cohort study. *Journal of Acquired Immune Deficiency Syndromes*. 2008; 48(4): 491–9.

246 Orlando G, Tanzi E, Beretta R et al. Human papillomavirus genotypes and anal-related lesions among HIV-1-infected men in Milan, Italy. *Journal of Acquired Immune Deficiency Syndromes*. 2008; 47(1): 129–31.

247 Moscicki AB, Schiffman M, Kjaer S et al. Updating the natural history of HPV and anogenital cancer. *Vaccine.* Chapter 5, 2006; 24(suppl 3): S3/42–51.

248 Johnson LG, Madeleine MM, Newcomer LM et al. Anal cancer incidence and survival: the surveillance, epidemiology, and end results experience, 1973–2000. *Cancer.* 2004; 101(2): 281–8.

249 Daling JR, Weiss NS, Hislop TG et al. Sexual practices, sexually transmitted diseases, and the incidence of anal cancer. *New England Journal of Medicine.* 1987; 317(16): 973–7.

250 Clark MA, Hartley A, Geh JI. Cancer of the anal canal. *Lancet Oncology.* 2004; 5(3): 149–57.

251 Chang GJ, Welton ML. Human papillomavirus, condylomata acuminata, and anal neoplasia. *Clinics in Colon and Rectal Surgery.* 2004; 17(4): 221–30.

252 Nyitray A, Nielson CM, Harris RB et al. Prevalence of and risk factors for anal human papillomavirus infection in heterosexual men. *Journal of Infectious Diseases.* 2008; 197(12): 1676–84.

253 Palefsky JM, Holly EA, Ralston ML et al. Prevalence and risk factors for anal human papillomavirus infection in human immunodeficiency virus (HIV)-positive and high-risk HIV-negative women. *Journal of Infectious Diseases.* 2001; 183(3): 383–91.

254 Nyitray A, Nielson CM, Harris RB et al. Prevalence of and risk factors for anal human papillomavirus infection in heterosexual men. *Journal of Infectious Diseases.* 2008; 197(12): 1676–84.

255 Holm R, Tanum G, Karlsen F et al. Prevalence and physical state of human papillomavirus DNA in anal carcinomas. *Modern Pathology.* 1994; 7(4): 449–53.

256 Bruland O, Fluge O, Immervoll H et al. Gene expression reveals two distinct groups of anal carcinomas with clinical implications. *British Journal of Cancer.* 2008; 98(7): 1264–73.

257 Daling JR, Madeleine MM, Johnson LG et al. Human papillomavirus, smoking, and sexual practices in the etiology of anal cancer. *Cancer.* 2004; 101(2): 270–80.

258 Steenbergen RD, de Wilde J, Wilting SM et al. HPV-mediated transformation of the anogenital tract. *Journal of Clinical Virology.* 2005; 32(suppl 1): S25–33.

259 Palefsky J, Handley J. *What Your Doctor May Not Tell You about HPV and Abnormal Pap Smears.* New York: Warner, 2002.

260 Frisch M, Fenger C, van den Brule AJ et al. Variants of squamous cell carcinoma of the anal canal and perianal skin and their relation to human papillomaviruses. *Cancer Research.* 1999; 59(3): 753–7.

261 Gervaz P, Hirschel B, Morel P. Molecular biology of squamous cell carcinoma of the anus. *British Journal of Surgery.* 2006; 93(5): 531–8.

262 Zbar AP, Fenger C, Efron J et al. The pathology and molecular biology of anal intraepithelial neoplasia: comparisons with cervical and vulvar intraepithelial carcinoma. *International Journal of Colorectal Disease.* 2002; 17(4): 203–15.

263 Chang GJ, Welton ML. Human papillomavirus, condylomata acuminata, and anal neoplasia. *Clinics in Colon and Rectal Surgery.* 2004; 17(4): 221–30.

264 Kreuter A, Brockmeyer NH, Hochdorfer B et al. Clinical spectrum and virologic characteristics of anal intraepithelial neoplasia in HIV infection. *Journal of the American Academy of Dermatology.* 2005; 52(4): 603–8.

265 Pereira A, Lacerda HR, Barros RR. Prevalence and factors associated with anal lesions mediated by human papillomavirus in men with HIV/AIDS. *International Journal of STD and AIDS*. 2008; 19(3): 192–6.
266 Orlando G, Tanzi E, Beretta R et al. Human papillomavirus genotypes and anal-related lesions among HIV-1-infected men in Milan, Italy. *Journal of Acquired Immune Deficiency Syndromes*. 2008; 47(1): 129–31.
267 Kreuter A, Brockmeyer NH, Altmeyer P et al. Anal intraepithelial neoplasia in HIV infection. *Journal of the German Society of Dermatology*. 2008; 6(11): 925–34.
268 Hessol NA, Holly EA, Efird JT et al. Anal intraepithelial neoplasia in a multisite study of HIV-infected and high-risk HIV-uninfected women. *AIDS*. 2009; 23(1): 59–70.
269 Gervaz P, Hirschel B, Morel P. Molecular biology of squamous cell carcinoma of the anus. *British Journal of Surgery*. 2006; 93(5): 531–8.
270 Zbar AP, Fenger C, Efron J et al. The pathology and molecular biology of anal intraepithelial neoplasia: comparisons with cervical and vulvar intraepithelial carcinoma. *International Journal of Colorectal Disease*. 2002; 17(4): 203–15.
271 Chin-Hong PV, Palefsky JM. Natural history and clinical management of anal human papillomavirus disease in men and women infected with human immunodeficiency virus. *Clinical Infectious Diseases*. 2002; 35(9): 1127–34.
272 Gervaz P, Hirschel B, Morel P. Molecular biology of squamous cell carcinoma of the anus. *British Journal of Surgery*. 2006; 93(5): 531–8.
273 Darragh TM. Anal cytology for anal cancer screening: is it time yet? *Diagnostic Cytopathology*. 2004; 30(6): 371–4.
274 Chiao EY, Giordano TP, Palefsky JM et al. Screening HIV-infected individuals for anal cancer precursor lesions: a systematic review. *Clinical Infectious Diseases*. 2006; 43(2): 223–33.
275 Piketty C, Darragh TM, Da Costa M et al. High prevalence of anal human papillomavirus infection and anal cancer precursors among HIV-infected persons in the absence of anal intercourse. *Annals of Internal Medicine*. 2003; 138(6): 453–9.
276 Patel HS, Silver AR, Northover JM. Anal cancer in renal transplant patients. *International Journal of Colorectal Disease*. 2007; 22(1): 1–5.
277 Adami J, Gabel H, Lindelof B et al. Cancer risk following organ transplantation: a nationwide cohort study in Sweden. *British Journal of Cancer*. 2003; 89(7): 1221–7.
278 Watson AJ, Smith BB, Whitehead MR et al. Malignant progression of anal intra-epithelial neoplasia. *ANZ Journal of Surgery*. 2006; 76(8): 715–7.
279 Scholefield JH, Castle MT, Watson NF. Malignant transformation of high-grade anal intraepithelial neoplasia. *British Journal of Surgery*. 2005; 92(9): 1133–6.
280 Drobacheff C, Dupont P, Mougin C et al. Anal human papillomavirus DNA screening by Hybrid Capture II in human immunodeficiency virus-positive patients with or without anal intercourse. *European Journal of Dermatology*. 2003; 13(4): 367–71.
281 Gervaz P, Hirschel B, Morel P. Molecular biology of squamous cell carcinoma of the anus. *British Journal of Surgery*. 2006; 93(5): 531–8.
282 Critchlow CW, Hawes SE, Kuypers JM et al. Effect of HIV infection on the natural history of anal human papillomavirus infection. *AIDS*. 1998; 12(10): 1177–84.

283 Moscicki AB, Durako SJ, Houser J et al. Human papillomavirus infection and abnormal cytology of the anus in HIV-infected and uninfected adolescents. *AIDS*. 2003; 17(3): 311–20.
284 Hernandez BY, McDuffie K, Zhu X et al. Anal human papillomavirus infection in women and its relationship with cervical infection. *Cancer Epidemiology, Biomarkers and Prevention*. 2005; 14(11 Pt 1): 2550–6.
285 Daling JR, Madeleine MM, Johnson LG et al. Human papillomavirus, smoking, and sexual practices in the etiology of anal cancer. *Cancer*. 2004; 101(2): 270–80.
286 Moscicki AB, Hills NK, Shiboski S et al. Risk factors for abnormal anal cytology in young heterosexual women. *Cancer Epidemiology, Biomarkers and Prevention*. 1999; 8(2): 173–8.
287 Critchlow CW, Hawes SE, Kuypers JM et al. Effect of HIV infection on the natural history of anal human papillomavirus infection. *AIDS*. 1998; 12(10): 1177–84.
288 Tsen HF, Morgenstern H, Mack T et al. Risk factors for penile cancer: results of a population-based case-control study in Los Angeles County (United States). *Cancer Causes and Control*. 2001; 12(3): 267–77.
289 Daling JR, Madeleine MM, Johnson LG et al. Human papillomavirus, smoking, and sexual practices in the etiology of anal cancer. *Cancer*. 2004; 101(2): 270–80.
290 Chang GJ, Welton ML. Human papillomavirus, condylomata acuminata, and anal neoplasia. *Clinics in Colon and Rectal Surgery*. 2004; 17(4): 221–30.
291 Edgren G, Sparen P. Risk of anogenital cancer after diagnosis of cervical intraepithelial neoplasia: a prospective population-based study. *Lancet Oncology*. 2007; 8(4): 311–6.
292 Nahas CS, Lin O, Weiser MR et al. Prevalence of perianal intraepithelial neoplasia in HIV-infected patients referred for high-resolution anoscopy. *Diseases of the Colon and Rectum*. 2006; 49(10): 1581–6.
293 Chaiyachati K, Cinti SK, Kauffman CA et al. HIV-infected patients with anal carcinoma who subsequently developed oral squamous cell carcinoma: report of 2 cases. *Journal of the International Association of Physicians in AIDS Care*. 2008; 7(6): 306–10.
294 Krueger H, McLean D, Williams D. *The Prevention of Second Primary Cancers*. Basel: Karger, 2008.
295 Balamurugan A, Ahmed F, Saraiya M et al. Potential role of human papillomavirus in the development of subsequent primary in situ and invasive cancers among cervical cancer survivors. *Cancer*. 2008; 113(suppl 10): 2919–25.
296 Krueger H, McLean D, Williams D. *The Prevention of Second Primary Cancers*. Basel: Karger, 2008.
297 Chaturvedi AK, Engels EA, Gilbert ES et al. Second cancers among 104,760 survivors of cervical cancer: evaluation of long-term risk. *Journal of the National Cancer Institute*. 2007; 99(21): 1634–43.
298 Schockaert S, Poppe W, Arbyn M et al. Incidence of vaginal intraepithelial neoplasia after hysterectomy for cervical intraepithelial neoplasia: a retrospective study. *American Journal of Obstetrics and Gynecology*. 2008; 199(2): 113 e1–5.
299 Gonzalez Bosquet E, Torres A, Busquets M et al. Prognostic factors for the development of vaginal intraepithelial neoplasia. *European Journal of Gynaecological Oncology*. 2008; 29(1): 43–5.

300 Hampl M, Wentzensen N, Vinokurova S et al. Comprehensive analysis of 130 multicentric intraepithelial female lower genital tract lesions by HPV typing and p16 expression profile. *Journal of Cancer Research and Clinical Oncology.* 2007; 133(4): 235–45.

301 Hemminki K, Dong C, Vaittinen P. Second primary cancer after in situ and invasive cervical cancer. *Epidemiology.* 2000; 11(4): 457–61.

302 Evans HS, Newnham A, Hodgson SV et al. Second primary cancers after cervical intraepithelial neoplasia III and invasive cervical cancer in Southeast England. *Gynecologic Oncology.* 2003; 90(1): 131–6.

303 Goodman MT, Shvetsov YB, McDuffie K et al. Acquisition of anal human papillomavirus (HPV) infection in women: the Hawaii HPV Cohort study. *Journal of Infectious Diseases.* 2008; 197(7): 957–66.

304 Veo CA, Saad SS, Nicolau SM et al. Study on the prevalence of human papillomavirus in the anal canal of women with cervical intraepithelial neoplasia grade III. *European Journal of Obstetrics and Gynecology and Reproductive Biology.* 2008; 140(1): 103–7.

305 Kreuter A, Brockmeyer NH, Weissenborn SJ et al. Penile intraepithelial neoplasia is frequent in HIV-positive men with anal dysplasia. *Journal of Investigative Dermatology.* 2008; 128(9): 2316–24.

306 Widschwendter A, Brunhuber T, Wiedemair A et al. Detection of human papillomavirus DNA in breast cancer of patients with cervical cancer history. *Journal of Clinical Virology.* 2004; 31(4): 292–7.

307 Hennig EM, Nesland JM, Di Lonardo A et al. Multiple primary cancers and HPV infection: are they related? *Journal of Experimental and Clinical Cancer Research.* 1999; 18(1): 53–4.

308 Rose Ragin CC, Taioli E. Second primary head and neck tumor risk in patients with cervical cancer—SEER data analysis. *Head and Neck.* 2008; 30(1): 58–66.

309 Georgieva S, Iordanov V. A woman with synchronous cervical, vaginal and laryngeal squamous cell carcinomas and positive human papillomavirus type 16; case presentation with literature review. *Journal of the Balkan Union of Oncology.* 2008; 13(1): 109–12.

310 Matsukura T, Sugase M. Pitfalls in the epidemiologic classification of human papillomavirus types associated with cervical cancer using polymerase chain reaction: driver and passenger. *International Journal of Gynecologic Cancer.* 2008; 18(5): 1042–50.

311 Giatromanolaki A, Sivridis E, Papazoglou D et al. Human papillomavirus in endometrial adenocarcinomas: infectious agent or a mere "passenger"? *Infectious Diseases in Obstetrics and Gynecology.* 2007; 2007: 60549.

312 Psyrri A, DiMaio D. Human papillomavirus in cervical and head-and-neck cancer. *Nature Clinical Practice Oncology.* 2008; 5(1): 24–31.

313 Applebaum KM, Furniss CS, Zeka A et al. Lack of association of alcohol and tobacco with HPV16-associated head and neck cancer. *Journal of the National Cancer Institute.* 2007; 99(23): 1801–10.

314 Gillison ML, Shah KV. Role of mucosal human papillomavirus in nongenital cancers. *Journal of the National Cancer Institute Monographs.* Chapter 9, 2003; (31): 57–65.

315 Hobbs CG, Sterne JA, Bailey M et al. Human papillomavirus and head and neck cancer: a systematic review and meta-analysis. *Clinical Otolaryngology.* 2006; 31(4): 259–66.

316 Haddad RI, Shin DM. Recent advances in head and neck cancer. *New England Journal of Medicine.* 2008; 359(11): 1143–54.
317 Venuti A, Manni V, Morello R et al. Physical state and expression of human papillomavirus in laryngeal carcinoma and surrounding normal mucosa. *Journal of Medical Virology.* 2000; 60(4): 396–402.
318 Boy S, Van Rensburg EJ, Engelbrecht S et al. HPV detection in primary intraoral squamous cell carcinomas—commensal, aetiological agent or contamination? *Journal of Oral Pathology and Medicine.* 2006; 35(2): 86–90.
319 Fakhry C, Gillison ML. Clinical implications of human papillomavirus in head and neck cancers. *Journal of Clinical Oncology.* 2006; 24(17): 2606–11.
320 Kreimer AR, Clifford GM, Boyle P et al. Human papillomavirus types in head and neck squamous cell carcinomas worldwide: a systematic review. *Cancer Epidemiology, Biomarkers and Prevention.* 2005; 14(2): 467–75.
321 Syrjanen S. Human papillomaviruses in head and neck carcinomas. *New England Journal of Medicine.* 2007; 356(19): 1993–5.
322 Devaraj K, Gillison ML, Wu TC. Development of HPV vaccines for HPV-associated head and neck squamous cell carcinoma. *Critical Reviews in Oral Biology and Medicine.* 2003; 14(5): 345–62.
323 Furniss CS, McClean MD, Smith JF et al. Human papillomavirus 6 seropositivity is associated with risk of head and neck squamous cell carcinoma, independent of tobacco and alcohol use. *Annals of Oncology.* 2009; 20(3): 534–41.
324 De Petrini M, Ritta M, Schena M et al. Head and neck squamous cell carcinoma: role of the human papillomavirus in tumour progression. *New Microbiologica.* 2006; 29(1): 25–33.
325 Ragin CC, Taioli E. Survival of squamous cell carcinoma of the head and neck in relation to human papillomavirus infection: review and meta-analysis. *International Journal of Cancer.* 2007; 121(8): 1813–20.
326 Fakhry C, Westra WH, Li S et al. Improved survival of patients with human papillomavirus-positive head and neck squamous cell carcinoma in a prospective clinical trial. *Journal of the National Cancer Institute.* 2008; 100(4): 261–9.
327 Armas GL, Su CY, Huang CC et al. The impact of virus in N3 node dissection for head and neck cancer. *European Archives of Oto-Rhino-Laryngology.* 2008; 265(11): 1379–84.
328 Zhang MQ, El-Mofty SK, Davila RM. Detection of human papillomavirus-related squamous cell carcinoma cytologically and by in situ hybridization in fine-needle aspiration biopsies of cervical metastasis: a tool for identifying the site of an occult head and neck primary. *Cancer.* 2008; 114(2): 118–23.
329 Braakhuis BJ, Snijders PJ, Keune WJ et al. Genetic patterns in head and neck cancers that contain or lack transcriptionally active human papillomavirus. *Journal of the National Cancer Institute.* 2004; 96(13): 998–1006.
330 Smith EM, Wang D, Kim Y et al. p16(INK4a) Expression, human papillomavirus, and survival in head and neck cancer. *Oral Oncology.* 2008; 44(2): 133–42.
331 Begum S, Westra WH. Basaloid squamous cell carcinoma of the head and neck is a mixed variant that can be further resolved by HPV status. *American Journal of Surgical Pathology.* 2008; 32(7): 1044–50.
332 Ritta M, De Andrea M, Mondini M et al. Cell cycle and viral and immunologic profiles of head and neck squamous cell carcinoma as predictable variables of tumor progression. *Head and Neck.* 2009; 31(3): 318–27.

333 Schlecht NF, Burk RD, Adrien L et al. Gene expression profiles in HPV-infected head and neck cancer. *Journal of Pathology.* 2007; 213(3): 283–93.
334 Strati K, Lambert PF. Role of Rb-dependent and Rb-independent functions of papillomavirus E7 oncogene in head and neck cancer. *Cancer Research.* 2007; 67(24): 11585–93.
335 Westra WH, Taube JM, Poeta ML et al. Inverse relationship between human papillomavirus-16 infection and disruptive p53 gene mutations in squamous cell carcinoma of the head and neck. *Clinical Cancer Research.* 2008; 14(2): 366–9.
336 Ragin CC, Modugno F, Gollin SM. The epidemiology and risk factors of head and neck cancer: a focus on human papillomavirus. *Journal of Dental Research.* 2007; 86(2): 104–14.
337 Gillison ML, D'Souza G, Westra W et al. Distinct risk factor profiles for human papillomavirus type 16-positive and human papillomavirus type 16-negative head and neck cancers. *Journal of the National Cancer Institute.* 2008; 100(6): 407–20.
338 Underbrink MP, Hoskins SL, Pou AM et al. Viral interaction: a possible contributing factor in head and neck cancer progression. *Acta Oto-Laryngologica.* 2008; 128(12): 1361–9.
339 Pica F, Volpi A. Transmission of human herpesvirus 8: an update. *Current Opinions in Infectious Diseases.* 2007; 20(2): 152–6.
340 D'Souza G, Fakhry C, Sugar EA et al. Six-month natural history of oral versus cervical human papillomavirus infection. *International Journal of Cancer.* 2007; 121(1): 143–50.
341 Gillison ML, Shah KV. Role of mucosal human papillomavirus in nongenital cancers. *Journal of the National Cancer Institute Monographs.* Chapter 9, 2003; (31): 57–65.
342 Smith EM, Ritchie JM, Summersgill KF et al. Age, sexual behavior and human papillomavirus infection in oral cavity and oropharyngeal cancers. *International Journal of Cancer.* 2004; 108(5): 766–72.
343 Furniss CS, McClean MD, Smith JF et al. Human papillomavirus 16 and head and neck squamous cell carcinoma. *International Journal of Cancer.* 2007; 120(11): 2386–92.
344 Giraldo P, Goncalves AK, Pereira SA et al. Human papillomavirus in the oral mucosa of women with genital human papillomavirus lesions. *European Journal of Obstetrics, Gynecology, and Reproductive Biology.* 2006; 126(1): 104–6.
345 Fakhry C, D'Souza G, Sugar E et al. Relationship between prevalent oral and cervical human papillomavirus infections in human immunodeficiency virus-positive and –negative women. *Journal of Clinical Microbiology.* 2006; 44(12): 4479–85.
346 Smith EM, Ritchie JM, Yankowitz J et al. HPV prevalence and concordance in the cervix and oral cavity of pregnant women. *Infectious Diseases in Obstetrics and Gynecology.* 2004; 12(2): 45–56.
347 Rintala M, Grenman S, Puranen M et al. Natural history of oral papillomavirus infections in spouses: a prospective Finnish HPV Family Study. *Journal of Clinical Virology.* 2006; 35(1): 89–94.
348 Giraldo P, Goncalves AK, Pereira SA et al. Human papillomavirus in the oral mucosa of women with genital human papillomavirus lesions. *European Journal of Obstetrics, Gynecology, and Reproductive Biology.* 2006; 126(1): 104–6.

349 Scully C. Oral cancer; the evidence for sexual transmission. *British Dental Journal.* 2005; 199(4): 203–7.
350 Smith EM, Swarnavel S, Ritchie JM et al. Prevalence of human papillomavirus in the oral cavity/oropharynx in a large population of children and adolescents. *Pediatric Infectious Disease Journal.* 2007; 26(9): 836–40.
351 Sinal SH, Woods CR. Human papillomavirus infections of the genital and respiratory tracts in young children. *Seminars in Pediatric Infectious Diseases.* 2005; 16(4): 306–16.
352 Sinclair KA, Woods CR, Kirse DJ et al. Anogenital and respiratory tract human papillomavirus infections among children: age, gender, and potential transmission through sexual abuse. *Pediatrics.* 2005; 116(4): 815–25.
353 Powell J, Strauss S, Gray J et al. Genital carriage of human papilloma virus (HPV) DNA in prepubertal girls with and without vulval disease. *Pediatric Dermatology.* 2003; 20(3): 191–4.
354 Padayachee A. Human papillomavirus (HPV) types 2 and 57 in oral verrucae demonstrated by in situ hybridization. *Journal of Oral Pathology and Medicine.* 1994; 23(9): 413–7.
355 Handley J, Hanks E, Armstrong K et al. Common association of HPV 2 with anogenital warts in prepubertal children. *Pediatric Dermatology.* 1997; 14(5): 339–43.
356 Clavel CE, Huu VP, Durlach AP et al. Mucosal oncogenic human papillomaviruses and extragenital Bowen disease. *Cancer.* 1999; 86(2): 282–7.
357 Smith EM, Ritchie JM, Yankowitz J et al. HPV prevalence and concordance in the cervix and oral cavity of pregnant women. *Infectious Diseases in Obstetrics and Gynecology.* 2004; 12(2): 45–56. Note that precisely this sort of autoinoculation has been suggested to explain the spread of oncogenic HPV from the anogenital region to the female breast. Kan CY, Iacopetta BJ, Lawson JS et al. Identification of human papillomavirus DNA gene sequences in human breast cancer. *British Journal of Cancer.* 2005; 93(8): 946–8.
358 Herrero R, Castellsague X, Pawlita M et al. Human papillomavirus and oral cancer: the International Agency for Research on Cancer multicenter study. *Journal of the National Cancer Institute.* 2003; 95(23): 1772–83.
359 Gillison ML. Human papillomavirus-associated head and neck cancer is a distinct epidemiologic, clinical, and molecular entity. *Seminars in Oncology.* 2004; 31(6): 744–54.
360 Slebos RJ, Yi Y, Ely K et al. Gene expression differences associated with human papillomavirus status in head and neck squamous cell carcinoma. *Clinical Cancer Research.* 2006; 12(3 Pt 1): 701–9.
361 Smeets SJ, Braakhuis BJ, Abbas S et al. Genome-wide DNA copy number alterations in head and neck squamous cell carcinomas with or without oncogene-expressing human papillomavirus. *Oncogene.* 2006; 25(17): 2558–64.
362 Anderson CE, McLaren KM, Rae F et al. Human papilloma virus in squamous carcinoma of the head and neck: a study of cases in south east Scotland. *Journal of Clinical Pathology.* 2007; 60(4): 439–41.
363 Speel EJM, Claessen SHM, Hopman AHN et al. Genomic analysis of oropharyngeal squamous cell carcinomas that contain or lack oncogenic HPV-16. *Clinical Otolaryngology.* 2007; 32: 158.
364 Badaracco G, Rizzo C, Mafera B et al. Molecular analyses and prognostic relevance of HPV in head and neck tumours. *Oncology Reports.* 2007; 17(4): 931–9.

365 El-Mofty SK, Lu DW. Prevalence of high-risk human papillomavirus DNA in nonkeratinizing (cylindrical cell) carcinoma of the sinonasal tract: a distinct clinicopathologic and molecular disease entity. *American Journal of Surgical Pathology.* 2005; 29(10): 1367–72.

366 El-Mofty SK, Patil S. Human papillomavirus (HPV)-related oropharyngeal nonkeratinizing squamous cell carcinoma: characterization of a distinct phenotype. *Oral Surgery, Oral Medicine, Oral Pathology, Oral Radiology, and Endodontics.* 2006; 101(3): 339–45.

367 Umudum H, Rezanko T, Dag F et al. Human papillomavirus genome detection by in situ hybridization in fine-needle aspirates of metastatic lesions from head and neck squamous cell carcinomas. *Cancer (Cancer Cytopathology).* 2005; 105(3): 171–7.

368 Hoffmann M, Orlamunder A, Sucher J et al. HPV16 DNA in histologically confirmed tumour-free neck lymph nodes of head and neck cancers. *Anticancer Research.* 2006; 26(1B): 663–70.

369 Begum S, Gillison ML, Nicol TL et al. Detection of human papillomavirus-16 in fine-needle aspirates to determine tumor origin in patients with metastatic squamous cell carcinoma of the head and neck. *Clinical Cancer Research.* 2007; 13(4): 1186–91.

370 Hafkamp HC, Speel EJ, Haesevoets A et al. A subset of head and neck squamous cell carcinomas exhibits integration of HPV 16/18 DNA and overexpression of p16INK4A and p53 in the absence of mutations in p53 exons 5–8. *International Journal of Cancer.* 2003; 107(3): 394–400.

371 Rose B, Li W, O'Brien C. Human papillomavirus: a cause of some head and neck cancer? *Medical Journal of Australia.* 2004; 181(18): 415–6.

372 Li G, Sturgis EM. The role of human papillomavirus in squamous carcinoma of the head and neck. *Current Oncology Reports.* 2006; 8(2): 130–9.

373 Major T, Szarka K, Sziklai I et al. The characteristics of human papillomavirus DNA in head and neck cancers and papillomas. *Journal of Clinical Pathology.* 2005; 58(1): 51–5.

374 Will C, Schewe C, Petersen I. Incidence of HPV in primary and metastatic squamous cell carcinomas of the aerodigestive tract: implications for the establishment of clonal relationships. *Histopathology.* 2006; 48(5): 605–7.

375 Sugiyama M, Bhawal UK, Kawamura M et al. Human papillomavirus-16 in oral squamous cell carcinoma: clinical correlates and 5-year survival. *British Journal of Oral and Maxillofacial Surgery.* 2007; 45(2): 116–22.

376 El-Mofty SK, Patil S. Human papillomavirus (HPV)-related oropharyngeal nonkeratinizing squamous cell carcinoma: characterization of a distinct phenotype. *Oral Surgery, Oral Medicine, Oral Pathology, Oral Radiology, and Endodontics.* 2006; 101(3): 339–45.

377 Rosenquist K, Wennerberg J, Annertz K et al. Recurrence in patients with oral and oropharyngeal squamous cell carcinoma: human papillomavirus and other risk factors. *Acta Oto-laryngologica.* 2007; 127(9): 980–7.

378 Kreimer AR, Clifford GM, Snijders PJ et al. HPV16 semiquantitative viral load and serologic biomarkers in oral and oropharyngeal squamous cell carcinomas. *International Journal of Cancer.* 2005; 115(2): 329–32.

379 Rosenquist K. Risk factors in oral and oropharyngeal squamous cell carcinoma: a population-based case-control study in southern Sweden. *Swedish Dental Journal. Supplement.* 2005; (179): 1–66.

380 Hansson BG, Rosenquist K, Antonsson A et al. Strong association between infection with human papillomavirus and oral and oropharyngeal squamous cell carcinoma: a population-based case-control study in southern Sweden. *Acta Oto-laryngologica.* 2005; 125(12): 1337–44.

381 Silva CE, Silva ID, Cerri A et al. Prevalence of human papillomavirus in squamous cell carcinoma of the tongue. *Oral Surgery, Oral Medicine, Oral Pahtology, Oral Radiology and Endodontics.* 2007; 104(4): 497–500.

382 Dahlgren L, Dahlstrand HM, Lindquist D et al. Human papillomavirus is more common in base of tongue than in mobile tongue cancer and is a favorable prognostic factor in base of tongue cancer patients. *International Journal of Cancer.* 2004; 112(6): 1015–9.

383 Liang XH, Lewis J, Foote R et al. Prevalence and significance of human papillomavirus in oral tongue cancer: the Mayo Clinic experience. *Journal of Oral and Maxillofacial Surgery.* 2008; 66(9): 1875–80.

384 Siebers TJ, Merkx MA, Slootweg PJ et al. No high-risk HPV detected in SCC of the oral tongue in the absolute absence of tobacco and alcohol—a case study of seven patients. *Oral and Maxillofacial Surgery.* 2008; 12(4): 185–8.

385 Soderberg C, Perez DS, Ukpo OC et al. Differential loss of expression of common fragile site genes between oral tongue and oropharyngeal squamous cell carcinomas. *Cytogenetic and Genome Research.* 2008; 121(3–4): 201–10.

386 Ha PK, Califano JA. The role of human papillomavirus in oral carcinogenesis. *Critical Reviews in Oral Biology and Medicine.* 2004; 15(4): 188–96.

387 Herrero R, Castellsague X, Pawlita M et al. Human papillomavirus and oral cancer: the International Agency for Research on Cancer multicenter study. *Journal of the National Cancer Institute.* 2003; 95(23): 1772–83.

388 Syrjanen S. Human papillomavirus (HPV) in head and neck cancer. *Journal of Clinical Virology.* 2005; 32(suppl 1): S59–66.

389 Termine N, Panzarella V, Falaschini S et al. HPV in oral squamous cell carcinoma vs head and neck squamous cell carcinoma biopsies: a meta-analysis (1988–2007). *Annals of Oncology.* 2008; 19(10): 1681–90.

390 Anaya-Saavedra G, Ramirez-Amador V, Irigoyen-Camacho ME et al. High association of human papillomavirus infection with oral cancer: a case-control study. *Archives of Medical Research.* 2008; 39(2): 189–97.

391 Fujita S, Senba M, Kumatori A et al. Human papillomavirus infection in oral verrucous carcinoma: genotyping analysis and inverse correlation with p53 expression. *Pathobiology.* 2008; 75(4): 257–64.

392 Luo CW, Roan CH, Liu CJ. Human papillomaviruses in oral squamous cell carcinoma and pre-cancerous lesions detected by PCR-based gene-chip array. *International Journal of Oral and Maxillofacial Surgery.* 2007; 36(2): 153–8.

393 Tsantoulis PK, Kastrinakis NG, Tourvas AD et al. Advances in the biology of oral cancer. *Oral Oncology.* 2007; 43(6): 523–34.

394 Giovannelli L, Campisi G, Colella G et al. Brushing of oral mucosa for diagnosis of HPV infection in patients with potentially malignant and malignant oral lesions. *Molecular Diagnosis and Therapy.* 2006; 10(1): 49–55.

395 Furrer VE, Benitez MB, Furnes M et al. Biopsy vs. superficial scraping: detection of human papillomavirus 6, 11, 16, and 18 in potentially malignant and malignant oral lesions. *Journal of Oral Pathology and Medicine.* 2006; 35(6): 338–44.

396 Simonato LE, Garcia JF, Sundefeld ML et al. Detection of HPV in mouth floor squamous cell carcinoma and its correlation with clinicopathologic variables, risk factors and survival. *Journal of Oral Pathology and Medicine.* 2008; 37(10): 593–8.

397 da Silva CE, da Silva ID, Cerri A et al. Prevalence of human papillomavirus in squamous cell carcinoma of the tongue. *Oral Surgery, Oral Medicine, Oral Pathology, Oral Radiology and Endodontics.* 2007; 104(4): 497–500.

398 Gheit T, Vaccarella S, Schmitt M et al. Prevalence of human papillomavirus types in cervical and oral cancers in central India. *Vaccine.* 2009; 27(5): 636–9.

399 Chen X, Sturgis EM, El-Naggar AK et al. Combined effects of the p53 codon 72 and p73 G4C14-to-A4T14 polymorphisms on the risk of HPV16-associated oral cancer in never-smokers. *Carcinogenesis.* 2008; 29(11): 2120–5.

400 Soares RC, Oliveira MC, Souza LB et al. Human papillomavirus in oral squamous cells carcinoma in a population of 75 Brazilian patients. *American Journal of Otolaryngology.* 2007; 28(6): 397–400.

401 Ha PK, Pai SI, Westra WH et al. Real-time quantitative PCR demonstrates low prevalence of human papillomavirus type 16 in premalignant and malignant lesions of the oral cavity. *Clinical Cancer Research.* 2002; 8(5): 1203–9.

402 Syrjanen S. PL7 Oral viral infections that could be transmitted oro-genitally. *Oral Diseases.* 2006; 12(suppl 1): 2.

403 Volter C, He Y, Delius H et al. Novel HPV types present in oral papillomatous lesions from patients with HIV infection. *International Journal of Cancer.* 1996; 66(4): 453–6.

404 Sugiyama M, Bhawal UK, Kawamura M et al. Human papillomavirus-16 in oral squamous cell carcinoma: clinical correlates and 5-year survival. *British Journal of Oral and Maxillofacial Surgery.* 2007; 45(2): 116–22.

405 Dahlstrom KR, Adler-Storthz K, Etzel CJ et al. Human papillomavirus type 16 infection and squamous cell carcinoma of the head and neck in never-smokers: a matched pair analysis. *Clinical Cancer Research.* 2003; 9(7): 2620–6.

406 Luo CW, Roan CH, Liu CJ. Human papillomaviruses in oral squamous cell carcinoma and pre-cancerous lesions detected by PCR-based gene-chip array. *International Journal of Oral and Maxillofacial Surgery.* 2007; 36(2): 153–8.

407 Campisi G, Panzarella V, Giuliani M et al. Human papillomavirus: its identity and controversial role in oral oncogenesis, premalignant and malignant lesions (review). *International Journal of Oncology.* 2007; 30(4): 813–23.

408 Acay R, Rezende N, Fontes A et al. Human papillomavirus as a risk factor in oral carcinogenesis: a study using in situ hybridization with signal amplification. *Oral Microbiology and Immunology.* 2008; 23(4): 271–4.

409 Campisi G, Panzarella V, Giuliani M et al. Human papillomavirus: its identity and controversial role in oral oncogenesis, premalignant and malignant lesions (review). *International Journal of Oncology.* 2007; 30(4): 813–23.

410 Koyama K, Uobe K, Tanaka A. Highly sensitive detection of HPV-DNA in paraffin sections of human oral carcinomas. *Journal of Oral Pathology and Medicine.* 2007; 36(1): 18–24.

411 Balderas-Loaeza A, Anaya-Saavedra G, Ramirez-Amador VA et al. Human papillomavirus-16 DNA methylation patterns support a causal association

of the virus with oral squamous cell carcinomas. *International Journal of Cancer*. 2007; 120(10): 2165–9.
412 Rivero ER, Nunes FD. HPV in oral squamous cell carcinomas of a Brazilian population: amplification by PCR. *Brazilian Oral Research*. 2006; 20(1): 21–4.
413 Chaturvedi AK, Engels EA, Anderson WF et al. Incidence trends for human papillomavirus-related and –unrelated oral squamous cell carcinomas in the United States. *Journal of Clinical Oncology*. 2008; 26(4): 612–9.
414 Cameron JE, Hagensee ME. Oral HPV complications in HIV-infected patients. *Current HIV/AIDS Reports*. 2008; 5(3): 126–31.
415 Passmore JA, Marais DJ, Sampson C et al. Cervicovaginal, oral, and serum IgG and IgA responses to human papillomavirus type 16 in women with cervical intraepithelial neoplasia. *Journal of Medical Virology*. 2007; 79(9): 1375–80.
416 Tsantoulis PK, Kastrinakis NG, Tourvas AD et al. Advances in the biology of oral cancer. *Oral Oncology*. 2007; 43(6): 523–34.
417 Lavelle CL, Scully C. Criteria to rationalize population screening to control oral cancer. *Oral Oncology*. 2005; 41(1): 11–6.
418 Hille JJ, Webster-Cyriaque J, Palefski JM et al. Mechanisms of expression of HHV8, EBV and HPV in selected HIV-associated oral lesions. *Oral Diseases*. 2002; 8(suppl 2): 161–8.
419 Balderas-Loaeza A, Anaya-Saavedra G, Ramirez-Amador VA et al. Human papillomavirus-16 DNA methylation patterns support a causal association of the virus with oral squamous cell carcinomas. *International Journal of Cancer*. 2007; 120(10): 2165–9.
420 Kansky AA, Seme K, Maver PJ et al. Human papillomaviruses (HPV) in tissue specimens of oral squamous cell papillomas and normal oral mucosa. *Anticancer Research*. 2006; 26(4B): 3197–201.
421 Lim KP, Hamid S, Lau SH et al. HPV infection and the alterations of the pRB pathway in oral carcinogenesis. *Oncology Reports*. 2007; 17(6): 1321–6.
422 Worden FP, Ha H. Controversies in the management of oropharynx cancer. *Journal of the National Comprehensive Cancer Network*. 2008; 6(7): 707–14.
423 Klozar J, Kratochvil V, Salakova M et al. HPV status and regional metastasis in the prognosis of oral and oropharyngeal cancer. *European Archives of Oto-Rhino-Laryngology*. 2008; 265(suppl 1): S75–82.
424 Worden FP, Ha H. Controversies in the management of oropharynx cancer. *Journal of the National Comprehensive Cancer Network*. 2008; 6(7): 707–14.
425 Ryerson AB, Peters ES, Coughlin SS et al. Burden of potentially human papillomavirus-associated cancers of the oropharynx and oral cavity in the US, 1998–2003. *Cancer*. 2008; 113(suppl 10): 2901–9.
426 Ernster JA, Sciotto CG, O'Brien MM et al. Rising incidence of oropharyngeal cancer and the role of oncogenic human papilloma virus. *Laryngoscope*. 2007; 117(12): 2115–28.
427 Sturgis EM, Cinciripini PM. Trends in head and neck cancer incidence in relation to smoking prevalence: an emerging epidemic of human papillomavirus-associated cancers? *Cancer*. 2007; 110(7): 1429–35.
428 Pintos J, Black MJ, Sadeghi N et al. Human papillomavirus infection and oral cancer: a case-control study in Montreal, Canada. *Oral Oncology*. 2008; 44(3): 242–50.

429 Ji X, Neumann AS, Sturgis EM et al. p53 codon 72 polymorphism associated with risk of human papillomavirus-associated squamous cell carcinoma of the oropharynx in never-smokers. *Carcinogenesis.* 2008; 29(4): 875–9.
430 Chen X, Sturgis EM, Etzel CJ et al. p73 G4C14-to-A4T14 polymorphism and risk of human papillomavirus-associated squamous cell carcinoma of the oropharynx in never smokers and never drinkers. *Cancer.* 2008; 113(12): 3307–14.
431 Psyrri A, Prezas L, Burtness B. Oropharyngeal cancer. *Clinical Advances in Hematology and Oncology.* 2008; 6(8): 604–12.
432 Romanitan M, Nasman A, Ramqvist T et al. Human papillomavirus frequency in oral and oropharyngeal cancer in Greece. *Anticancer Research.* 2008; 28(4B): 2077–80.
433 Closmann JJ. The human papilloma virus, the vaccines, and oral and oropharyngeal squamous cell carcinoma: what every dentist should know. *General Dentistry.* 2007; 55(3): 252–4.
434 Andrews E, Seaman WT, Webster-Cyriaque J. Oropharyngeal carcinoma in non-smokers and non-drinkers: a role for HPV. *Oral Oncology.* 2009; 45(6): 486–91.
435 Tran N, Rose BR, O'Brien CJ. Role of human papillomavirus in the etiology of head and neck cancer. *Head and Neck.* 2007; 29(1): 64–70.
436 Chen R, Aaltonen LM, Vaheri A. Human papillomavirus type 16 in head and neck carcinogenesis. *Reviews in Medical Virology.* 2005; 15(6): 351–63.
437 Frisch M, Biggar RJ. Aetiological parallel between tonsillar and anogenital squamous-cell carcinomas. *The Lancet.* 1999; 354(9188): 1442–3.
438 Hemminki K, Dong C, Frisch M. Tonsillar and other upper aerodigestive tract cancers among cervical cancer patients and their husbands. *European Journal of Cancer Prevention.* 2000; 9(6): 433–7.
439 Syrjanen S. HPV infections and tonsillar carcinoma. *Journal of Clinical Pathology.* 2004; 57(5): 449–55.
440 Dahlstrand HM, Dalianis T. Presence and influence of human papillomaviruses (HPV) in tonsillar cancer. *Advances in Cancer Research.* 2005; 93: 59–89.
441 Venuti A, Badaracco G, Rizzo C et al. Presence of HPV in head and neck tumours: high prevalence in tonsillar localization. *Journal of Experimental and Clinical Cancer Research.* 2004; 23(4): 561–6.
442 Puscas L. The role of human papilloma virus infection in the etiology of oropharyngeal carcinoma. *Current Opinion in Otolaryngology and Head and Neck Surgery.* 2005; 13(4): 212–6.
443 Kim SH, Koo BS, Kang S et al. HPV integration begins in the tonsillar crypt and leads to the alteration of p16, EGFR and c-myc during tumor formation. *International Journal of Cancer.* 2007; 120(7): 1418–25.
444 Begum S, Cao D, Gillison M et al. Tissue distribution of human papillomavirus 16 DNA integration in patients with tonsillar carcinoma. *Clinical Cancer Research.* 2005; 11(16): 5694–9.
445 Li W, Tran N, Lee SC et al. New evidence for geographic variation in the role of human papillomavirus in tonsillar carcinogenesis. *Pathology.* 2007; 39(2): 217–22.
446 Chien CY, Su CY, Fang FM et al. Lower prevalence but favorable survival for human papillomavirus-related squamous cell carcinoma of tonsil in Taiwan. *Oral Oncology.* 2008; 44(2): 174–9.

447 Shiboski CH, Schmidt BL, Jordan RC. Tongue and tonsil carcinoma: increasing trends in the U.S. population ages 20–44 years. *Cancer.* 2005; 103(9): 1843–9.
448 Golas SM. Trends in palatine tonsillar cancer incidence and mortality rates in the United States. *Community Dentistry and Oral Epidemiology.* 2007; 35(2): 98–108.
449 Hammarstedt L, Dahlstrand H, Lindquist D et al. The incidence of tonsillar cancer in Sweden is increasing. *Acta Oto-laryngologica.* 2007; 127(9): 988–92.
450 Hammarstedt L, Lindquist D, Dahlstrand H et al. Human papillomavirus as a risk factor for the increase in incidence of tonsillar cancer. *International Journal of Cancer.* 2006; 119(11): 2620–3.
451 El-Mofty SK, Lu DW. Prevalence of human papillomavirus type 16 DNA in squamous cell carcinoma of the palatine tonsil, and not the oral cavity, in young patients: a distinct clinicopathologic and molecular disease entity. *American Journal of Surgical Pathology.* 2003; 27(11): 1463–70.
452 Dahlgren L, Mellin H, Wangsa D et al. Comparative genomic hybridization analysis of tonsillar cancer reveals a different pattern of genomic imbalances in human papillomavirus-positive and –negative tumors. *International Journal of Cancer.* 2003; 107(2): 244–9.
453 Klussmann JP, Weissenborn SJ, Wieland U et al. Human papillomavirus-positive tonsillar carcinomas: a different tumor entity? *Medical Microbiology and Immunology.* 2003; 192(3): 129–32.
454 D'Souza G, Kreimer AR, Viscidi R et al. Case-control study of human papillomavirus and oropharyngeal cancer. *New England Journal of Medicine.* 2007; 356(19): 1944–56.
455 El-Mofty SK, Patil S. Human papillomavirus (HPV)-related oropharyngeal nonkeratinizing squamous cell carcinoma: characterization of a distinct phenotype. *Oral Surgery, Oral Medicine, Oral Pathology, Oral Radiology, and Endodontics.* 2006; 101(3): 339–45.
456 Hafkamp HC, Manni JJ, Haesevoets A et al. Marked differences in survival rate between smokers and nonsmokers with HPV 16-associated tonsillar carcinomas. *International Journal of Cancer.* 2008; 122(12): 2656–64.
457 Chien CY, Su CY, Fang FM et al. Lower prevalence but favorable survival for human papillomavirus-related squamous cell carcinoma of tonsil in Taiwan. *Oral Oncology.* 2008; 44(2): 174–9.
458 Charfi L, Jouffroy T, de Cremoux P et al. Two types of squamous cell carcinoma of the palatine tonsil characterized by distinct etiology, molecular features and outcome. *Cancer Letters.* 2008; 260(1–2): 72–8.
459 Weinberger PM, Yu Z, Haffty BG et al. Molecular classification identifies a subset of human papillomavirus-associated oropharyngeal cancers with favorable prognosis. *Journal of Clinical Oncology.* 2006; 24(5): 736–47.
460 Wittekindt C, Gultekin E, Weissenborn SJ et al. Expression of p16 protein is associated with human papillomavirus status in tonsillar carcinomas and has implications on survival. *Advances in Otorhinolaryngology.* 2005; 62: 72–80.
461 Li W, Thompson CH, O'Brien CJ et al. Human papillomavirus positivity predicts favourable outcome for squamous carcinoma of the tonsil. *International Journal of Cancer.* 2003; 106(4): 553–8.

462 Cohen MA, Basha SR, Reichenbach DK et al. Increased viral load correlates with improved survival in HPV-16-associated tonsil carcinoma patients. *Acta Oto-Laryngologica*. 2008; 128(5): 583–9.

463 Rosenquist K, Wennerberg J, Annertz K et al. Recurrence in patients with oral and oropharyngeal squamous cell carcinoma: human papillomavirus and other risk factors. *Acta Oto-laryngologica*. 2007; 127(9): 980–7.

464 Licitra L, Perrone F, Bossi P et al. High-risk human papillomavirus affects prognosis in patients with surgically treated oropharyngeal squamous cell carcinoma. *Journal of Clinical Oncology*. 2006; 24(36): 5630–6.

465 Chung YL, Lee MY, Horng CF et al. Use of combined molecular biomarkers for prediction of clinical outcomes in locally advanced tonsillar cancers treated with chemoradiotherapy alone. *Head and Neck*. 2009; 31(1): 9–20.

466 Hashibe M, Brennan P, Benhamou S et al. Alcohol drinking in never users of tobacco, cigarette smoking in never drinkers, and the risk of head and neck cancer: pooled analysis in the International Head and Neck Cancer Epidemiology Consortium. *Journal of the National Cancer Institute*. 2007; 99(10): 777–89.

467 Ragin CC, Modugno F, Gollin SM. The epidemiology and risk factors of head and neck cancer: a focus on human papillomavirus. *Journal of Dental Research*. 2007; 86(2): 104–14.

468 Perrone F, Mariani L, Pastore E et al. p53 codon 72 polymorphisms in human papillomavirus-negative and human papillomavirus-positive squamous cell carcinomas of the oropharynx. *Cancer*. 2007; 109(12): 2461–5.

469 Na, II, Kang HJ, Cho SY et al. EGFR mutations and human papillomavirus in squamous cell carcinoma of tongue and tonsil. *European Journal of Cancer*. 2007; 43(3): 520–6.

470 Chen R, Sehr P, Waterboer T et al. Presence of DNA of human papillomavirus 16 but no other types in tumor-free tonsillar tissue. *Journal of Clinical Microbiology*. 2005; 43(3): 1408–10.

471 do Sacramento PR, Babeto E, Colombo J et al. The prevalence of human papillomavirus in the oropharynx in healthy individuals in a Brazilian population. *Journal of Medical Virology*. 2006; 78(5): 614–8.

472 Mammas IN, Sourvinos G, Michael C et al. Human papilloma virus in hyperplastic tonsillar and adenoid tissues in children. *Pediatric Infectious Disease Journal*. 2006; 25(12): 1158–62.

473 Syrjanen S. HPV infections and tonsillar carcinoma. *Journal of Clinical Pathology*. 2004; 57(5): 449–55.

474 D'Souza G, Kreimer AR, Viscidi R et al. Case-control study of human papillomavirus and oropharyngeal cancer. *New England Journal of Medicine*. 2007; 356(19): 1944–56.

475 Hammarstedt L, Lindquist D, Dahlstrand H et al. Human papillomavirus as a risk factor for the increase in incidence of tonsillar cancer. *International Journal of Cancer*. 2006; 119(11): 2620–3.

476 Dahlstrand HM, Dalianis T. Presence and influence of human papillomaviruses (HPV) in tonsillar cancer. *Advances in Cancer Research*. 2005; 93: 59–89.

477 Sturgis EM, Cinciripini PM. Trends in head and neck cancer incidence in relation to smoking prevalence: an emerging epidemic of human papillomavirus-associated cancers? *Cancer*. 2007; 110(7): 1429–35.

478 Aaltonen LM, Rihkanen H, Vaheri A. Human papillomavirus in larynx. *Laryngoscope*. 2002; 112(4): 700–7.
479 Torrente MC, Ampuero S, Abud M et al. Molecular detection and typing of human papillomavirus in laryngeal carcinoma specimens. *Acta Oto-Laryngologica*. 2005; 125(8): 888–93.
480 Manjarrez ME, Ocadiz R, Valle L et al. Detection of human papillomavirus and relevant tumor suppressors and oncoproteins in laryngeal tumors. *Clinical Cancer Research*. 2006; 12(23): 6946–51.
481 de Oliveira DE, Bacchi MM, Macarenco RS et al. Human papillomavirus and Epstein-Barr virus infection, p53 expression, and cellular proliferation in laryngeal carcinoma. *American Journal of Clinical Pathology*. 2006; 126(2): 284–93.
482 Hobbs CG, Sterne JA, Bailey M et al. Human papillomavirus and head and neck cancer: a systematic review and meta-analysis. *Clinical Otolaryngology*. 2006; 31(4): 259–66.
483 Rees L, Birchall M, Bailey M et al. A systematic review of case-control studies of human papillomavirus infection in laryngeal squamous cell carcinoma. *Clinical Otolaryngology and Allied Sciences*. 2004; 29(4): 301–6.
484 Torrente MC, Ampuero S, Abud M et al. Molecular detection and typing of human papillomavirus in laryngeal carcinoma specimens. *Acta Oto-Laryngologica*. 2005; 125(8): 888–93.
485 Licitra L, Bernier J, Grandi C et al. Cancer of the larynx. *Critical Reviews in Oncology / Hematology*. 2003; 47(1): 65–80.
486 Balukova OV, Shcherbak LN, Savelov NA et al. Papilloma virus infection in pretumor and tumor masses of the larynx. *Vestnik Rossiiskoi Akademii Meditsinskikh Nauk*. 2004; (12): 36–9.
487 Aaltonen LM, Rihkanen H, Vaheri A. Human papillomavirus in larynx. *Laryngoscope*. 2002; 112(4): 700–7.
488 Lele SM, Pou AM, Ventura K et al. Molecular events in the progression of recurrent respiratory papillomatosis to carcinoma. *Archives of Pathology and Laboratory Medicine*. 2002; 126(10): 1184–8.
489 Syrjanen S. Human papillomavirus (HPV) in head and neck cancer. *Journal of Clinical Virology*. 2005; 32(suppl 1): S59–66.
490 Licitra L, Bernier J, Grandi C et al. Cancer of the larynx. *Critical Reviews in Oncology / Hematology*. 2003; 47(1): 65–80.
491 Venuti A, Manni V, Morello R et al. Physical state and expression of human papillomavirus in laryngeal carcinoma and surrounding normal mucosa. *Journal of Medical Virology*. 2000; 60(4): 396–402.
492 Balukova OV, Shcherbak LN, Savelov NA et al. Papilloma virus infection in pretumor and tumor masses of the larynx. *Vestnik Rossiiskoi Akademii Meditsinskikh Nauk*. 2004; (12): 36–9.
493 Laco J, Slaninka I, Jirasek M et al. High-risk human papillomavirus infection and p16INK4a protein expression in laryngeal lesions. *Pathology, Research and Practice*. 2008; 204(8): 545–52.
494 Hobbs CG, Sterne JA, Bailey M et al. Human papillomavirus and head and neck cancer: a systematic review and meta-analysis. *Clinical Otolaryngology*. 2006; 31(4): 259–66.

495 Liu HC, Chen GG, Vlantis AC et al. Inhibition of apoptosis in human laryngeal cancer cells by E6 and E7 oncoproteins of human papillomavirus 16. *Journal of Cellular Biochemistry*. 2008; 103(4): 1125–43.

496 Venuti A, Manni V, Morello R et al. Physical state and expression of human papillomavirus in laryngeal carcinoma and surrounding normal mucosa. *Journal of Medical Virology*. 2000; 60(4): 396–402.

497 Rees L, Birchall M, Bailey M et al. A systematic review of case-control studies of human papillomavirus infection in laryngeal squamous cell carcinoma. *Clinical Otolaryngology and Allied Sciences*. 2004; 29(4): 301–6.

498 Torrente MC, Ojeda JM. Exploring the relation between human papilloma virus and larynx cancer. *Acta Oto-laryngologica*. 2007; 127(9): 900–6.

499 Syrjanen S. Human papillomavirus (HPV) in head and neck cancer. *Journal of Clinical Virology*. 2005; 32(suppl 1): S59–66.

500 El-Mofty SK, Lu DW. Prevalence of high-risk human papillomavirus DNA in nonkeratinizing (cylindrical cell) carcinoma of the sinonasal tract: a distinct clinicopathologic and molecular disease entity. *American Journal of Surgical Pathology*. 2005; 29(10): 1367–72.

501 Syrjanen KJ. HPV infections in benign and malignant sinonasal lesions. *Journal of Clinical Pathology*. 2003; 56(3): 174–81.

502 Hoffmann M, Klose N, Gottschlich S et al. Detection of human papillomavirus DNA in benign and malignant sinonasal neoplasms. *Cancer Letters*. 2006; 239(1): 64–70.

503 Katori H, Nozawat A, Tsukuda M. Relationship between p21 and p53 expression, human papilloma virus infection and malignant transformation in sinonasal-inverted papilloma. *Clinical Oncology*. 2006; 18(4): 300–5.

504 McKay SP, Gregoire L, Lonardo F et al. Human papillomavirus (HPV) transcripts in malignant inverted papilloma are from integrated HPV DNA. *Laryngoscope*. 2005; 115(8): 1428–31.

505 Katori H, Nozawa A, Tsukuda M. Markers of malignant transformation of sinonasal inverted papilloma. *European Journal of Surgical Oncology*. 2005; 31(8): 905–11.

506 Kim JY, Yoon JK, Citardi MJ et al. The prevalence of human papilloma virus infection in sinonasal inverted papilloma specimens classified by histological grade. *American Journal of Rhinology*. 2007; 21(6): 664–9.

507 Kamangar F, Qiao YL, Schiller JT et al. Human papillomavirus serology and the risk of esophageal and gastric cancers: results from a cohort in a high-risk region in China. *International Journal of Cancer*. 2006; 119(3): 579–84.

508 Yao PF, Li GC, Li J et al. Evidence of human papilloma virus infection and its epidemiology in esophageal squamous cell carcinoma. *World Journal of Gastroenterology*. 2006; 12(9): 1352–5.

509 Gao GF, Roth MJ, Wei WQ et al. No association between HPV infection and the neoplastic progression of esophageal squamous cell carcinoma: result from a cross-sectional study in a high-risk region of China. *International Journal of Cancer*. 2006; 119(6): 1354–9.

510 Souto Damin AP, Guedes Frazzon AP, de Carvalho Damin D et al. Detection of human papillomavirus DNA in squamous cell carcinoma of the esophagus by auto-nested PCR. *Diseases of the Esophagus*. 2006; 19(2): 64–8.

511 Si HX, Tsao SW, Poon CS et al. Viral load of HPV in esophageal squamous cell carcinoma. *International Journal of Cancer.* 2003; 103(4): 496–500.
512 Rai N, Jenkins GJ, McAdam E et al. Human papillomavirus infection in Barrett's oesophagus in the UK: an infrequent event. *Journal of Clinical Virology.* 2008; 43(2): 250–2.
513 Will C, Schewe C, Petersen I. Incidence of HPV in primary and metastatic squamous cell carcinomas of the aerodigestive tract: implications for the establishment of clonal relationships. *Histopathology.* 2006; 48(5): 605–7.
514 Lu XM, Monnier-Benoit S, Mo LZ et al. Human papillomavirus in esophageal squamous cell carcinoma of the high-risk Kazakh ethnic group in Xinjiang, China. *European Journal of Surgical Oncology.* 2008; 34(7): 765–70.
515 Miller BA, Davidson M, Myerson D et al. Human papillomavirus type 16 DNA in esophageal carcinomas from Alaska Natives. *International Journal of Cancer.* 1997; 71(2): 218–22.
516 Koh JS, Lee SS, Baek HJ et al. No association of high-risk human papillomavirus with esophageal squamous cell carcinomas among Koreans, as determined by polymerase chain reaction. *Diseases of the Esophagus.* 2008; 21(2): 114–7.
517 Awerkiew S, Bollschweiler E, Metzger R et al. Esophageal cancer in Germany is associated with Epstein-Barr-virus but not with papillomaviruses. *Medical Microbiology and Immunology.* 2003; 192(3): 137–40.
518 Pantelis A, Pantelis D, Ruemmele P et al. p53 Codon 72 polymorphism, loss of heterozygosity and high-risk human papillomavirus infection in a low-incidence German esophageal squamous cell carcinoma patient cohort. *Oncology Reports.* 2007; 17(5): 1243–8.
519 Far AE, Aghakhani A, Hamkar R et al. Frequency of human papillomavirus infection in oesophageal squamous cell carcinoma in Iranian patients. *Scandinavian Journal of Infectious Diseases.* 2007; 39(1): 58–62.
520 Matsha T, Donninger H, Erasmus RT et al. Expression of p53 and its homolog, p73, in HPV DNA positive oesophageal squamous cell carcinomas. *Virology.* 2007; 369(1): 182–90.
521 Dreilich M, Bergqvist M, Moberg M et al. High-risk human papilloma virus (HPV) and survival in patients with esophageal carcinoma: a pilot study. *BMC Cancer.* 2006; 6: 94.
522 Castillo A, Aguayo F, Koriyama C et al. Human papillomavirus in esophageal squamous cell carcinoma in Colombia and Chile. *World Journal of Gastroenterology.* 2006; 12(38): 6188–92.
523 Lyronis ID, Baritaki S, Bizakis I et al. K-ras mutation, HPV infection and smoking or alcohol abuse positively correlate with esophageal squamous carcinoma. *Pathology Oncology Research.* 2008; 14(3): 267–73.
524 Yang W, Zhang Y, Tian X et al. p53 Codon 72 polymorphism and the risk of esophageal squamous cell carcinoma. *Molecular Carcinogenesis.* 2008; 47(2): 100–4.
525 Shuyama K, Castillo A, Aguayo F et al. Human papillomavirus in high- and low-risk areas of oesophageal squamous cell carcinoma in China. *British Journal of Cancer.* 2007; 96(10): 1554–9.
526 Sjo NC, von Buchwald C, Cassonnet P et al. Human papillomavirus in normal conjunctival tissue and in conjunctival papilloma: types and frequencies in a large series. *British Journal of Ophthalmology.* 2007; 91(8): 1014–5.

527 Karcioglu ZA, Issa TM. Human papilloma virus in neoplastic and non-neoplastic conditions of the external eye. *British Journal of Ophthalmology.* 1997; 81(7): 595–8.
528 Nakamura Y, Mashima Y, Kameyama K et al. Detection of human papillomavirus infection in squamous tumours of the conjunctiva and lacrimal sac by immunohistochemistry, in situ hybridisation, and polymerase chain reaction. *British Journal of Ophthalmology.* 1997; 81(4): 308–13.
529 Toth J, Karcioglu ZA, Moshfeghi AA et al. The relationship between human papillomavirus and p53 gene in conjunctival squamous cell carcinoma. *Cornea.* 2000; 19(2): 159–62.
530 Basti S, Macsai MS. Ocular surface squamous neoplasia: a review. *Cornea.* 2003; 22(7): 687–704.
531 Tornesello ML, Duraturo ML, Waddell KM et al. Evaluating the role of human papillomaviruses in conjunctival neoplasia. *British Journal of Cancer.* 2006; 94(3): 446–9.
532 Reszec J, Sulkowski S. The expression of P53 protein and infection of human papilloma virus in conjunctival and eyelid neoplasms. *International Journal of Molecular Medicine.* 2005; 16(4): 559–64.
533 Ateenyi-Agaba C, Weiderpass E, Tommasino M et al. Papillomavirus infection in the conjunctiva of individuals with and without AIDS: an autopsy series from Uganda. *Cancer Letters.* 2006; 239(1): 98–102.
534 de Koning MN, Waddell K, Magyezi J et al. Genital and cutaneous human papillomavirus (HPV) types in relation to conjunctival squamous cell neoplasia: a case-control study in Uganda. *Infectious Agents and Cancer.* 2008; 3: 12.
535 Sen S, Sharma A, Panda A. Immunohistochemical localization of human papilloma virus in conjunctival neoplasias: a retrospective study. *Indian Journal of Ophthalmology.* 2007; 55(5): 361–3.
536 Scott IU, Karp CL, Nuovo GJ. Human papillomavirus 16 and 18 expression in conjunctival intraepithelial neoplasia. *Ophthalmology.* 2002; 109(3): 542–7.
537 Tulvatana W, Bhattarakosol P, Sansopha L et al. Risk factors for conjunctival squamous cell neoplasia: a matched case-control study. *British Journal of Ophthalmology.* 2003; 87(4): 396–8.
538 Nakamura Y, Mashima Y, Kameyama K et al. Detection of human papillomavirus infection in squamous tumours of the conjunctiva and lacrimal sac by immunohistochemistry, in situ hybridisation, and polymerase chain reaction. *British Journal of Ophthalmology.* 1997; 81(4): 308–13.
539 Ateenyi-Agaba C, Weiderpass E, Smet A et al. Epidermodysplasia verruciformis human papillomavirus types and carcinoma of the conjunctiva: a pilot study. *British Journal of Cancer.* 2004; 90(9): 1777–9.
540 Sjo NC, von Buchwald C, Cassonnet P et al. Human papillomavirus in normal conjunctival tissue and in conjunctival papilloma: types and frequencies in a large series. *British Journal of Ophthalmology.* 2007; 91(8): 1014–5.
541 Palazzi MA, Yunes JA, Cardinalli IA et al. Detection of oncogenic human papillomavirus in sporadic retinoblastoma. *Acta Ophthalmologica Scandinavica.* 2003; 81(4): 396–8.
542 Gillison ML, Chen R, Goshu E et al. Human retinoblastoma is not caused by known pRb-inactivating human DNA tumor viruses. *International Journal of Cancer.* 2007; 120(7): 1482–90.

543 Gerein V, Rastorguev E, Gerein J et al. Incidence, age at onset, and potential reasons of malignant transformation in recurrent respiratory papillomatosis patients: 20 years experience. *Otolaryngology—Head and Neck Surgery*. 2005; 132(3): 392–4.
544 Fakhry C, Gillison ML. Clinical implications of human papillomavirus in head and neck cancers. *Journal of Clinical Oncology*. 2006; 24(17): 2606–11.
545 Hording U, Nielsen HW, Daugaard S et al. Human papillomavirus types 11 and 16 detected in nasopharyngeal carcinomas by the polymerase chain reaction. *Laryngoscope*. 1994; 104(1 Pt 1): 99–102.
546 Krishna SM, James S, Kattoor J et al. Human papilloma virus infection in Indian nasopharyngeal carcinomas in relation to the histology of tumour. *Indian Journal of Pathology and Microbiology*. 2004; 47(2): 181–5.
547 Mirzamani N, Salehian P, Farhadi M et al. Detection of EBV and HPV in nasopharyngeal carcinoma by in situ hybridization. *Experimental and Molecular Pathology*. 2006; 81(3): 231–4.
548 Tung YC, Lin KH, Chu PY et al. Detection of human papilloma virus and Epstein-Barr virus DNA in nasopharyngeal carcinoma by polymerase chain reaction. *Kaohsiung Journal of Medical Sciences*. 1999; 15(5): 256–62.
549 Gerein V, Rastorguev E, Gerein J et al. Incidence, age at onset, and potential reasons of malignant transformation in recurrent respiratory papillomatosis patients: 20 years experience. *Otolaryngology—Head and Neck Surgery*. 2005; 132(3): 392–4.
550 Lopez-Lizarraga E, Sanchez-Corona J, Montoya-Fuentes H et al. Human papillomavirus in tonsillar and nasopharyngeal carcinoma: isolation of HPV subtype 31. *Ear, Nose, and Throat Journal*. 2000; 79(12): 942–4.
551 Syrjanen KJ. HPV infections and lung cancer. *Journal of Clinical Pathology*. 2002; 55(12): 885–91.
552 Chen YC, Chen JH, Richard K et al. Lung adenocarcinoma and human papillomavirus infection. *Cancer*. 2004; 101(6): 1428–36.
553 Park MS, Chang YS, Shin JH et al. The prevalence of human papillomavirus infection in Korean non-small cell lung cancer patients. *Yonsei Medical Journal*. 2007; 48(1): 69–77.
554 Will C, Schewe C, Petersen I. Incidence of HPV in primary and metastatic squamous cell carcinomas of the aerodigestive tract: implications for the establishment of clonal relationships. *Histopathology*. 2006; 48(5): 605–7.
555 Fei Y, Yang J, Hsieh WC et al. Different human papillomavirus 16/18 infection in Chinese non-small cell lung cancer patients living in Wuhan, China. *Japanese Journal of Clinical Oncology*. 2006; 36(5): 274–9.
556 Castillo A, Aguayo F, Koriyama C et al. Human papillomavirus in lung carcinomas among three Latin American countries. *Oncology Reports*. 2006; 15(4): 883–8.
557 Nadji SA, Mokhtari-Azad T, Mahmoodi M et al. Relationship between lung cancer and human papillomavirus in north of Iran, Mazandaran province. *Cancer Letters*. 2007; 248(1): 41–6.
558 Klein F, Kotb WF, Petersen I. Incidence of human papilloma virus in lung cancer. *Lung Cancer*. 2009; 65(1): 13–8.
559 Zhao X, Rasmussen S, Perry J et al. The human papillomavirus as a possible cause of squamous cell carcinoma: a case study with a review of the medical literature. *American Surgeon*. 2006; 72(1): 49–50.

560 Chen YC, Chen JH, Richard K et al. Lung adenocarcinoma and human papillomavirus infection. *Cancer.* 2004; 101(6): 1428–36.

561 Carlson JW, Nucci MR, Brodsky J et al. Biomarker-assisted diagnosis of ovarian, cervical and pulmonary small cell carcinomas: the role of TTF-1, WT-1 and HPV analysis. *Histopathology.* 2007; 51(3): 305–12.

562 Aguayo F, Castillo A, Koriyama C et al. Human papillomavirus-16 is integrated in lung carcinomas: a study in Chile. *British Journal of Cancer.* 2007; 97(1): 85–91.

563 Wang Y, Wang A, Jiang R et al. Human papillomavirus type 16 and 18 infection is associated with lung cancer patients from the central part of China. *Oncology Reports.* 2008; 20(2): 333–9.

564 Boscolo-Rizzo P, Da Mosto MC, Fuson R et al. HPV-16 E6 L83V variant in squamous cell carcinomas of the upper aerodigestive tract. *Journal of Cancer Research and Clinical Oncology.* 2009; 135(4): 559–66.

565 Giuliani L, Favalli C, Syrjanen K et al. Human papillomavirus infections in lung cancer. Detection of E6 and E7 transcripts and review of the literature. *Anticancer Research.* 2007; 27(4C): 2697–704.

566 Park MS, Chang YS, Shin JH et al. The prevalence of human papillomavirus infection in Korean non-small cell lung cancer patients. *Yonsei Medical Journal.* 2007; 48(1): 69–77.

567 Giuliani L, Jaxmar T, Casadio C et al. Detection of oncogenic viruses (SV40, BKV, JCV, HCMV, HPV) and p53 codon 72 polymorphism in lung carcinoma. *Lung Cancer.* 2007; 57(3): 273–81.

568 Buyru N, Altinisik J, Isin M et al. p53 codon 72 polymorphism and HPV status in lung cancer. *Medical Science Monitor.* 2008; 14(9): CR493–7.

569 Hsu NY, Cheng YW, Chan IP et al. Association between expression of human papillomavirus 16/18 E6 oncoprotein and survival in patients with stage I non-small cell lung cancer. *Oncology Reports.* 2009; 21(1): 81–7.

570 Cheng YW, Wu TC, Chen CY et al. Human telomerase reverse transcriptase activated by E6 oncoprotein is required for human papillomavirus-16/18-infected lung tumorigenesis. *Clinical Cancer Research.* 2008; 14(22): 7173–9.

571 Cheng YW, Lee H, Shiau MY et al. Human papillomavirus type 16/18 up-regulates the expression of interleukin-6 and antiapoptotic Mcl-1 in non-small cell lung cancer. *Clinical Cancer Research.* 2008; 14(15): 4705–12.

572 Jin YT, Tsai ST, Li C et al. Prevalence of human papillomavirus in middle ear carcinoma associated with chronic otitis media. *American Journal of Pathology.* 1997; 150(4): 1327–33.

573 Tsai ST, Li C, Jin YT et al. High prevalence of human papillomavirus types 16 and 18 in middle-ear carcinomas. *International Journal of Cancer.* 1997; 71(2): 208–12.

574 Wang M, Hu M, Liu C et al. The study of human papillomavirus (HPV) DNA expression in middle-ear carcinomas. *Journal of Clinical Otorhinolaryngology.* 2001; 15(7): 293–5.

575 Santos Torres Sde M, Castro TW, Bento RF et al. Middle ear papilloma. *Revista Brasileira de Otorrinolaringologia* 2007; 73(3): 431.

576 Syrjanen KJ. HPV infections in benign and malignant sinonasal lesions. *Journal of Clinical Pathology.* 2003; 56(3): 174–81.

577 Sjo NC, von Buchwald C, Cassonnet P et al. Human papillomavirus: cause of epithelial lacrimal sac neoplasia? *Acta Ophthalmologica Scandinavica.* 2007; 85(5): 551–6.

578 Buchwald C, Skoedt V, Tos M. An expansive papilloma of the nasolachrymal drainage system harbouring human papilloma virus. *Rhinology.* 1996; 34(3): 184–5.
579 Wu QJ, Guo M, Lu ZM et al. Detection of human papillomavirus-16 in ovarian malignancy. *British Journal of Cancer.* 2003; 89(4): 672–5.
580 Yang HJ, Liu VW, Tsang PC et al. Comparison of human papillomavirus DNA levels in gynecological cancers: implication for cancer development. *Tumour Biology.* 2003; 24(6): 310–6.
581 Konidaris S, Kouskouni EE, Panoskaltsis T et al. Human papillomavirus infection in malignant and benign gynaecological conditions: a study in Greek women. *Health Care for Women International.* 2007; 28(2): 182–91.
582 Quirk JT, Kupinski JM, DiCioccio RA. Analysis of ovarian tumors for the presence of human papillomavirus DNA. *Journal of Obstetrics and Gynaecology Research.* 2006; 32(2): 202–5.
583 Kuscu E, Ozdemir BH, Erkanli S et al. HPV and p53 expression in epithelial ovarian carcinoma. *European Journal of Gynaecological Oncology.* 2005; 26(6): 642–5.
584 Giordano G, D'Adda T, Gnetti L et al. Detection of human papillomavirus in organs of upper genital tract in women with cervical cancer. *International Journal of Gynecological Cancer.* 2006; 16(4): 1601–7.
585 Elishaev E, Gilks CB, Miller D et al. Synchronous and metachronous endocervical and ovarian neoplasms: evidence supporting interpretation of the ovarian neoplasms as metastatic endocervical adenocarcinomas simulating primary ovarian surface epithelial neoplasms. *American Journal of Surgical Pathology.* 2005; 29(3): 281–94.
586 O'Leary JJ, Landers RJ, Crowley M et al. Human papillomavirus and mixed epithelial tumors of the endometrium. *Human Pathology.* 1998; 29(4): 383–9.
587 Gingelmaier A, Gutsche S, Mylonas I et al. Expression of HPV, steroid receptors (ERalpha, ERbeta, PR-A and PR-B) and inhibin/activin subunits (alpha, betaA and betaB) in adenosquamous endometrial carcinoma. *Anticancer Research.* 2007; 27(4A): 2011–7.
588 Sutcliffe S, Giovannucci E, Gaydos CA et al. Plasma antibodies against Chlamydia trachomatis, human papillomavirus, and human herpesvirus type 8 in relation to prostate cancer: a prospective study. *Cancer Epidemiology, Biomarkers and Prevention.* 2007; 16(8): 1573–80.
589 Korodi Z, Dillner J, Jellum E et al. Human papillomavirus 16, 18, and 33 infections and risk of prostate cancer: a Nordic nested case-control study. *Cancer Epidemiology, Biomarkers and Prevention.* 2005; 14(12): 2952–5.
590 Leiros GJ, Galliano SR, Sember ME et al. Detection of human papillomavirus DNA and p53 codon 72 polymorphism in prostate carcinomas of patients from Argentina. *BMC Urology.* 2005; 5: 15.
591 Kong DB, Zheng XY, Xie LP et al. Is prostate cancer an HPV-associated lesion? *Medical Hypotheses.* 2009; 72(1): 101.
592 Gunter J. Genital and perianal warts: new treatment opportunities for human papillomavirus infection. *American Journal of Obstetrics and Gynecology.* 2003; 189(suppl 3): S3–11.
593 Hodges A, Talley L, Gokden N. Human Papillomavirus DNA and P16INK4A are not detected in renal tumors with immunohistochemistry and signal-amplified in situ hybridization in paraffin-embedded tissue. *Applied Immunohistochemistry and Molecular Morphology.* 2006; 14(4): 432–5.

594 Kong CS, Welton ML, Longacre TA. Role of human papillomavirus in squamous cell metaplasia-dysplasia-carcinoma of the rectum. *American Journal of Surgical Pathology.* 2007; 31(6): 919–25.

595 Damin DC, Caetano MB, Rosito MA et al. Evidence for an association of human papillomavirus infection and colorectal cancer. *European Journal of Surgical Oncology.* 2007; 33(5): 569–74.

596 Gutierrez J, Jimenez A, de Dios Luna J et al. Meta-analysis of studies analyzing the relationship between bladder cancer and infection by human papillomavirus. *Journal of Urology.* 2006; 176(6 Pt 1): 2474–81.

597 Youshya S, Purdie K, Breuer J et al. Does human papillomavirus play a role in the development of bladder transitional cell carcinoma? A comparison of PCR and immunohistochemical analysis. *Journal of Clinical Pathology.* 2005; 58(2): 207–10.

598 Barghi MR, Hajimohammadmehdiarbab A, Moghaddam SM et al. Correlation between human papillomavirus infection and bladder transitional cell carcinoma. *BMC Infectious Diseases.* 2005; 5: 102.

599 Yang H, Yang K, Khafagi A et al. Sensitive detection of human papillomavirus in cervical, head/neck, and schistosomiasis-associated bladder malignancies. *Proceedings of the National Academy of Sciences of the United States of America.* 2005; 102(21): 7683–8.

600 Helal Tel A, Fadel MT, El-Sayed NK. Human papilloma virus and p53 expression in bladder cancer in Egypt: relationship to schistosomiasis and clinicopathologic factors. *Pathology Oncology Research.* 2006; 12(3): 173–8.

601 Damin AP, Karam R, Zettler CG et al. Evidence for an association of human papillomavirus and breast carcinomas. *Breast Cancer Research and Treatment.* 2004; 84(2): 131–7.

602 Yasmeen A, Bismar TA, Kandouz M et al. E6/E7 of HPV type 16 promotes cell invasion and metastasis of human breast cancer cells. *Cell Cycle.* 2007; 6(16): 2038–42.

603 de Cremoux P, Thioux M, Lebigot I et al. No evidence of human papillomavirus DNA sequences in invasive breast carcinoma. *Breast Cancer Research and Treatment.* 2008; 109(1): 55–8.

604 Lindel K, Forster A, Altermatt HJ et al. Breast cancer and human papillomavirus (HPV) infection: no evidence of a viral etiology in a group of Swiss women. *Breast.* 2007; 16(2): 172–7.

605 Amarante MK, Watanabe MA. The possible involvement of virus in breast cancer. *Journal of Cancer Research and Clinical Oncology.* 2009; 135(3): 329–37.

606 Choi YL, Cho EY, Kim JH et al. Detection of human papillomavirus DNA by DNA chip in breast carcinomas of Korean women. *Tumour Biology.* 2007; 28(6): 327–32.

607 Kan CY, Iacopetta BJ, Lawson JS et al. Identification of human papillomavirus DNA gene sequences in human breast cancer. *British Journal of Cancer.* 2005; 93(8): 946–8.

608 de Villiers EM, Sandstrom RE, zur Hausen H et al. Presence of papillomavirus sequences in condylomatous lesions of the mamillae and in invasive carcinoma of the breast. *Breast Cancer Research.* 2005; 7(1): R1–11.

609 Widschwendter A, Brunhuber T, Wiedemair A et al. Detection of human papillomavirus DNA in breast cancer of patients with cervical cancer history. *Journal of Clinical Virology.* 2004; 31(4): 292–7.

610 Hennig EM, Suo Z, Thoresen S et al. Human papillomavirus 16 in breast cancer of women treated for high grade cervical intraepithelial neoplasia (CIN III). *Breast Cancer Research and Treatment.* 1999; 53(2): 121–35.
611 Liang W, Tian H. Hypothetic association between human papillomavirus infection and breast carcinoma. *Medical Hypotheses.* 2008; 70(2): 305–7.
612 Yasmeen A, Bismar TA, Kandouz M et al. E6/E7 of HPV type 16 promotes cell invasion and metastasis of human breast cancer cells. *Cell Cycle.* 2007; 6(16): 2038–42.
613 Shai A, Pitot HC, Lambert PF. p53 Loss synergizes with estrogen and papillomaviral oncogenes to induce cervical and breast cancers. *Cancer Research.* 2008; 68(8): 2622–31.
614 Yasmeen A, Bismar TA, Dekhil H et al. ErbB-2 receptor cooperates with E6/E7 oncoproteins of HPV type 16 in breast tumorigenesis. *Cell Cycle.* 2007; 6(23): 2939–43.
615 Subhawong AP, Subhawong T, Nassar H et al. Most basal-like breast carcinomas demonstrate the same Rb-/p16+ immunophenotype as the HPV-related poorly differentiated squamous cell carcinomas which they resemble morphologically. *American Journal of Surgical Pathology.* 2009; 33(2): 163–75.
616 Akil N, Yasmeen A, Kassab A et al. High-risk human papillomavirus infections in breast cancer in Syrian women and their association with Id-1 expression: a tissue microarray study. *British Journal of Cancer.* 2008; 99(3): 404–7.
617 Mendizabal-Ruiz AP, Morales JA, Ramirez-Jirano LJ et al. Low frequency of human papillomavirus DNA in breast cancer tissue. *Breast Cancer Research and Treatment.* 2009; 114(1): 189–94.
618 Kahn JA, Lan D, Kahn RS. Sociodemographic factors associated with high-risk human papillomavirus infection. *Obstetrics and Gynecology.* 2007; 110(1): 87–95.
619 Cazzaniga M, Gheit T, Casadio C et al. Analysis of the presence of cutaneous and mucosal papillomavirus types in ductal lavage fluid, milk and colostrum to evaluate its role in breast carcinogenesis. *Breast Cancer Research and Treatment.* 2009; 114(3): 599–605.
620 Viscidi RP, Shah KV. Cancer. A skin cancer virus? *Science.* 2008; 319(5866): 1049–50.
621 Nindl I, Rosl F. Molecular concepts of virus infections causing skin cancer in organ transplant recipients. *American Journal of Transplantation.* 2008; 8(11): 2199–204.
622 Ulrich C, Hackethal M, Meyer T et al. Skin infections in organ transplant recipients. *Journal of the German Society of Dermatology.* 2008; 6(2): 98–105.
623 Tan HH, Goh CL. Viral infections affecting the skin in organ transplant recipients: epidemiology and current management strategies. *American Journal of Clinical Dermatology.* 2006; 7(1): 13–29.
624 Molho-Pessach V, Lotem M. Viral carcinogenesis in skin cancer. *Current Problems in Dermatology.* 2007; 35: 39–51.
625 Hengge UR. Role of viruses in the development of squamous cell cancer and melanoma. *Advances in Experimental Medicine and Biology.* 2008; 624: 179–86.
626 van Seters M, ten Kate FJ, van Beurden M et al. In the absence of (early) invasive carcinoma, vulvar intraepithelial neoplasia associated with lichen

sclerosus is mainly of undifferentiated type: new insights in histology and aetiology. *Journal of Clinical Pathology.* 2007; 60(5): 504-9.
627 Kessler GM, Ackerman AB. Nomenclature for very superficial squamous cell carcinoma of the skin and of the cervix: A critique in historical perspective. *American Journal of Dermatopathology.* 2006; 28(6): 537-45.
628 The condition is known as Bowenoid papulosis.
629 Hama N, Ohtsuka T, Yamazaki S. Detection of mucosal human papilloma virus DNA in bowenoid papulosis, Bowen's disease and squamous cell carcinoma of the skin. *Journal of Dermatology.* 2006; 33(5): 331-7.
630 Nindl I, Gottschling M, Stockfleth E. Human papillomaviruses and non-melanoma skin cancer: basic virology and clinical manifestations. *Disease markers.* 2007; 23(4): 247-59.
631 Jenson AB, Geyer S, Sundberg JP et al. Human papillomavirus and skin cancer. *Journal of Investigative Dermatology.* 2001; 6(3): 203-6.
632 Akgul B, Cooke JC, Storey A. HPV-associated skin disease. *Journal of Pathology.* 2006; 208(2): 165-75.
633 Jenson AB, Geyer S, Sundberg JP et al. Human papillomavirus and skin cancer. *Journal of Investigative Dermatology.* 2001; 6(3): 203-6.
634 Alam M, Ratner D. Cutaneous squamous-cell carcinoma. *New England Journal of Medicine.* 2001; 344(13): 975-83.
635 Cassarino DS, Derienzo DP, Barr RJ. Cutaneous squamous cell carcinoma: a comprehensive clinicopathologic classification. Part one. *Journal of Cutaneous Pathology.* 2006; 33(3): 191-206.
636 Cassarino DS, Derienzo DP, Barr RJ. Cutaneous squamous cell carcinoma: a comprehensive clinicopathologic classification. Part two. *Journal of Cutaneous Pathology.* 2006; 33(4): 261-79.
637 Feltkamp MC, de Koning MN, Bavinck JN et al. Betapapillomaviruses: innocent bystanders or causes of skin cancer. *Journal of Clinical Virology.* 2008; 43(4): 353-60.
638 Chen Z, Schiffman M, Herrero R et al. Human papillomavirus (HPV) types 101 and 103 isolated from cervicovaginal cells lack an E6 open reading frame (ORF) and are related to gamma-papillomaviruses. *Virology.* 2007; 360(2): 447-53.
639 Forslund O. Genetic diversity of cutaneous human papillomaviruses. *Journal of General Virology.* 2007; 88(Pt 10): 2662-9.
640 This information is drawn from the fuller picture of HPV disease associations offered in the table appending Chapter 2.
641 Forslund O, Ly H, Reid C et al. A broad spectrum of human papillomavirus types is present in the skin of Australian patients with non-melanoma skin cancers and solar keratosis. *British Journal of Dermatology.* 2003; 149(1): 64-73.
642 Iftner A, Klug SJ, Garbe C et al. The prevalence of human papillomavirus genotypes in nonmelanoma skin cancers of nonimmunosuppressed individuals identifies high-risk genital types as possible risk factors. *Cancer Research.* 2003; 63(21): 7515-9.
643 Dell'Oste V, Azzimonti B, De Andrea M et al. High beta-HPV DNA loads and strong seroreactivity are present in epidermodysplasia verruciformis. *Journal of Investigative Dermatology.* 2009; 129(4): 1026-34.
644 Forslund O, Iftner T, Andersson K et al. Cutaneous human papillomaviruses found in sun-exposed skin: beta-papillomavirus species 2 predominates in squamous cell carcinoma. *Journal of Infectious Diseases.* 2007; 196(6): 876-83.

645 Chen AC, McMillian NA, Antonsson A. Human papillomavirus type spectrum in normal skin of individuals with or without a history of frequent sun exposure. *Journal of General Virology.* 2008; 89: 2891–97.

646 Mahe E, Bodemer C, Descamps V et al. High frequency of detection of human papillomaviruses associated with epidermodysplasia verruciformis in children with psoriasis. *British Journal of Dermatology.* 2003; 149(4): 819–25.

647 Li YH, Chen G, Dong XP et al. Detection of epidermodysplasia verruciformis-associated human papillomavirus DNA in nongenital seborrhoeic keratosis. *British Journal of Dermatology.* 2004; 151(5): 1060–5.

648 Cronin JG, Mesher D, Purdie K et al. Beta-papillomaviruses and psoriasis: an intra-patient comparison of human papillomavirus carriage in skin and hair. *British Journal of Dermatology.* 2008; 159(1): 113–9.

649 Carlson JA, Cribier B, Nuovo G et al. Epidermodysplasia verruciformis-associated and genital-mucosal high-risk human papillomavirus DNA are prevalent in nevus sebaceus of Jadassohn. *Journal of the American Academy of Dermatology.* 2008; 59(2): 279–94.

650 Nindl I, Gottschling M, Stockfleth E. Human papillomaviruses and non-melanoma skin cancer: basic virology and clinical manifestations. *Disease markers.* 2007; 23(4): 247–59.

651 Harwood CA, Surentheran T, Sasieni P et al. Increased risk of skin cancer associated with the presence of epidermodysplasia verruciformis human papillomavirus types in normal skin. *British Journal of Dermatology.* 2004; 150(5): 949–57.

652 Akgul B, Lemme W, Garcia-Escudero R et al. UV-B irradiation stimulates the promoter activity of the high-risk, cutaneous human papillomavirus 5 and 8 in primary keratinocytes. *Archives of Virology.* 2005; 150(1): 145–51.

653 Vasiljevic N, Nielsen L, Doherty G et al. Differences in transcriptional activity of cutaneous human papillomaviruses. *Virus Research.* 2008; 137(2): 213–9.

654 Patel AS, Karagas MR, Perry AE et al. Exposure profiles and human papillomavirus infection in skin cancer: an analysis of 25 genus beta-types in a population-based study. *Journal of Investigative Dermatology.* 2008; 128(12): 2888–93.

655 Forslund O, Iftner T, Andersson K et al. Cutaneous human papillomaviruses found in sun-exposed skin: beta-papillomavirus species 2 predominates in squamous cell carcinoma. *Journal of Infectious Diseases.* 2007; 196(6): 876–83.

656 Waterboer T, Abeni D, Sampogna F et al. Serological association of beta and gamma human papillomaviruses with squamous cell carcinoma of the skin. *British Journal of Dermatology.* 2008; 159(2): 457–9.

657 Asgari MM, Kiviat NB, Critchlow CW et al. Detection of human papillomavirus DNA in cutaneous squamous cell carcinoma among immunocompetent individuals. *Journal of Investigative Dermatology.* 2008; 128(6): 1409–17.

658 Kullander J, Handisurya A, Forslund O et al. Cutaneous human papillomavirus 88: remarkable differences in viral load. *International Journal of Cancer.* 2008; 122(2): 477–80.

659 Massimi P, Thomas M, Bouvard V et al. Comparative transforming potential of different human papillomaviruses associated with non-melanoma skin cancer. *Virology.* 2008; 371(2): 374–9.

660 Dang C, Koehler A, Forschner T et al. E6/E7 expression of human papillomavirus types in cutaneous squamous cell dysplasia and carcinoma in immunosuppressed organ transplant recipients. *British Journal of Dermatology*. 2006; 155(1): 129–36.

661 The table references are Luron L, Avril MF, Sarasin A et al. Prevalence of human papillomavirus in skin tumors from repair deficient xeroderma pigmentosum patients. *Cancer Letters*. 2007; 250(2): 213–9; Schaller J, Rohwedder A, Burgdorf WH et al. Identification of human papillomavirus DNA in cutaneous lesions of Cowden syndrome. *Dermatology*. 2003; 207(2): 134–40; Weber F, Fuchs PG, Pfister HJ et al. Human papillomavirus infection in Netherton's syndrome. *British Journal of Dermatology*. 2001; 144(5): 1044–9; Ochiai T, Honda A, Morishima T et al. Human papillomavirus types 16 and 39 in a vulval carcinoma occurring in a woman with Hailey-Hailey disease. *British Journal of Dermatology*. 1999; 140(3): 509–13; and Kutler DI, Wreesmann VB, Goberdhan A et al. Human papillomavirus DNA and p53 polymorphisms in squamous cell carcinomas from Fanconi anemia patients. *Journal of the National Cancer Institute*. 2003; 95(22): 1718–21.

662 Weissenborn SJ, De Koning MN, Wieland U et al. Intrafamilial transmission and family-specific spectra of cutaneous betapapillomaviruses. *Journal of Virology*. 2009; 83(2): 811–6.

663 Kusters-Vandevelde HV, de Koning MN, Melchers WJ et al. Expression of P14(Arf), P16(Ink4a) and P53 in Relation to Hpv in (Pre) Malignant Squamous Skin Tumors. *Journal of Cellular and Molecular Medicine*. 2008: Epublished ahead of print.

664 Pfister H. Human papillomavirus and skin cancer. *Journal of the National Cancer Institute Monograph*. Chapter 8, 2003; (31): 52–6.

665 Akgul B, Cooke JC, Storey A. HPV-associated skin disease. *Journal of Pathology*. 2006; 208(2): 165–75.

666 Majewski S, Jablonska S. Current views on the role of human papillomaviruses in cutaneous oncogenesis. *International Journal of Dermatology*. 2006; 45(3): 192–6.

667 Nindl I, Gottschling M, Stockfleth E. Human papillomaviruses and non-melanoma skin cancer: basic virology and clinical manifestations. *Disease markers*. 2007; 23(4): 247–59.

668 Termorshuizen F, Feltkamp MC, Struijk L et al. Sunlight exposure and (sero)prevalence of epidermodysplasia verruciformis-associated human papillomavirus. *Journal of Investigative Dermatology*. 2004; 122(6): 1456–62.

669 Simmonds M, Storey A. Identification of the regions of the HPV 5 E6 protein involved in Bak degradation and inhibition of apoptosis. *International Journal of Cancer*. 2008; 123(10): 2260–6.

670 Underbrink MP, Howie HL, Bedard KM et al. E6 proteins from multiple human betapapillomavirus types degrade Bak and protect keratinocytes from apoptosis after UVB irradiation. *Journal of Virology*. 2008; 82(21): 10408–17.

671 Gabet AS, Accardi R, Bellopede A et al. Impairment of the telomere/telomerase system and genomic instability are associated with keratinocyte immortalization induced by the skin human papillomavirus type 38. *FASEB Journal*. 2008; 22(2): 622–32.

672 Cordano P, Gillan V, Bratlie S et al. The E6E7 oncoproteins of cutaneous human papillomavirus type 38 interfere with the interferon pathway. *Virology.* 2008; 377(2): 408–18.
673 Akgul B, Ghali L, Davies D et al. HPV8 early genes modulate differentiation and cell cycle of primary human adult keratinocytes. *Experimental Dermatology.* 2007; 16(7): 590–9.
674 Orth G. Host defenses against human papillomaviruses: lessons from epidermodysplasia verruciformis. *Current Topics in Microbiology and Immunology.* 2008; 321: 59–83.
675 Patel AS, Karagas MR, Pawlita M et al. Cutaneous human papillomavirus infection, the EVER2 gene and incidence of squamous cell carcinoma: a case-control study. *International Journal of Cancer.* 2008; 122(10): 2377–9.
676 Zheng S, Adachi A, Shimizu M et al. Human papillomaviruses of the mucosal type are present in some cases of extragenital Bowen's disease. *British Journal of Dermatology.* 2005; 152(6): 1243–7.
677 Iftner A, Klug SJ, Garbe C et al. The prevalence of human papillomavirus genotypes in nonmelanoma skin cancers of nonimmunosuppressed individuals identifies high-risk genital types as possible risk factors. *Cancer Research.* 2003; 63(21): 7515–9.
678 Sun JD, Barr RJ. Papillated Bowen disease, a distinct variant. *American Journal of Dermatopathology.* 2006; 28(5): 395–8.
679 Murao K, Kubo Y, Takiwaki H et al. Bowen's disease on the sole: p16INK4a overexpression associated with human papillomavirus type 16. *British Journal of Dermatology.* 2005; 152(1): 170–3.
680 Zheng S, Adachi A, Shimizu M et al. Human papillomaviruses of the mucosal type are present in some cases of extragenital Bowen's disease. *British Journal of Dermatology.* 2005; 152(6): 1243–7.
681 Dell'oste V, Azzimonti B, Mondini M et al. Altered expression of UVB-induced cytokines in human papillomavirus-immortalized epithelial cells. *Journal of General Virology.* 2008; 89(Pt 10): 2461–6.
682 Where lesions are still prone to regression; this is a histological presentation essentially equivalent to actinic keratosis, by one definition.
683 Daher A, Simbulan-Rosenthal CM, Rosenthal DS. Apoptosis induced by ultraviolet B in HPV-immortalized human keratinocytes requires caspase-9 and is death receptor independent. *Experimental Dermatology.* 2006; 15(1): 23–34.
684 Erb P, Ji J, Kump E et al. Apoptosis and pathogenesis of melanoma and non-melanoma skin cancer. *Advances in Experimental Medicine and Biology.* 2008; 624: 283–95.
685 Mouret S, Favier A, Beani JC et al. Differential p53-mediated responses to solar-simulated radiation in human papillomavirus type 16-infected keratinocytes. *Experimental Dermatology.* 2007; 16(6): 476–84.
686 Leverrier S, Bergamaschi D, Ghali L et al. Role of HPV E6 proteins in preventing UVB-induced release of pro-apoptotic factors from the mitochondria. *Apoptosis.* 2007; 12(3): 549–60.
687 Struijk L, van der Meijden E, Kazem S et al. Specific betapapillomaviruses associated with squamous cell carcinoma of the skin inhibit UVB-induced apoptosis of primary human keratinocytes. *Journal of General Virology.* 2008; 89(Pt 9): 2303–14.

688 Karagas MR, Nelson HH, Sehr P et al. Human papillomavirus infection and incidence of squamous cell and basal cell carcinomas of the skin. *Journal of the National Cancer Institute.* 2006; 98(6): 389–95.

689 Hazard K, Karlsson A, Andersson K et al. Cutaneous human papillomaviruses persist on healthy skin. *Journal of Investigative Dermatology.* 2007; 127(1): 116–9.

690 Masini C, Fuchs PG, Gabrielli F et al. Evidence for the association of human papillomavirus infection and cutaneous squamous cell carcinoma in immunocompetent individuals. *Archives of Dermatology.* 2003; 139(7): 890–4.

691 Boxman IL, Russell A, Mulder LH et al. Case-control study in a subtropical Australian population to assess the relation between non-melanoma skin cancer and epidermodysplasia verruciformis human papillomavirus DNA in plucked eyebrow hairs. The Nambour Skin Cancer Prevention Study Group. *International Journal of Cancer.* 2000; 86(1): 118–21.

692 Ambretti S, Venturoli S, Mirasoli M et al. Assessment of the presence of mucosal human papillomaviruses in malignant melanomas using combined fluorescent in situ hybridization and chemiluminescent immunohistochemistry. *British Journal of Dermatology.* 2007; 156(1): 38–44.

693 Sterling JC. Human papillomaviruses and skin cancer. *Journal of Clinical Virology.* 2005; 32(suppl 1): S67–71.

6

HUMAN PAPILLOMAVIRUS: DETECTION OF INFECTION AND DISEASE

> In addition to testing the feasibility of various optional screening tools in early detection...[and] ongoing clinical trials with prophylactic HPV vaccines, another major focus of current HPV research includes the intense screening of new biomarkers as potential predictors of disease progression and outcome of oncogenic HPV infections.[1]

Disease prompted or promoted by HPV tends to develop slowly. The development of cancer is commonly a multistage process, and precursors of malignancies often take a long time to emerge. The benefit of a gradual natural history is that multiple opportunities are afforded for screening and intervention before HPV-related disease is fully expressed.

In this chapter, conventional screening methodologies for HPV-related disease and new detection and monitoring approaches based on HPV DNA and other biomarkers will be reviewed. In the following chapter, primary prevention approaches related to HPV will be covered.

While addressing a secondary prevention topic such as screening before dealing with primary prevention seems logically out of order, it does reflect the historical progression of interventions related to HPV. The earliest population approaches were dominated by screening programs, notably based on the well-known Pap smear (as discussed later) for the detection of cervical dysplasia now known to be caused by HPV. On the other hand, vaccination represents a more recent innovation, and one that has relevance for a wider range of HPV disease sites. Therefore, the ordering of the last two chapters on HPV—screening first and vaccination and other prevention efforts second—makes sense chronologically. It also anticipates the growing understanding of the scope of diseases caused by HPV, which has increased the demand for novel prevention efforts that go beyond Pap smears and cervical cancer. Nonetheless, it will become evident that cervical cancer continues to dominate even within the emerging story of screening and prevention, reflecting the relative importance of this disease in the world.

INTRODUCTION TO DETECTION AND SCREENING: A SUCCESS STORY

There are a number of reasons why public health leaders, clinicians, and researchers want to detect HPV infection. It is important to note that the various motivations of these domains, from population health screening to diagnostic/prognostic testing to follow-up after treatment, represent related but distinct aims. Monitoring HPV for epidemiological research purposes arguably defines a further domain in the world of viral detection.

The ultimate objective of screening for cervical cancer or other HPV-related conditions is to reduce the incidence of advanced disease and the morbidity and mortality associated with it. In general, screening has historically been accomplished by identifying the precursor lesions associated with HPV infection, which then prompts various intervention measures. There is extensive and strong evidence that the identification of abnormal or suspicious cells can be achieved by cytology-based screening programs. These efforts continue to be the foundation of global prevention efforts, despite service delivery challenges that seem to be especially relevant in resource-poor settings. Indeed, there are many countries in the world where the majority of women have never had a pelvic examination.[2]

The great majority of developed countries, including the United States and Canada, clearly promote screening for HPV-related cervical disease; but, even in these settings, real-world practice can be inconsistent. Adding to the difficulty of maintaining adequate screening programs is the lack of consensus between medical bodies on specific screening guidelines, a challenge that has only increased with the advent of new technologies.[3,4] Variation in population health practices is also a concern. For example, screening protocols differ among Canadian provinces and territories; similarly, inter- and intrastate variation in selection and use of screening guidelines has been reported in the United States.[5] Not surprisingly, the Pap smear uptake rate in the United States is lowest among women with no health insurance; on the other hand, screening rates are highest among those with private insurance.[6] Proactive campaigns among health management organizations and Medicaid may explain the counterintuitive evidence that Pap test rates in the United States are actually higher than those in Canada for all ages, that is, despite the existence of a universal health plan in Canada.[7]

Most of the cervical cancer screening in Canada is opportunistic. Recommendations exist that encourage women to have Pap smears every 1–3 years, but few population health measures are in place to ensure that these guidelines are followed. Commonly, it is up to the individual to keep track of their own records and to make efforts to update their testing. This leads to population underscreening, thereby increasing the risk of disease progression and resulting in higher societal costs for medical treatment. Some form of registry and recall system could potentially increase utilization of screening and further reduce disease incidence. It could also facilitate adequate screening among high-risk women, though such groups are sometimes difficult to contact and track. Adding to the many calls for a registry system, Franco et al. recently suggested that the advent of routine HPV-DNA testing could help to launch a program that comprehensively tracks women and their screening history over time.[8] It is not immediately clear how HPV-DNA testing, with its high false positive rate (discussed later), will provide the extra incentive needed to create a comprehensive cervical cancer surveillance program. For example, moving from the current administrative record systems maintained by Canadian provinces to a population-level HPV infection registry would require a very large infusion of new resources; a cost–benefit analysis would likely be a prerequisite for any such initiative.

As suggested earlier, cervical cancer screening based on the techniques of cytology (i.e., examination of cellular structure) has had a much longer history than the development of HPV-DNA testing, vaccination against the virus, and other prevention innovations. Despite the challenges of client uptake, this arena of public health represents a well-known "good news" story. Pap smear programs have substantially reduced the incidence of cervical cancer. One recent UK report concluded that screening prevented an epidemic that would have killed about 1 in 65 British women born since 1950. At least 100,000 women born between 1951 and 1970 have been spared premature death in that country.[9]

In Canada, the reduction in deaths due to cervical cancer is just as striking as in the UK, the United States, and elsewhere in the developed world. In recent decades, the rates of both incidence and mortality related to cervical cancer in Canada have declined steeply, as detailed in Chapter 4. The largest decrease occurred in the 1970s and early 1980s (apparently correlating with the expected latency period following the advent of screening programs).[10,11]

CERVICAL PAP SMEAR

Other than a basic gynecologic examination, the most common screening test related to cervical HPV infection is the so-called Pap smear. "Pap" is an abbreviation based on the surname of its originator, G.N. Papanicolaou.[12] He published a foundational paper in 1941 that demonstrated a correlation between cervical cancer onset and abnormalities observed microscopically in scraped cells. The eventual result of the relatively simple screening test that followed involved saving "millions of women who would otherwise discover their cancer of the cervix uteri at a noncurable stage."[13] As already noted, precursor lesions usually appear a considerable length of time before any carcinoma; thus, early detection and prompt management can lead to effective prevention of the disease. The reduced morbidity and mortality in developed countries over the past few decades may be directly attributed to the invention of the Pap smear and the development of conventional cytology programs.

Pap smears should be thought of as a screening method rather than a full diagnostic test. This means that the detection of any abnormal cells, from various types of dysplasia to cervical intraepithelial neoplasia (CIN), generally must be followed up with further tests or examinations. The aim of any follow-up is to more precisely determine whether cancer or its precursors are present or threatening to appear. Depending on additional information, an abnormal Pap smear can be managed in a variety of ways. These may include conservative monitoring over a period of months to see if the affected part of the cervix returns to a normal state, cryosurgery that freezes and destroys affected cells, or other procedures that lead to the excision of diseased tissue.

Test Accuracy

Despite the remarkable impact of Pap smears on population health, there has been steady motivation to advance the deployment of HPV-DNA testing and/or vaccination strategies. The quest for alternatives or improvements to conventional cytology is partly attributable to the false-negative rate of 5–30% found with Pap smears.[14] The relatively low sensitivity of the test contributes to the significant number of routinely screened women who still are eventually diagnosed with cervical cancer.

It is important to emphasize that such experiences do not negate the value of the Pap test. The incidence of cervical cancer is far lower in those who are regularly screened than in those who have never, or rarely, had a Pap test. In the United States, Leyden et al. found that

56% of invasive cervical cancers were due to inadequate screening, 32% due to Pap test detection failure, and 13% due to follow-up failure.[15] The pattern is very similar in Canada, where about 70–80% of women aged 18–69 years report receiving a Pap test at least once every 3 years (Figure 6.1); approximately 60% of invasive cervical cancers occur in the remaining 20–30% who do not receive adequate screening.[16] Consistent with these results, Nygard and colleagues found that inadequate screening increased the risk of invasive cervical cancer by 3.4 times among Norwegian women.[17] A recent study in Australia showed that even irregular screening can significantly reduce the risk of developing invasive cervical cancer.[18]

In addition to perceived problems with test accuracy, there are a number of specific technical issues related to Pap smears. For instance, cervical adenocarcinomas in younger women are especially hard to detect by means of conventional cytology.[19,20] This fact may account for the increased incidence for this subset of cervical cancer in the United States, Canada, and other countries in recent years.[21,22] Undetected cancer, which is the most serious sequelae of false negative results in Pap smears, has generated significant litigation and large court awards in recent decades.[23]

False-positive results with Pap smears, though occurring less frequently, are also of concern. It is true that some degree of anxiety is produced by any kind of positive medical test. In the case of Pap smears, this consequence pertains whether the positive test result is true or false. Fear and stigma are common experiences, even though, in the vast majority of cases, both HPV infection and any cellular changes resolve spontaneously. Of course, challenges related to psychosocial management of a positive screening or diagnostic result apply equally to the other HPV tests that will be introduced in this chapter.[24,25]

Innovations

Practitioners may have reached the limit of human ability to derive appropriate and reproducible information from the microscopic examination of cervical tissue; some element of subjective interpretation will always be involved, and thus some degree of potential inaccuracy. This may explain why recent technical efforts to increase the sensitivity of Pap screening have focused on the collection, handling, and processing of specimens. For example, a Cochrane review of over 40 studies confirmed that extended tip spatulas appeared to be superior for collecting samples from the cervix, especially when combined with a cytobrush.[26]

Innovations such as thin-layer or liquid-based cytology (LBC) involve collecting material with a soft brush and then rinsing it into a special fluid preservative; a thin-layer slide may then be prepared that offers several improvements in terms of the quality of examination results. This method also promises to provide useable material for any subsequent HPV DNA test or other forms of bioassay, though technical challenges still need to be overcome.[27] Some comparisons of LBC with conventional Pap have confirmed the advantages of the new technology, though not consistently across all populations.[28-30] A recent systematic review and meta-analysis raised serious questions about whether LBC is more sensitive and specific than conventional Pap smears.[31] Another important concern is that LBC is more expensive than conventional cytology and requires more highly trained laboratory staff.[32,33]

Notwithstanding the risks and consequences of false-negative test results, there may also be drawbacks to devising the "perfect" Pap smear; in short, the methodology may simply become too sophisticated or costly to deploy at a population health level, particularly in low-resource settings. There is a potential for reduced screening accessibility if the currently inexpensive Pap smear protocol becomes superseded by more specialized specimen collection and preparation, computerized rescreening, etc. The outcome may paradoxically be increased cancer incidence.[34] A crucial fact should be recalled in this context: more women experience the development of cancer because of the failure to have a regular Pap smear than because of any errors or misinterpretations in cytological testing.[35] A similar public health concern pertains to the potential for lower screening rates in a postvaccination era.

It should also be noted that the moderate physical irritation produced by the Pap smear appears to generate an immune response that itself affords some protection against cervical cancer development,[36,37] which could offer another reason to maintain conventional screening. Other methods of collecting samples for testing (e.g., urinalysis), or dependence on vaccination, would not offer this extra protective benefit.

An extended application of Pap smears has been investigated that coincides with the broader theme of this book, namely, the prevention of cancers related to infections other than HPV. Several of the microbes indirectly detectable through Pap smears have been implicated as factors or cofactors in carcinogenesis. These include *Chlamydia trachomatis* and herpes simplex viruses. At this point, Pap testing does not appear to be a strong contender as a primary screening methodology for such infections.[38] On the other hand, there may be a public health benefit in combining specialized tests for agents such as *Chlamydia* with scheduled Pap smears.[39,40] Finally, some researchers are investigating the possibility of screening for osteopenia and osteoporosis in women by means of Pap tests, based on the fact that atrophic smear patterns are correlated with these conditions.[41]

Self-collection of samples for Pap smear testing may be an attractive option in public health, especially because of its potential to improve screening rates in any population with inadequate uptake rates due to low resources or other barriers (see the following section).[42] However, as described later, most research seems to be directed toward the role of self-collection for HPV-DNA testing rather than for Pap evaluations per se.[43] The evidence for the utility of self-collection for traditional cytological analysis remains mixed.[44,45]

Cervical Cancer Screening Disparities

While both incidence and mortality rates of cervical cancer in the United States and other developed countries have decreased dramatically with the advent of Pap screening in the 1940s, the results have not been identical across groups within these countries.[46] A growing body of evidence suggests that immigrants and ethnic minorities are particularly vulnerable to disparities in screening.[47] This is a likely explanation for the fact that more than half of cervical cancer mortality occurs among foreign-born women in the United States.[48] The public health response to this situation must take into account the fact that disparities differ among immigrant populations according to country of origin, duration in the United States, and so on.[49-51]

In Canada as a whole, Pap smears have been an effective screening tool, as evidenced by the decrease in incidence and mortality rates related to cervical cancer (see Chapter 4).[52] Nonetheless, there are provinces that exhibit substandard screening levels, and no region is exempt from the challenge of improving on the current rate of women receiving regular Pap smears. Data from June 2005 show that 11.5% (1.3 million) of all women in the country between the ages of 18 and 69 have never had a Pap smear. The shortfall in screening uptake was largest for the youngest women.[53] While this may partly reflect the lower cumulative years of opportunity to be tested, another study based on 2002–2003 data confirmed that Canadian women aged 18–29 years also report the lowest rate of being screened less than 3 years ago.[54] Also of concern is the fact that women over 50 years, even though they are at the greatest risk of developing cervical cancer, have consistently demonstrated less compliance with screening guidelines than middle-aged women.[55]

Data from a number of countries demonstrate that factors other than age have an influence on screening trends. For instance, cultural and/or socioeconomic barriers to testing are thought to account for disparate cervical cancer incidence in the United States[56-60] Such barriers and related disparities seem to have been mitigated to some degree in Canada, probably due to the universal health insurance system.[61] Despite apparent improvements in prevention services to underserved groups, however, evidence of lower screening and higher disease rates does persist among low income, poorly educated, and (possibly) rural populations in various regions and in Canada as a whole.[62,63] Ethnic groups also demonstrate variation in Pap smear participation, with lower rates seen, for example, among Vancouver Chinese groups and Nova Scotian Black communities.[64,65]

The situation for Aboriginal peoples in Canada appears to be more complex. There is some evidence that Pap screening rates are lower for Aboriginal people in certain provinces.[66,67] This pattern correlates with some older evidence of higher cervical cancer incidence and mortality rates among native women (see Chapter 4).[68] For example, one study suggested the mortality rate in the past for Aboriginal women has been six times higher than that for the general population in British Columbia, though other provinces suggest more modest disparities.[69,70] It is perhaps not surprising to discover that Hislop et al. reported lower-than-average cervical cancer screening rates for Aboriginal women in all age categories in that province (albeit using data from a few years later).[71] In contrast, a 1994 study of an Inuit population in what is now Nunavut found a higher screening rate than the average seen among Quebec women.[72] This result was attributed to an organized program of tracking and recall, which may in fact be more feasible in remote communities and reserves than in large cities. The circumstantial evidence for the efficiency of mounting screening programs in close-knit communities (such as those in the north of Canada) is borne out by provincial and territorial self-reported screening data from 2002 to 2005. As Figure 6.1 demonstrates, all three northern territories in Canada (Yukon, Northwest Territory, and Nunavut) had higher screening rates than most other provinces in that country. However, further research is required to see whether apparent screening advantages in certain populations in the country have actually translated into lower rates of cervical cancer. As a counterpoint to the argument about the advantage of living in a highly bounded community, Hislop et al. observed (in their study cited earlier) that there was no clear difference in screening rates for aboriginal women living on or off reserve in British Columbia, including for those residing in downtown Vancouver.[73]

Any proven instance of underscreening is a cause for concern,[74,75] especially given that roughly half of all cervical cancer occurs in the subset of women who have not had regular Pap smears. Even making allowances for the high proportion of false negatives, the clear protective value of Pap smears as a screening modality should prompt an increased focus on reaching all groups of women with appropriate

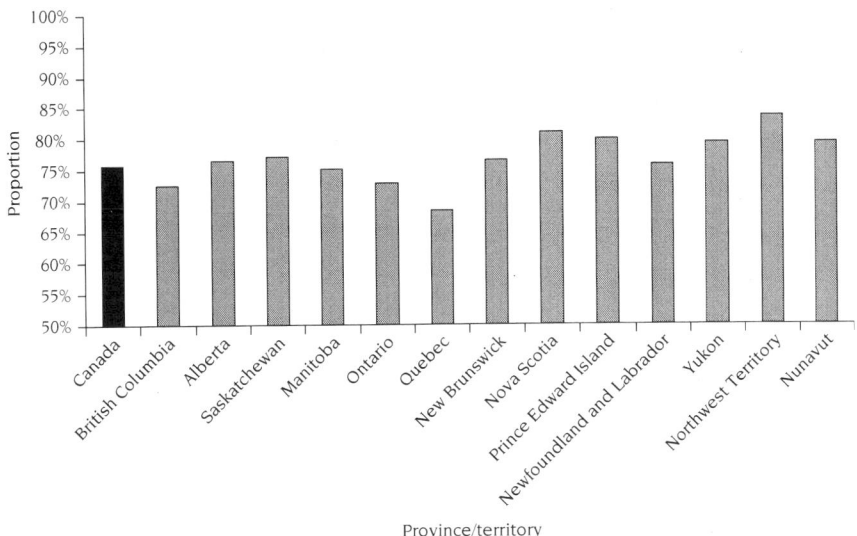

Figure 6.1. Regional variation in cervical cancer screening: proportion* of females aged 18–69 years receiving pap smears within last 3 years Cancada and its provinces and territories. *Source: Canadian Community Health Survey*, 2005. *Not age-standardized.

screening.[76] In this regard, the relevant Cochrane review identified the following potential approaches to improve screening rates[77]:

- general invitations (letters, calls, etc.), plus reminders to those overdue
- education (materials, home visits, etc.) and counseling
- risk factor assessment during other health care encounters
- economic incentives

In all, 35 studies were identified in the Cochrane review (including 27 randomized controlled trials). The only extensive and strong evidence was for invitation letters; there was also limited support for educational interventions being effective in increasing rates of screening.

As one Canadian authority remarked over 10 years ago, "if the incidence of cervical cancer is reduced, the savings in treatment and long-term care will quickly result in a net cost savings to the health care system, quite apart from preventing unnecessary suffering for hundreds of women and their families."[78] The same sort of perspective helps to explain the intense interest in an augmented prevention program involving prophylactic vaccines.

HPV-DNA TESTING

There has been considerable debate concerning the potential utility of enhancing (or even replacing) conventional cytological screening for cervical cancer with an HPV DNA test.[79] As one study noted in the context of cancers of the cervix, "the extreme rarity of HPV-negative cancers reinforces the rationale for HPV testing in addition to, or even instead of, cervical cytology in routine cervical screening."[80] However, the extra cost of HPV testing is viewed by some authorities as being prohibitive. At the same time, research has revealed favorable results for HPV testing, adding weight to any suggestions that this approach should be widely adopted in public health.[81,82] As well, pressure to consider HPV-DNA testing continues to arise in light of the perceived deficiencies of current routine screening methods. Indeed, recent studies have confirmed that HPV-DNA testing is significantly (and substantially) more sensitive for detecting high-grade CIN when compared with conventional cytology.[83] On the other hand, the test is not as specific as the Pap smear, with the resulting false positives leading to instances of overtreatment, especially in younger women.[84]

The topic of HPV-DNA testing is complicated by the multitude of technologies available and their variable applicability to viral typing. Some HPV-testing methods do not provide information on specific HPV type. Approaches that do detect high-risk or oncogenic HPV types may be of particular value in a screening program; however, cost and other issues related to the more precise technologies must be factored into the final planning equation.[85]

The World Health Organization (WHO) recently published results from a collaborative study underlining the differences between HPV tests. It recommended the creation of international guidelines and standards for HPV testing that would be similar to those created for hepatitis and other infectious agents.[86,87] The suggested development process would not be simple; it is especially complicated by the variety in HPV type distributions in different population groups around the world (see Chapter 2).[88]

In April 2005, the American College of Obstetricians and Gynecologists released a practice bulletin that acknowledged the high sensitivity of HPV-DNA testing in terms of ruling out cervical cancer. That same year the International Agency for Research on Cancer concluded that HPV-DNA testing is at least as effective as conventional cytology for detecting cervical precursor lesions.[89,90]

An ongoing Canadian trial is assessing the different findings of Pap cytology and HPV testing among nearly 10,000 women in two major cities. All women in the RCT are being screened by both methods. Data released to date show that the HPV tests resulted in a higher number of true abnormal results in all age groups when compared with Pap smears.[91] This confirms that HPV-DNA testing can feasibly identify women at high risk (i.e., those infected with oncogenic HPV types) who could then be closely monitored for dysplasia.[92,93] A trial comparing LBC with HPV testing is currently underway at the University of British Columbia, and is expected to be completed in March 2014. This study is in response to the recommendation from the Pan-Canadian Cervical Cancer Forum to establish LBC as the standard of preventive care in Canada.[94]

Essentially, if HPV is not present (as determined by a DNA test), women can be assured, with a very high degree of certainty, that they are free of cervical cancer or its precursor lesions. Driving the test in the opposite direction is when problems arise. It is challenging to decide the appropriate response when an HPV infection (even with high risk types) is detected but there is no cervical abnormality present; should such women be closely followed and perhaps even treated?[95] It is clear that the presence of HPV by itself cannot be equated with detecting cancer. For this reason, it is recommended by some researchers that HPV testing only be used in women over age 30 (i.e., 10–15 years after sexual debut) so that the many cases of HPV infection that resolve on their own are not treated unnecessarily.[96]

One proposal in the U.S. context for integrating HPV-DNA testing and Pap smears is outlined in Figure 6.2.[97]

Specific Populations

In addition to the general evidence for HPV testing, there are clinical circumstances that require special consideration. For example, HPV infection is more common in HIV-positive individuals or those who are otherwise immunosuppressed; usually the intervals between tests in such populations should be shorter than in general populations.[98]

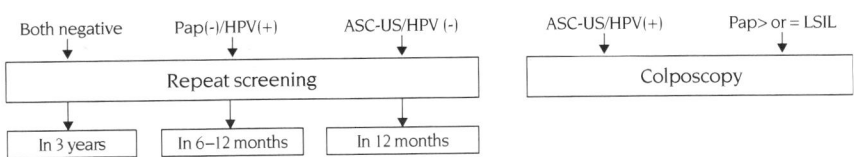

Figure 6.2. Combining results for cytology (pap smears) and HPV testing. *Source*: National Cancer Institute as adapted by Cox et al., *Obstetrical and Gynecological Survey*, 2006. Note: ASC-US = atypical squamous cells of undertermined significance; LSIL = low-grade squamous intraepithelial lesions.

These recommendations for specific target populations must be more fully researched, with any new information informing cost-effectiveness models.

Another potential application of HPV testing is rapid intermediate evaluation of treatments for precancerous lesions.[99–101] This must be contrasted with alternate approaches for tracking disease development and monitoring the effectiveness of therapies; the alternate methods essentially depend on surveillance of other biomarkers associated with the natural history of HPV infection and pathogenesis (discussed later).[102]

Despite the ongoing debate on the optimal usage of HPV-DNA testing, a survey of U.S. clinicians in 2004 found that almost all were aware of the technology, and 67% were already employing it. The data also showed that a large number of physicians had used such testing in both men and women without appropriate indications, underlining the need for improved guideline development and dissemination.[103]

Issues Related to Sample Source and Collection

Self-collection has been identified as a possible advantage of HPV-DNA testing. As the name suggests, self-collection allows women to collect their own sample and provide it to the laboratory for testing. The suggestion is that the combination of enhanced privacy and convenience could increase the number of women who participate in screening.[104,105] A 2007 Canadian meta-analysis indicated that there is little evidence supporting a self-collection strategy and further investigation was recommended.[106] A Swiss study from the same year and 2008 research among U.S. Hispanics came to the opposite conclusion, suggesting that the investigation in this area is far from complete, and that results for such maneuvers may differ among ethnic groups.[107,108]

The rate of unusable samples and overall test reliability are two of the outstanding research issues related to collection of samples.[109] The evaluation of methods to collect cervical samples has become quite technical, even reaching the level of comparing different types of sponges.[110]

Another testing methodology under consideration involves urine samples. Samples may be self-collected in private, or acquired in a clinical setting. Payan et al. found that using urine is feasible for HPV-DNA testing, and that this approach could facilitate higher screening rates in women who want to avoid invasive procedures.[111] This form of sampling also increases the appropriateness of including children and adolescents in screening; it may even make the process more appealing to men. While requiring validation in a larger population, a urine-based HPV DNA test has been shown to be effective in initial investigations.[112,113] In contrast, while HPV DNA can be detected in the peripheral blood of infected individuals, results are not consistent enough to form the basis of a screening or diagnostic strategy.[114]

Viral Load, DNA Integration, and Transcripts

Beyond identifying the presence of HPV, a quantitative analysis of the amount of viral DNA in a specimen is also potentially relevant. This measure is sometimes referred to as the viral load. Several studies in the 1990s suggested that viral load could be an important risk factor for progression from infection to cervical cancer.[115] The development of new techniques to estimate the amount of HPV in clinical samples has allowed such conclusions to be fine-tuned. For instance, high-risk HPV viral load has been found to be significantly associated with cervical cancer precursors, especially higher grade CIN and larger lesions.[116-120] This measurement approach appears to have some limitations further along the disease pathway. While the load of HPV-16 is a clear determinant for the development of invasive cervical cancer, the same relationship has not been consistently observed for other high-risk viral types.[121-126]

As was briefly described in Chapter 3, a potentially important step in HPV-related carcinogenesis is the shift of viral DNA from an episomal state to integration in the host genome. A variety of methods may be used to estimate the degree of integration, with fluorescence in situ hybridization being particularly sensitive.[127] Integration seems to be mainly a marker for high-grade dysplasia and invasive cancers, and therefore testing for the physical status of HPV DNA will not necessarily qualify as a primary prevention methodology; instead, it may find use as a predictor of potential disease development after diagnosis.[128,129] However, even as a progression marker, detecting the percentage of integrated HPV DNA in host cells appears to produce mixed results as an aid in clinical evaluations.[130-132]

An alternative to DNA assay involves the detection of transcripts (messenger RNA, or mRNA) for HPV proteins (such as E7).[133] A recent comparison of DNA-based and mRNA-based methods for the detection of high-grade CIN indicated that the transcript method demonstrated some utility but did not surpass the accuracy of DNA testing.[134] Similar to measurements of DNA integration, mRNA may be most appropriate in evaluating the risk of progression rather than in primary screening.[135]

SERUM ANTIBODY TESTING

HPV DNA can only be detected while the virus is in the host; this limits the value of such a marker in an epidemiological study that is interested in whether an infection has ever been present. Serum testing that assesses HPV infection indirectly through systemic immune markers (i.e., antibodies or other signs of immune response) sometimes offers a viable alternative to either DNA testing or examination of cytomorphology. As with any test, serum testing is not perfect, and the supporting evidence is mixed. In some instances, individuals with proven HPV-related cancer have been measured as seronegative. Conversely, the association between seropositivity and current or past HPV infection has been shown to be very high.[136-138]

Seroprevalence is not identical to positive infection status.[139] Although it demonstrates limited applicability to screening or diagnosis, serum testing is still valuable as an epidemiological research tool. For example, it could help to determine the optimal age to administer vaccinations in specific populations.[140] Using serum antibody testing to check for cumulative HPV infection rates in children is more acceptable than more invasive approaches (e.g., genital samples). Countries are utilizing this method to determine the average and the earliest age at which HPV infections appear. These sorts of data are important, as the efficacy evaluation of current HPV vaccines is directly tied to whether the vaccinated population is HPV-naive.[141] Thus, serum testing can play a role in the assessment of HPV vaccines, especially in determining the mitigating impact of any preexisting HPV antibodies.

VISUAL SCREENING AND OTHER EMERGING APPROACHES

Screening technologies continue to be developed and evaluated. This includes the use of cervical spectroscopy, which permits discrimination of low- and high-grade lesions from normal cervical tissue.[142] This technology is beginning to come on-stream, at least for secondary testing following an abnormal Pap smear.[143] The use of high-resolution photographs of the cervix (so-called cervicography) also continues to be explored.[144]

In some areas of the world, financial and other barriers stand in the way of implementing HPV-DNA testing and even Pap smears widely in the population. The cost of testing and lack of resources in the community result in many women never having a single screening test performed in their lifetime. This situation has propelled low-tech, relatively accessible approaches to screening to the center of the stage. The methods are for the most part different types of visual inspection (VI). By applying either an acetic acid solution (shorthand: VIA) or Lugol's iodine (shorthand: VILI), healthcare professionals can detect areas of abnormal tissue according to the resulting color change.[145] VI has several advantages. Highly specialized laboratory equipment and staff are not required, results are available immediately, and further treatment and diagnosis can begin at the same appointment; the latter features can be very beneficial in regions where medical treatment is normally a long journey from home.[146-148] In fact, such concerns may even be relevant in developed countries such as Canada that have remote communities.[149]

VI methods are less reliable than Pap smears in ruling out disease. Ultimately, these approaches are dependent on the skill and ability of the person performing the examination, though this same caveat applies to any screening program. Of the two well-known types, VILI has demonstrated less observer variability than VIA, but unfortunately its accuracy has traditionally been low.[150,151] Recently, a cluster-randomized trial in India demonstrated that VIA screening was an effective method to prevent cervical cancer, given good staff training and a system of quality assurance.[152] This sort of result is important for south Asia, as one-third of the world cervical cancer burden is found in India, Bangladesh, Nepal, and Sri Lanka.[153]

Summary of Screening Strategies

One of the challenges involved with comparing different approaches to detecting HPV is that innovations are being pursued across the entire spectrum of technologies. This means that any comparative study has to engage a series of moving targets. Table 6.1 offers a current snapshot of the various forms of secondary screening described in this chapter.

SCREENING AT OTHER SITES

Anal Pap Smears

Although practice and research related to Pap smears is dominated by the detection of abnormal cervical (and vaginal) cells, there are other uses for the basic collection and examination techniques in both women and men. Anal cancer is a growing concern, with incidence rising in the United States by over 95% for men and around 40% for women over the last few decades. Mixed evidence has been generated concerning the effectiveness of Pap smears in screening high-risk individuals for anal squamous intraepithelial lesions.[154] In fact, anoscopy has been shown to be more accurate in some jurisdictions.[155,156] Annual screening using smears among HIV-positive men who have sex with men has been found to be cost-effective compared with colon cancer screening and

Table 6.1. Characteristics of Screening Methods for Cervical Cancer

Test	Procedure	Strengths	Limitations	Status
Conventional cytology (Pap smear)	Sample of cervical cells taken by provider and examined by trained cytotechnicians in a laboratory	• History of long use • Widely accepted • Permanent record of test • Training and mechanisms for quality control established • Modest investments in existing programs can improve services • High specificity	• Results not immediately available • Systems needed to ensure timely communication of test results and follow-up of women • Transport required for specimen to laboratory and for results to clinic • Requires laboratory quality assurance • Moderate sensitivity	• Available in many countries since 1950s • Cytology-based programs have reduced cancer mortality in developed countries
Liquid-based cytology (LBC)	Sample of cervical cells is obtained with a small brush, immersed in special liquid and sent to laboratory for processing and screening	• Fewer inadequate or unsatisfactory samples requiring patient call-back and rescreening • Once cytotechnicians are proficient, LBC samples take less time to review • Samples can be used for molecular analysis (such as HPV DNA testing)	• Results not immediately available • Supplies and laboratory facilities more expensive than for conventional cytology • No controlled studies, to date, comparing sensitivity and specificity with conventional cytology	• Selected as screening method in some developed countries (e.g., UK)

		Advantages	Disadvantages	
HPV DNA testing	Molecular testing for HPV- swab taken by provider or woman herself and sent to laboratory	• Collection of specimen simple • Automated processing • Can be combined with Pap smear to increase the sensitivity, but this also increases the cost • A negative test means no HPV or related morbidity is present • The assay result is a permanent record • High specificity in women over age 35	• Results not immediately available • High unit cost • Complex laboratory requirements and specimen transport • Low specificity in young women leading to overtreatment • Storage of reagents problematic	• Commercially available and used in some developed countries in addition to cytology • Lower-cost tests in development
Visual methods (VIA and VILI)	Trained provider examines cervix after staining with vinegar (in VIA) or with Lugol's iodine (in VILI)	• Relatively simple and inexpensive • Results available immediately • Can be performed by wide range of personnel after short training • Low level of infrastructure required • Can be combined with offer of immediate treatment in single-visit approach	• High provider variability • Lower specificity resulting in high referral rate and overtreatment • No permanent record of test • Not appropriate for postmenopausal women • Lack of standardization • Frequent retraining needed	• Limited evidence available • Only recommended at this time for use in demonstration projects • Large randomized controlled trials under way to determine effect on cancer incidence and mortality

Source: WHO Comprehensive Cervical Cancer Control: A Guide to Essential Practice, 2006. Used by permission.

other widely accepted secondary prevention procedures[157]; other recent research has generated the opposite conclusion with respect to the reference case.[158] A discussion similar to cervical cancer screening has been initiated concerning the pros and cons of self-collected anal cytology samples.[159]

While clearly more work remains to be done in this area, the likely targets for this type of screening are already clear: any individuals undergoing receptive anal intercourse, people who are HIV-positive, and women with cervical HPV infection. Unfortunately, many members of these subgroups are not aware of their increased risk for anal cancer. Formal guidelines for anal cancer screening are lacking in Canada and other jurisdictions, a situation which can easily exacerbate undertesting.[160-162]

HPV Detection in Men

Men are not routinely screened for HPV infection or related diseases. However, a modest literature has developed related to male HPV detection that coincides with the growing interest in the prevalence and impact of the virus in men.[163] Analysis of male HPV infection has been challenging because of the lack of consistency in collection methods, low accuracy of cytological analysis, and the inability to obtain samples that allow full results to be derived from molecular methods.[164,165] The continuing methodological questions have prompted recent studies of various collection strategies.[166] Recently, a Florida-based research team specializing in male HPV infections demonstrated that a swab method to collect skin exfoliated cells is adequate for obtaining a sample to be used in DNA testing.[167] Another U.S. study supported the value of self-collected samples in men,[168] whereas recent research in British Columbia, Canada, suggested that there are "continued opportunities" to improve such techniques.[169]

As well, in contrast to the well-established anatomic target in Pap sampling in women, it has been unclear how to optimally localize the collection of cells from the male anogenital region; it seems that inconsistency in site of collection has contributed to heterogeneous data on HPV prevalence.[170] Research at the same Florida center noted earlier has led to a suggestion that the most accurate sampling protocol will involve multiple anogenital sites in men, including different parts of the penis.[171]

As noted earlier, seropositivity for HPV represents an alternate approach for detection of the virus, albeit inadequate to assess whether an infection is currently present and active. One study has shown that there is a difference between men and women in terms of behaviors and other biomarkers associated with seropositivity; in particular, researchers need to be aware that tonsillar HPV infection can impact seroprevalence in men.[172] Finally, as was seen in the case of women, there is interest in exploring the use of urine samples in men as an alternate means of testing for HPV infection.[173,174]

Emerging technologies in HPV testing may allow men to be included in screening more easily. A 2006 study that tested both men and women for HPV found that the males actually demonstrated a higher proportion of oncogenic viral types in their genital tract.[175] Although HPV-related cancer in males is rarer than in women, there are suggestions that men should be drawn more fully into HPV prevention programs for the sake of both male health and that of their sexual partners.[176,177] In particular, the male sexual partners of women with HPV-related disease exhibit a high risk of infection, and therefore could benefit from targeted screening.[178]

Head and Neck Surveillance

Surveillance of head and neck sites for cancers and other abnormalities possibly related to HPV infection can be accomplished by a general practitioner or, in the case of the oral cavity, by a dentist. However, even though a comprehensive examination only takes about 5 min, many cancers of the head and neck are not diagnosed until they are at a late stage. There is good evidence, at least in the case of oral cavity cancers, that this may be explained by the fact that those at highest risk due to alcohol and cigarette consumption, poor nutrition exacerbated by poverty, etc. rarely present for examination.

HPV infection in oral mucosa can appear as distinct flat, white areas, as elevated patches or plaques with erythematous presentation, and as verrucous lesions. When abnormal tissue is detected, a sample of affected cells (for further testing) can be extracted by spatula scraping, cytobrush, mouthwash rinse, or biopsy.[179,180]

Early detection or diagnosis of oral cavity carcinoma is actually difficult to achieve.[181] Technologies to enhance visual detection do exist, but they have not yet been validated for a true screening program.[182,183] The U.S. Preventive Services Task Force has concluded that the evidence is insufficient to recommend for or against routine screening of adults for oral cancer.[184] Likewise, the relevant Cochrane review did not find enough evidence to support a universal screening program for oral cancer.[185]

In fact, no population-based screening programs for oral cancer have been established in developed countries, though various organizations have advocated opportunistic approaches.[186] For instance, dentists in the

MOLECULAR BIOMARKERS: LEADING EDGE OF DETECTION AND MONITORING

The discussion of detection methods will end with a brief review of biomarkers for HPV infection and disease. As discussed in the section "Introduction to Detection and Screening: A Success Story," this is part of an important and rapidly growing field within oncology. The extensive investigation of molecular biomarkers for HPV found in the literature will serve as a paradigm of what may be possible for all the infectious agents of cancer.

While still the most prevalent means of screening for HPV, the high dependence of the Pap smear on the skills of the specimen collector and examiner limits the accuracy and consistency of the test; this reality continues to drive the quest for new biomarkers of infection and disease.[189] More specific and reproducible assays are aimed at improving current screening programs and avoiding "unnecessary medical intervention and psychological distress for the affected women."[190] A growing understanding of the carcinogenic mechanisms related to HPV infection has generated a host of potential molecular markers beyond the two best-known ones introduced earlier in this chapter (i.e., viral DNA and mRNA).[191,192] One of the candidate biomarkers could ultimately augment Pap smears, and even act as an alternative to HPV-DNA testing. While almost a dozen forms of viral DNA measurement are available, only a few have been clinically validated. Thus, the door to developing other effective detection and/or monitoring tools remains wide open as a potential avenue to control anogenital and other HPV-related cancers.[193]

Representative Biomarker: p16(INK4a)

The tumor suppressor protein p16(INK4a) is the most intensively studied marker of HPV infection and disease activity outside of viral DNA itself. Some research has shown p16(INK4a) to be more reliable in identifying cervical dysplasia and carcinogenesis than other biomarkers.[194,195] The protein can be found in epithelial cells that are infected with high-risk HPV; p16(INK4a) is also strongly observed in cervical dysplasia and carcinoma.[196,197] The overexpression of p16(INK4a) has been associated with a variety of other malignancies, including anogenital cancers (e.g., vulvar, penile) and head and neck cancers (e.g., tonsillar).[198–202]

Many studies have shown that p16(INK4a) is strongly expressed in cases of high-grade cervical dysplasia.[203] There is also an association with low-grade cervical dysplasia caused by high-risk HPV types (thereby representing cases at increased risk for progression to cancer).[204,205]

p16(INK4a) can be detected in the laboratory using immunohistochemical methods.[206] The protein is one of the biomarkers that can be detected in LBC samples.[207] Although p16(INK4a) is yet to be clinically validated, recent evidence suggests that current HPV screening practices may be enhanced when used in combination with detection of the protein.[208,209] For example, the identification of p16(INK4a) may confirm the diagnosis of cervical dysplasia in certain ambiguous Pap smears.[210]

Establishing new biomarker detection methods should lower the rate of false-positive and false-negative results from current testing methods, "gaining thereby great advantages for patients and for cost-efficiency."[211]

Other Investigational Biomarkers

A spectrum of other biomarkers for HPV infection has been explored, though not to the same extent as p16(INK4a). For convenience, key recent investigative results have been summarized in Table 6.2. It is a remarkable list, representing a large volume of research activity. However, the general consensus on novel biomarkers is that "their usefulness in routinely collected exfoliated cells remains uncertain."[212]

Table 6.2. Selected Investigational Biomarkers for HPV-related Disease

Biomarker	Role in HPV Disease	Sites Studied	Detection	Stage of Application	Lead Authors and Date
Viral Expression Markers					
E4	HPV protein, expression correlated with viral genome amplification		Assay, such as for mRNA	Found to be expressed at higher levels than E7	Middleton (2003)
E6	HPV oncoprotein, causes multiple changes in cell mechanisms, most notably interruption of p53 mechanism		Assay, such as for mRNA	Found in the majority of cervical carcinomas; ratio of E2 and E6 can differentiate between high-grade and low-grade SILs	Cricca (2007), Castle (2007), Kraus (2006)
E7	HPV oncoprotein, causes multiple changes in cell mechanisms, most notably interruption of pRb mechanism		Assay, such as for mRNA	Found in the majority of cervical carcinomas	Castle (2007), Kraus (2006), Scheurer (2007)
Host Cell Functional Markers					
p16 (or p16[INK4a])	Tumor suppressor protein that affects cell cycle by inhibiting Cyclin D; overexpressed in HPV-infected epithelial cells, especially in high-grade CIN and low-grade CIN with high-risk HPV	Cervix, vulva, anorectal region, tonsils, pharynx, other head and neck	Immunohisto-chemistry	The best novel test for detection of cervical lesions; not yet fully validated, but showing promise to improve accuracy of Pap smears; considered the most reliable prognostic marker for cervical and oropharyngeal dysplasia	Reimers (2007), Nemes (2006), Murphy (2005), Lorenzato (2005)

p53	Tumor suppressor protein that detects DNA damage and promotes p21 expression; degraded by HPV oncoprotein E6	Cervix, anorectal region, penis, aerodigestive tract, and mouth	Immunohisto-chemistry	The related gene is the most frequently mutated in human neoplasms and, as such, p53 is less useful as a specific HPV disease marker than p16; further, mutations of p53 gene may not serve a major role in HPV-induced carcinogenesis	Queiroz (2006), Gentile (2006), Lu (2003), Nemes (2006), Caputi (1998)
pRb (retinoblastoma protein)	Tumor suppressor protein, degraded through formation of a complex with HPV oncoprotein E7	Cervix and anorectal region	Immunohisto-chemistry	Expression (but not function) increased in squamous cell carcinoma; useful surrogate biomarker for early HPV-related events	Lu (2003), Nemes (2006)
p21 (CDKN1A)	Cyclin-dependent kinase inhibitor, specifically affecting Cyclin D; blocked directly by E7 and indirectly by E6 through p53 interaction; (counterintuitively) is overexpressed in many HPV-related carcinomas	Cervix and anorectal region	Immunohisto-chemistry	Overexpressed in invasive carcinoma and high-grade CIN, but not in low-grade CIN	Bahnassy (2007), Keating (2001), Holm (2001)

(Continued)

Table 6.2. (Continued)

Biomarker	Role in HPV Disease	Sites Studied	Detection	Stage of Application	Lead Authors and Date
p27 (CDKN1B)	Cyclin-dependent kinase inhibitor, specifically affecting Cyclin E; blocked directly by E7 and underexpressed in HPV related carcinomas	Cervix and anorectal region	Immunohistochemistry	Significantly decreased in carcinoma and early HPV-related events	Keating (2001), Holm (2001)
DNA ploidy	Degree of repetition of number of chromosomes within a cell; normal human cells are diploid (two sets), while cancerous cells can be diploid, tetraploid (four sets), or aneuploid (uneven number of chromosomes)		Flow cytometry	Diploid cancers are more similar to normal human cells and are often less harmful and more responsive to therapies; tetraploid and aneuploid cancers are more dangerous	Ochatt (2006)
ICBP90	Cell cycle regulator protein; downregulated by p53; overexpressed in cancer cells	Cervix	Immunohistochemistry	Found to be one of the most accurate tests distinguishing high- and low-grade SIL	Lorenzato (2005)
EGFR (epidermal growth factor receptor)	Elevated levels in HPV-positive sinonasal inverted papilloma; decreased expression in HPV- and p16-positive oropharyngeal squamous cell carcinomas	Nose, sinuses, and pharynx	Flow cytometry; immunohistochemistry	Low levels indicate increased likelihood of survival in oropharyngeal squamous cell carcinomas	Katori (2005), Reimers (2007)

Ki67	Proliferation marker, mutated expression (through interaction with oncoproteins E6 and E7) in high-risk HPV-related carcinomas	Cervix, anus, and penis	Immunohistochemistry	One of the most accurate tests distinguishing high- and low-grade SIL; possibly a useful adjunct in the diagnosis and grading of anal intraepithelial neoplasia	Gentile (2006), Walts (2006), Keating (2001), Lorenzato (2005)
Cyclin A	Cell cycle regulating protein functioning in synthesis phase of cell cycle; upregulated by E7		Immunohistochemistry	Higher levels associated with some HPV types	Mansour (2007)
Cyclin D	Cell cycle regulating protein; overexpression factor in the development of many cancers		Immunohistochemistry	Less useful than p16 as a marker of late HPV-related events	Bahnassy (2007), Queiroz (2006)
Cyclin E	Cell cycle regulating protein; allows cell to enter synthesis phase, thereby controlling viral replication; upregulated by E7		Immunohistochemistry	Associated with both high- and low-grade squamous intraepithelial lesions of the cervix and, in general, early HPV-related events	Bahnassy (2007), Keating (2001)
Cyclin G	May play an important role in the genesis of CIN and cervical squamous cell carcinoma by high-risk HPV infection		Immunohistochemistry	Possibly useful for detecting CIN and squamous cell carcinoma; overexpressed in both lesions	Liang (2006)

(Continued)

Table 6.2. (Continued)

Biomarker	Role in HPV Disease	Sites Studied	Detection	Stage of Application	Lead Authors and Date
TGF-α (transforming growth factor-α)	Induces epithelial development; upregulated in some HPV-related cancers	Cervix, nose, sinuses, head, and neck	Immunohistochemistry	Overexpressed in malignant and premalignant tissues	Katori (2005)
MCM-2, -5, -6, -7	Chromosome maintenance proteins; overexpressed as a result of HPV infection and subsequent uncontrolled activation of gene transcription	Cervix	Immunohistochemistry	Expected to play a role in improving the screening and detection of cervical disease	Malinowski (2005), Murphy (2005)
CDC6 (cell division cycle)	Protein essential for DNA replication; preferentially expressed in high-grade lesions and invasive squamous cell carcinoma	Cervix	Immunohistochemistry	Possibly useful in detection of high-grade and invasive lesions of the cervix; limited utility for low grade dysplasia	Murphy (2005)
S100A8	Cell cycle regulating protein; upregulated and overexpressed in HPV-18-positive oral squamous cell carcinoma	Mouth	Suppression subtractive hybridization; immunohistochemistry	Suspected to play an important role in oral carcinogenesis following HPV-18 infection; thus potentially a powerful biomarker and even a therapeutic target in patients	Lo (2007)

PCNA (proliferating cell nuclear antigen)	Protein factor in DNA synthesis, increasing speed up to 1000×; overexpressed in precancerous epithelial inflammations	Cervix	Immunohisto-chemistry	Positivity for marker slightly precedes accumulation of viral DNA	Keating (2001)
Mitotic frequency (MPM-2)	Labels proteins related to cell cycle, specifically mitosis		Flow cytometry		
MMP (metallo-proteinases)	Expression increased in precancerous sinonasal lesions of inverted papilloma	Nose and sinuses	Immunohisto-chemistry	MMP-2 and 9 overexpression found to predict tumor aggressiveness and invasiveness	Katori (2006)
Telomerases	Ribonucleoprotein enzymes; support tumor growth by allowing cells to divide repeatedly without DNA corruption	Premalignant and malignant tissues	Immunohisto-chemistry	Limited clinical utility due to low expression levels; difficult to detect using conventional methods	Keating (2001)
Antiapoptotic markers	Protect cells (including damaged/mutated ones) from death; allow tumor formation		Immunohisto-chemistry	Overexpressed in cancers	
CEA (carcino-embryonic antigen)	Glycoprotein found in embryos during development; produced by some cancers		Blood tests	Positivity combined with high Ki67 only found in malignant tumors	Keating (2001)

(Continued)

Table 6.2. (Continued)

Biomarker	Role in HPV Disease	Sites Studied	Detection	Stage of Application	Lead Authors and Date
MN/CA9 (carbonic anhydrase IX)	Tumor-associated antigen; exact relationship with HPV not understood	Cervix	Immunohistochemistry	Identifies low- and high-grade SILs, invasive carcinomas, and adenocarcinomas at rates of 65%, 77%, 92%, and 100%, respectively	Keating (2001)
CDK4 (Cyclin-dependent kinase)	Affects growth and synthesis stages of cell cycle; regulated by Cyclin D; overexpressed in HPV-related carcinoma	Cervix	Immunohistochemistry	Significantly increased in squamous cell carcinoma and early HPV-related events	Bahnassy (2007)
COX-2	Inflammation protein; expressed in premalignant lesions	Cervix	Immunohistochemistry	No significant relationship to HPV positivity found; further trials suggested	Saldivar (2007)
Host Cell Structural Markers					
Cytokeratins (CK)	Provide cell structure; expression varies by cell type, and can be altered by HPV infection	Cervix and mouth	Immunohistochemistry	Expression of CK8, 16 and 17 is useful marker of high-grade CIN; changes in CK1, 10, 13, 14, 15, 18 and 19 are also measurable	Carrilho (2005), Regauer (2007), Akgul (2007)

Involucrin	Provides structure in epithelial cells; expression altered by HPV infection	Squamous epithelium	Immunohistochemistry	May help distinguish benign from malignant neoplasms
CD44	Cell-surface glycoprotein; downregulated during transition from CIN to invasive squamous carcinoma	Cervix	Immunohistochemistry	Awaiting further studies	Keating (2001)
Integrin α6	Transmembrane protein, with a role in cellular shape and mobility; expression increased in HPV-infected cells		Microfluidic screening	Investigational method of HPV detection	Wankhede (2006)

BIBLIOGRAPHY FOR TABLE 6.2

Akgul B, Ghali L, Davies D et al. HPV8 early genes modulate differentiation and cell cycle of primary human adult keratinocytes. *Experimental Dermatology.* 2007; 16(7): 590–9.

Bahnassy AA, Zekri AR, Saleh M et al. The possible role of cell cycle regulators in multistep process of HPV-associated cervical carcinoma. *BMC Clinical Pathology.* 2007; 7: 4.

Caputi M, Esposito V, Baldi A et al. p21waf1/cip1mda-6 expression in non-small-cell lung cancer: relationship to survival. *American Journal of Respiratory Cell and Molecular Biology.* 1998; 18(2): 213–7.

Carrilho C, Cirnes L, Alberto M et al. Distribution of HPV infection and tumour markers in cervical intraepithelial neoplasia from cone biopsies of Mozambican women. *Journal of Clinical Pathology.* 2005; 58(1): 61–8.

Castle PE, Dockter J, Giachetti C et al. A cross-sectional study of a prototype carcinogenic human papillomavirus E6/E7 messenger RNA assay for detection of cervical precancer and cancer. *Clinical Cancer Research.* 2007; 13(9): 2599–605.

Cricca M, Morselli-Labate AM, Venturoli S et al. Viral DNA load, physical status and E2/E6 ratio as markers to grade HPV16 positive women for high-grade cervical lesions. *Gynecologic Oncology.* 2007; 106(3): 549–57.

Gentile V, Vicini P, Giacomelli L et al. Detection of human papillomavirus DNA, p53 and ki67 expression in penile carcinomas. *International Journal of Immunopathology and Pharmacology.* 2006; 19(1): 209–15.

Holm R, Skovlund E, Skomedal H et al. Reduced expression of p21WAF1 is an indicator of malignant behaviour in anal carcinomas. *Histopathology.* 2001; 39(1): 43–9.

Katori H, Nozawa A, Tsukuda M. Markers of malignant transformation of sinonasal inverted papilloma. *European Journal of Surgical Oncology.* 2005; 31(8): 905–11.

Katori H, Nozawa A, Tsukuda M. Increased expression of matrix metalloproteinase-2 and 9 and human papilloma virus infection are associated with malignant transformation of sinonasal inverted papilloma. *Journal of Surgical Oncology.* 2006; 93(1): 80–5.

Keating JT, Ince T, Crum CP. Surrogate biomarkers of HPV infection in cervical neoplasia screening and diagnosis. *Advances in Anatomic Pathology.* 2001; 8(2): 83–92.

Kraus I, Molden T, Holm R et al. Presence of E6 and E7 mRNA from human papillomavirus types 16, 18, 31, 33, and 45 in the majority of cervical carcinomas. *Journal of Clinical Microbiology.* 2006; 44(4): 1310–7.

Liang J, Bian ML, Chen QY et al. Relationship between cyclin G1 and human papilloma virus infection in cervical intraepithelial neoplasia and cervical carcinoma. *Chinese Medical Sciences Journal.* 2006; 21(2): 81–5.

Lo WY, Lai CC, Hua CH et al. S100A8 is identified as a biomarker of HPV18-infected oral squamous cell carcinomas by suppression subtraction hybridization, clinical proteomics analysis, and immunohistochemistry staining. *Journal of Proteome Research.* 2007; 6(6): 2143–51.

Lorenzato M, Caudroy S, Bronner C et al. Cell cycle and/or proliferation markers: what is the best method to discriminate cervical high-grade lesions? *Human Pathology.* 2005; 36(10): 1101–7.

Lu DW, El-Mofty SK, Wang HL. Expression of p16, Rb, and p53 proteins in squamous cell carcinomas of the anorectal region harboring human papillomavirus DNA. *Modern Pathology*. 2003; 16(7): 692–9.

Malinowski DP. Molecular diagnostic assays for cervical neoplasia: emerging markers for the detection of high-grade cervical disease. *BioTechniques*. 2005; 38(suppl 4): 17–23.

Mansour M, Touka M, Hasan U et al. E7 properties of mucosal human papillomavirus types 26, 53 and 66 correlate with their intermediate risk for cervical cancer development. *Virology*. 2007; 367(1): 1–9.

Middleton K, Peh W, Southern S et al. Organization of human papillomavirus productive cycle during neoplastic progression provides a basis for selection of diagnostic markers. *Journal of Virology*. 2003; 77(19): 10186–201.

Murphy N, Ring M, Heffron CC et al. p16INK4A, CDC6, and MCM5: predictive biomarkers in cervical preinvasive neoplasia and cervical cancer. *Journal of Clinical Pathology*. 2005; 58(5): 525–34.

Nemes JA, Deli L, Nemes Z et al. Expression of p16(INK4A), p53, and Rb proteins are independent from the presence of human papillomavirus genes in oral squamous cell carcinoma. *Oral Surgery, Oral Medicine, Oral Pathology, Oral Radiology, and Endodontics*. 2006; 102(3): 344–52.

Ochatt SJ. Flow cytometry (ploidy determination, cell cycle analysis, DNA content per nucleus). In: Mathesius U, Journet EP, Sumner LW, eds. *Medicago Truncatula Handbook*. Version November 2006. Available at http://www.noble.org/medicagohandbook/pdf/FlowCytometry.pdf. Accessed April 2008.

Queiroz C, Silva TC, Alves VA et al. Comparative study of the expression of cellular cycle proteins in cervical intraepithelial lesions. *Pathology, Research and Practice*. 2006; 202(10): 731–7.

Regauer S, Reich O. CK17 and p16 expression patterns distinguish (atypical) immature squamous metaplasia from high-grade cervical intraepithelial neoplasia (CIN III). *Histopathology*. 2007; 50(5): 629–35.

Reimers N, Kasper HU, Weissenborn SJ et al. Combined analysis of HPV-DNA, p16 and EGFR expression to predict prognosis in oropharyngeal cancer. *International Journal of Cancer*. 2007; 120(8): 1731–8.

Saldivar JS, Lopez D, Feldman RA et al. COX-2 overexpression as a biomarker of early cervical carcinogenesis: a pilot study. *Gynecologic Oncology*. 2007; 107(1 suppl 1): S155–62.

Scheurer ME, Guillaud M, Tortolero-Luna G et al. Human papillomavirus-related cellular changes measured by cytometric analysis of DNA ploidy and chromatin texture. *Cytometry*. 2007; 72(5): 324–31.

Sotlar K, Stubner A, Diemer D et al. Detection of high-risk human papillomavirus E6 and E7 oncogene transcripts in cervical scrapes by nested RT-polymerase chain reaction. *Journal of Medical Virology*. 2004; 74(1): 107–16.

Walts AE, Lechago J, Bose S. P16 and Ki67 immunostaining is a useful adjunct in the assessment of biopsies for HPV-associated anal intraepithelial neoplasia. *American Journal of Surgical Pathology*. 2006; 30(7): 795–801.

Wankhede SP, Du Z, Berg JM et al. Cell detachment model for an antibody-based microfluidic cancer screening system. *Biotechnology Progress*. 2006; 22(5): 1426–33.

NOTES

1. Syrjanen K. PL8: the causal role of genital human papillomavirus (hpv) infections in cervical carcinogenesis. *Oral Diseases.* 2006; 12(suppl 1): 2.
2. Gakidou E, Nordhagen S, Obermeyer Z. Coverage of cervical cancer screening in 57 countries: low average levels and large inequalities. *PLoS Medicine.* 2008; 5(6): e132.
3. Cox JT. Human papillomavirus testing in primary cervical screening and abnormal Papanicolaou management. Obstetrical and Gynecological Survey. 2006; 61(6 suppl 1): S15–25.
4. *Summary Tables of Cervical Cancer Screening Guidelines and Recommendations for New Technologies.* 2004. Centers for Disease Control and Prevention. Available at http://www.cdc.gov/std/hpv/ScreeningTables.pdf. Accessed June 2007.
5. Rathore SS, McGreevey JD, 3rd, Schulman KA et al. Mandated coverage for cancer-screening services: whose guidelines do states follow? *American Journal of Preventive Medicine.* 2000; 19(2): 71–8.
6. StatBite: percentage screened for cancer by insurance status. *Journal of National Cancer Institute.* 2008; 100(11): 772.
7. Blackwell DL, Martinez ME, Gentleman JF. Women's compliance with public health guidelines for mammograms and pap tests in Canada and the United States: an analysis of data from the Joint Canada/United States Survey Of Health. *Women's Health Issues.* 2008; 18(2): 85–99.
8. Franco EL, Cuzick J, Hildesheim A et al. Issues in planning cervical cancer screening in the era of HPV vaccination. *Vaccine.* Chapter 20, 2006; 24(suppl 3): S171–7.
9. Peto J, Gilham C, Fletcher O et al. The cervical cancer epidemic that screening has prevented in the UK. *The Lancet.* 2004; 364(9430): 249–56.
10. Ng E, Wilkins R, Fung MF et al. Cervical cancer mortality by neighbourhood income in urban Canada from 1971 to 1996. *Canadian Medical Association Journal.* 2004; 170(10): 1545–9.
11. Liu S, Semenciw R, Probert A et al. Cervical cancer in Canada: changing patterns in incidence and mortality. *International Journal of Gynecological Cancer.* 2001; 11(1): 24–31.
12. Alternate terminology includes Pap test, Papanicolaou smear, cervical smear, cervical/vaginal cytology.
13. Michalas SP. The Pap test: George N. Papanicolaou (1883–1962). A screening test for the prevention of cancer of uterine cervix. *European Journal of Obstetrics and Gynecology and Reproductive Biology.* 2000; 90(2): 135–8.
14. Foulks MJ. The Papanicolaou smear: its impact on the promotion of women's health. *Journal of Obstetric, Gynecologic and Neonatal Nursing.* 1998; 27(4): 367–73.
15. Leyden WA, Manos MM, Geiger AM et al. Cervical cancer in women with comprehensive health care access: attributable factors in the screening process. *Journal of the National Cancer Institute.* 2005; 97(9): 675–83.
16. Health Canada. *Cervical Cancer Screening in Canada: 1998 Surveillance Report.* 2002. Available at http://www.phac-aspc.gc.ca/publicat/ccsic-dccuac/pdf/cervical-e3.pdf. Accessed April 2008.

17. Nygard JF, Nygard M, Skare GB, Thoresen SO. Screening histories of women with CIN 2/3 compared with women diagnosed with invasive cervical cancer: a retrospective analysis of the Norwegian Coordinated Cervical Cancer Screening Program. *Cancer Causes and Control.* 2005; 16: 463–74.
18. Yang B, Morrell S, Zuo Y et al. A case-control study of the protective benefit of cervical screening against invasive cervical cancer in NSW women. *Cancer Causes and Control.* 2008; 19(6): 569–76.
19. Crum CP. The beginning of the end for cervical cancer? *New England Journal of Medicine.* 2002; 347(21): 1703–5.
20. Pak SC, Martens M, Bekkers R et al. Pap smear screening history of women with squamous cell carcinoma and adenocarcinoma of the cervix. *Australian and New Zealand Journal of Obstetrics and Gynaecology.* 2007; 47(6): 504–7.
21. Vinh-Hung V, Bourgain C, Vlastos G et al. Prognostic value of histopathology and trends in cervical cancer: a SEER population study. *BioMed Central Cancer.* 2007; 7: 164.
22. Liu S, Semenciw R, Probert A et al. Cervical cancer in Canada: changing patterns in incidence and mortality. *International Journal of Gynecological Cancer.* 2001; 11(1): 24–31.
23. Coleman DV, Poznansky JJ. Review of cervical smears from 76 women with invasive cervical cancer: cytological findings and medicolegal implications. *Cytopathology.* 2006; 17: 127–36.
24. Nijhuis ER, Reesink-Peters N, Wisman GB et al. An overview of innovative techniques to improve cervical cancer screening. *Cellular Oncology.* 2006; 28(5–6): 233–46.
25. Waller J, McCaffery KJ, Forrest S et al. Human papillomavirus and cervical cancer: issues for biobehavioral and psychosocial research. *Annals of Behavioral Medicine.* 2004; 27(1): 68–79.
26. Martin-Hirsch P, Jarvis G, Kitchener H et al. Collection devices for obtaining cervical cytology samples. *Cochrane Database of Systematic Reviews (Online).* 2006.
27. Schiller CL, Nickolov AG, Kaul KL et al. High-risk human papillomavirus detection: a split-sample comparison of hybrid capture and chromogenic in situ hybridization. *American Journal of Clinical Pathology.* 2004; 121(4): 537–45.
28. Taylor S, Kuhn L, Dupree W et al. Direct comparison of liquid-based and conventional cytology in a South African screening trial. *International Journal of Cancer.* 2006; 118(4): 957–62.
29. Hussein T, Desai M, Tomlinson A et al. The comparative diagnostic accuracy of conventional and liquid-based cytology in a colposcopic setting. *BJOG.* 2005; 112(11): 1542–6.
30. Guo M, Hu L, Martin L et al. Accuracy of liquid-based Pap tests: comparison of concurrent liquid-based tests and cervical biopsies on 782 women with previously abnormal Pap smears. *Acta Cytologica.* 2005; 49(2): 132–8.
31. Arbyn M, Bergeron C, Klinkhamer P et al. Liquid compared with conventional cervical cytology: a systematic review and meta-analysis. *Obstetrics and Gynecology.* 2008; 111(1): 167–77.
32. Michalas SP. The Pap test: George N. Papanicolaou (1883–1962). A screening test for the prevention of cancer of uterine cervix. *European Journal of Obstetrics and Gynecology and Reproductive Biology.* 2000; 90(2): 135–8.

33 Hayanga AJ. Distribution of human papillomavirus types in ThinPrep papanicolaou tests classified according to the Bethesda 2001 terminology and correlations with patient age and biopsy outcomes. *Cancer.* 2006; 107(4): 883–4.
34 DeMay RM. Common problems in Papanicolaou smear interpretation. *Archives of Pathology and Laboratory Medicine.* 1997; 121(3): 229–38.
35 Boronow RC. Death of the Papanicolaou smear? A tale of three reasons. *American Journal of Obstetrics and Gynecology.* 1998; 179(2): 391–6.
36 Shapiro S, Carrara H, Allan BR et al. Hypothesis: the act of taking a Papanicolaou smear reduces the prevalence of human papillomavirus infection: a potential impact on the risk of cervical cancer. *Cancer Causes and Control.* 2003; 14(10): 953–7.
37 Passmore JA, Morroni C, Shapiro S et al. Papanicolaou smears and cervical inflammatory cytokine responses. *Journal of Inflammation.* 2007; 4: 8.
38 Fitzhugh VA, Heller DS. Significance of a diagnosis of microorganisms on pap smear. *Journal of Lower Genital Tract Disease.* 2008; 12(1): 40–51.
39 Bowden FJ, Currie MJ, Toyne H et al. Screening for *Chlamydia trachomatis* at the time of routine Pap smear in general practice: a cluster randomised controlled trial. *Medical Journal of Australia.* 2008; 188(2): 76–80.
40 Oehme A, Gaschler G, Straube E. Genotyping of *Chlamydia trachomatis* strains from cultured isolates and nucleic acid amplification test-positive specimens. *International Journal of Medical Microbiology.* 2003; 293(2–3): 225–8.
41 Repse-Fokter A, Fokter SK. Osteopenia and osteoporosis can be predicted from Pap test. *Acta Cytologica.* 2008; 52(1): 8–13.
42 De Alba I, Anton-Culver H, Hubbell FA et al. Self-sampling for human papillomavirus in a community setting: feasibility in Hispanic women. *Cancer Epidemiology, Biomarkers and Prevention.* 2008; 17(8): 2163–8.
43 Ogilvie G, Krajden M, Maginley J et al. Feasibility of self-collection of specimens for human papillomavirus testing in hard-to-reach women. *Canadian Medical Association Journal.* 2007; 177(5): 480–3.
44 Pengsaa P, Sriamporn S, Kritpetcharat O et al. A comparison of cytology with Pap smears taken by a gynecologist and with a self-sampling device. *Asian Pacific Journal of Cancer Prevention.* 2003; 4(2): 99–102.
45 Budge M, Halford J, Haran M et al. Comparison of a self-administered tampon ThinPrep test with conventional pap smears for cervical cytology. *Australian and New Zealand Journal of Obstetrics and Gynaecology.* 2005; 45(3): 215–9.
46 Safaeian M, Solomon D, Castle PE. Cervical cancer prevention—cervical screening: science in evolution. *Obstetrics and Gynecology Clinics of North America.* 2007; 34(4): 739–60, ix.
47 Johnson CE, Mues KE, Mayne SL et al. Cervical cancer screening among immigrants and ethnic minorities: A systematic review using the Health Belief Model. *Journal of Lower Genital Tract Disease.* 2008; 12(3): 232–41.
48 Seeff LC, McKenna MT. Cervical cancer mortality among foreign-born women living in the United States, 1985 to 1996. *Cancer Detection and Prevention.* 2003; 27(3): 203–8.
49 Rogoza RM, Ferko N, Bentley J et al. Optimization of primary and secondary cervical cancer prevention strategies in an era of cervical cancer vaccination: a multi-regional health economic analysis. *Vaccine.* 2008; 26(suppl 5): F46–58.

50 Tsui J, Saraiya M, Thompson T et al. Cervical cancer screening among foreign-born women by birthplace and duration in the United States. *Journal of Women's Health*. 2007; 16(10): 1447–57.
51 Owusu GA, Eve SB, Cready CM et al. Race and ethnic disparities in cervical cancer screening in a safety-net system. *Maternal and Child Health Journal*. 2005; 9(3): 285–95.
52 Liu S, Semenciw R, Probert A et al. Cervical cancer in Canada: changing patterns in incidence and mortality. *International Journal of Gynecological Cancer*. 2001; 11(1): 24–31.
53 Statistics Canada. *Table 105–0442 - Pap smear, by age group, females aged 18 to 69 years, Canada, provinces, territories, health regions (June 2005 boundaries) and peer groups, every 2 years, CANSIM (database)*. Available at http://cansim2.statcan.ca/cgi-win/cnsmcgi.exe?Lang=E&RootDir=CII/&ResultTemplate=CII/CII___&Array_Pick=1&ArrayId=1050442. Accessed March 2009.
54 Blackwell DL, Martinez ME, Gentleman JF. Women's compliance with public health guidelines for mammograms and pap tests in Canada and the United States: an analysis of data from the Joint Canada/United States Survey Of Health. *Womens Health Issues*. 2008; 18(2): 85–99.
55 Lee J, Parsons GF, Gentleman JF. Falling short of Pap test guidelines. *Health Reports*. 1998; 10(1): 9–19(ENG); 9–21(FRE).
56 Fact Sheet : HPV Vaccine: Implementation and Financing Policy. 2007. Henry J. Kaiser Family Foundation. Available at www.kff.org/womenshealth/7602.cfm. Accessed July 2007.
57 Akers AY, Newmann SJ, Smith JS. Factors underlying disparities in cervical cancer incidence, screening, and treatment in the United States. *Current Problems in Cancer*. 2007; 31(3): 157–81.
58 Taylor VM, Nguyen TT, Jackson JC et al. Cervical cancer control research in Vietnamese American communities. *Cancer Epidemiology Biomarkers and Prevention*. 2008; 17(11): 2924–30.
59 McDougall JA, Madeleine MM, Daling JR et al. Racial and ethnic disparities in cervical cancer incidence rates in the United States, 1992–2003. *Cancer Causes and Control*. 2007; 18(10): 1175–86.
60 Smith JS. Ethnic disparities in cervical cancer illness burden and subsequent care: a prospective view in managed care. *American Journal of Managed Care*. 2008; 14(6 suppl 1): S193–9.
61 Ng E, Wilkins R, Fung MF et al. Cervical cancer mortality by neighbourhood income in urban Canada from 1971 to 1996. *Canadian Medical Association Journal*. 2004; 170(10): 1545–9.
62 Johnston GM, Boyd CJ, MacIsaac MA. Community-based cultural predictors of Pap smear screening in Nova Scotia. *Canadian Journal of Public Health*. 2004; 95(2): 95–8.
63 Bosch FX, Qiao YL, Castellsague X. CHAPTER 2 The epidemiology of human papillomavirus infection and its association with cervical cancer. *International Journal of Gynaecology and Obstetrics*. 2006; 94(suppl 1): S8–21.
64 Hislop TG, Deschamps M, Teh C et al. Facilitators and barriers to cervical cancer screening among Chinese Canadian women. *Canadian Journal of Public Health*. 2003; 94(1): 68–73.

65 Johnston GM, Boyd CJ, MacIsaac MA. Community-based cultural predictors of Pap smear screening in Nova Scotia. *Canadian Journal of Public Health.* 2004; 95(2): 95–8.
66 Young TK, Kliewer E, Blanchard J et al. Monitoring disease burden and preventive behavior with data linkage: cervical cancer among aboriginal people in Manitoba, Canada. *Amercian Journal of Public Health.* 2000; 90(9): 1466–8.
67 Johnston GM, Boyd CJ, MacIsaac MA. Community-based cultural predictors of Pap smear screening in Nova Scotia. *Canadian Journal of Public Health.* 2004; 95(2): 95–8.
68 Gallagher RP, Elwood JM. Cancer mortality among Chinese, Japanese, and Indians in British Columbia, 1964–73. *National Cancer Institute Monograph.* 1979; (53): 89–94.
69 Band PR, Gallagher RP, Threlfall WJ et al. Rate of death from cervical cancer among native Indian women in British Columbia. *Canadian Medical Association Journal.* 1992; 147(12): 1802–4.
70 Clarke EA. Screening for cervical cancer. *Canadian Medical Association Journal.* 1998; 158(3): 301–2.
71 Hislop TG, Clarke HF, Deschamps M et al. Cervical cytology screening. How can we improve rates among First Nations women in urban British Columbia? *Canadian Family Physician.* 1996; 42: 1701–8.
72 Jetté M, Thibault J. Faits saillants—Enquête Santé Québec Inuit, 1992/ Highlights - Santé Québec Health Survey Inuit, 1992, 1994; Montréal, Santé Québec, Gouvernement du Québec.
73 Hislop TG, Clarke HF, Deschamps M et al. Cervical cytology screening. How can we improve rates among First Nations women in urban British Columbia? *Canadian Family Physician.* 1996; 42: 1701–8.
74 Spayne J, Ackerman I, Milosevic M et al. Invasive cervical cancer: a failure of screening. *European Journal of Public Health.* 2008; 18(2): 162–5.
75 Andrae B, Kemetli L, Sparen P et al. Screening-preventable cervical cancer risks: evidence from a nationwide audit in Sweden. *Journal of the National Cancer Institute.* 2008; 100(9): 622–9.
76 Benedet JL, Bertrand MA, Matisic JM et al. Costs of colposcopy services and their impact on the incidence and mortality rate of cervical cancer in Canada. *Journal of Lower Genital Tract Disease.* 2005; 9(3): 160–6.
77 Forbes C, Jepson R, Martin-Hirsch P. Interventions targeted at women to encourage the uptake of cervical screening. *Cochrane Database of Systematic Reviews.* 2002.
78 Clarke EA. Screening for cervical cancer. *Canadian Medical Association Journal.* 1998; 158(3): 301–2.
79 Wright TC, Jr. Cervical cancer screening in the 21st century: is it time to retire the PAP smear? *Clinical Obstetrics and Gynecology.* 2007; 50(2): 313–23.
80 Walboomers JM, Jacobs MV, Manos MM et al. Human papillomavirus is a necessary cause of invasive cervical cancer worldwide. *Journal of Pathology.* 1999; 189(1): 12–9.
81 Cuzick J, Mayrand MH, Ronco G et al. New dimensions in cervical cancer screening. *Vaccine.* Chapter 10, 2006; 24(suppl 3): S90–7.
82 Cuzick J, Clavel C, Petry KU et al. Overview of the European and North American studies on HPV testing in primary cervical cancer screening. *International Journal of Cancer.* 2006; 119(5): 1095–101.

83 Proca DM, Williams JD, Rofagha S et al. Improved rate of high-grade cervical intraepithelial neoplasia detection in human papillomavirus DNA hybrid capture testing. *Analytical and Quantitative Cytology and Histology.* 2007; 29(4): 264–70.
84 Solomon D, Davey D, Kurman R et al. The 2001 Bethesda System: terminology for reporting results of cervical cytology. *Journal of the American Medical Association.* 2002; 287: 2114–9.
85 Franco EL, Cuzick J, Hildesheim A et al. Issues in planning cervical cancer screening in the era of HPV vaccination. *Vaccine.* Chapter 20, 2006; 24(suppl 3): S171–7.
86 Quint WG, Pagliusi SR, Lelie N et al. Results of the first World Health Organization international collaborative study of detection of human papillomavirus DNA. *Journal of Clinical Microbiology.* 2006; 44(2): 571–9.
87 Ferguson M, Heath A, Johnes S et al. Results of the first WHO international collaborative study on the standardization of the detection of antibodies to human papillomaviruses. *International Journal of Cancer.* 2006; 118(6): 1508–14.
88 Chan PK, Cheung TH, Tam AO et al. Biases in human papillomavirus genotype prevalence assessment associated with commonly used consensus primers. *International Journal of Cancer.* 2006; 118(1): 243–5.
89 Summary available at http://investor.digene.com/phoenix.zhtml?c=82439&p=irol-newsArticle_Print&ID= 695453&highlight=. Accessed June 2005.
90 Cox T, Cuzick J. HPV DNA testing in cervical cancer screening: from evidence to policies. *Gynecologic Oncology.* 2006; 103(1): 8–11.
91 Mayrand MH, Duarte-Franco E, Coutlee F et al. Randomized controlled trial of human papillomavirus testing versus Pap cytology in the primary screening for cervical cancer precursors: design, methods and preliminary accrual results of the Canadian cervical cancer screening trial (CCCaST). *International Journal of Cancer.* 2006; 119(3): 615–23.
92 Nijhuis ER, Reesink-Peters N, Wisman GB et al. An overview of innovative techniques to improve cervical cancer screening. *Cellular Oncology.* 2006; 28(5–6): 233–46.
93 Bulkmans NW, Berkhof J, Bulk S et al. High-risk HPV type-specific clearance rates in cervical screening. *British Journal of Cancer.* 2007; 96(9): 1419–24.
94 Pungpapong S, Kim WR, Poterucha JJ. Natural history of hepatitis B virus infection: an update for clinicians. *Mayo Clinic Proceedings.* 2007; 82(8): 967–75.
95 Franceschi S, Mahe C. Human papillomavirus testing in cervical cancer screening. *British Journal of Cancer.* 2005; 92(9): 1591–2.
96 Meijer CJ, Snijders PJ, Castle PE. Clinical utility of HPV genotyping. *Gynecologic Oncology.* 2006; 103(1): 12–7.
97 Summary information from U.S. National Cancer Institute, as adapted by Cox JT. Human papillomavirus testing in primary cervical screening and abnormal Papanicolaou management. *Obstetrical and Gynecological Survey.* 2006; 61(6 suppl 1): S15–25.
98 Cox JT. Human papillomavirus testing in primary cervical screening and abnormal Papanicolaou management. *Obstetrical and Gynecological Survey.* 2006; 61(6 suppl 1): S15–25.

99 Elfgren K, Jacobs M, Walboomers JM et al. Rate of human papillomavirus clearance after treatment of cervical intraepithelial neoplasia. *Obstetrics and Gynecology.* 2002; 100(5 Pt 1): 965–71.
100 Paraskevaidis E, Arbyn M, Sotiriadis A et al. The role of HPV DNA testing in the follow-up period after treatment for CIN: a systematic review of the literature. *Cancer Treatment Reviews.* 2004; 30(2): 205–11.
101 Bodner K, Bodner-Adler B, Wierrani F et al. Is therapeutic conization sufficient to eliminate a high-risk HPV infection of the uterine cervix? A clinicopathological analysis. *Anticancer Research.* 2002; 22(6B): 3733–6.
102 Padilla-Paz LA. Emerging technology in cervical cancer screening: status of molecular markers. *Clinical Obstetrics and Gynecology.* 2005; 48(1): 218–25.
103 Jain N, Irwin K, Carlin L et al. Use of DNA tests for human papillomavirus infection by US clinicians, 2004. *Journal of Infectious Diseases.* 2007; 196(1): 76–81.
104 Stenvall H, Wikstrom I, Backlund I et al. Accuracy of HPV testing of vaginal smear obtained with a novel self-sampling device. *Acta Obstetricia et Gynecologica Scandinavica.* 2007; 86(1): 16–21.
105 Morris BJ, Rose BR. Cervical screening in the 21st century: the case for human papillomavirus testing of self-collected specimens. *Clinical Chemistry and Laboratory Medicine.* 2007; 45(5): 577–91.
106 Stewart DE, Gagliardi A, Johnston M et al. Self-collected samples for testing of oncogenic human papillomavirus: a systematic review. *Journal of Obstetrics and Gynaecology Canada.* 2007; 29(10): 817–28.
107 Petignat P, Faltin DL, Bruchim I et al. Are self-collected samples comparable to physician-collected cervical specimens for human papillomavirus DNA testing? A systematic review and meta-analysis. *Gynecologic Oncology.* 2007; 105(2): 530–5.
108 De Alba I, Anton-Culver H, Hubbell FA et al. Self-sampling for human papillomavirus in a community setting: feasibility in Hispanic women. *Cancer Epidemiology, Biomarkers and Prevention.* 2008; 17(8): 2163–8.
109 Sherris J, Castro W, Levin C et al. The Case for Investing in Cervical Cancer Prevention. 2004. Alliance for Cervical Cancer Prevention. Available at http://www.path.org/files/RH_accp_case.pdf. Accessed June 2007.
110 Kemp TJ, Hildesheim A, Falk RT et al. Evaluation of two types of sponges used to collect cervical secretions and assessment of antibody extraction protocols for recovery of neutralizing anti-human papillomavirus type 16 antibodies. *Clinical and Vaccine Immunology.* 2008; 15(1): 60–4.
111 Payan C, Ducancelle A, Aboubaker MH et al. Human papillomavirus quantification in urine and cervical samples by using the Mx4000 and LightCycler general real-time PCR systems. *Journal of Clinical Microbiology.* 2007; 45(3): 897–901.
112 Szarewski A, Cadman L, Mallett S et al. Human papillomavirus testing by self-sampling: assessment of accuracy in an unsupervised clinical setting. *Journal of Medical Screening.* 2007; 14(1): 34–42.
113 Gupta A, Arora R, Gupta S et al. Human papillomavirus DNA in urine samples of women with or without cervical cancer and their male partners compared with simultaneously collected cervical/penile smear or biopsy specimens. *Journal of Clinical Virology.* 2006; 37(3): 190–4.

114 Ho CM, Yang SS, Chien TY et al. Detection and quantitation of human papillomavirus type 16, 18 and 52 DNA in the peripheral blood of cervical cancer patients. *Gynecologic Oncology.* 2005; 99(3): 615–21.
115 Josefsson AM, Magnusson PK, Ylitalo N et al. Viral load of human papilloma virus 16 as a determinant for development of cervical carcinoma in situ: a nested case-control study. *The Lancet.* 2000; 355(9222): 2189–93.
116 Wu Y, Chen Y, Li L et al. Associations of high-risk HPV types and viral load with cervical cancer in China. *Journal of Clinical Virology.* 2006; 35(3): 264–9.
117 Tsai HT, Wu CH, Lai HL et al. Association between quantitative high-risk human papillomavirus DNA load and cervical intraepithelial neoplasm risk. *Cancer Epidemiology, Biomarkers and Prevention.* 2005; 14(11 Pt 1): 2544–9.
118 Santos AL, Derchain SF, Martins MR et al. Human papillomavirus viral load in predicting high-grade CIN in women with cervical smears showing only atypical squamous cells or low-grade squamous intraepithelial lesion. *São Paulo Medical Journal.* 2003; 121(6): 238–43.
119 Dalstein V, Riethmuller D, Pretet JL et al. Persistence and load of high-risk HPV are predictors for development of high-grade cervical lesions: a longitudinal French cohort study. *International Journal of Cancer.* 2003; 106(3): 396–403.
120 Sun CA, Lai HC, Chang CC et al. The significance of human papillomavirus viral load in prediction of histologic severity and size of squamous intraepithelial lesions of uterine cervix. *Gynecologic Oncology.* 2001; 83(1): 95–9.
121 Ylitalo N, Sorensen P, Josefsson AM et al. Consistent high viral load of human papillomavirus 16 and risk of cervical carcinoma in situ: a nested case-control study. *The Lancet.* 2000; 355(9222): 2194–8.
122 Zerbini M, Venturoli S, Cricca M et al. Distribution and viral load of type specific HPVs in different cervical lesions as detected by PCR-ELISA. *Journal of Clinical Pathology.* 2001; 54(5): 377–80.
123 Moberg M, Gustavsson I, Gyllensten U. Type-specific associations of human papillomavirus load with risk of developing cervical carcinoma in situ. *International Journal of Cancer.* 2004; 112(5): 854–9.
124 Lai HC, Peng MY, Nieh S et al. Differential viral loads of human papillomavirus 16 and 58 infections in the spectrum of cervical carcinogenesis. *International Journal of Gynecological Cancer.* 2006; 16(2): 730–5.
125 Snijders PJ, Hogewoning CJ, Hesselink AT et al. Determination of viral load thresholds in cervical scrapings to rule out CIN 3 in HPV 16, 18, 31 and 33-positive women with normal cytology. *International Journal of Cancer.* 2006; 119(5): 1102–7.
126 Khouadri S, Villa LL, Gagnon S et al. Viral load of episomal and integrated forms of human papillomavirus type 33 in high-grade squamous intraepithelial lesions of the uterine cervix. *International Journal of Cancer.* 2007; 121(12): 2674–81.
127 Hopman AH, Kamps MA, Smedts F et al. HPV in situ hybridization: impact of different protocols on the detection of integrated HPV. *International Journal of Cancer.* 2005; 115(3): 419–28.
128 Vinokurova S, Wentzensen N, von Knebel Doeberitz M. Analysis of p16INK4a and integrated HPV genomes as progression markers. *Methods in Molecular Medicine.* 2005; 119: 73–83.

129 Manavi M, Hudelist G, Fink-Retter A et al. Human papillomavirus DNA integration and messenger RNA transcription in cervical low- and high-risk squamous intraepithelial lesions in Austrian women. *International Journal of Gynecological Cancer.* 2008; 18(2): 285–94.

130 Hudelist G, Manavi M, Pischinger KI et al. Physical state and expression of HPV DNA in benign and dysplastic cervical tissue: different levels of viral integration are correlated with lesion grade. *Gynecologic Oncology.* 2004; 92(3): 873–80.

131 Fontaine J, Hankins C, Mayrand MH et al. High levels of HPV-16 DNA are associated with high-grade cervical lesions in women at risk or infected with HIV. *AIDS.* 2005; 19(8): 785–94.

132 Rousseau MN, Costes V, Konate I et al. Viral load and genomic integration of HPV 16 in cervical samples from HIV-1-infected and uninfected women in Burkina Faso. *Journal of Medical Virology.* 2007; 79(6): 766–70.

133 Scheurer ME, Dillon LM, Chen Z et al. Absolute quantitative real-time polymerase chain reaction for the measurement of human papillomavirus E7 mRNA in cervical cytobrush specimens. *Infectious Agents and Cancer.* 2007; 2: 8.

134 Lie AK, Risberg B, Borge B et al. DNA- versus RNA-based methods for human papillomavirus detection in cervical neoplasia. *Gynecologic Oncology.* 2005; 97(3): 908–15.

135 Steinau M, Rajeevan MS, Lee DR et al. Evaluation of RNA markers for early detection of cervical neoplasia in exfoliated cervical cells. *Cancer Epidemiology, Biomarkers and Prevention.* 2007; 16(2): 295–301.

136 Tabrizi SN, Frazer IH, Garland SM. Serologic response to human papillomavirus 16 among Australian women with high-grade cervical intraepithelial neoplasia. *International Journal of Gynecological Cancer.* 2006; 16(3): 1032–5.

137 Naucler P, Chen HC, Persson K et al. Seroprevalence of human papillomaviruses and *Chlamydia trachomatis* and cervical cancer risk: nested case-control study. *Journal of General Virology.* 2007; 88(Pt 3): 814–22.

138 Pintos J, Black MJ, Sadeghi N et al. Human papillomavirus infection and oral cancer: a case-control study in Montreal, Canada. *Oral Oncology.* 2008; 44(3): 242–50.

139 Andersson K, Waterboer T, Kirnbauer R et al. Seroreactivity to cutaneous human papillomaviruses among patients with nonmelanoma skin cancer or benign skin lesions. *Cancer Epidemiology, Biomarkers and Prevention.* 2008; 17(1): 189–95.

140 Di Bonito P, Grasso F, Mochi S et al. Serum antibody response to Human papillomavirus (HPV) infections detected by a novel ELISA technique based on denatured recombinant HPV16 L1, L2, E4, E6 and E7 proteins. *Infectious Agents and Cancer.* 2006; 1: 6.

141 Dunne EF, Karem KL, Sternberg MR et al. Seroprevalence of human papillomavirus type 16 in children. *Journal of Infectious Diseases.* 2005; 191(11): 1817–9.

142 Marin NM, Milbourne A, Rhodes H et al. Diffuse reflectance patterns in cervical spectroscopy. *Gynecologic Oncology.* 2005; 99(3 suppl 1): S116–20.

143 Kendrick JE, Huh WK, Alvarez RD. LUMA cervical imaging system. *Expert Review of Medical Devices.* 2007; 4(2): 121–9.

144 Moscicki AB, Durako SJ, Ma Y et al. Utility of cervicography in HIV-infected and uninfected adolescents. *Journal of Adolescent Health*. 2003; 32(3): 204–13.
145 Use of Lugol's iodine is also known as the Schiller test.
146 Ashford L, Collymore Y. *Preventing Cervical Cancer Worldwide*. 2004. Population Reference Bureau. Available at http://www.prb.org/pdf05/PreventCervCancer_Eng.pdf. Accessed June 2007.
147 Sherris J, Castro W, Levin C et al. *The Case for Investing in Cervical Cancer Prevention*. 2004. Alliance for Cervical Cancer Prevention. Available at http://www.path.org/files/RH_accp_case.pdf. Accessed June 2007.
148 Abdel-Hady ES, Emam M, Al-Gohary A et al. Screening for cervical carcinoma using visual inspection with acetic acid. *International Journal of Gynaecology and Obstetrics*. 2006; 93(2): 118–22.
149 Healey SM, Aronson KJ, Mao Y et al. Oncogenic human papillomavirus infection and cervical lesions in aboriginal women of Nunavut, Canada. *Sexually Transmitted Diseases*. 2001; 28(12): 694–700.
150 Wright TC, Jr., Denny L, Kuhn L et al. Use of visual screening methods for cervical cancer screening. *Obstetrics and Gynecology Clinics of North America*. 2002; 29(4): 701–34.
151 Heatley MK. A critical evaluation of the use of the Schiller test in selecting blocks from the uterine cervix in suspected intraepithelial neoplasia. *Ulster Medical Journal*. 1995; 64(2): 147–50.
152 Sankaranarayanan R, Esmy PO, Rajkumar R et al. Effect of visual screening on cervical cancer incidence and mortality in Tamil Nadu, India: a cluster-randomised trial. *The Lancet*. 2007; 370: 398–406.
153 Sankaranarayanan R, Bhatla N, Gravitt PE et al. Human papillomavirus infection and cervical cancer prevention in India, Bangladesh, Sri Lanka and Nepal. *Vaccine*. 2008; 26(suppl 12): M43–52.
154 Gohy L, Gorska I, Rouleau D et al. Genotyping of human papillomavirus DNA in anal biopsies and anal swabs collected from HIV-seropositive men with anal dysplasia. *Journal of Acquired Immune Deficiency Syndromes*. 2008; 49(1): 32–9.
155 Pereira AC, de Lacerda HR, Barros RC. Diagnostic methods for prevention of anal cancer and characteristics of anal lesions caused by HPV in men with HIV/AIDS. *Brazilian Journal of Infectious Diseases*. 2002; 12(4): 293–9.
156 Chin-Hong PV, Berry JM, Cheng SC et al. Comparison of patient- and clinician-collected anal cytology samples to screen for human papillomavirus-associated anal intraepithelial neoplasia in men who have sex with men. *Annals of Internal Medicine*. 2008; 149(5): 300–6.
157 Chiao EY, Giordano TP, Palefsky JM et al. Screening HIV-infected individuals for anal cancer precursor lesions: a systematic review. *Clinical Infectious Diseases*. 2006; 43(2): 223–33.
158 Karnon J, Jones R, Czoski-Murray C et al. Cost-utility analysis of screening high-risk groups for anal cancer. *Journal of Public Health*. 2008; 30(3): 293–304.
159 Chin-Hong PV, Berry JM, Cheng SC et al. Comparison of patient- and clinician-collected anal cytology samples to screen for human papillomavirus-associated anal intraepithelial neoplasia in men who have sex with men. *Annals of Internal Medicine*. 2008; 149(5): 300–6.

160 Pitts MK, Fox C, Willis J et al. What do gay men know about human papillomavirus? Australian gay men's knowledge and experience of anal cancer screening and human papillomavirus. *Sexually Transmitted Diseases.* 2007; 34(3): 170–3.

161 Hernandez BY, McDuffie K, Zhu X et al. Anal human papillomavirus infection in women and its relationship with cervical infection. *Cancer Epidemiology, Biomarkers and Prevention.* 2005; 14(11 Pt 1): 2550–6.

162 Hayanga AJ. When to test women for human papillomavirus: take this opportunity to screen for anal cancer too. *British Medical Journal.* 2006; 332(7535): 237.

163 Giuliano AR, Lazcano E, Villa LL et al. Circumcision and sexual behavior: factors independently associated with human papillomavirus detection among men in the HIM study. *International Journal of Cancer.* 2009; 124(6): 1251–7.

164 de Lima Rocha MG, Faria FL, Souza MD et al. Detection of human papillomavirus infection in penile samples through liquid-based cytology and polymerase chain reaction. *Cancer.* 2008; 114(6): 489–93.

165 Aynaud O, Ionesco M, Barrasso R. Cytologic detection of human papillomavirus DNA in normal male urethral samples. *Urology.* 2003; 61(6): 1098–101.

166 Giovannelli L, Migliore MC, Capra G et al. Penile, urethral, and seminal sampling for diagnosis of human papillomavirus infection in men. *Journal of Clinical Microbiology.* 2007; 45(1): 248–51.

167 Flores R, Abalos AT, Nielson CM et al. Reliability of sample collection and laboratory testing for HPV detection in men. *Journal of Virological Methods.* 2008; 149(1): 136–43.

168 Hernandez BY, McDuffie K, Goodman MT et al. Comparison of physician- and self-collected genital specimens for detection of human papillomavirus in men. *Journal of Clinical Microbiology.* 2006; 44(2): 513–7.

169 Ogilvie G, Taylor D, Krajden M et al. Self collection of genital human papillomavirus in heterosexual men. *Sexually Transmitted Infections.* 2009; 85(3): 221–5.

170 Moscicki AB, Schiffman M, Kjaer S et al. Updating the natural history of HPV and anogenital cancer. *Vaccine.* Chapter 5, 2006; 24(suppl 3): S3/42–51.

171 Giuliano AR, Nielson CM, Flores R et al. The optimal anatomic sites for sampling heterosexual men for human papillomavirus (HPV) detection: the HPV detection in men study. *Journal of Infectious Diseases.* 2007; 196(8): 1146–52.

172 Kreimer AR, Alberg AJ, Viscidi R et al. Gender differences in sexual biomarkers and behaviors associated with human papillomavirus-16, -18, and -33 seroprevalence. *Sexually Transmitted Diseases.* 2004; 31(4): 247–56.

173 Gupta A, Arora R, Gupta S et al. Human papillomavirus DNA in urine samples of women with or without cervical cancer and their male partners compared with simultaneously collected cervical/penile smear or biopsy specimens. *Journal of Clinical Virology.* 2006; 37(3): 190–4.

174 D'Hauwers K, Depuydt C, Bogers JP et al. Urine versus brushed samples in human papillomavirus screening: study in both genders. *Asian Journal of Andrology.* 2007; 9(5): 705–10.

175 Carestiato FN, Silva KC, Dimetz T et al. Prevalence of human papillomavirus infection in the genital tract determined by hybrid capture assay. *Brazilian Journal of Infectious Diseases.* 2006; 10(5): 331–6.
176 Palefsky JM. HPV infection in men. *Disease Markers.* 2007; 23(4): 261–72.
177 D'Hauwers KW, Tjalma WA. HPV in men. *European Journal of Gynaecological Oncology.* 2008; 29(4): 338–40.
178 Giraldo PC, Eleuterio J, Jr., Cavalcante DI et al. The role of high-risk HPV-DNA testing in the male sexual partners of women with HPV-induced lesions. *European Journal of Obstetrics, Gynecology, and Reproductive Biology.* 2008; 137(1): 88–91.
179 Furrer VE, Benitez MB, Furnes M et al. Biopsy vs. superficial scraping: detection of human papillomavirus 6, 11, 16, and 18 in potentially malignant and malignant oral lesions. *Journal of Oral Pathology and Medicine.* 2006; 35(6): 338–44.
180 Lawton G, Thomas S, Schonrock J et al. Human papillomaviruses in normal oral mucosa: a comparison of methods for sample collection. *Journal of Oral Pathology and Medicine.* 1992; 21(6): 265–9.
181 Robinson PN, Mickelson AR. Early diagnosis of oral cavity cancers. *Otolaryngologic Clinics of North America.* 2006; 39(2): 295–306.
182 Lingen MW, Kalmar JR, Karrison T et al. Critical evaluation of diagnostic aids for the detection of oral cancer. *Oral Oncology.* 2008; 44(1): 10–22.
183 Patton LL, Epstein JB, Kerr AR. Adjunctive techniques for oral cancer examination and lesion diagnosis: a systematic review of the literature. *Journal of the American Dental Association.* 2008; 139(7): 896–905.
184 U.S. Preventive Services Task Force. *Screening for Oral Cancer: Recommendation Statement.* 2004. Agency for Healthcare Research and Quality. Available at http://www.ahrq.gov/clinic/3rduspstf/oralcan/oralcanrs.pdf. Accessed April 2008.
185 Kujan O, Glenny AM, Oliver RJ et al. Screening programmes for the early detection and prevention of oral cancer. Cochrane Database of Systematic Reviews (Online). 2006.
186 National Cancer Institute. *Oral Cancer Screening.* Available at http://www.cancer.gov/cancertopics/pdq/screening/oral/HealthProfessional/page3. Accessed January 2009.
187 Lehew CW, Kaste LM. Oral cancer prevention and early detection knowledge and practices of Illinois dentists—a brief communication. *Journal of Public Health Dentistry.* 2007; 67(2): 89–93.
188 Clovis JB, Horowitz AM, Poel DH. Oral and pharyngeal cancer: practices and opinions of dentists in British Columbia and Nova Scotia. *Journal of the Canadian Dental Association.* 2002; 68(7): 421–5.
189 Gravitt PE, Coutlee F, Iftner T et al. New technologies in cervical cancer screening. *Vaccine.* 2008; 26(suppl 10): K42–52.
190 von Knebel Doeberitz M. New molecular tools for efficient screening of cervical cancer. *Disease Markers.* 2001; 17(3): 123–8.
191 Branca M, Ciotti M, Giorgi C et al. Predicting high-risk human papillomavirus infection, progression of cervical intraepithelial neoplasia, and prognosis of cervical cancer with a panel of 13 biomarkers tested in multivariate modeling. *International Journal of Gynecological Pathology.* 2008; 27(2): 265–73.

192 Chung YL, Lee MY, Horng CF et al. Use of combined molecular biomarkers for prediction of clinical outcomes in locally advanced tonsillar cancers treated with chemoradiotherapy alone. *Head and Neck.* 2009; 31(1): 9–20.
193 Muneer A, Kayes O, Ahmed HU et al. Molecular prognostic factors in penile cancer. *World Journal of Urology.* 2009; 27(2): 161–7.
194 Murphy N, Ring M, Heffron CC et al. p16INK4A, CDC6, and MCM5: predictive biomarkers in cervical preinvasive neoplasia and cervical cancer. *Journal of Clinical Pathology.* 2005; 58(5): 525–34.
195 Queiroz C, Silva TC, Alves VA et al. Comparative study of the expression of cellular cycle proteins in cervical intraepithelial lesions. *Pathology, Research and Practice.* 2006; 202(10): 731–7.
196 Walts AE, Lechago J, Bose S. P16 and Ki67 immunostaining is a useful adjunct in the assessment of biopsies for HPV-associated anal intraepithelial neoplasia. *American Journal of Surgical Pathology.* 2006; 30(7): 795–801.
197 Mao C, Balasubramanian A, Yu M et al. Evaluation of a new p16(INK4A) ELISA test and a high-risk HPV DNA test for cervical cancer screening: results from proof-of-concept study. *International Journal of Cancer.* 2007; 120(11): 2435–8.
198 Nemes JA, Deli L, Nemes Z et al. Expression of p16(INK4A), p53, and Rb proteins are independent from the presence of human papillomavirus genes in oral squamous cell carcinoma. *Oral Surgery, Oral Medicine, Oral Pathology, Oral Radiology, and Endodontics.* 2006; 102(3): 344–52.
199 Mellin Dahlstrand H, Lindquist D, Bjornestal L et al. P16(INK4a) correlates to human papillomavirus presence, response to radiotherapy and clinical outcome in tonsillar carcinoma. *Anticancer Research.* 2005; 25(6C): 4375–83.
200 Lu DW, El-Mofty SK, Wang HL. Expression of p16, Rb, and p53 proteins in squamous cell carcinomas of the anorectal region harboring human papillomavirus DNA. *Modern Pathology.* 2003; 16(7): 692–9.
201 Rufforny I, Wilkinson EJ, Liu C et al. Human papillomavirus infection and p16(INK4a) protein expression in vulvar intraepithelial neoplasia and invasive squamous cell carcinoma. *Journal of Lower Genital Tract Disease.* 2005; 9(2): 108–13.
202 Prowse DM, Ktori EN, Chandrasekaran D et al. Human papillomavirus-associated increase in p16INK4A expression in penile lichen sclerosus and squamous cell carcinoma. *British Journal of Dermatology.* 2008; 158(2): 261–5.
203 O'Neill CJ, McCluggage WG. p16 expression in the female genital tract and its value in diagnosis. *Advances in Anatomic Pathology.* 2006; 13(1): 8–15.
204 Dehn D, Torkko KC, Shroyer KR. Human papillomavirus testing and molecular markers of cervical dysplasia and carcinoma. *Cancer.* 2007; 111(1): 1–14.
205 Kalof AN, Cooper K. p16INK4a immunoexpression: surrogate marker of high-risk HPV and high-grade cervical intraepithelial neoplasia. *Advances in Anatomic Pathology.* 2006; 13(4): 190–4.
206 Kong CS, Balzer BL, Troxell ML et al. p16INK4A immunohistochemistry is superior to HPV in situ hybridization for the detection of high-risk HPV in atypical squamous metaplasia. *American Journal of Surgical Pathology.* 2007; 31(1): 33–43.

207 Wentzensen N, Bergeron C, Cas F et al. Evaluation of a nuclear score for p16INK4a-stained cervical squamous cells in liquid-based cytology samples. *Cancer.* 2005; 105(6): 461–7.
208 Dehn D, Torkko KC, Shroyer KR. Human papillomavirus testing and molecular markers of cervical dysplasia and carcinoma. *Cancer.* 2007; 111(1): 1–14.
209 Ekalaksananan T, Pientong C, Sriamporn S et al. Usefulness of combining testing for p16 protein and human papillomavirus (HPV) in cervical carcinoma screening. *Gynecologic Oncology.* 2006; 103(1): 62–6.
210 Bose S, Evans H, Lantzy L et al. p16(INK4A) is a surrogate biomarker for a subset of human papilloma virus-associated dysplasias of the uterine cervix as determined on the Pap smear. *Diagnostic Cytopathology.* 2005; 32(1): 21–4.
211 Dallenbach-Hellweg G, Trunk MJ, von Knebel Doeberitz M. Traditional and new molecular methods for early detection of cervical cancer. *(Archives of Pathology) Arkhiv Patologii.* 2004; 66(5): 35–9.
212 Steinau M, Rajeevan MS, Lee DR et al. Evaluation of RNA markers for early detection of cervical neoplasia in exfoliated cervical cells. *Cancer Epidemiology, Biomarkers and Prevention.* 2007; 16(2): 295–301.

7

HUMAN PAPILLOMAVIRUS: PREVENTION OF INFECTION AND DISEASE

> The relevance and high level of scientific interest surrounding HPVs are related to the oncogenic potential of some viral types belonging to this family and the possibility to influence the incidence of various tumour forms like cervical carcinoma, improving the efficacy of specific screening programs or defining preventive strategies like vaccination.[1]

The topic of preventing HPV infection and cancers caused by the virus has recently received substantial attention in both academic journals and the popular press. Although dealing with cervical cancer has been at the forefront of the discussion, it should be recognized that HPV is associated with many different genital and nongenital diseases, both malignant and nonmalignant, and affecting both men and women. Nonetheless, as the prevention picture related to HPV is examined, an emphasis on cervical cancer will once again be very apparent.

A rationale for the prominent position of cervical cancer becomes clearer as one grasps the basic levers of prevention. There is a primary prevention "logic" that relates directly to the transmission of a disease-causing microbe. In short, to interrupt the infection is to interrupt the disease. The logic as applied to HPV is particularly compelling in the case of cervical cancer, where the proven burden attributable to viral infection approaches 100%. This means that dealing directly with the virus as a necessary etiologic agent is virtually equivalent to dealing with the cancer itself—an almost unique scenario in the world of oncology.[2] This mechanism may be summed up in the following terms: "Cervical cancer as a preventable disease process hinges on the concept that it is fundamentally a sexually transmitted disease with a known causative agent."[3] As will be seen, the first prevention category (avoiding exposure) flows naturally from this perspective; in the case of HPV, exposure control overlaps strongly with protection against sexually transmitted infections (STIs) in general.

Although further innovations are very likely to emerge, powerful tools are already available to combat HPV infection and cervical cancer. These include sexual health initiatives, cytology assessment (i.e., Pap smears), HPV-DNA testing, ablative procedures, and, now, prophylactic vaccination.[4] But the story has definitely moved beyond the uterine cervix. Apart from the surgeries and other treatments specific to cervical cancer management, all the tools in the list are also relevant to the other HPV-related malignancies.

PREVENTION APPROACHES

A flowchart of prevention options available along the pathogenic pathway was presented in the "Introduction" to the book. An explanation of the suggested prevention categories may be found there. For convenience, the flowchart is reproduced in Figure 7.1. In this chapter, the key information on HPV infection and cancer relevant to each category will be reviewed.

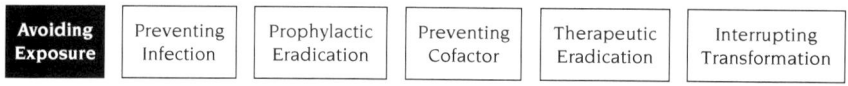

1. Avoiding Exposure to the Agent

The literature related to sexual health promotion, and especially to the prevention of STIs, is vast. Because of the scope of this book, the key approaches that come under this category of primary prevention will only be briefly reviewed.

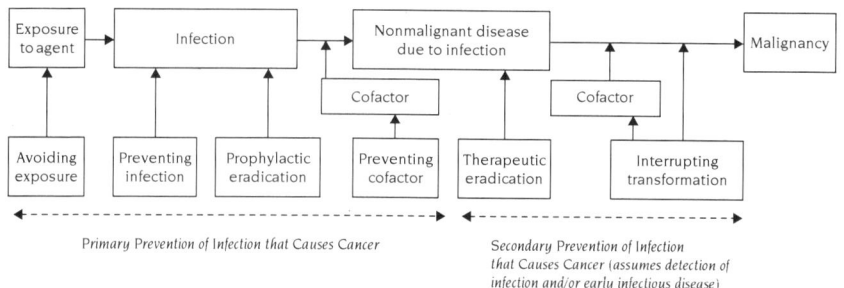

Figure 7.1. Prevention options in infection-related carcinogenesis.

In strictly logical terms, the most straightforward way to eliminate the risk of genital HPV infections is to refrain from all genital contact with another person. The next most certain approach is to be sexually active only within a mutually monogamous relationship with an uninfected partner.[5] Reducing the number of potentially risky sexual partners by any means is also an obvious preventive measure, though less certain than the two approaches just mentioned. However, in light of the apparent inability to consistently prevent HPV transmission through condom use, any version of proactive "partner management" is very useful.[6,7]

Despite the acceptance of the preceding arguments among most health care providers, advice about using condoms tends to be more common than any recommendations about abstinence and monogamy. A recent Canadian report suggested that the latter two approaches were "not reliable."[8] Table 7.1 highlights the results from a survey of U.S. clinicians on the effectiveness of the various primary prevention measures, and the professional opinion on their application in practice.[9] Clearly, for some interventions there is a disconnection between theoretical effectiveness (which should properly be called efficacy) and effectiveness in the real world (probably mediated by factors such as acceptability and adherence).

Research concerning the effectiveness of condoms continues to evolve. It has been accepted that a major limitation of their ability to prevent HPV infection is that the virus seems to be transmitted from (and to) genital areas left exposed by condoms.[10] In line with this, several earlier studies suggested that condoms were not effective in limiting

Table 7.1. Strategies to Prevent HPV Infection or HPV-related Conditions: Opinions of Clinicians in the United States, 2004

Prevention Strategy	Agree that Strategy Is Highly Effective		Agree that Strategy Is Usually Worth Recommending to the Sexually Active	
	%	95% CI*	%	95% CI
1. Monogamy	95	(94–97)	81[†]	(78–83)
2. Limiting number of sexual partners	95	(94–96)	—	—
3. Abstinence	91	(89–92)	45	(42–47)
4. Consistent condom use	78	(76–80)	89	(87–91)

Source: Centers for Disease Control and Prevention, *Morbidity and Mortality Weekly Report*, 2006.

*Confidence interval.

[†]Response for strategy 1 and 2 combined.

the spread of HPV.[11] However, a recent U.S. study did indicate that regular use of condoms reduced the risk of male-to-female transmission, a phenomenon which may have particular significance for cervical cancer prevention.[12] In contrast, a 2008 study suggested that the use of a diaphragm by women who also received risk counseling and condoms did not affect HPV incidence or clearance.[13] Beyond the impact on infection per se, other studies have identified an association between condom use and reduced occurrence of HPV-related disease, improved regression of neoplasia, and/or faster clearance of infection.[14–18] Whatever new research may show, it is unlikely that condom use for preventing HPV infection will ever achieve the level of efficacy demonstrated in the control of, for example, HIV transmission.[19] Condoms do not seem poised to rival the promise of vaccines in the prevention of infection.[20,21]

Building on the logical and evidence-based understanding of exposure prevention strategies, there are extensive reports on the best community-level applications of approaches to STIs. Again, the large volume literature on this topic can only be cursorily reviewed.

Population-based interventions to reduce STIs. Several strategies to maximize the impact of sexual health promotion have been identified and studied at the population level. These include the following:

- education and media campaigns for safer sexual behavior
- integration of case-finding into routine health care
- mass treatment of persons in at-risk communities, even if they are asymptomatic
- improved STI treatment services following disease diagnosis

The review by the Cochrane group relevant to this area of public health was restricted to randomized controlled trials (RCTs); the unit of randomization was either a community or treatment facility (rather than individual patients). Only five studies met the inclusion criteria. The research was based in developing countries, and none of the studies focused on HPV infection. The programs reviewed were mostly unsuccessful in reducing STI incidence rates.[22] While the Cochrane review group assigned to this area continues to examine the literature related to community-level STI programs in both developed and developing countries, their various review projects were still at the protocol stage at the time of this writing.[23–25]

A 2005 systematic review of interventions to prevent STIs examined three of the same community-based studies identified by the Cochrane review (including the one trial that showed some measure of success). In fact, all the identified population-level studies were based in the same

African communities covered by Cochrane.[26] There apparently has been no experimental research concerning STI prevention at the population level in developed countries. This is surprising given the common understanding that STI interventions need to be implemented beyond the classic clinical setting in order to have any real impact.[27]

The one exception to this research gap involves abstinence education geared to preventing HIV infection. Implementation settings range from schools to community centers to health care facilities. The special focus on such topics likely reflect global and especially U.S. political priorities. The relevant Cochrane work on approaches to prevent HIV infection is more recent than the reviews related to STIs in general. The reviewers indicate that programs combining abstinence and safer sex messages appear to reduce short- and long-term risk behavior; confirmation based on biological evidence, on the other hand, was lacking. Messages that are restricted to the abstinence theme appear to have a null effect, neither reducing nor exacerbating HIV risk.[28]

Individual and group approaches to STI control. The majority of the studies identified in the 2005 systematic review noted earlier actually dealt with individual approaches, with a smaller number (n = 9) focusing on group-based programs.[29] A third of the group-based interventions involved counseling and skills building that led to significant decreases in STI transmission. One study showed that counseling focused on skills training (8.6% STI incidence over 12 months) was superior to a health education model (15.4% STI incidence).[30] The most recent literature has supported the efficacy of cognitive-behavioral group interventions for STI control.[31] Overall, a large percentage of these group projects demonstrated significant success, a conclusion mirrored by earlier reviews of the literature.[32] A Cochrane review completed in 2000 confirmed that small-scale health promotion projects directed at groups of women can reduce sexual risk behaviors—especially with respect to increased use of condoms for vaginal intercourse—though none of the studies focused on the control of cervical cancer as an end point.[33]

Summary. Commenting on STI control in general, Johnson and colleagues acknowledged that "the evidence base for many interventions is sparse and randomized trials of interventions are in their early days."[34] Moreover, the studies specifically focusing on exposure prevention of HPV are even rarer. This is not to say that lessons may not be drawn from more general research. Results from several studies have found that the most effective STI prevention programs were based on social cognition or other such theoretical models; also, successful approaches tended to be developed by and for specific subpopulations.[35,36] Targeted

264 HPV and Other Infectious Agents in Cancer

health promotion programs indeed may be worth pursuing. Promising results from one U.S. study revealed that an HPV-specific protocol was highly effective in increasing knowledge about the virus and its sequelae in adolescents.[37]

Despite the weak evidence of effectiveness, primary care continues to be advanced as an important arena of primary prevention. The challenge is for physicians to introduce patient counseling with respect to risk factors for HPV infection and their possible consequences. Initiating a "nonjudgmental discussion" about matters such as multiple sex partners and (with adolescent patients) early sexual debut is suggested, along with advice on how to control such behaviors.[38]

Whatever the ultimate effectiveness of STI control related specifically to HPV, the apparent unreliability of the component strategies (i.e., abstinence, monogamy, and other aspects of healthy sexual expression, condom usage) has certainly intensified interest in HPV vaccination (see the following subsection). Questions have been raised about whether introducing vaccines will create complacency around behavioral interventions, reducing their already limited positive impact.

Finally, the relative importance of the measures examined earlier may change as information continues to emerge about HPV transmission routes that do not involve sexual contact. Of course, any newly identified route would likely prompt a quest for another set of exposure prevention measures.

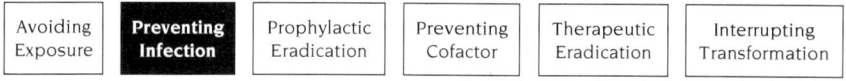

2. Preventing Infection after Exposure to the Agent

The classic approach to primary prevention that protects individuals in the face of probable exposure to infection is prophylactic vaccination. As indicated elsewhere in this book, this is an arena marked by a steady stream of research and reviews. This subsection begins with a definition of the different vaccine categories.

Categories of vaccines. To understand the true prevention options, it is important to distinguish three types of vaccines:

- Prophylactic—refers to a vaccine that prevents the establishment of infection and, presumably, protects against the diseases (such as cancer) directly caused by the infection. Two prophylactic HPV vaccines have been approved in various countries, as will be reviewed later[39]
- Therapeutic—refers to a vaccine that treats an existing infection and/or infection-related disease. No therapeutic HPV vaccines

have been approved to date, though research is ongoing (see the relevant subsection later).[40] Even if such measures were implemented, they would not be relevant to the topic of primary prevention of infection (as this supercategory has been defined in Figure 7.1), but could accomplish primary prevention of cancer
- Chimeric—refers to a vaccine that comprises components used in both prophylactic and therapeutic vaccines. No chimeric HPV vaccines have been approved to date, though research is once again ongoing.[41]

Approved prophylactic vaccines. Gardasil™ was the first HPV vaccine to receive government approvals, and the only one licensed for use in the United States and Canada at the time of this writing. The relatively rapid market licensing of Gardasil™ was based on trials indicating that it is highly efficacious, particularly for vaccine-specific HPV types in HPV-naive women who receive three doses over 6 months; as well, it has a good safety profile.[42]

Gardasil™, developed by Merck, is a quadrivalent vaccine targeting: (i) HPV-16 and -18, the oncogenic types responsible for at least 70% of cervical cancer, plus a substantial number of other cancers; and (ii) HPV-6 and 11, the causes of almost all cases of anogenital warts. It is the product receiving the most attention in the literature. GlaxoSmithKline (GSK), on the other hand, is promoting a bivalent HPV vaccination, trade name Cervarix™, that targets just HPV-16 and 18.

Both vaccines are based on virus-like particle (VLP) technology. VLPs are formed from self-assembling proteins derived from the capsid of a virus; they mimic the virus and in general are highly immunogenic. VLPs do not contain viral genetic material, and therefore do not constitute a "live virus" vaccine. HPV vaccine researchers in fact were inspired by a VLP strategy first developed for hepatitis B.[43]

Gardasil™ and Cervarix™ demonstrate similar levels of efficacy in preventing type-specific HPV infection and cancer precursors; they also enjoy comparable safety profiles. These two vaccines are compared at a qualitative level in Table 7.2.

Bottom line: efficacy and effectiveness. Efficacy information represents a ratio, which can be expressed as a fraction or (more commonly) as a percentage, that is, the number of cases prevented by the intervention divided by the number of cases without the intervention. But both the end point and the population on which the data are based can dramatically affect the results. This was highlighted by Ault et al. in their combined analysis of four randomized clinical trials assessing the efficacy and effectiveness of HPV vaccines (summarized in Table 7.3).[44] These

Table 7.2. Key Results from HPV Vaccine Trials

	Gardasil	Cervarix
Vaccine Description		
Time of follow-up (Phase III)	36 months	15 months (interim)
Target HPV types	6, 11, 16, 18	16, 18
VLP source	Yeast (*Saccharomyces cerevisiae*)	Baculovirus expression
Adjuvant	Aluminum hydroxyphosphate sulfate (proprietary Merck aluminum adjuvant)	Aluminum hydroxide plus 3-deacylated monophosphoryl lipid A (proprietary GSK AS04 adjuvant)
Vaccine Evaluation		
Efficacy: Persistent HPV infection	Proven	Proven
HPV 16 or 18 CIN 2+	Proven	Proven
HPV 16 or 18 CIN 3	Proven	Not proven
VIN or VaIN 2+	Proven	Not reported
Genital warts	Proven	Not in target
Therapeutic efficacy	None	None
Safety at 6 years	Demonstrated	Demonstrated
Cross protection (persistent HPV infection)	6 months	12 months
Cross protection (lesions)	Reported	Not reported
Duration of protection (as of 2007)	5–6 years	5–6 years
Adolescent immunogenicity/safety trials	Females 9–15 years Males 9–15 years	Females 10–14 years Males 10–18 years
Immunogenicity in preadolescents	Proven	Proven
Immunogenicity in older women	Proven	Proven
Phase III trial locations	North America (25%); Latin America (27%); Europe (44%); Asia-Pacific (4%)	North America (12%); Latin America (34%); Europe (30%); Asia-Pacific (25%)
Phase II trial locations	Brazil (34%); Europe (21%); USA (45%)	Brazil (>50%); North America (<50%)

Table 7.3. Gardasil Phase III Trial Information

Population	Efficacy/Effectiveness Against High-Grade Cervical Lesions (95% CI) Caused by the Target Types
Protocol population	
Subjects naive to target HPV types at enrolment and through month 7, no protocol deviations	99% (93–100%)
Unrestricted population	
Subjects naive to target HPV types at enrolment, receiving at least one dose	98% (93–100%)
General population	
All subjects, regardless of baseline status with respect to HPV infection and cervical neoplasia	44% (31–55%)
	Effectiveness Against High-Grade Cervical Lesions, Regardless of Causal HPV Type
General population	
All subjects, regardless of baseline status with respect to HPV infection and cervical neoplasia	17% (7–29%)

Source: Future II Study Group, *The Lancet*, 2007. Used by permission.

four studies enrolled 20,583 healthy women aged 15–26. Exclusion criteria included a previous abnormal Pap smear, a lifetime history of five or more sex partners, and pregnancy.

This summary clearly indicates that the efficacy of the current HPV vaccines is very high (approaching 100%) against high-grade cervical lesions caused by HPV-16 and -18 in women who were not infected with either of these HPV types when they were vaccinated. The effectiveness of the vaccines in the general female population, which includes women who have previously been infected with HPV-16 and/or -18, is much lower at 18%. This low effectiveness in the general population has led to a focus on vaccinating young girls prior to their sexual debut and, presumably, prior to HPV exposure. Vaccination in a school setting also enhances the probability of receiving all three doses. In the Ault et al. review noted earlier, 21% of enrolled women had evidence of either HPV-16 or 18 infections at baseline, and 12% had abnormal cervical cytology at enrolment.

The equivalent trial results for Cervarix™ in an unrestricted population were only 90%, suggesting a slight edge for Gardasil™.[45] This is in addition to the advantage Gardasil™ enjoys in providing protection against anogenital warts. Assertions about the comparative strengths of the two vaccines have focused on duration of protection,[46] level of cross-protection,[47] and selection of adjuvant.[48]

Many other types of trials have been announced or already launched for both Gardasil™ and Cervarix™, including efficacy, immunogenicity bridging, safety in older women, safety and immunogenicity in HIV-infected individuals, and efficacy in males.[49] Naturally, the vaccine manufacturers are motivated to see the licensed target populations expand. The results of the various studies will no doubt be closely monitored by health care planners, especially data from any head-to-head comparisons between the two vaccine products.[50]

HPV vaccine launch: one national example. Health Canada licensed Gardasil™ for use across the country on July 10, 2006. In its 2007 budget, the Canadian federal government allocated $300 million toward the implementation of an HPV vaccine program. This initiative did not address the issue of program sustainability once the grant was spent. One analysis of HPV vaccinations in British Columbia suggested that the promised federal funding might cover 2–3 years of vaccinations, assuming an 80% uptake among 12-year-old girls.[51] Some Canadian provinces decided to roll out the vaccine as early as the 2007 school year. At the same time, several jurisdictions in the country have committed to developing further evidence with respect to Gardasil™.[52]

Canada's National Advisory Committee on Immunization provided a position statement related to Gardasil™ early in 2007.[53] The majority of their document covered background information on HPV infection and cervical cancer, with the final section reviewing the Gardasil™ trial results and offering a list of recommendations and issues for further research. The key conclusions were as follows:

- Gardasil™ is recommended for females between 9 and 13 years of age. *Rationale:* The age period is before the onset of sexual intercourse for most females in Canada; immunogenicity data also imply high efficacy (in the absence of direct evidence for this age group).
- Gardasil™ is recommended for females between ages 14 and 26. *Rationale:* Whether or not females are sexually active or have shown cervical abnormalities, it is unlikely they have been infected with all four HPV types covered by the vaccine, so a certain degree of efficacy would be expected; an important caveat is that there is no evidence that the vaccine will have a therapeutic effect on existing cervical lesions.

- Gardasil™ is not recommended for females less than 9 or over 26 years of age, or for males. *Rationale:* Efficacy data are not available for these groups, and for younger girls and boys the duration of protection of the vaccine is also not known.
- Current guidelines for cervical cancer screening should stay in force. *Rationale:* Vaccinated females (if already sexually active before they receive the vaccine) may have already contracted one of the high-risk HPV types covered by the vaccine, and of course all individuals continue to be susceptible to the various oncogenic HPV types not covered by the vaccine; it is important to remember that about 30% of cervical cancer cases are attributed to types other than HPV-16 and 18.

Vaccination in the context of cervical screening programs. The HPV vaccine is being implemented in the context of one of the most effective cancer prevention initiatives in history, namely, cervical cancer screening using the Pap test (see Chapter 6).

In the absence of screening, the lifetime risk of cervical cancer (based on data from the United States, Australia, and the United Kingdom) is 2.19%.[54-56] Implementing a cervical cancer screening program reduces this risk to 0.75%, based on the analyses in the same three studies just noted. By introducing a vaccination program in addition to the screening program, the lifetime risk can be further reduced to 0.30%.[57] The overall change from 2.19% to 0.30% represents an 86% reduction in the lifetime risk of cervical cancer for a combined screening and vaccination program, as summarized in Table 7.4. Another way to interpret this table is that, in the absence of any intervention, 219 out of every 10,000 females would contract cervical cancer in developed countries. Current screening programs reduce this risk to 75/10,000, whereas the addition of a vaccination program to current screening programs would further reduce the risk to 30/10,000.

A number of studies assessing the economic aspect of implementing an HPV vaccination program suggest that cost-effectiveness could be enhanced by modifying current screening practices.[58-60] It seems

Table 7.4. Impact of Prevention Modalities on Cervical Cancer Risk

Lifetime Cervical Cancer Risk		% Reduction	
With no intervention	2.19%	66%	86%
With current screening	0.75%		
With current screening & vaccination	0.30%	60%	

reasonable that a declining prevalence of oncogenic HPV types in the postvaccination era could permit a lower intensity of screening. There are, however, at least three factors that prompt some caution about changing cervical cancer secondary prevention regimes too quickly.

First, cancer precursors caused by HPV-16 and -18, as well as other oncogenic types, will of course still develop among (older) women not currently targeted for vaccination. The pool of vaccinated individuals who were not naive for one of the target viruses when they were vaccinated are also expected to continue to have normal levels of disease susceptibility to those HPV types. This is because vaccination is only effective against a targeted HPV type prior to infection with that type.

Second, though the vaccines offer a high level of vaccine protection against HPV-16 and 18 in HPV-naive individuals, there are at least 13 additional oncogenic HPV types that currently cause up to 30% of all cervical cancers. This explains the fact that second-generation vaccines are already under development, based on various formulations with increased polyvalency.[61,62]

Finally, screening itself is a moving target, starting with emerging improvements in Pap smear collection and evaluation. This makes decisions about the value of screening, and how best to integrate it with vaccination, difficult to finalize. Indeed, the same innovation in molecular-level technologies that have made vaccine development possible in the first place also promises to change the face of cervical cancer screening. Ultimately, it may include a range of biomarkers (beginning with HPV DNA) that provide a window on the state and stage of HPV-related disease development (see Chapter 6).[63]

There are several other challenges that may be encountered while maintaining a screening program in the postvaccination era.

1. Removing the most threatening oncogenic types through vaccination will likely result in fewer abnormal smears and possibly a higher proportion of equivocal results during Pap screening. This could introduce a number of unpredictable human factors into the equation, including boredom among screening personnel, resulting in reduced attention, less professional satisfaction related to making a public health difference, and an overall compromise of quality. Organizational measures may need to be instituted to counteract these effects.
2. Another collateral effect of HPV vaccination would be a structural decrease in test accuracy and cost-effectiveness for this aspect of the prevention effort, as the Pap smear program would be responsible for a lower rate of avoided precursors and cancers.

HPV: Prevention of Infection and Disease   271

This simply reinforces the importance of treating any economic analysis as an integrated exercise comprising both screening and vaccination.

3. There are questions about how vaccination will alter client attitudes concerning the importance of screening. Vaccinated women may feel that the necessity or urgency of screening is reduced. Such a development could paradoxically lead to an increase in cervical cancers. Clearly, a robust public education program about the essential role of ongoing screening will need to be maintained alongside vaccination for the foreseeable future.

It is clear that the independent and overlapping benefits of both vaccination and screening must be maintained in an integrated prevention strategy.[64] The cautions discussed earlier ought to motivate a program of careful monitoring prior to any substantial changes in screening protocols. In some at-risk populations, there may be a need for concerted attempts to improve screening uptake rates, especially if vaccination effectiveness proves to be less than optimal in real-world contexts. A case in point is sexually active adolescent females, where the rate of cervical cancer screening is low (only 12–45%).[65] Data that gradually emerge from the vaccination experience in real-world populations will provide better insight on how to enhance or moderate screening practices in light of both cost and clinical factors. This suggests the need for a vaccination registry that is linkable to both screening and cancer registries. Such registries are necessary for evaluation and surveillance, and for eventually helping to answer a number of outstanding questions.

Areas requiring further study. There are several areas of investigation that could influence future HPV vaccine implementation and other aspects of prevention policy. The following issues should be noted:

- The natural history of HPV is still being elucidated. Infectious agents are rarely static; the various HPV types are likely to have differing and perhaps even changing transmission dynamics.
- Even what is already known about HPV presents challenges for mathematical modeling. It is difficult to simulate the effect of sexual contact patterns among groups of people. The natural history of multiple HPV infections is also very complex.
- The understanding of approaches related to HPV and a variety of cancers is still evolving.
- There is a question as to whether persistent HPV infections in older women represent a reactivation of a latent HPV acquired

earlier, or a brand new infection. Insights on this topic may influence decisions about expanding the vaccine indications to include older populations.
- There is a need to understand the costs and value of including older women and boys in a vaccination program.
- Research continues on alternate methods of vaccine delivery, which is of special relevance in the developing world. The inconvenience and expense of parenteral injections has increased interest in vaccines that can, for example, be administered nasally (i.e., by aerosol spray).[66]

Additional unanswered questions associated with HPV vaccination were recently summarized by Haug:[67]

1. Will the vaccine ultimately prevent not only cervical lesions but also cervical cancers and death?
2. How long will vaccine protection last?
3. Will the vaccine have the same effect on preadolescent girls as on the main 16- to 26-year-old trial subjects?
4. Will other HPV strains emerge as significant oncogenic serotypes if HPV-16 and -18 are effectively suppressed?[68]
5. Will vaccinated women continue to regularly access screening?
6. Will vaccination affect natural immunity against HPV?

The answers to these questions will substantially affect both the effectiveness and cost-effectiveness of any HPV vaccination program.

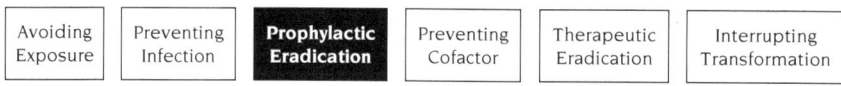

3. Prophylactic Eradication or Suppression

In the literature, there was no mention of prophylactic eradication or suppression of HPV infection that parallels the universal and/or targeted approaches employed with hepatitis B and *Helicobacter pylori* (see Chapters 8 and 9). A long latency period and well-established screening for preventable HPV disease suggests that any more complex measures developed to eliminate infection (e.g., gene therapy[69]) will likely be restricted to investigational groups or special cases rather than being deployed at a population level.

HPV: Prevention of Infection and Disease   273

| Avoiding Exposure | Preventing Infection | Prophylactic Eradication | **Preventing Cofactor** | Therapeutic Eradication | Interrupting Transformation |

4. Cofactor Prevention

Smoking is a proven risk factor for cervical cancer, which puts the disease in the same company as many other malignancies. There have been suggestions in the past that the observed association may be an artifact of smokers having, on average, more lifetime sexual partners.[70] However, as detailed in Chapter 4, more recent analysis has confirmed the role of smoking as a cofactor in the development of cervical cancer. Evidence of the biological effects of smoking supports this conclusion. For instance, women who smoke do not seem to clear an HPV infection as quickly as nonsmokers. As well, a 2007 study confirmed that exposure to secondhand smoke is a risk factor for developing cervical intraepithelial neoplasia (CIN), which is suggestive of a causal impact for tobacco smoke.[71]

In addition to the primary prevention potential of cessation (or not smoking in the first place), the positive impacts on secondary prevention have been demonstrated. In short, tobacco use seems to decrease the effectiveness of treatments for cervical cancer precursors.[72] In a recent survey of general practitioners in the United States, most respondents underestimated the role of smoking as a risk factor related to cervical cancer, suggesting an opportunity for improved clinical education.[73]

Beyond smoking control, exposure to STIs other than HPV should be avoided in order to reduce synergistic effects that elevate the risk of progressing to cervical cancer. Fortunately, the same behavioral changes already advised for preventing HPV infection would automatically be protective against other agents. In particular, primary prevention measures against HIV infection (and its attendant immunosuppression) will have collateral benefits in terms of reducing cancer incidence, even though the impact on HPV infection rates is less clear.[74] The importance of STI control implies that there is a strong overlap between sexual health behaviors that protect against HPV infection (see earlier discussion) and those that reduce progression to cervical cancer; such recognition will not necessarily increase the utility of interventions in this area. Nonetheless, the delay of intercourse until age 21 in particular affords additional protection against cancer development because it allows maturation of the transformation zone, making it less vulnerable to the consequences of HPV exposure.[75]

Women who have used oral contraceptives (OCs) are found to be at higher risk for persistent infection and cancer development, though the relationship may not be causal but rather related to lower condom usage or other risky sexual behaviors.[76] While avoidance of OCs may be a feasible option, it is less clear how to counteract other types of reproductive risk factors (e.g., higher parity).

In some countries, risk factors for cervical cancer seem to include lower family income and lower levels of education.[77] However, the association does not seem to pertain to the Canadian setting.[78] Although there once were differences in cervical cancer mortality based upon income, these disparities have diminished dramatically since universal health care coverage was introduced in the country.[79] Recent U.S. results in this regard have suggested mixed effects: lower education and higher poverty conferred increased risk of cervical, vaginal, and penile cancer, whereas higher education was associated with increased incidence of vulvar cancer, as well as excess anal and head and neck cancers in both men and women.[80] The conclusion seems to be that investigation of the effects of socioeconomic status does not offer an immediate way forward as a prevention strategy.

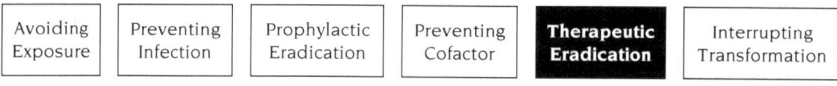

5. Therapeutic Eradication or Suppression

This category of prevention refers to an intervention that more or less directly addresses an established infection, but prior to the onset of any clinical disease. This should be distinguished from the next and final category in the typology, that is, where the focus is the carcinogenic transformation process (rather than the infection per se). Admittedly, categories 5 and 6 (and the disease processes to which they refer) logically and practically overlap to some extent. For example, both types of prevention presuppose that HPV infection has been detected. The affinity between the categories, reflecting the intimate relationship between infection and carcinogenesis, means that locating a particular therapy appropriately within them is sometimes debatable.

The concept of eradication is most applicable to microbes that are not protected within host cells, for example, a bacterium such as *H. pylori*. When a virus is housed in a cell and/or some of its products are integrated into host cellular mechanisms, eradication seems less feasible. In such cases, it may be better to think in terms of the suppression of infectious processes. On the other hand, eradication may be the correct rubric for interventions designed to detect and actually destroy only HPV-infected cells. An intermediate impact would be one where the infection was not eliminated, but at least production and transmission of new viruses were prevented.

The fact is that treatment is generally not recommended for subclinical genital HPV infection. The diagnosis of subclinical genital HPV infection may not become common until HPV-DNA testing is routinely implemented. Not only is diagnosis rarely definitive, but no therapy has yet been identified that can eliminate HPV infection.[81,82] This gap has been confirmed in one of the most common eradication contexts, namely, following ablative treatments for cervical dysplasia. Likewise, though approaches are available for the treatment of genital warts, HPV infection generally cannot be cured, and the recurrence of lesions is common.[83]

Despite the obstacles noted earlier, researchers continue to pursue measures that could eliminate an HPV infection. The most popular investigational approach is therapeutic vaccines.[84,85] Earlier, this strategy was distinguished from prophylactic vaccination (see "Preventing Infection after Exposure to the Agent"). In the case of HPV, therapeutic vaccines generally involve immune system modulation in individuals already infected with HPV. The aim of such vaccines is to interrupt some element of the infectious process, and thereby stop the progression to serious forms of disease such as cancer. Boosting immunity has the potential to be efficacious, especially given the fact that HPV infection in the mucosal surfaces of the female genital region of the body normally elicits a weak immune response.[86]

Essentially, there are three points in the natural history of HPV infection where the host's immune system may be enhanced in order to combat the virus[87]:

- Before infection of the epithelium, interrupting mucosal entry of the virus (i.e., classic prophylaxis)
- During viral replication, eliminating cells expressing late genes and thus interrupting the formation of new virions
- After viral integration, aiming to control or stop the growth of tumors by targeting oncoproteins generated by HPV genes E6 and E7

There are many components to consider in the development of therapeutic HPV vaccination, beginning with biological sources[88] and basic vaccine technology. The various approaches include peptide/protein, DNA, VLPs, dendritic and Langerhans cells, and recombinant viruses.[89-93] The antigen target of the vaccine is also critical; the key options comprise the protein products coded by viral DNA. Unlike the current prophylactic vaccines that are targeted at the capsid protein L1, therapeutic agents have been developed for the capsid proteins, for E7, and for a combination of E6 and E7. The oncoproteins E6 and E7 currently dominate the research agenda.[94-99]

Initial results from small phase I trials of therapeutic vaccines have been mixed,[100] although more recent research has shown more promise,[101-103] and a variety of innovations are being pursued to increase efficacy. For example, encouraging results have emerged from investigations of ways to enhance vaccine potency by linking HPV antigens to other proteins.[104,105] Other research is exploring the potential of broadly protective vaccines that neutralize a diverse set of HPV types, usually based on the L2 capsid antigen.[106,107]

While most of the trials on therapeutic vaccines in humans have focused on genital diseases (including vulval and vaginal dysplasia[108]), researchers hope that there will be benefits for other parts of the body, such as HPV-related tumors in the head and neck.[109,110] Given the burden of cancer caused by HPV, and the fact that the full benefits of prophylactic vaccination will not be seen for some years, the quest for a therapeutic breakthrough will continue. One of the "holy grails" for researchers is a chimeric vaccine, which combines the properties of prophylactic and therapeutic approaches.[111] This vaccination strategy generally targets a combination of early and late viral proteins.[112]

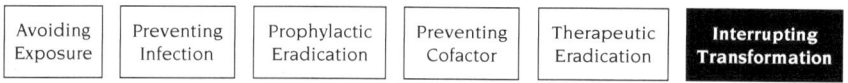

6. Interrupting Transformation Related to Infection

It is understandable that the immunotherapies targeting HPV infection may overlap with the final prevention topic, which focuses on viral or cellular processes that lead to cancer. There is a fine line between these categories; in some cases, the distinctions may even begin to blur between these therapies and treatments for premalignant lesions.

It has been already suggested during the discussion of HPV eradication that interventions directly targeting the virus and its processes are very limited. This was confirmed in the only systematic review located, which dates to 2000.[113] While effective antiviral therapies for subclinical HPV infection are not yet available in practice, progress continues to be made at a research level.[114]

In this regard, recombinant human interferon gamma has shown good results in terms of the regression of precancerous cells, sometimes even leading to complete remission of HPV infection.[115,116] As well, an earlier study suggested that the highly active antiretroviral therapy used with HIV/AIDS can have a positive effect on cervical precancer (though the impact on HPV clearance was not reported).[117] The ultimate quest is for a targeted antiviral, rather than simply the induction of nonspecific inflammation that in turn generates a "bystander immune response."[118] Antivirals for HPV are especially important for the substantial population of immunosuppressed individuals who may not benefit from novel immunotherapies, including the therapeutic vaccines described in the previous subsection.

The skin is also a common site of HPV infection, which sometimes leads to squamous cell cancer. While no traditional cutaneous antiviral therapies have demonstrated superior results, certain immunomodulatory compounds have been shown to achieve both HPV clearance and low recurrence rates.[119]

The remaining conservative (i.e., nonsurgical) approaches to HPV infection and its associated precancerous lesions include a wide range of strategies examined in the laboratory. Whether involving dietary nutrients (e.g., retinoids, beta-carotenes) or topical medications such as cidofovir, the results have been, at best, mixed.[120–122] A 2007 Cochrane review of the effectiveness of retinoids in treating CIN concluded that these agents were not effective in preventing progression.[123] The authors also found that retinoids were ineffective in promoting regression of CIN3, though some positive effects on CIN2 were noted.

Data from the limited RCTs investigating the effectiveness of potential chemopreventive agents on the prevention of cervical cancer have not been very promising.[124,125] While modest results have been shown for a few agents, further testing has been impeded, due in large part to side effects.

Nonsteroidal antiinflammatories and gene therapies are also at an early stage of investigation.[126–128] Finally, an experimental treatment for HPV infection, photodynamic therapy, has so far shown variable efficacy.[129]

The growing understanding of the molecular biology of HPV infection has guided innovation in the arena of anti-infection and anticancer strategies. With the exception of E1, the oncogenic proteins of HPV lack enzymatic activity; they generally achieve their effects by interacting with cellular proteins. While protein–protein interactions are difficult to suppress using conventional drugs, they "are amenable to inhibition using intracellular antibodies or intrabodies, which bind the viral proteins and sterically inhibit their association with cellular partners. The lack of homology between viral and cellular proteins, and the fact that HPV infections can be treated topically, makes them particularly well suited to the intrabody approach."[130]

CONCLUSION: HPV AND PREVENTION IN THE FUTURE

The prevention picture related to HPV and the diseases caused by this virus is currently dominated by prophylactic vaccination. This is understandable, as effective vaccines are perceived as the pinnacle of primary prevention of diseases caused by infections.

In the end, HPV vaccine effectiveness (and, ultimately, cost-effectiveness) will be proven by reductions in HPV-related disease burden. Given the long pathogenic latency periods associated with HPV infection and cancer development, assessing the validity of mathematical simulation models based on results in the real world will require a certain amount of patience. Confirmation of estimates with actual outcomes data may be decades away.

From a certain perspective, the development of the vaccine Gardasil™ reveals a picture of intense scientific study and an apparent narrowing of vaccination options. Thus, one dominant vaccine (and one possible competitor) has emerged onto the stage of public health policy at the present time; on the other hand, other approaches have been practically eclipsed. For example, Merck's earlier work on a monovalent vaccine targeting HPV-16 appears to have been superseded. While the results for the latter approach were actually quite impressive,[131,132] the discussion is now focused on polyvalent HPV vaccines and their expanded prevention power.

The recent extensive academic and media attention received by Gardasil™ (and, increasingly, by Cervarix™) has expanded general interest in the arena of HPV prophylactic vaccination. This could in turn lead to new ideas and energy around alternate vaccination approaches. Beyond the VLP technology employed with Gardasil™, Cervarix™, and several monovalent formulations, both DNA and plasmid DNA vaccine models have also been tested.[133] It is unclear whether any of the alternate approaches will gain traction in the years to come, but it is possible that revolutionary insights may still emerge. It is also likely that the lessons learned from other infectious agents of cancer may also bear positively on the cause of HPV prevention, as has already occurred in the adaptation of the hepatitis vaccine technology to HPV vaccine development.

NOTES

1   Lillo FB. Human papillomavirus infection and its role in the genesis of dysplastic and neoplastic lesions of the squamous epithelia. *New Microbiologica.* 2005; 28(2): 111–8.

2. "Almost unique" is the appropriate phrase because, as will be shown later in the book, other, albeit rarer cancers also enjoy a one-to-one relationship with an infectious cause.
3. Schoell WM, Janicek MF, Mirhashemi R. Epidemiology and biology of cervical cancer. *Seminars in Surgical Oncology*. 1999; 16(3): 203–11.
4. Bosch FX, Munoz N. The viral etiology of cervical cancer. *Virus Research*. 2002; 89(2): 183–90.
5. *Report to Congress: Prevention of Genital Human Papillomavirus Infection*. Centers for Disease Control and Prevention; 2004. Available at http://www.cdc.gov/std/HPV/2004HPV%20Report.pdf. Accessed May 2005.
6. Olatunbosun O. Human papillomavirus vaccine, teen sex and politics. *Journal of Family Planning and Reproductive Health Care*. 2006; 32(2): 74.
7. Frazer IH, Cox JT, Mayeaux EJ, Jr. et al. Advances in prevention of cervical cancer and other human papillomavirus-related diseases. *Pediatric Infectious Disease Journal*. 2006; 25(2 suppl): S65–81.
8. Kaplan-Myrth N, Dollin J. Cervical cancer awareness and HPV prevention in Canada. *Canadian Family Physician*. 2007; 53(4): 693–7.
9. Keeffe EB, Dieterich DT, Han SH et al. A treatment algorithm for the management of chronic hepatitis B virus infection in the United States: an update. *Clinical Gastroenterology and Hepatology*. 2006; 4(8): 936–62.
10. Frazer IH, Cox JT, Mayeaux EJ, Jr. et al. Advances in prevention of cervical cancer and other human papillomavirus-related diseases. *Pediatric Infectious Disease Journal*. 2006; 25(2 suppl): S65–81.
11. Scheurer ME, Tortolero-Luna G, Adler-Storthz K. Human papillomavirus infection: biology, epidemiology, and prevention. *International Journal of Gynecological Cancer*. 2005; 15(5): 727–46.
12. Winer RL, Hughes JP, Feng Q et al. Condom use and the risk of genital human papillomavirus infection in young women. *New England Journal of Medicine*. 2006; 354(25): 2645–54.
13. Sawaya GF, Chirenje MZ, Magure MT et al. Effect of diaphragm and lubricant gel provision on human papillomavirus infection among women provided with condoms: a randomized controlled trial. *Obstetrics and Gynecology*. 2008; 112(5): 990–7.
14. Shew ML, Fortenberry JD, Tu W et al. Association of condom use, sexual behaviors, and sexually transmitted infections with the duration of genital human papillomavirus infection among adolescent women. *Archives of Pediatrics and Adolescent Medicine*. 2006; 160(2): 151–6.
15. Hogewoning CJ, Bleeker MC, van den Brule AJ et al. Condom use promotes regression of cervical intraepithelial neoplasia and clearance of human papillomavirus: a randomized clinical trial. *International Journal of Cancer*. 2003; 107(5): 811–6.
16. Epstein RJ. Primary prevention of human papillomavirus-dependent neoplasia: no condom, no sex. *European Journal of Cancer*. 2005; 41(17): 2595–600.
17. Giles S. Transmission of HPV. *Canadian Medical Association Journal*. 2003; 168(11): 1391.
18. Manhart LE, Koutsky LA. Do condoms prevent genital HPV infection, external genital warts, or cervical neoplasia? A meta-analysis. *Sexually Transmitted Diseases*. 2002; 29(11): 725–35.

19 Weller SC, Davis-Beaty K. Condom effectiveness in reducing heterosexual HIV transmission. *Cochrane Database of Systematic Reviews.* 2001.
20 Miksis S. A review of the evidence comparing the human papillomavirus vaccine versus condoms in the prevention of human papillomavirus infections. *Journal of Obstetric, Gynecologic and Neonatal Nursing.* 2008; 37(3): 329–37.
21 Plummer M, Franceschi S. Strategies for HPV prevention. *Virus Research.* 2002; 89(2): 285–93.
22 Sangani P, Rutherford G, Kennedy Gail E. Population-based interventions for reducing sexually transmitted infections, including HIV infection. *Cochrane Database of Systematic Reviews.* 2004.
23 Myer L, Morroni C, Mathews C et al. Structural and community-level interventions for increasing condom use to prevent HIV and other sexually transmitted infections (protocol). *Cochrane Database of Systematic Reviews.* 2009.
24 Mukoma W, Kagee A, Flisher AJ et al. School-based interventions to postpone sexual intercourse and promote condom use among adolescents (protocol). *Cochrane Database of Systematic Reviews.* 2009.
25 Bailey JV, Murray E, Rait G et al. Interactive computer-based interventions for sexual health promotion (protocol). *Cochrane Database of Systematic Reviews.* 2007.
26 Manhart LE, Holmes KK. Randomized controlled trials of individual-level, population-level, and multilevel interventions for preventing sexually transmitted infections: what has worked? *Journal of Infectious Diseases.* 2005; 191(suppl 1): S7–24.
27 Sangani P, Rutherford G, Kennedy Gail E. Population-based interventions for reducing sexually transmitted infections, including HIV infection. *Cochrane Database of Systematic Reviews.* 2004.
28 Underhill K, Montgomery P, Operario D. Abstinence-plus programs for HIV infection prevention in high-income countries. *Cochrane Database of Systematic Reviews.* 2007.
29 Manhart LE, Holmes KK. Randomized controlled trials of individual-level, population-level, and multilevel interventions for preventing sexually transmitted infections: what has worked? *Journal of Infectious Diseases.* 2005; 191(suppl 1): S7–24.
30 Baker SA, Beadnell B, Stoner S et al. Skills training versus health education to prevent STDs/HIV in heterosexual women: a randomized controlled trial utilizing biological outcomes. *AIDS Education and Prevention.* 2003; 15(1): 1–14.
31 Boyer CB, Shafer MA, Shaffer RA et al. Evaluation of a cognitive-behavioral, group, randomized controlled intervention trial to prevent sexually transmitted infections and unintended pregnancies in young women. *Preventive Medicine.* 2005; 40(4): 420–31.
32 Elwy AR, Hart GJ, Hawkes S et al. Effectiveness of interventions to prevent sexually transmitted infections and human immunodeficiency virus in heterosexual men: a systematic review. *Archives of Internal Medicine.* 2002; 162(16): 1818–30.
33 Shepherd JJ, Peersman G, Napuli I. Interventions for encouraging sexual lifestyles and behaviours intended to prevent cervical cancer. *Cochrane Database of Systematic Reviews.* 1999.
34 Johnson AM, Fenton KA, Mercer C. Phase specific strategies for the prevention, control, and elimination of sexually transmitted diseases: background

country profile, England and Wales. *Sexually Transmitted Infections.* 2002; 78(suppl 1): i125–32.
35 Ward DJ, Rowe B, Pattison H et al. Reducing the risk of sexually transmitted infections in genitourinary medicine clinic patients: a systematic review and meta-analysis of behavioural interventions. *Sexually Transmitted Infections.* 2005; 81(5): 386–93.
36 van Kesteren NM, Hospers HJ, Kok G. Sexual risk behavior among HIV-positive men who have sex with men: a literature review. *Patient Education and Counseling.* 2007; 65(1): 5–20.
37 Wetzel C, Tissot A, Kollar LM et al. Development of an HPV educational protocol for adolescents. *Journal of Pediatric and Adolescent Gynecology.* 2007; 20(5): 281–7.
38 Herbert J, Coffin J. Reducing patient risk for human papillomavirus infection and cervical cancer. *Journal of the American Osteopathic Association.* 2008; 108(2): 65–70.
39 Szarewski A. Prophylactic HPV vaccines. *European Journal of Gynaecological Oncology.* 2007; 28(3): 165–9.
40 Brinkman JA, Hughes SH, Stone P et al. Therapeutic vaccination for HPV induced cervical cancers. *Disease Markers.* 2007; 23(4): 337–52.
41 Scheurer ME, Tortolero-Luna G, Adler-Storthz K. Human papillomavirus infection: biology, epidemiology, and prevention. *International Journal of Gynecological Cancer.* 2005; 15(5): 727–46.
42 Villa LL, Costa RL, Petta CA et al. Prophylactic quadrivalent human papillomavirus (types 6, 11, 16, and 18) L1 virus-like particle vaccine in young women: a randomised double-blind placebo-controlled multicentre phase II efficacy trial. *Lancet Oncology.* 2005; 6(5): 271–8.
43 Ludwig C, Wagner R. Virus-like particles-universal molecular toolboxes. *Current Opinion in Biotechnology.* 2007; 18(6): 537–45.
44 Ault KA. The Future II Study Group. Effect of prophylactic human papillomavirus L1 virus-like-particle vaccine on risk of cervical intraepithelial neoplasia grade 3, grade 3, and adenocarcinoma in situ: a combined analysis of four randomized clinical trials. *The Lancet.* 2007; 369: 1861–68.
45 Paavonen J. Human papillomavirus infection and the development of cervical cancer and related genital neoplasias. *International Journal of Infectious Diseases.* 2007; 11(suppl 2): S3–9.
46 Zhou Y, Nabeshima K, Koga K et al. Comparison of Epstein-Barr virus genotypes and clinicohistopathological features of nasopharyngeal carcinoma between Guilin, China and Fukuoka, Japan. *Oncology Reports.* 2008; 19(6): 1413–20.
47 2nd Cervical Cancer Vaccine on the Way? Study Shows Cervarix Protects Against Virus That Can Cause Cervical Cancer. 2007. Available at http://www.webmd.com/sexual-conditions/hpv-genital-warts/news/20070627/2nd-cervical-cancer-vaccine-on-the-way. Accessed April 2008.
48 de Boer MA, Jordanova ES, Kenter GG et al. High human papillomavirus oncogene mRNA expression and not viral DNA load is associated with poor prognosis in cervical cancer patients. *Clinical Cancer Research.* 2007; 13(1): 132–8.
49 Cutts FT, Franceschi S, Goldie S et al. Human papillomavirus and HPV vaccines: a review. *Bulletin of the World Health Organization.* 2007; 85(9): 719–26.

50 Gardasil and Cervarix Go Head-To-Head. 2007. Available at http://www.natap.org/2007/newsUpdates/012207_04.htm. Accessed April 2008.
51 Gish RG. Hepatocellular carcinoma: overcoming challenges in disease management. *Clinical Gastroenterology and Hepatology.* 2006; 4(3): 252–61.
52 Eggertson L. Three provinces to study 2-dose HPV vaccine. *Canadian Medical Association Journal.* 2007; 177(5): 444–5.
53 National Advisory Committee on Immunization Statement on Human Papillomavirus Vaccine. 2007. Available at http://www.phac-aspc.gc.ca/publicat/ccdr-rmtc/07vol33/acs-02/index_e.html. Accessed April 2007.
54 Goldhaber-Fiebert JD, Stout NK, Salomon JA et al. Cost-effectiveness of cervical cancer screening with human papillomavirus DNA testing and HPV-16,18 vaccination. *Journal of the National Cancer Institute.* 2008; 100(5): 308–20.
55 Kulasingam S, Connelly L, Conway E et al. A cost-effectiveness analysis of adding a human papillomavirus vaccine to the Australian National Cervical Cancer Screening Program. *Sexual Health.* 2007; 4(3): 165–75.
56 Kulasingam SL, Benard S, Barnabas RV et al. Adding a quadrivalent human papillomavirus vaccine to the UK cervical cancer screening programme: a cost-effectiveness analysis. *Cost Effectiveness and Resource Allocation.* 2008; 6(1): 4.
57 This reduction is estimated based on a review of cost-effectiveness studies published to November 2008 by Krueger H. Implementing a Human Papillomavirus Program: Evidence on Cost-Effectiveness. December 31, 2008. Available at www.krueger.ca.
58 See, for example, Goldhaber-Fiebert JD, Stout NK, Salomon JA et al. Cost-effectiveness of cervical cancer screening with human papillomavirus DNA testing and HPV-16,18 vaccination. *Journal of the National Cancer Institute.* 2008; 100(5): 308–20.
59 Rogoza RM, Ferko N, Bentley J et al. Optimization of primary and secondary cervical cancer prevention strategies in an era of cervical cancer vaccination: a multi-regional health economic analysis. *Vaccine.* 2008; 26(suppl 5): F46–58.
60 Kim JJ, Goldie SJ. Health and economic implications of HPV vaccination in the United States. *New England Journal of Medicine.* 2008; 359(8): 821–32.
61 Roden RB, Monie A, Wu TC. Opportunities to improve the prevention and treatment of cervical cancer. *Current Molecular Medicine.* 2007; 7(5): 490–503.
62 Stanley M, Gissmann L, Nardelli-Haefliger D. Immunobiology of human papillomavirus infection and vaccination - implications for second generation vaccines. *Vaccine.* 2008; 26(suppl 10): K62–7.
63 Lowy DR, Solomon D, Hildesheim A et al. Human papillomavirus infection and the primary and secondary prevention of cervical cancer. *Cancer.* 2008; 113(suppl 7): 1980–93.
64 Stanley M. Human papillomavirus vaccines versus cervical cancer screening. *Clinical Oncology.* 2008; 20(6): 388–94.
65 Frega A, Stentella P, De Ioris A et al. Young women, cervical intraepithelial neoplasia and human papillomavirus: risk factors for persistence and recurrence. *Cancer Letters.* 2003; 196(2): 127–34.
66 Schiller JT, Davies P. Delivering on the promise: HPV vaccines and cervical cancer. Nature Reviews. *Microbiology.* 2004; 2(4): 343–7.
67 Haug CJ. Human papillomavirus vaccination—reasons for caution. *New England Journal of Medicine.* 2008; 359(8): 861–2.

68 Type replacement may be occurring with, for example, the 7-valent pneumococcal conjugate vaccine. See Singleton RJ, Hennessy TW, Bulkow LR et al. Invasive pneumococcal disease caused by nonvaccine serotypes among Alaska native children with high levels of 7-valent pneumococcal conjugate vaccine coverage. *Journal of the American Medical Association.* 2007; 297(16): 1784–92.

69 Carson A, Wang Z, Xiao X et al. A DNA recombination-based approach to eliminate papillomavirus infection. *Gene Therapy.* 2005; 12(6): 534–40.

70 Kalliala I, Nieminen P, Dyba T et al. Cancer free survival after CIN treatment: comparisons of treatment methods and histology. *Gynecologic Oncology.* 2007; 105(1): 228–33.

71 Tsai HT, Tsai YM, Yang SF et al. Lifetime cigarette smoke and second-hand smoke and cervical intraepithelial neoplasm—a community-based case-control study. *Gynecologic Oncology.* 2007; 105(1): 181–8.

72 Acladious NN, Sutton C, Mandal D et al. Persistent human papillomavirus infection and smoking increase risk of failure of treatment of cervical intraepithelial neoplasia (CIN). *International Journal of Cancer.* 2002; 98(3): 435–9.

73 Baay MF, Verhoeven V, Peremans L et al. General practitioners' perception of risk factors for cervical cancer development: consequences for patient education. *Patient Education and Counseling.* 2006; 62(2): 277–81.

74 Viscidi RP, Ahdieh-Grant L, Schneider MF et al. Serum immunoglobulin A response to human papillomavirus type 16 virus-like particles in human immunodeficiency virus (HIV)-positive and high-risk HIV-negative women. *Journal of Infectious Diseases.* 2003; 188(12): 1834–44.

75 Diaz ML. Human papilloma virus: prevention and treatment. *Obstetrics and Gynecology Clinics of North America.* 2008; 35(2): 199–217.

76 Sellors JW, Mahony JB, Kaczorowski J et al. Prevalence and predictors of human papillomavirus infection in women in Ontario, Canada. Survey of HPV in Ontario Women (SHOW) Group. *Canadian Medical Association Journal.* 2000; 163(5): 503–8.

77 Kliucinskas M, Nadisauskiene RJ, Minkauskiene M. Prevalence and risk factors of HPV infection among high-risk rural and urban Lithuanian women. *Gynecologic and Obstetric Investigation.* 2006; 62(3): 173–80.

78 Sellors JW, Mahony JB, Kaczorowski J et al. Prevalence and predictors of human papillomavirus infection in women in Ontario, Canada. Survey of HPV in Ontario Women (SHOW) Group. *Canadian Medical Association Journal.* 2000; 163(5): 503–8.

79 Ng E, Wilkins R, Fung MF et al. Cervical cancer mortality by neighbourhood income in urban Canada from 1971 to 1996. *Canadian Medical Association Journal.* 2004; 170(10): 1545–9.

80 Benard VB, Johnson CJ, Thompson TD et al. Examining the association between socioeconomic status and potential human papillomavirus-associated cancers. *Cancer.* 2008; 113(suppl 10): 2910–8.

81 As reported on the CDC website at http://www.cdc.gov/STD/treatment/6-2002TG.htm#SubclinicalGenitalHPV Infection. Accessed June 2005.

82 Stanley M. Chapter 17: Genital human papillomavirus infections—current and prospective therapies. *Journal of the National Cancer Institute Monograph.* 2003; (31): 117–24.

83 Doorbar J, Griffin H. Intrabody strategies for the treatment of human papillomavirus-associated disease. *Expert Opinion on Biological Therapy.* 2007; 7(5): 677–89.
84 These drugs may be less confusingly referred to as immunotherapeutic agents, given that "vaccine" is firmly fixed in the minds of many people as referring to a prophylactic strategy.
85 Psyrri A, Tsiodras S. Optimizing approaches to head-and-neck cancers. Viruses in head-and-neck cancers: prevention and therapy. *Annals of Oncology.* 2008; 19(suppl 7): vii189–94.
86 Hoglund P, Karre K, Klein G. The uterine cervix—a new member of the family of immunologically exceptional sites? *Cancer Immunity.* 2003; 3: 6.
87 Scheurer ME, Tortolero-Luna G, Adler-Storthz K. Human papillomavirus infection: biology, epidemiology, and prevention. *International Journal of Gynecological Cancer.* 2005; 15(5): 727–46.
88 Massa S, Franconi R, Brandi R et al. Anti-cancer activity of plant-produced HPV16 E7 vaccine. *Vaccine.* 2007; 25(16): 3018–21.
89 Crosbie EJ, Kitchener HC. Human papillomavirus in cervical screening and vaccination. *Clinical Science.* 2006; 110(5): 543–52.
90 Jung WW, Chun T, Sul D et al. Strategies against human papillomavirus infection and cervical cancer. *Journal of Microbiology.* 2004; 42(4): 255–66.
91 Stern PL. Immune control of human papillomavirus (HPV) associated anogenital disease and potential for vaccination. *Journal of Clinical Virology.* 2005; 32(suppl 1): S72–81.
92 Bellone S, Pecorelli S, Cannon MJ et al. Advances in dendritic-cell-based therapeutic vaccines for cervical cancer. *Expert Review of Anticancer Therapy.* 2007; 7(10): 1473–86.
93 Santin AD, Hermonat PL, Ravaggi A et al. Induction of human papillomavirus-specific CD4(+) and CD8(+) lymphocytes by E7-pulsed autologous dendritic cells in patients with human papillomavirus type 16- and 18-positive cervical cancer. *Journal of Virology.* 1999; 73(7): 5402–10.
94 Peng S, Ji H, Trimble C et al. Development of a DNA vaccine targeting human papillomavirus type 16 oncoprotein E6. *Journal of Virology.* 2004; 78(16): 8468–76.
95 Scheurer ME, Tortolero-Luna G, Adler-Storthz K. Human papillomavirus infection: biology, epidemiology, and prevention. *International Journal of Gynecological Cancer.* 2005; 15(5): 727–46.
96 Wu TC. Therapeutic human papillomavirus DNA vaccination strategies to control cervical cancer. *European Journal of Immunology.* 2007; 37(2): 310–4.
97 Brulet JM, Maudoux F, Thomas S et al. DNA vaccine encoding endosome-targeted human papillomavirus type 16 E7 protein generates CD4+ T cell-dependent protection. *European Journal of Immunology.* 2007; 37(2): 376–84.
98 Kim SW, Yang JS. Human papillomavirus type 16 E5 protein as a therapeutic target. *Yonsei Medical Journal.* 2006; 47(1): 1–14.
99 Brinkman JA, Xu X, Kast WM. The efficacy of a DNA vaccine containing inserted and replicated regions of the E7 gene for treatment of HPV-16 induced tumors. *Vaccine.* 2007; 25(17): 3437–44.
100 Stanley M. Chapter 17: Genital human papillomavirus infections—current and prospective therapies. *Journal of the National Cancer Institute Monograph.* 2003; (31): 117–24.

101 Crosbie EJ, Kitchener HC. Human papillomavirus in cervical screening and vaccination. *Clinical Science*. 2006; 110(5): 543–52.
102 Fox PA, Tung MY. Human papillomavirus: burden of illness and treatment cost considerations. *American Journal of Clinical Dermatology*. 2005; 6(6): 365–81.
103 Brinkman JA, Hughes SH, Stone P et al. Therapeutic vaccination for HPV induced cervical cancers. *Disease Markers*. 2007; 23(4): 337–52.
104 McDougall JA, Madeleine MM, Daling JR et al. Racial and ethnic disparities in cervical cancer incidence rates in the United States, 1992–2003. *Cancer Causes and Control*. 2007; 18(10): 1175–86.
105 Huang CY, Chen CA, Lee CN et al. DNA vaccine encoding heat shock protein 60 co-linked to HPV16 E6 and E7 tumor antigens generates more potent immunotherapeutic effects than respective E6 or E7 tumor antigens. *Gynecologic Oncology*. 2007; 107(3): 404–12.
106 Gambhira R, Karanam B, Jagu S et al. A protective and broadly cross-neutralizing epitope of human papillomavirus L2. *Journal of Virology*. 2007; 81(24): 13927–31.
107 Gambhira R, Jagu S, Karanam B et al. Protection of rabbits against challenge with rabbit papillomaviruses by immunization with the N terminus of human papillomavirus type 16 minor capsid antigen L2. *Journal of Virology*. 2007; 81(21): 11585–92.
108 Baldwin PJ, van der Burg SH, Boswell CM et al. Vaccinia-expressed human papillomavirus 16 and 18 e6 and e7 as a therapeutic vaccination for vulval and vaginal intraepithelial neoplasia. *Clinical Cancer Research*. 2003; 9(14): 5205–13.
109 Devaraj K, Gillison ML, Wu TC. Development of HPV vaccines for HPV-associated head and neck squamous cell carcinoma. *Critical Reviews in Oral Biology and Medicine*. 2003; 14(5): 345–62.
110 Badaracco G, Venuti A. Human papillomavirus therapeutic vaccines in head and neck tumors. *Expert Review of Anticancer Therapy*. 2007; 7(5): 753–66.
111 Snoeck R. Papillomavirus and treatment. *Antiviral Research*. 2006; 71(2–3): 181–91.
112 Scheurer ME, Tortolero-Luna G, Adler-Storthz K. Human papillomavirus infection: biology, epidemiology, and prevention. *International Journal of Gynecological Cancer*. 2005; 15(5): 727–46.
113 Russomano F, Reis A, de Camargo MJ et al. Efficacy in treatment of subclinical cervical HPV infection without intraepithelial neoplasia: systematic review. *Sao Paulo Medical Journal*. 2000; 118(4): 109–15.
114 Fradet-Turcotte A, Archambault J. Recent advances in the search for antiviral agents against human papillomaviruses. *Antiviral Therapy*. 2007; 12(4): 431–51.
115 Stanley M. Genital human papillomavirus infections—current and prospective therapies. *Journal of the National Cancer Institute Monograph*. Chapter 17, 2003; (31): 117–24.
116 Sikorski M, Zrubek H. Recombinant human interferon gamma in the treatment of cervical intraepithelial neoplasia (CIN) associated with human papillomavirus (HPV) infection. *European Journal of Gynaecological Oncology*. 2003; 24(2): 147–50.
117 Heard I, Tassie JM, Kazatchkine MD et al. Highly active antiretroviral therapy enhances regression of cervical intraepithelial neoplasia in HIV-seropositive women. *AIDS*. 2002; 16(13): 1799–802.

118 Stanley M. Genital human papillomavirus infections—current and prospective therapies. *Journal of the National Cancer Institute Monograph.* Chapter 17, 2003; (31): 117–24.
119 Rivera A, Tyring SK. Therapy of cutaneous human papillomavirus infections. *Dermatologic Therapy.* 2004; 17(6): 441–8.
120 Stanley M. Genital human papillomavirus infections—current and prospective therapies. *Journal of the National Cancer Institute Monograph.* Chapter 17, 2003; (31): 117–24.
121 Manetta A, Schubbert T, Chapman J et al. Beta-carotene treatment of cervical intraepithelial neoplasia: a phase II study. *Cancer Epidemiology, Biomarkers and Prevention.* 1996; 5(11): 929–32.
122 Keefe KA, Schell MJ, Brewer C et al. A randomized, double blind, Phase III trial using oral beta-carotene supplementation for women with high-grade cervical intraepithelial neoplasia. *Cancer Epidemiology, Biomarkers and Prevention.* 2001; 10(10): 1029–35.
123 Helm CW, Lorenz DJ, Meyer NJ et al. Retinoids for preventing the progression of cervical intra-epithelial neoplasia. *Cochrane Database of Systematic Reviews.* 2007.
124 Sasieni P. Chemoprevention of cervical cancer. *Best Practice and Research. Clinical Obstetrics and Gynaecology.* 2006; 20(2): 295–305.
125 Follen M, Meyskens FL, Jr., Alvarez RD et al. Cervical cancer chemoprevention, vaccines, and surrogate endpoint biomarkers. *Cancer.* 2003; 98(9 suppl): 2044–51.
126 Shariff Osman M, Wulff Judith L, Helm CW. Anti-inflammatory agents for preventing the progression of cervical intraepithelial neoplasia. *Cochrane Database of Systematic Reviews.* 2008.
127 Sethi N, Palefsky J. Treatment of human papillomavirus (HPV) type 16-infected cells using herpes simplex virus type 1 thymidine kinase-mediated gene therapy transcriptionally regulated by the HPV E2 protein. *Human Gene Therapy.* 2003; 14(1): 45–57.
128 Shillitoe EJ. Papillomaviruses as targets for cancer gene therapy. *Cancer Gene Therapy.* 2006; 13(5): 445–50.
129 Stanley M. Genital human papillomavirus infections—current and prospective therapies. *Journal of the National Cancer Institute Monograph.* Chapter 17, 2003; (31): 117–24.
130 Doorbar J, Griffin H. Intrabody strategies for the treatment of human papillomavirus-associated disease. *Expert Opinion on Biological Therapy.* 2007; 7(5): 677–89.
131 Koutsky LA, Ault KA, Wheeler CM et al. A controlled trial of a human papillomavirus type 16 vaccine. *New England Journal of Medicine.* 2002; 347(21): 1645–51.
132 For example, Mao C, Koutsky LA, Ault KA et al. Efficacy of human papillomavirus-16 vaccine to prevent cervical intraepithelial neoplasia: a randomized controlled trial. *Obstetrics and Gynecology.* 2006; 107(1): 18–27.
133 Scheurer ME, Tortolero-Luna G, Adler-Storthz K. Human papillomavirus infection: biology, epidemiology, and prevention. *International Journal of Gynecological Cancer.* 2005; 15(5): 727–46.

8

HEPATITIS VIRUSES

HCV is the most important risk factor for hepatocellular carcinoma in western European and North American countries... [while] the World Health Organization has reported HBV to be second only to tobacco as a known human carcinogen.[1]

INTRODUCTION

Jaundice was recognized as a disease symptom as long ago as the fifth century BC, and an infectious cause was already suspected by the eighth century AD.[2] The viral origin of certain forms of hepatic disease was confirmed in the last 50 years; more recently, two hepatitis viruses have been specifically linked to the development of liver cancer. Worldwide, it is estimated that 400 million people are chronically infected with hepatitis B virus (HBV), and chronic hepatitis C virus (HCV) infection affects approximately 170 million people.[3]

Infection with either virus elevates the risk of developing primary liver cancer. Hepatocellular carcinoma (HCC) is the most common form of liver cancer[4]; it is the fifth most common malignancy in the world, and the most rapidly increasing cancer in the United States.[5] The incidence of HCC has also increased in Canada in the last two decades.[6,7] The high burden of liver disease has focused attention on all known causes, including infections and alcoholic cirrhosis. Adding to the concern about cancer is the substantial burden of "benign" and premalignant disease, attributable to the two main viral agents. In this light, it is not surprising that prevention efforts related to HBV and HCV have steadily intensified.[8-10]

Despite the attention being paid to the recent introduction of a prophylactic vaccine against human papillomavirus (HPV), it is important to recall that the first true cancer vaccine is now over 25 years old. Indeed, the implementation of highly efficacious and safe childhood vaccination programs for HBV around the world has dramatically reduced the global prevalence of hepatitis B.[11] On the other hand, drug therapy for patients chronically infected with HBV does not eradicate the virus but only slows down replication. This underscores the importance of primary prevention through means such as vaccination. Even more importantly, the current absence of a vaccine for HCV highlights the need to maximize any other prevention measures deemed to be useful in the short or long term. The urgency is even greater among medically underserved populations and ethnic and other at-risk groups, including Aboriginal peoples in Canada.[12]

THE VIRUSES

The hepatitis viruses are so named not because of genetic or other structural similarities, but due to their common connection with hepatic disease. In fact, hepatitis B and C belong to different viral families, and are thus sometimes treated separately in textbooks on infectious causes of cancer.[13] Classically, viruses labeled with the term hepatitis are hepatotropic, that is, they replicate in hepatocytes and thus cause acute or chronic hepatitis.[14] Hepatitis simply means "inflammation of the liver." A term such as "hepatitis C" is used to name the inflammation caused by a particular virus, and as shorthand for the virus itself. The limitations of this usage are immediately evident when one considers that HCV in particular has been linked to a broad range of extrahepatic manifestations. Reflecting this reality, some authorities have introduced the term "HCV syndrome" to cover the entire set of HCV-related diseases.[15]

As indicated in Table 8.1, six types of virus have been identified and named as hepatitis so far, though one form does not warrant that identification.[16,17]

This inventory continues to be fine-tuned by new research. For instance, hepatitis G does not appear to be hepatotropic or a cause of liver cancer, so another label, GB virus type C (GBV-C), is sometimes preferred.[18] One intriguing aspect of GBV-C is that it appears to reduce the impact of human immunodeficiency virus (HIV) in cases of coinfection.[19] Hepatitis F has not yet been confirmed, but it has been reserved

Table 8.1. Summary of Hepatitis Viruses

Hepatitis Type	Year Identified	Nucleic Acid	Transmission	Risk Groups	Chronic Hepatitis	Vaccine Available
A	1973	RNA	Fecal–oral	5- to 14-year olds	No	Yes
B	1965	DNA	Blood borne	25- to 39-year olds	Yes	Yes
C	1988	RNA	Blood borne	20- to 39-year olds with high risk behaviors	Yes	No
D	1977	RNA	Blood borne	Multiple blood transfusion recipients (e.g., hemophiliacs); injection drug users	Yes (as a co- or super-infection)	No
E	1983	RNA	Fecal–oral	15- to 40-year olds	No	No
G	1995	RNA	Blood borne	None	Unclear	No

Source: Fry, American Surgeon, 2007; Gillcrist, Journal of the American Dental Association, 1999.

as the label for a novel blood-borne infection detected in different parts of the world.[20,21] Other hepatotropic viruses (e.g., TTV, SENV) have been isolated, notably in transfusion patients, but their disease associations are unclear.[22–24] Even with the sophisticated detection methods now available, all clinical cases of viral hepatitis have not been linked to a known virus; it is likely that other hepatotropic viruses remain to be identified.

Hepatitis B Virus

A member of the Hepadnaviridae virus family, HBV was discovered in 1965, an achievement that later garnered the Nobel Prize. The virus contains double-stranded circular DNA that replicates via an RNA intermediate. The DNA is enclosed by an icosahedral capsid, as well as a lipid envelope.[25]

Eight HBV genotypes have been identified to date (labeled A–H, an unfortunate confusion with hepatitis A, B, etc.). Each genotype seems to demonstrate characteristic geographical distributions and clinical outcomes.[26] For example, while genotype A is more prevalent in North America and Europe, genotypes B and C are more commonly found in Asia.[27,28] Subtype A1 is endemic in South Africa, and has been associated with a higher risk for development of HCC.[29,30] Genotype C also appears to be common in cases of HCC. Recently, the same pattern was found to be true for genotype F among Alaskan Native people.[31] However, the exact clinical implication of each genotype and its geographical connection remains controversial.[32,33]

One molecular factor that has been investigated in the context of genotypes is hepatitis B antigen e (HBeAg). As a marker of an immune tolerance phase in the HBV natural history, it tends to be expressed in chronically infected children or young adults prior to an effective antibody response (the latter known as seroconversion). Early HBeAg seroconversion has been considered to be a positive sign in terms of disease outcome, whereas late or absent emergence of anti-HBe indicated a poorer prognosis. In Asian contexts, genotype B demonstrates earlier HBeAg seroconversion than genotype C; in other words, the latter genotype may confer a higher risk of chronic liver diseases, including cancer.[34] In a recent study among Alaskan Natives, the age at which 50% of persons infected as children with genotypes A, B, and D managed to clear HBeAg was <20 years, but almost 48 years in the case of genotype C. This sort of "delayed" seroconversion has been associated with a higher risk of progression to cirrhosis.[35] Finally, genotype F also cleared the antigen relatively early, but showed a greater tendency to revert to the HBeAg-positive state.[36]

This entire topic remains an active area of investigation. The utility of HBeAg as a prognostic marker has been questioned; in fact, there is evidence that a patient in a reactivated, HBeAG-negative chronic state may have a higher risk of progression to cirrhosis (see the section "Disease Mechanism and Process").[37] Thus, other factors may need to be examined to explain any differential associations of genotypes with disease outcome. Further, while genotype C may prompt earlier progression to cirrhosis and HCC, it may not always be true that the risk of developing liver cancer is higher (or survival rates lower) for any particular genotype of HBV.[38]

Hepatitis C Virus

HCV is a member of the Flaviviridae virus family. It contains a single-stranded RNA genome, housed within an icosahedral capsid and a lipid envelope.[39] Viral replication occurs in the cytoplasm following entry of viral RNA into the hepatocyte, with the RNA being used as a direct template in protein synthesis.[40]

There are six major HCV genotypes, and several subtypes.[41] Similar to HBV, each genotype is associated with a characteristic geographical distribution and clinical course.[42,43] In North America and western Europe, genotype 1 is the most common, whereas genotypes 2 and 3 have been found less frequently.[44] The genotypes appear to work differently in the pathogenesis of liver disease, particularly related to the process of lipid accumulation (or steatosis). Thus, in "genotype 3-infected patients, steatosis is likely viral-induced, and represents a direct cytopathic effect of HCV, whereas in patients infected with other genotypes, host metabolic risk factors for insulin resistance such as obesity, type 2 diabetes and hyperlipidemia play a major role."[45] In this sense, obesity and diabetes act as cofactors in the development of certain cases of hepatic steatosis, which can lead to sequelae such as cirrhosis and HCC.[46]

In this chapter, the established and emerging information concerning HBV and HCV is elucidated, especially regarding their involvement in liver cancer. The information is organized around the following topics: evidence of associated cancers, disease mechanism and process (including cofactors), transmission and occurrence of the agents, detection methods, and prevention approaches.

EVIDENCE OF ASSOCIATED CANCERS

Liver Cancer

In 1994, the International Agency for Research on Cancer (IARC) classified both HBV and HCV as human carcinogens.[47] The designation of HBV was based on over 20 years of evidence showing that the virus is an etiological agent for HCC.[48] Based on the studies reviewed by IARC, an HBV-positive individual appears to be 5–30 times more likely to develop liver cancer than those without infection. In a comparable review of the research based on newer detection tests, the relative risk for HCC due to HCV exposure ranged from 1.1 to 52.0.[49]

Accepting the best-supported data, an estimated 50–55% of the most common liver cancers are attributable to HBV infection, whereas HCV has been identified in approximately 25–30% of cases.[50,51] This suggests that, globally, at least three-quarters of the HCC burden has a viral cause. In the United States and Canada, because of the relative contributions of alcoholic cirrhosis and nonalcoholic steatohepatitis to the equation,[52] the proportion linked to viruses may be lower.

The exact epidemiologic profile can vary greatly from region to region. This may be largely due to differences in both viral load and viral prevalence. For instance, one study has demonstrated a geographic variation in viral load among hepatitis B carriers, with a concomitant impact on cancer development rates.[53] The more important driver may be the prevalence of the viruses in the population of interest. For example, in Egypt, with the highest prevalence of HCV worldwide, over 60% of HCC cases are attributable to HCV infection alone.[54] By comparison, an estimated 21% of HCC in the United States is due to HCV and 10% to HBV, and as many as 40% of the cases are presently classified as idiopathic.[55]

As suggested by the U.S. and Egyptian examples, the relative contribution of the two viruses to HCC can also vary. A 2007 meta-analysis of 90 studies confirmed that HBV predominates in the HCC cases in most Asian, African, and Latin American countries (Figure 8.1). However, similar to the situation in Egypt, HCV can be the more common cause of HCC in specific countries in these regions, including Japan, Pakistan, and Mongolia.[56] What is true in these specific countries holds across the developed world; thus, the prevalence of HCV generally exceeds that of HBV in the United States, Canada, and Europe. The one exception may be urban areas, such as Vancouver and Toronto in Canada, where immigration patterns may tip the balance toward HBV as the main viral cause of liver cancer.[57,58]

Liver cancer rates are increasing in both the United States and Canada, with a concomitant growth in the economic burden of illness.[59] Viral agency has been suspected as contributing to these trends. Given the long course of carcinogenesis, increasing incidence of liver cancer may be traceable to factors that came into effect as long as two or three

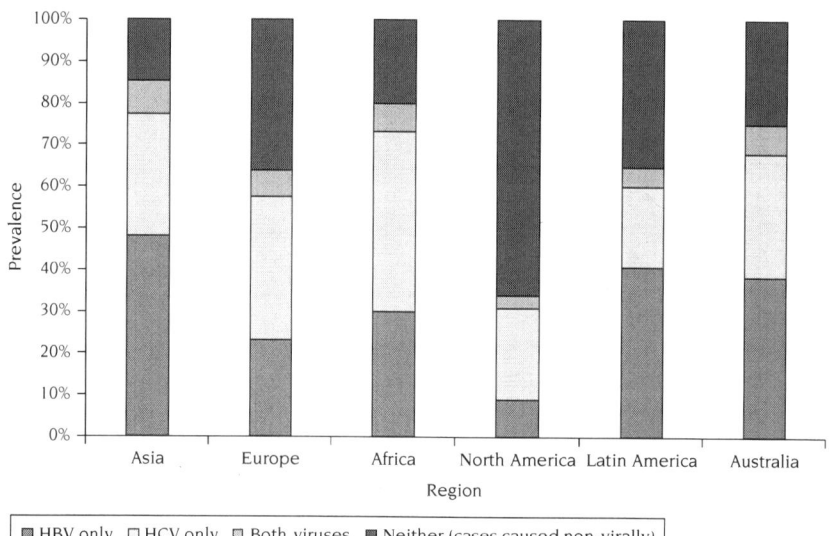

Figure 8.1. Hepatitis virus prevalence in hepatocellular carcinoma cases by region. *Source*: Raza et al., *British Journal of Cancer*, 2007. Used by permission.

decades ago. This would include infection through intravenous drug use and, as already suggested, expanded immigration from endemic regions of the world.[60,61]

Other Malignant Associations

The role of hepatitis B and C is clearly established in the development of liver cancer, especially HCC. Rarer forms of liver cancer, such as primary lymphomas and lymphoepithelioma-like carcinoma (LELC), have also been linked to HCV,[62-64] though the majority of cases of hepatic LELC actually seem to be associated with Epstein-Barr virus.[65]

Cholangiocarcinoma (cancer of the bile duct), especially the intrahepatic type, offers a complex picture. While the epidemiology of intrahepatic cholangiocarcinoma (ICC) differs from HCC in some respects, there is evidence that HCV and probably HBV infections play an etiologic role.[66,67] The evidence for HCV involvement seems to be strongest in developed countries of the West,[68-70] whereas HBV may be the predominant cause of ICC in Asian nations such as South Korea and China.[71,72] Although still rare, ICC incidence has been increasing in some countries, including the United States.[73] As a final note, the hepatitis viruses appear not to be involved with extrahepatic cholangiocarcinoma.[74]

In addition to hepatic malignancies, the hepatitis viruses are strongly associated with nonmalignant liver disease. HBV and HCV both cause chronic hepatitis and cirrhosis, which can lead to liver cancer. Hepatitis infections have also been connected to metabolic processes that cause nonalcoholic fatty liver disease (and perhaps early atherosclerosis).[75-77]

Although hepatitis viruses are primarily associated with the liver, HBV and especially HCV have been implicated in various nonmalignant extrahepatic diseases. Demonstrating direct viral involvement, however, has sometimes proven to be elusive.[78]

More pertinently, evidence of associations between the viruses and malignancies outside of the liver has been emerging. The greatest research attention has been paid to non-Hodgkin's lymphoma (NHL), driven in part by the fact that this is one of the few malignancies demonstrating increasing global incidence.[79] The concern is that hepatitis infections may be playing a role in this growing population health issue.

HBV infection has been implicated in certain forms of extrahepatic NHL.[80-84] The association appears to hold for B-cell NHL rather than the T-cell variety.[85] HCV has also been strongly connected to a spectrum of NHLs outside the liver.[86-91] The prevalence of HCV detected in investigations of NHL has ranged from 7% to 37%.[92]

The mediator between infection and both lymphomas and nonmalignant diseases outside the liver seems to be the body's immune system.

For example, circulating immune complexes are believed to play a causal role in HBV-related arthritis.[93] In addition to inflammatory arthropathies, HBV infection has been linked to polyarteritis nodosa, glomerulonephritis, and dermatitis.[94] While HBV replication has been demonstrated in a variety of extrahepatic tissues and cell types, including in endothelia, there are still doubts about the viral etiology of the diseases involved.[95,96] For instance, data from one study raised questions about whether HBV actually replicates in human lymphatic tissue.[97]

It is also difficult to consider HCV-related carcinogenesis without referring to various nonmalignant or premalignant disorders occurring outside the liver.[98,99] A sizeable percentage of patients with chronic HCV infection may develop such diseases.[100] Confirmed or suspected extrahepatic manifestations of the virus include mixed cryoglobulinemia (MC), glomerulonephritis, and Sjögren's syndrome (or sicca complex).[101] Associations with HCV have also been posited for diabetes, arthritis, and thyroid disease.[102–105] The pathophysiologic basis for most of these disorders again seems to involve immunological (possibly autoimmune) processes that can lead to some form of lymphoproliferation.[106–108] Thus, it is specifically the autoimmune types of thyroid disease that have been linked to HCV.[109] As noted earlier, an understanding of this sort of systemic impact of HCV[110,111] has led to the suggestion that its associated conditions should be identified as a formal syndrome.[112]

As a systemic phenomenon involving lymphatic tissues, one might expect multiple parts of the body to be affected. Notable within the spectrum of extrahepatic manifestations related to HCV are cutaneous conditions such as porphyria cutanea tarda and lichen planus.[113–115] The relationship between HCV infection and lichen planus is controversial, but the disease continues to be investigated as a potentially useful overt marker of chronic liver disease. A less contentious condition is MC, a systemic small-vessel vasculitis that usually includes a cutaneous presentation as well.[116] HCV infection is known to be the main causative factor of MC and related disorders, acting through a "multifactorial and multistep pathogenetic process."[117] B-cell expansion has been shown to be the biological foundation of the disease. Essentially, MC is a nonmalignant lymphoproliferative disorder that sometimes evolves into full NHL.[118,119]

Again, consistent with the concept of systemic conditions, many of the diseases noted so far in connection with hepatitis viruses actually occur in combination. For example, Sjögren's syndrome sometimes presents in association with other autoimmune disorders such as MC and polyarteritis nodosa, as well as systemic lupus erythematosus, rheumatoid arthritis, and scleroderma. Sjögren's syndrome has in fact generated special interest among HCV and cancer researchers. The disease is characterized by lymphocytic infiltration of exocrine glands, specifically salivary and lachrymal glands, leading to the characteristic "sicca complex" symptoms of dry mouth and dry eye.[120] Importantly, a subset of cases presenting with symptoms similar to Sjögren's syndrome have been connected to both HCV infection and various B-cell lymphomas.[121]

The latter combination of clinical features has further sharpened the focus on "suspected links between autoimmunity, infection, and cancer."[122] Patients with Sjögren-like characteristics in particular demonstrate a predominance of mucosa-associated lymphoid tissue (MALT) lymphomas.[123] This type of malignancy occurs in a variety of organs, including the conjunctiva, lachrymal glands, salivary glands, skin, thyroid gland, lungs, stomach, and (rarely) liver.[124,125] The MALT lymphomas associated specifically with Sjögren's syndrome occur extranodally in organs where HCV is also known to replicate, such as exocrine glands and the stomach.[126,127] This may be coincidental, purely a matter of "molecular mimicry," rather than proof of identical etiology.[128,129] Indeed, many questions remain concerning the role of HCV in lymphomagenesis, including interpreting the studies that have failed to show HCV infection in malignant cells.[130] This type of evidence raises the possibility that HCV infection acts as an exogenous trigger rather than as a direct agent of transformation.[131]

The uncertainty about the overlap of pathogenic pathways in the constellation of diseases under consideration does not detract from the main conclusion: HCV infection has been implicated in malignancies beyond the liver, and especially in MALT lymphomas in organs such as salivary glands and the stomach.[132-134] The inventory of cancers associated with HCV also includes other conditions with an immune system connection, including splenic large B-cell lymphomas, nodal marginal zone lymphomas, and thyroid gland cancer.[135-138]

An additional line of evidence supporting the overlap of diverse HCV-related conditions has emerged from research on second primary cancer (SPC).[139] Based on a study of 109,000 patients in 13 cancer registries, Brennan and colleagues demonstrated that there was a 55% higher risk of liver cancer in patients who have had NHL compared with the general population.[140] HCV infection as a common link between HCC and B-cell lymphoma may be part of the explanation. The same study also demonstrated that the risk of thyroid gland cancer was more than twice as high following NHL. As already noted, HCV is associated with autoimmune thyroid disease, suggesting that this again may be a factor in the SPC story.[141]

Finally, though there continues to be questions about the association between hepatitis viruses and cancers found outside the liver, a strong indication of the connection to HCV in particular has been offered by research on treatments.[142] For example, HCV-related marginal zone lymphomas have been shown to respond to antiviral therapy.[143]

In summary, there is compelling evidence of HBV and HCV involvement in a subset of NHL, though precise mechanisms are still being elucidated. A condition such as MC may be a paradigm of HCV-related B-cell proliferation, which in turn represents "an important model of virus-driven autoimmune/neoplastic disorder."[144]

TRANSMISSION AND OCCURRENCE OF THE AGENTS

More is known about the transmission of HBV and HCV than many of the infectious agents in this book. This understanding is crucial in the development of the first category of primary prevention, namely, avoiding exposure.

Hepatitis B

Transmission of HBV occurs primarily through parenteral exposure to blood and blood products. While other body fluids (e.g., saliva, semen, vaginal fluids, tears, breast milk, and urine) have been implicated as carriers of infection, the lower levels of HBV found in them seem to ensure that transmission remains inefficient.[145,146]

According to a helpful summary offered by UK public health authorities, HBV can be transmitted via the following pathways that permit contact with the host bloodstream[147]:

- From infected mother to her baby (known as vertical transmission)
- Use of contaminated equipment during injection drug use
- Sexual activity
- Receiving infected blood or blood products for medical reasons (e.g., transfusion)
- Occupational injuries involving infected needles and other sharp objects (e.g., in the health care setting)
- Other accidental trauma
- Tattooing and body piercing

HBV infection in developed countries occurs most commonly in young adults in high-risk groups (e.g., those with multiple sex partners, men who have sex with men, and injection drug users). However, specific transmission patterns vary greatly from country to country.[148,149] Thus, among infected persons in the United States, high-risk sexual activity has been reported as the most frequent behavioral factor, followed by injection drug use.[150] In northern Europe, injection drug use accounts for most infections; by contrast, high-risk sexual activity appears to be the most common mode of transmission in western and southern Europe.[151]

In Africa and Asia, where HBV is endemic, transmission typically occurs in the first five years of life.[152] Horizontal transmission through familial contact in early childhood appears to be a common mode of infection in Africa, though precise mechanisms are not well understood.[153] Some studies have suggested that normal, casual contact between parent and child may be part of the overall story.[154] Finally, in East and Southeast Asia, vertical transmission (i.e., mother-to-child during birth) used to be considered the main mode of pediatric acquisition.[155] This finding is now disputed based on evidence from Taiwan's HBV vaccination program. Research has shown that while 50% of infections were still traceable to the perinatal period, the other half occurred after the perinatal period (usually before the age of six).[156]

HBV infection of unvaccinated surgeons and other health care workers has been documented. Among developed countries, vaccination of medical personnel has been effective in preventing HBV transmission via equipment used in the health care setting.[157] In the developing world, transmission through contaminated needles and syringes continues to be a problem, due to both an inadequate supply of equipment and poor sterilization procedures.[158]

In developed countries, transmission through blood transfusions or tissue transplantation is now rare due to effective screening of donations.[159] For example, the risk of acquiring HBV from donated blood components that test negative for HBV is just 1 in 200,000–500,000 in the United States.[160,161] Since blood banks in many endemic regions of the world do not screen for HBV, transfusions are much more likely to be a source of transmission.[162] For any country, long latency ensures that chronic hepatitis originating from transfusions and transplantations in eras with less stringent testing will continue to be a concern for some time.

Transmission of HBV seems to occur infrequently through breastfeeding.[163] Likewise, while there is evidence of intrauterine transmission of HBV, it is a rare occurrence.[164,165] Infection via this route may occur following leakage of infected maternal blood across the placenta; this may be caused by, for example, contractions during delivery.[166] Risks associated with such acquisition can be virtually eliminated through pediatric vaccination.

The age of acquisition of the virus influences the geographic pattern of HBV prevalence. Infection rates are highest in regions where transmission typically occurs during the perinatal or early childhood period.[167,168]

The prevalence in countries is usually classified as high, intermediate, or low based on seroprevalence rates. Each of these categories is reflected in Table 8.2.[169]

Understanding the disease patterns behind Table 8.2 reinforces the key prevention challenge. Children tend to become chronic carriers (and are therefore at higher risk for HCC), whereas adults infected with HBV develop chronic disease at a rate of less than 5%.[170] The chronicity rate of the perinatally infected is the highest of all, over 90% according to research in Taiwan; this is why it is so critical to provide passive vaccination to newborns of infected mothers (see section "Prophylactic Eradication or Suppression").[171] In sum, childhood transmission of hepatitis B is the major concern with respect to chronic infection everywhere in the world.

Geographical variation of genotypes may also enter the endemicity equation. It was noted earlier that genotype C is more common in Asia and infection with this variant of HBV tends to allow an HBeAg-positive state to persist for a much longer time. Further, rates of transmission to children are >90% in HBeAg-positive mothers, but 25% or even less after seroconversion (i.e., after host-immune response to antigen e).[172] Even worse, passive–active immunoprophylaxis with hepatitis B immunoglobulin and hepatitis B vaccine (as discussed later) is apparently not as effective in the case of HBeAg-positive mothers.[173]

Because of immigration and travel from endemic regions, prevalence of HBV is increasing in the developed world.[174] This fact has been

Table 8.2. Global HBV Prevalence by Age of Infection and Geographical Location

Typical Age of Infection	Geographic Region	Chronically Infected (%)	Serologic Evidence of Past Infection (%)
Perinatal/ early childhood	Southeast Asia, sub-Saharan Africa	8	70–90
Mixed*	Eastern Europe, Middle East, Russia	1–7	10–60
Adults engaging in high-risk behavior†	United States, Western Europe, Australia	<1	5–7

*Infant, early childhood, adult transmission patterns.

†injection drug users, persons with multiple heterosexual partners, MSM.

Source: Alter, Journal of Hepatology, 2003.

implicated in the increasing rate of virus-related deaths, cancers, and hospitalizations in the United States in the past decade.[175] Countries in Europe, including the UK, Netherlands, and Iceland, have detected a relatively high frequency of HBV infections among immigrants.[176–178] In Iceland, for instance, immigrants from endemic countries account for an estimated 80–90% of reported HBV cases.[179]

With its very active immigration program, HBV infection will likely remain a health concern in Canada for some time.[180] The current number of individuals in Canada chronically infected with HBV is not known with any accuracy; based on a variety of assumptions, the estimates range from 250,000 to 600,000.[181,182] This compares with reported totals of 2 million chronically infected with HBV in the United States.[183]

Hepatitis C

Similar to HBV, transmission of HCV occurs primarily through contaminated blood or blood products. In low-prevalence countries, HCV is typically acquired by adolescents or adults, usually through injection drug use and high-risk sexual activity.[184]

Using intravenously administered drugs predominates as a risk factor, accounting for over 40% of HCV cases (or three times the proportion due to sexual activity)[185,186]; one authority has suggested that up to 60% of HCV infections in Canada may be traced to drug abuse.[187] Reinforcing this conclusion, almost 80% of injecting-drug users in the United States are known to be infected with HCV.[188] As a final note, an association between noninjection drug use (e.g., cocaine, methamphetamines) and HCV infection has not been established.[189] Nonetheless, there have been attempts to encourage safer noninjection drug use practices, including a project developed in Vancouver, Canada.[190]

Based on the preceding information, sexual activity appears to be a relatively minor route of HCV transmission. Groups at special risk in this regard include individuals who have multiple sexual partners and men who have sex with men (MSM).[191] Specific behaviors of concern are those that cause mucosal trauma, such as fisting.[192,193] Higher transmission rates have been associated with the presence of other sexually transmitted infections (STIs), such as syphilis, HIV, and herpes simplex virus. Because of shared transmission routes, individuals infected with HIV are commonly coinfected with HBV and/or HCV.[194,195] This is a matter of some importance in the marshalling of health care resources related to HIV/AIDS patients.

The prevalence of important behavioral risk factors in certain urban areas of the developed world means that residential location may be associated with HCV infection. Thus, injection drug use is inordinately high in the Downtown Eastside neighborhood of Vancouver, Canada, contributing to elevated HCV rates among the local population.[196,197]

In HCV-endemic regions of the world, infection occurs mainly in infants and young children through vertical and horizontal transmission.[198] Blood transfusions and unsafe injection practices (notably, reusing improperly sterilized needles and syringes in mass vaccination campaigns), however, can also lead to infections in such countries.[199]

An estimated 5% of infants born to HCV-infected mothers are themselves infected.[200] If the mother is coinfected with HIV, the risk of an affected offspring appears to be elevated.[201] The possibility of intrauterine transmission has been suggested by research detecting the presence of HCV in newborn serum samples. A 2005 study revealed that one-third to one-half of children infected with HCV acquired the virus in utero.[202] Although some studies have detected the presence of HCV RNA in breast milk, breastfeeding is not considered to be an important vehicle of transmission.[203–206]

The implementation of procedures in the early 1990s for screening blood donations lowered the risk of HCV infection via transfusions.[207] The introduction of nucleic acid amplification testing in 1998–2000 in the United States, Canada, Australia, Japan, and other developed countries further reduced the risk related to blood products.[208] According to one U.S. estimate, the odds of acquiring HCV from donated blood that tests negative for the virus are now about one in 2 million.[209] Contracting HCV through other inadvertent blood exposure does remain a possibility. For example, since a vaccine for HCV is currently unavailable, infection through occupational exposure in health care settings can occur; however, transmission under these circumstances appears to be rare.[210]

Among the general adult population, the prevalence of chronic HCV infection varies from 0.5% to 2% in western Europe, North America, and nonendemic regions of Asia to 5% to 15% in high-prevalence parts of Africa.[211] The highest infection rates have been reported in Egypt (15–20%), whereas the United Kingdom and Nordic countries demonstrate some of the lowest prevalence rates (<0.1%).[212] Despite extremes in the data, the average global HCV prevalence (at 3%, or about half that seen for HBV) is close to the rate within developed countries.[213] This implies that, unlike HBV, the urgency of controlling HCV is consistent around the world. Reinforcing this fact in the context of developed countries, it is often noted that HCV is the most common blood-borne infection in the United States[214]

In Canada, an estimated 250,000 people are infected with HCV (the same number as seen with HBV), which equates to a prevalence rate of about 0.76%.[215] This estimate for all of Canada is similar to recent data from the province of Alberta that indicated the seroprevalence of HCV in tissue and organ donors to be 0.48%; by comparison, the rate for HBV in that study was only 0.09%.[216] Of special concern, the incidence among Aboriginal people in Canada is several times higher than in the general population. In 2004, the incidence of new HCV infections among non-Aboriginals over age 14 years was 2.8 per 100,000, whereas for Aboriginal people it was 18.9.[217]

In sum, the HCV-positive population in Canada can be overwhelmingly attributed to injection drug use within society (about 60% of cases), combined with immigration from endemic regions of the world (about 30%).[218] Injection drug use also is the main force behind the over 3 million individuals chronically infected with HCV in the United States[219]

DISEASE MECHANISM AND PROCESSES

In this section, the specific pathogenic elements involved with HBV- and HCV-related cancer will be briefly reviewed.

Among the hepatitis viruses, only HBV and HCV are able to persist in the host as a single infection and cause chronic hepatitis. By comparison, hepatitis D only contributes to chronic disease as a coinfection or super-infection along with HBV.[220,221] It should be noted that HCC is actually uncommon with HDV infection because patients die of progressive liver disease before cancer develops.

In the course of persistent infection, inflammation becomes the foundation of chronic hepatitis that can in turn initiate the progression to nodular fibrosis, cirrhosis, and, ultimately, HCC.[222] As described in an earlier section, HBV and HCV have other cancer associations, notably with B-cell lymphomas. While this expanding area of research holds great interest for basic scientists and lymphoma specialists, the relative rarity of such cancers must still be acknowledged. As such, the focus in the rest of the chapter will be on HCC.

Hepatitis B

Chronic HBV infection can lead to the development of cirrhosis and/or HCC.[223] At least one of these diseases will eventually manifest itself in an estimated 15–40% of chronically infected, untreated patients.[224] In fact, cirrhosis usually precedes the onset of HCC.[225] Annually, 1–5% of chronic HBV carriers who have cirrhosis will progress to cancer.[226]

The potential for HBV clearance can differ from the pattern seen in HPV infection. Regardless of the age of acquisition, the great majority of HPV infections are known to clear relatively quickly. By contrast, infants and children infected with HBV demonstrate a high risk for chronicity. This may be compared with the more acute and self-limiting type of infection typically seen in those acquiring HBV during adulthood.[227,228] Notably, the pattern with HCV is reversed: the chronicity rate appears to be lower in individuals acquiring the virus at a younger age.[229]

The explanation for the sometimes dramatic difference in outcomes among HBV carriers is not always clear. Potential drivers include a number of sometimes overlapping factors[230]:

- Infection clearance
- Viral replication/degree of hepatocellular injury
- Disease clearance

As suggested earlier, there is some evidence that viral genotype influences the outcome of HBV infection.[231] One study revealed an association between genotype A1 and HCC risk; genotype C was correlated with increased cancer risk in other research.[232,233] Even stronger evidence has suggested that high viral load, as manifested by elevated levels of viral DNA in sera, increases HCC risk.[234,235]

The natural history of HBV infection has been elucidated in some detail. There are various states and transitions related to chronic HBV infection, including immunotolerance; immunoactive prior to HBeAg seroconversion; inactive carrier status (generally following seroconversion); and reactivation.[236,237] The classic phases of HBV chronic infection are outlined in Figure 8.2, reflecting the changes in prevailing levels of HBV antigen e and DNA.[238] The first three states represent potentially successive stages in liver disease progression. Note that reactivation from an inactive carrier state can move in one of two directions, with HBeAG levels either re-elevating or remaining negative. As indicated earlier, an HBeAg-negative chronic state may confer particularly high risk of cirrhosis and/or HCC development.

In the immunotolerant patient, serum HBV DNA is very high, but there are no disease symptoms. By contrast, the immunoactive process is marked both by symptoms and declining serum HBV DNA.[239] Initial immunoactivity (or some form of reactivation) presents the most serious risks. It may be accompanied by an inflammatory response, hepatic tissue injury, and, eventually, the onset of HCC.[240] On the other hand, the inactive carrier phase is marked by low- or nonreplicative virus; it can last for a long time prior to reactivation. Because of this latency period, cancer often takes decades to appear, a factor that must be taken into account when explaining the apparent rising incidence of HCC in the United States and Canada.[241,242]

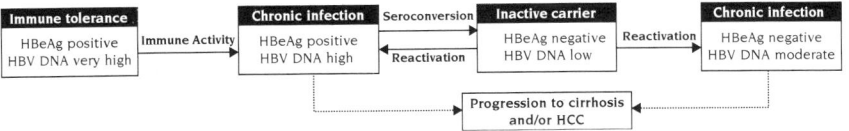

Figure 8.2. Natural history of chronic HBV infection. *Source*: Pungpapong et al., *Mayo Clinic Proceedings*, 2007. Used by permission.

Clearly, the preferred state from the perspective of disease prevention is that of virus clearance and/or full immunity. As discussed later, this may be achieved through vaccination and immunotherapies.

Hepatitis C

Carcinogenesis driven by HCV overlaps substantially with the process seen for HBV. Chronicity characterizes the majority of individuals who acquire HCV.[243,244] As is the case for HBV, chronic carriers of HCV are at risk for developing cirrhosis and HCC; cirrhosis generally precedes any progression to cancer.[245]

There is evidence that HCV causes HCC through oxidative stress, mutation of growth-regulatory genes, and disruption of cell proliferation signaling processes.[246] Molecular research has shown that the HCV genome does not become integrated with host DNA as part of cell transformation.[247,248] Viral genotype may also be an important factor influencing carcinogenesis.[249,250]

Once an HCV-positive patient progresses to HCC, prognosis is poor. The median survival following diagnosis is 6–12 months.[251]

Disease Risk Factors

Table 8.3 outlines some proposed modifiable risk factors (other than viral infection) for liver cancer development.[252] For the most part, the cancer of interest is HCC; occupational vinyl chloride exposure appears to be linked to angiosarcoma in the liver, with evidence for HCC remaining unclear.[253,254]

The evidence for several influences on liver cancer risk is very weak. Even the long-accepted role of the *Schistosoma* parasite in liver cancer requires reassessment,[255] partly because earlier research in countries such as Egypt predated the contemporary understanding of HCV involvement in HCC. Both types of infection occur at a high rate in Egypt, possibly producing a confounding effect in epidemiologic research. Alternately, there is evidence that the presence of schistosomal infection may influence HCV (specifically genotype 4) coinfection, accelerating progression to cirrhosis, and possibly to HCC.[256–258] The immunosuppressive effects

Table 8.3. Selected Risk Factors for Liver Cancer

Evidence	Decreases Risk	Increases Risk
Convincing		Aflatoxin exposure (in HBV-positive individuals), alcohol intake, hemochromatosis
Probable	Vegetable consumption	High serum iron, diabetes mellitus, obesity, vinyl chloride exposure (angiosarcoma)
Possible	Selenium, green tea	Tobacco use, anabolic steroid exposure, androgen levels, parity, schistosomiasis
Unclear		Arsenic exposure

Source: McGlynn and London, *Best Practice & Research. Clinical Gastroenterology*, 2004. Used by permission.

of *Schistosoma* infection may also play an indirect role in the persistence of hepatitis infection and disease development.[259] In sum, the role of schistosomiasis in HCC development remains controversial.[260]

Some risk factors demonstrate geographical variation in terms of absolute or proportional impact. For example, exposure to the aflatoxin found in poorly stored grains is a special concern in areas endemic for liver cancer, whereas alcohol consumption is more important in low-risk regions of the world.[261,262] It should be noted that aflatoxin is now considered an "unnecessary" cofactor by some authorities; by this they mean that aflatoxin increases the risk of liver cancer only in HBV-positive individuals,[263] though evidence of an independent effect for the factor continues to be put forward.[264]

Unlike aflatoxin's connection to HBV, which is reminiscent of the relationship between HPV (a necessary cause of cervical cancer) and smoking (a dependent cofactor), alcohol consumption definitely causes cirrhosis and liver cancer independent of infection. However, there are synergies when both causal agencies are at work. Thus, excessive alcohol consumption interacts with viral infection to increase the rate of HCC development. For example, adjusting for hepatitis B and C infection, one study revealed a two- to threefold increase in HCC risk due to heavy alcohol consumption.[265] This was similar to an odds ratio of 4.5 (C.I. 1.4–14.8) for the cancer risk of heavy drinking (≥80 mL of ethanol per day) found by other researchers; however, they also found that the combined presence of chronic viral infection and heavy alcohol intake produced an odds ratio of 53.9 (C.I. 7.0–415.7).[266]

As suggested earlier, coinfections (acquired at the same time) and super-infections (a second infection happening later) are phenomena of interest in liver disease. Apart from cases involving multiple hepatitis viruses, the main coinfection of interest involves one or more hepatitis viruses and HIV.

It has already been noted that HBV and/or HCV coinfection is common in HIV-positive individuals. While it is not clear that coinfection with HIV increases the incidence of liver cancer (explaining its absence in Table 8.3), the virus does seem to have an impact on the course of disease. Thus, coinfection with HIV accelerates progression of hepatitis-related diseases. HCC, for example, may occurs at a younger age in HIV-positive individuals; as well, HIV infection can lead to complications during treatment of hepatitis.[267-271] There is also evidence that HBV vaccination is less effective in HIV-positive populations.[272,273] One reason that the expected increase in HCC incidence has not materialized so far in cases of HIV coinfection is that such patients may simply die before cancer can develop. Finally, a unique clinical challenge related to this topic is the fact that HIV drug treatments can themselves be hepatotoxic.[274]

VIRAL DETECTION METHODS

Similar to vaccination and other primary prevention measures, the ultimate aim of treatment in the event of known infection is to prevent the development of chronic diseases, including cancer. As there are some drawbacks to hepatitis therapies, the importance of primary prevention will continue to be emphasized. On the other hand, secondary prevention efforts related to HBV and HCV continue to improve. As defined earlier, secondary prevention in the context of this book presupposes a confirmed viral infection (and signs of early infectious disease). Certain forms of universal and targeted prophylaxis also depend on the detection of infection. The latter category includes the confirmation of HBV-positivity in pregnant women before initiating prophylactic measures in newborns.

Effective tests for detecting HBV and HCV infection do exist; most strategies were originally developed in the context of blood donation screening. Initial tests have traditionally been based on enzyme immunoassay. Since this approach generates a large percentage of false positives, confirmatory assays are part of the protocol.[275] Testing approaches continue to evolve, including the use of molecular methods for viral genome quantification, genotyping, and even the identification of specific mutations that may confer drug resistance.[276-278]

The oldest and most basic detection methods, based on different serum markers for each virus, are still useful. Thus, HBV is routinely diagnosed by means of circulating surface antigen, whereas antibodies against HCV offer a highly sensitive marker of infection.[279] Molecular testing is used to follow up a positive result from HCV antibody testing, both to confirm that an infection is current and to guide the treatment.[280, 281]

The sensitivity of tests for the detection of HCV RNA has improved in recent years, which has implications for assessing the efficacy of antiviral therapy directed at eradication.[282] It is important to note that quantitative HCV RNA does not correlate with disease severity or risk of progression.[283] On the other hand, a patient's HCV viral load and the rate of virus decline during therapy do seem to correlate with the likelihood of long-term positive response to antiviral therapy.[284]

PREVENTION APPROACHES

As with other infectious causes of malignancies, HBV and HCV are potentially important targets for cancer prevention. In fact, various public health interventions have been very effective in reducing the prevalence of HBV in particular.[285] Continued planning around prevention strategies should be calibrated to prevailing epidemiologic conditions. For example, a fundamental consideration in setting prevention priorities is the fact that, while HCV has a lower global prevalence than HBV, HCV is proportionately more prevalent in economically developed regions and thus may cause the larger proportion of HCC.[286] This general pattern may need to be amended in urban contexts due to tendency of immigrants to settle in metropolitan areas. Thus, the effect of newcomers from HBV-endemic countries may elevate the HCC prevalence related to the virus in the larger cities of the United States and Canada; the result is that HBV may account for up to 50% of HCC in such settings.[287]

A further consideration is the fact that the impact of transmission routes is variable over time, which can affect prevention priorities. For example, the risk of acquiring hepatitis infection through blood transfusions is now extremely low in developed nations and thus no longer represents a prevention target offering any real gains. It is important to note that the usual latency period means that improvements in blood donation screening introduced in the 1990s should translate into an even lower rate of liver cancer from this source in coming decades.[288]

Such success does not mean that further technological improvements would be unwelcome (including any efficiency in testing for multiple contaminants); likewise, even maintaining current safety programs requires some vigilance. However, while an ongoing concern in developing countries, it does seem that protecting the blood supply has been well addressed, at least for HBV, in public health programs of developed nations.

These comments aside, with up to half a million infected individuals in Canada and millions more in the United States, there is no doubt that disease prevention related to HBV and HCV is still very much a priority in the developed world, both in terms of exposure prevention and reducing the risk of disease progression once infected.

The six prevention categories developed with respect to HPV will be reviewed in the context of hepatitis viruses in this last section.

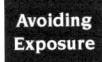 | Preventing Infection | Prophylactic Eradication | Preventing Cofactor | Therapeutic Eradication | Interrupting Transformation |

1. Avoiding Exposure to the Agent

The prevention of exposure to the hepatitis viruses is guided by the basic understanding of the main transmission routes. In the most general terms, this means protecting against blood-to-blood contact. Because the relative importance of the specific modes and settings of transmission differ from country to country, the most relevant control strategies for each setting need to be carefully selected.[289] Given the effective controls now offered through newborn prophylaxis (see section "Prophylactic Eradication or Suppression"), the most notable remaining route for HBV transmission in developed countries is sexual activity. But this does not depict the whole story. As noted earlier, HBV acquired by any means in adults does not lead to appreciable chronicity. This suggests that exposure prevention for HBV in adults may be quite limited in terms of the ultimate impact on HCC rates. In short, though transmission of hepatitis B between adults continues to occur, the vast majority of these infections will resolve spontaneously and thus are not a factor in HCC risk.

In contrast, the main route of acquiring HCV in developed countries is injection drug use, where well-known exposure prevention options do exist. It is outside the scope of this book to systematically describe and evaluate the multitude of drug control programs in use around the world. Although there is a large volume of studies on the topic, the fact is that evaluations have rarely been tied to the end-points of reduced hepatitis prevalence and/or lower cancer rates. Generally, it is true that specific interventions such as needle and syringe exchange programs have shown some promise in limiting the growth of (if not reversing) HCV prevalence.[290] The greatest hope may still lie in more comprehensive programs that integrate multiple strategies, though admittedly the evidence for these has been mixed.[291,292]

It has been observed that injection drug use is notoriously high in the "Downtown Eastside" neighborhood of Vancouver, British Columbia; this contributes to a high prevalence of HCV. There is recent evidence that comprehensive health programs incorporating multiple interventions, including a needle exchange program, may be effective in preventing HCV transmission in such an environment.[293]

Since more than simple skin-to-skin contact and superficial trauma are required for transmission, the hepatitis viruses are not as easily acquired through sexual activity as is HPV. Although the risk of chronic hepatitis (and thus HCC) related to sexual transmission seems to be low, it is not zero. This means that promotion of sexual health may have some modest effect on HCC incidence. The prevention strategies related to sexually transmitted infections are of course not unique to the hepatitis viruses. The various sexual health approaches were already introduced in the context of HPV (see Chapter 7); a review of them here is not required. One assumption could be noted: strategies such as condom use should be more effective for HBV and HCV than for HPV.

Beyond the broad arenas of injection drug use and sexual activity, strategies for more specific risk settings are also important. For example, preventing occupational infection among health care workers by wearing adequate protective gear and instituting other safety protocols will limit the risk of puncture by surgical and other instruments.[294]

By definition, the remaining prevention approaches for hepatitis viruses and related cancer (discussed later) are classified as postexposure.[295] The response to hepatitis viral exposure follows one of two basic plans: preventing infection from taking root or eradicating the agent before substantial disease develops. Eradication can also be divided into two categories: targeted and universal. A third approach following exposure to a hepatitis virus involves some sort of neutralization of any disease process. This classically involves tackling one or more of the cofactors (other than infection) that are necessary for disease initiation or progression. Each of these other prevention categories will be reviewed in the following subsections.

| Avoiding Exposure | **Preventing Infection** | Prophylactic Eradication | Preventing Cofactor | Therapeutic Eradication | Interrupting Transformation |

2. Preventing Infection after Exposure to the Agent

The classic measure brought into effect upon exposure is prophylactic vaccination. The efficacy and safety of HBV vaccines have been clearly demonstrated in terms of infection control, with very promising signs of HCC prevention from the "natural experiments" created by national vaccine programs (as discussed next).

Among immunocompetent persons, a complete course of pediatric vaccine may result in lifelong protection from HBV infection.[296] Therefore, some authorities project that booster doses are generally not

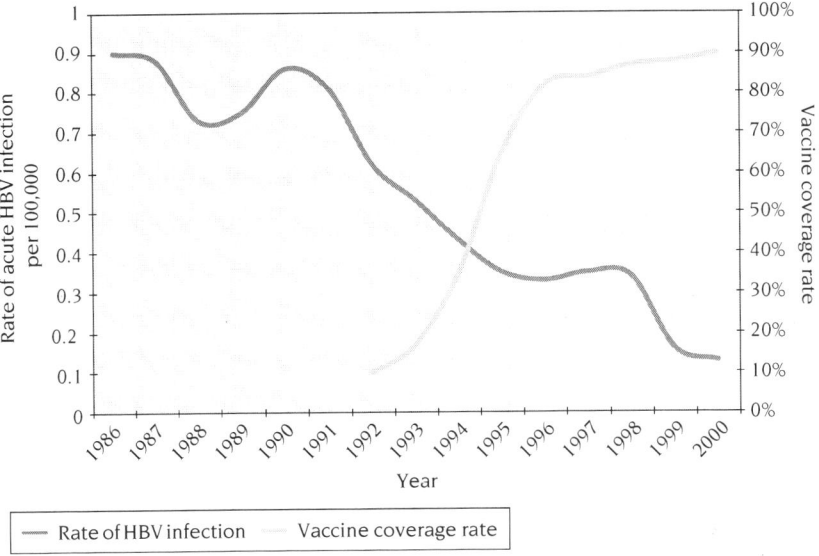

Figure 8.3. Effects of child HBV vaccination United States, 1986–2000. *Source*: CDC, *Morbidity and Mortality Weekly Report*, 2002.

required for those who have received full vaccination.[297] Others, pointing out the evidence of waning immunogenicity, suggest that a booster will be required, perhaps as early as 10 years after vaccination.[298]

Efficacy trials need to be confirmed by data from real-world applications. Results from a number of jurisdictions support the effectiveness of the HBV vaccine. In British Columbia, for example, the introduction of HBV immunization has reduced acute hepatitis B infections in children to almost zero.[299] A similar pattern has been observed in the United States, as seen in Figure 8.3.[300]

The early results concerning chronic disease control have also been encouraging. For example, a long-term study in Taiwan revealed a 75% decrease in the incidence of pediatric HCC following implementation of a national HBV vaccination program.[301,302]

The encouraging success of HBV and other childhood vaccines has prompted major global movements to extend the benefits of immunization to developing countries.[303,304] Among WHO member states, 154 of 192 reported universal pediatric HBV vaccination programs as of 2006. HBV vaccine coverage has increased dramatically since 1990, not only due to countries introducing vaccination programs, but also because of enhancements and increased uptake within existing programs.[305]

Notwithstanding the general progress, there are still advances to be made in securing full coverage across populations, even within developed countries. One Cochrane Collaboration review directly addresses immunization program enhancements, specifically patient reminder and patient recall systems. In 2002, 41 studies met the inclusion requirements, and 5 more were added in a 2005 update.[306] The conclusion of the authors was that patient reminder and recall systems in primary care are effective in improving immunization rates. This topic has natural linkages with population-based information systems. A U.S. study in 2002 noted that, though most physicians agreed on the utility of computerized systems to track immunizations in their practices, few had purchased and used them.[307] The practice setting may exert an influence on the enthusiasm for such systems. Successful application of patient reminder/recall can be elusive in populations marked by low socioeconomic status; the main obstacle appears to be the unreliability of getting in contact with clients.[308]

While patient reminder and recall systems tend to dominate the agenda in terms of interventions in primary care, other approaches to improving immunization coverage have been identified and supported, including standing orders to vaccinate patients in clinic or hospital settings, performance feedback, the involvement of multidisciplinary primary care teams, and continuing education.[309-311]

Although the World Health Organization recommends the implementation of universal programs, several countries have opted for an HBV vaccination strategy that targets at-risk populations such as immigrants from endemic regions.[312,313] Low general prevalence rates and continuing questions regarding the cost-effectiveness of universal vaccination are among the reasons for more limited implementation.[314] In contrast, one recent mathematical modeling study suggested that universal administration of HBV vaccine to children and/or adolescents has a greater impact on lowering population-wide prevalence than does a policy focusing on specific at-risk groups.[315]

A universal vaccination program may also generate potential collateral benefits. For example, immunizing children, who are relatively accessible as a cohort, may be superior to attempting full coverage for high-risk adult populations. Population-wide pediatric prevention may also be of particular use among medically underserved indigenous groups that are often subject to higher rates of chronic disease combined with sometimes high barriers to receiving adult health services. An important focus in this regard would be the Canadian North; the rate of HBV infection is estimated to be 20 times higher among Inuit populations compared with non-Aboriginals.[316] Finally, data indicating that HBV vaccination becomes less efficacious with older recipient age provide further support for implementing childhood vaccination programs.[317]

There are new cases of pediatric HBV infection every year, including in countries with universal childhood vaccination programs. This is partly attributable to a vaccination failure rate of around 5%.[318] In the United States, a large proportion of incident cases of childhood infection occur in immigrant children.[319] For example, among cases of pediatric HBV infection reviewed in 2005 at Mount Sinai Hospital in New York, close to half of the children originated from other countries.[320]

The discussion so far has been restricted to vaccination for HBV. Despite promising results from animal studies, a vaccine for HCV is currently not available.[321] Impediments to vaccine development include the existence of multiple HCV genotypes and a high viral mutation rate that permits escape from immune control.[322,323] The absence of a vaccine underscores the importance of pursuing HCC prevention through other means.

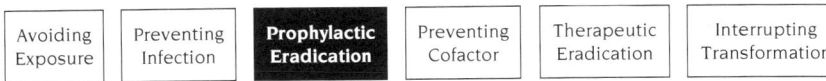

3. Prophylactic Eradication or Suppression

The universal eradication of an existing infection prior to the development of any symptoms is often proposed for agents such as *Helicobacter pylori* but not for hepatitis viruses. On the other hand, targeted eradication or suppression is employed with hepatitis viruses, as will be described later.

Universal screening and treatment. Universal screening and eradication programs for hepatitis infections have not been instituted for a number of reasons. While reliable viral detection is possible, the broad application of antiviral treatments is hindered by high costs, sometimes modest efficacy, and/or substantial side effects. The most common reason for not instituting a universal treatment program for HBV or HCV is the lack of evidence for better patient outcomes at the population level.[324,325] Given the reluctance to mandate follow-up treatment, the agencies tasked with making recommendations about clinical prevention services have been understandably equivocal about general screening as well, even among groups at elevated risk for infection. A specific hesitation about a "high-risk" strategy is that it is sometimes difficult to calibrate risk with general lifestyle factors. For instance, 20% of HCV-positive individuals do not have any easily identifiable risk factors.[326]

Targeted screening and prophylaxis: HBV. While universal screening for hepatitis viruses is not recommended, targeted screening does receive support from official agencies. The most established intervention of this sort in the public health arena involves the unique situation where the carrier is screened, but the potential recipient of infection is treated. The reference here is to the testing of pregnant women for HBV (preferably at the first prenatal visit), followed by treatment of the infants involved.[327]

Administering hepatitis B–immune globulin (HBIG) in the first 24 h postpartum—known as passive immunization—combined with active immunization with HBV vaccine has demonstrated high efficacy against chronic infection among such infants.[328] HBIG is an expensive therapy, leading countries with constrained resources and/or low HBV prevalence to sometimes limit screening to pregnant mothers at high risk of infection, for example, intravenous drug users or sex trade workers. Other jurisdictions use a treatment depending on the vaccine alone rather than in combination with HBIG.[329,330]

Other risk categories related to known HBV exposure were specified by one study as follows[331]:

- People in contact with blood that is known or suspected to be infected with HBV through being poked with a used injection needle; being splashed in the mouth, nose, or eyes with infected blood; being bitten by someone with hepatitis B; or coming into contact with contaminated household articles such as a toothbrush, dental floss, or a razor
- People who have had intimate sexual contact with a person with hepatitis B
- Victims of sexual assault

It would seem prudent to enhance this list in the context of immigration. Thus, children from endemic regions, or born to immigrant parents originating from such areas, probably should be monitored for infection.

Prophylactic administration of HBIG may be indicated in at-risk groups in order to prevent the development of infection. Where it is appropriate and feasible, the use of HBIG is well supported by evidence. Regimens involving HBIG are 70–90% efficacious in preventing the HBV carrier state; when combined with an HBV vaccination series, the efficacy achieved is between 85% and 95%.[332] Pertinent to this topic, some individuals (of any age) who receive the HBV vaccine do not develop immunity and, therefore, remain vulnerable to infection.[333] For these "nonresponders," it may be effective to apply passive immunization with HBIG immediately after any exposure to the virus; the challenge is to identify the candidates for such an intervention quickly enough.[334]

In sum, the fact that adult HBV infection is modest in terms of both chronicity and HCC development needs to be reemphasized. The priority has to be squarely on preventing or counteracting pediatric infection.

Targeted screening and prophylaxis: HCV. With respect to HBV, part of the caution around any adult screening (outside of pregnant women) relates to the fact that acute infection usually resolves without intervention.[335] HCV infection also spontaneously clears, though at a highly variable rate (10–60%).[336] Clearance seems to occur more readily in pediatric patients and young adults compared with older patients.[337]

Official government positions on HCV prevention, which feature a mostly conservative approach to screening, have generated controversy. The seriousness of chronic liver disease and the presumed positive impact of interventions have prompted advocacy groups such as the American Liver Foundation to call for more widespread and robust screening protocols around HCV. They further point out that government agencies such as the Centers for Disease Control (CDC) take a somewhat stronger position than the U.S. Preventive Services Task Force (USPSTF).[338] The USPSTF is an independent panel of experts in primary care and prevention that systematically reviews the evidence of effectiveness and develops recommendations for clinical preventive services. It is important to note that there is more agreement than disagreement between the CDC and USPSTF positions. Thus, both bodies advocate against routine HCV screening and eradication in asymptomatic populations but for screening when markers for liver disease are present (i.e., essentially a recommendation about a secondary prevention measure). The main difference is that the CDC, along with the U.S. National Institutes of Health, the American Association for the Study of Liver Diseases, and the American College of Preventive Medicine, also recommends HCV screening among high-risk groups prior to any disease indications.[339]

Various groups at risk for HCV infection have been identified by U.S. agencies as follows[340]:

- Persons who ever injected illegal drugs
- Persons with selected medical conditions, including persons who received clotting factor concentrates produced before 1987; persons who were ever on long-term hemodialysis; or persons with persistently abnormal alanine aminotransferase levels
- Prior recipients of transfusions or organ transplants, including persons who were notified that they received blood, where the donor later tested positive for HCV infection; persons who received a transfusion of blood or blood components before July 1992; or persons who received an organ transplant before July 1992

- Health care, emergency medical, and public safety workers experiencing needle sticks, cuts during procedures, or mucosal exposures to HCV-positive blood

Immigrants from endemic infection areas should also be added to such a list. It is not clear whether there will be strong movements toward instituting primary prevention measures among any of these subpopulations. If this is mandated, then the sort of interventions that could be used in cases of detected infection coincides with viral treatment options (see Prevention Categories 5 and 6).

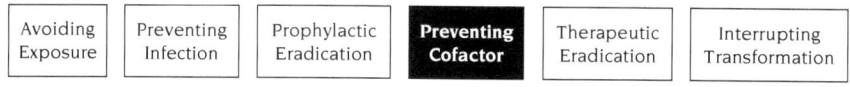

4. Cofactor Prevention

Identification of risk factors (other than viral infection) that are amenable to intervention should be a high priority in the prevention of HCC. It is clear that mechanisms other than hepatitis infection can cause liver cancer. As important as these are as a prevention target, the main interest in the context of this book is any cofactors that act along side viral infection in the development of HCC. This includes risk factors that do not act independently of HBV/HCV in carcinogenesis as well as those that can act independently but also demonstrate a synergistic impact on the risk associated with the viruses. In both cases, controlling the cofactor among infected populations raises the potential for reducing HCC. There appear to be few studies that have directly tested this hypothesis.

The candidate risk factors of most interest in the developed world are excessive alcohol intake, tobacco use, and diabetes/obesity. While smoking does not seem to initiate HCC, it does enhance the risks associated with viral infection (perhaps through interaction with host genetic susceptibility factors).[341,342] As noted earlier, diabetes and/or obesity act as cofactors in some liver disease, appearing to enhance the impact of HBV/HCV. Thus, these well-known aspects of the metabolic syndrome are suitable targets to prevent HCC, including reducing any synergistic effects in populations infected with hepatitis viruses.[343]

It is important to note that other, very compelling health objectives exist to prompt control efforts with all these risk factors. This is especially true of excessive alcohol intake, which has indirect implications for HCC due to synergies with hepatitis virus infection, as well as direct effects on liver disease and many other chronic conditions.[344] In sum, at least in the context of developed countries, there are few, if any, modifiable cofactors where the predominant health impact relates to HCC caused by infection. Thus, any reduction in liver cancer attributable to well-established prevention targets, such as alcohol consumption, may be considered to be a collateral benefit of a generally healthy lifestyle.[345] In terms of targeting HCC due to HBV/HCV, a frontal attack on infection emerges as the most pertinent prevention option.

| Avoiding Exposure | Preventing Infection | Prophylactic Eradication | Preventing Cofactor | **Therapeutic Eradication** | Interrupting Transformation |

5. Therapeutic Eradication or Suppression

This prevention category assumes that both infection and signs of early disease have been detected. In such situations, the ideal objective of HBV or HCV treatment is the eradication of the virus (clearance of the infection); this in turn allows for a reduction or prevention of hepatic injury and disease progression.[346, 347] Technically, eradication may be defined as the post-treatment absence of HBV DNA or HCV RNA according to the most sensitive tests currently available. Suppression on the other hand is best understood as a reduction in detectable levels of viral genetic material.[348] It should be distinguished from eradication, which is potentially permanent; in contrast, suppression, even so-called "complete suppression," may be temporary, lasting only as long as drugs are being applied.

HBV and HCV control is a complex and even controversial topic because of inconsistent eradication results, high costs, side effects, and imperfect outcomes in terms of the ultimate end-point of HCC prevention.[349] One important negative sequela is the development of resistant viral types when suppression is not completely achieved.[350]

A true eradication measure for HBV does not yet seem to exist, leaving suppression as the realistic expectation for now. A number of approved agents have demonstrated HBV DNA suppression. The class of drugs known as nucleoside/nucleotide analogues (NAs) offers the greatest potential to achieve complete HBV suppression, at least in the short term.[351] In the meantime, these and other compounds continue to be explored for their ability to moderate disease progression, with or without viral suppression. The topic will be revisited in the next section.

The story related to HCV eradication is more encouraging. Some therapy trials have achieved a "sustained virologic response" (SVR), defined as the absence of HCV RNA 6 months after treatment completion. Taking into account other evidence, there is a strong suggestion that HCV infection has been truly cleared in many such patients.[352,353]

Approved HCV treatment includes combination therapy with pegylated[354] interferon-alpha and ribavirin (a nucleoside analogue).[355,356] While demonstrating some success, the eradication rate of the current standard treatment does vary substantially across genotypes, from as high as 90% with genotypes 2 and 3, to closer to 50% with genotypes 1 and 4.[357] Beyond genotype, treatment response also depends on viral load and the extent of hepatic fibrosis.[358-360]

Because of the sometimes moderate efficacy, substantial side effects, high cost, and extended treatment period, combination therapy is not appropriate for all HCV-positive patients.[361] Adverse outcomes, including fever, headache, loss of appetite, and chronic fatigue, can reduce adherence to the prescribed interferon regimen.[362,363]

Even in the absence of eradication, therapies may slow disease progression and delay the complications of chronic HCV infection.[364] However, the ultimate aim of prevention in the context of this book is the control of HCC; in this respect, the evidence related to viral eradication remains mixed. While there are indications that liver cancer risk can be reduced with antiviral therapies,[365,366] studies have shown that some patients may still develop HCC even after SVR.[367,368]

The development and testing of drugs and combination therapies that can achieve true eradication of HBV/HCV and manifest reduction of HCC risk remains an active area of research.[369,370]

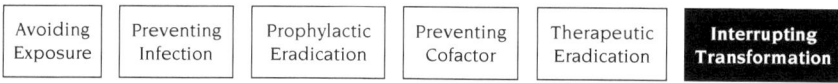

6. Interrupting Transformation Related to Infection

Since this book is ultimately aimed at preventing malignancies, the focus in this section will be avoidance of chronic hepatitis, which is understood to be the usual precursor to carcinogenesis. Unlike the previous section, here the end-point may or may not include reduction or elimination of the virus. In fact, there is evidence that control of chronic HCV complications does depend on a sustained virologic response. This topic was already discussed earlier; thus, discussion of the final prevention category can be restricted to HBV.

The typical strategic questions about HBV treatments include the following:

- Which patients should be treated, and at what stage of infection?
- Which drug or combination of drugs should be used, and for how long?

- Under what conditions should patients continue, stop, or switch therapies?

Clinical investigation of current therapies continues on all these fronts, along with efforts to develop new interventions of improved efficacy.

Treating symptoms is not the main objective of the therapy for HBV, as few symptoms are exhibited over the natural history of infection until the actual onset of serious liver disease.[371] Since current drug therapy does not eradicate infection, the immediate goal of treatment is to prevent the development of cirrhosis and HCC by suppressing viral replication.[372] In other words, the aim is to moderate chronic disease progression, and in this way to interrupt malignant transformation.

There are a number of therapies for chronic hepatitis B that have received approval in developed countries, including two formulations of interferon (standard and pegylated) and a variety of nucleoside and NAs.[373] Although effective in reducing disease in approximately one-third of patients, interferon therapy has several drawbacks, including high costs, the requirement for subcutaneous injection, and reported side effects.[374] NAs are orally administered, have more limited side effects, and are effective at inhibiting HBV replication.[375] In order for the benefit to be maintained, however, NAs must be used over an extended period, increasing the likelihood of drug resistance.[376]

Interferon-alpha and lamivudine (a nucleoside analogue) are the two antiviral drugs that have been approved by the U.S. FDA for the treatment of chronic HBV infection in children.[377] U.S. reviews have noted an efficacy rate of 20–58% (vs 8–17% for controls) for interferon-alpha, and around 23% for lamivudine (vs 13% for controls).[378,379] Other pediatric medications for HBV infection are expected to be tested in the next few years.[380] In fact, focusing substantial clinical attention on pediatric HBV infection may not be warranted. Although infected children manifest high viral loads, many do not experience active disease, and the risk of HCC is low compared to cases where active disease emerges in adulthood. A recent Taiwanese study questioned whether there was any real advantage in applying interferon-alpha therapy to perinatal or pediatric infections.[381]

By comparison, there are currently no FDA-approved drugs for treating HCV infection in children.[382] Although therapeutic options have not been investigated in large randomized controlled trials, a few smaller studies of standard interferon therapy have shown promising results.[383–385] Current Canadian consensus guidelines suggest that "there is insufficient information to make any specific recommendations about treating children with hepatitis C."[386]

CONCLUSION

Here it is beneficial to lay two additional oncogenic viruses, HBV and HCV, alongside the one that dominated the discussion up to now, that is, HPV. A key similarity is immediately clear: HPV and the hepatitis viruses are both related to cancers that currently stand out in terms of health and health care burden—cervical cancer and liver cancer, respectively. Whatever other cancer connections are proven or suspected, these two cancer sites will remain as important motivators of prevention efforts.

The fundamental disease processes related to HBV and HCV that affect multiple organs of the body, and sometimes lead to cancer, are similar to the widespread impact of HPV on keratinocytes in squamous epithelial tissues at many different sites. The main distinction is the systemic and multitargeted nature of hepatitis infection, allowing for various and even simultaneous disease manifestations.[387,388] Thus, while HPV appears to be exclusively epitheliotropic, HCV demonstrates at least three seemingly distinct tropisms: for hepatocytes, salivary gland cells, and lymphocytes.[389-391] Malignancies with demonstrated HCV involvement are found in the areas of the body related to these cells. While the rarer cancers involved with hepatitis (and other viruses to be introduced in this book) are of less importance in terms of prevention, they have benefited the cause of basic scientific exploration. In short, investigating the multisite dimension of agents related to cancer has generated insights in terms of the biology of oncogenic processes.

The primary prevention of hepatitis infection may be seen as a paradigm for the challenges encountered with many infectious agents of cancer. The obstacles to developing effective strategies include:

- The general challenges of vaccine development
- The phenomenon of asymptomatic carriers
- Long latency before cancer development
- The influence of socioeconomic forces on the uptake of risky behaviors
- The fact that transmission routes such as injection drug use are difficult to overcome, especially given the complexity of related psychological problems, mental illness, poverty, etc.
- Concerns about privacy and discrimination (e.g., regarding test results)

The urgency for preventive measures related to the hepatitis viruses arises not just from current and increasing rates of liver cancer and its poor survival rate, but from the impact of other serious diseases such as cirrhosis. In this way, hepatitis viruses stand apart from HPV—whereas both types of agents are implicated in a combination of (prevalent) non-malignant and (rarer) malignant conditions, cirrhosis would generally be considered more serious than genital warts.

However, HPV, HBV, and HCV become realigned when considering the similarly vast "reservoirs" of viral carriers around the world. Exacerbating this scenario is the fact that HBV, HCV, and HIV have similar transmission routes, leading to high coinfection rates.[392] These viruses interact synergistically, with the potential for "a major health care catastrophe in the coming years."[393] The risk of coinfection and increased disease development also seems to apply to HIV and HPV, though possibly to a lesser extent. Generally, this set of circumstances should motivate a concerted effort to control all these viral threats in the developed and especially the developing world.

NOTES

1. Gomaa AI, Khan SA, Toledano MB et al. Hepatocellular carcinoma: epidemiology, risk factors and pathogenesis. *World Journal of Gastroenterology.* 2008; 14(27): 4300–8.
2. Castiglia PT. Hepatitis in children. *Journal of Pediatric Health Care.* 1996; 10(6): 286–8.
3. Leemans WF, Janssen HL, de Man RA. Future prospectives for the management of chronic hepatitis B. *World Journal of Gastroenterology.* 2007; 13(18): 2554–67.
4. McGlynn KA, London WT. Epidemiology and natural history of hepatocellular carcinoma. *Best Practice and Research Clinical Gastroenterology.* 2005; 19(1): 3–23.
5. El-Serag HB, Rudolph KL. Hepatocellular carcinoma: epidemiology and molecular carcinogenesis. *Gastroenterology.* 2007; 132(7): 2557–76.
6. Dyer Z, Peltekian K, van Zanten SV. Review article: the changing epidemiology of hepatocellular carcinoma in Canada. *Alimentary Pharmacology and Therapeutics.* 2005; 22(1): 17–22.
7. elSaadany S, Tepper M, Mao Y et al. An epidemiologic study of hepatocellular carcinoma in Canada. *Canadian Journal of Public Health.* 2002; 93(6): 443–6.
8. Perz JF, Armstrong GL, Farrington LA et al. The contributions of hepatitis B virus and hepatitis C virus infections to cirrhosis and primary liver cancer worldwide. *Journal of Hepatology.* 2006; 45(4): 529–38.
9. Trinchet JC, Ganne-Carrie N, Nahon P et al. Hepatocellular carcinoma in patients with hepatitis C virus-related chronic liver disease. *World Journal of Gastroenterology.* 2007; 13(17): 2455–60.

10 Schwartz M, Roayaie S, Konstadoulakis M. Strategies for the management of hepatocellular carcinoma. *Nature Clinical Practice Oncology.* 2007; 4(7): 424–32.
11 Shepard CW, Simard EP, Finelli L et al. Hepatitis B virus infection: epidemiology and vaccination. *Epidemiologic Reviews.* 2006; 28: 112–25.
12 Minuk GY, Uhanova J. Viral hepatitis in the Canadian Inuit and First Nations populations. *Canadian Journal of Gastroenterology.* 2003; 17(12): 707–12.
13 See, for example, zur Hausen H. *Infections Causing Human Cancer.* Heidelberg: Wiley-VCH; 2006.
14 Berzsenyi MD, Bowden DS, Roberts SK. GB virus C: insights into co-infection. *Journal of Clinical Virology.* 2005; 33(4): 257–66.
15 Tennant F. Hepatitis C, B, D, and A: contrasting features and liver function abnormalities in heroin addicts. *Journal of Addictive Diseases.* 2001; 20(1): 9–17.
16 Fry DE. Occupational risks of blood exposure in the operating room. *American Surgeon.* 2007; 73(7): 637–46.
17 Gillcrist JA. Hepatitis viruses A, B, C, D, E and G: implications for dental personnel. *Journal of the American Dental Association.* 1999; 130(4): 509–20.
18 Berzsenyi MD, Bowden DS, Roberts SK. GB virus C: insights into co-infection. *Journal of Clinical Virology.* 2005; 33(4): 257–66.
19 Souza IE, Zhang W, Diaz RS et al. Effect of GB virus C on response to antiretroviral therapy in HIV-infected Brazilians. *HIV Medicine.* 2006; 7(1): 25–31.
20 Ellett ML. Hepatitis C, E, F, G, and non-A-G. *Gastroenterology Nursing.* 2000; 23(2): 67–72.
21 Bowden S. New hepatitis viruses: contenders and pretenders. *Journal of Gastroenterology and Hepatology.* 2001; 16(2): 124–31.
22 Zaki Mel S, el-Hady NA. Molecular detection of transfusion transmitted virus coinfection with some hepatotropic viruses. *Archives of Pathology and Laboratory Medicine.* 2006; 130(11): 1680–3.
23 Hsu HY, Ni YH, Chiang CL et al. SEN virus infection in children in Taiwan: transmission route and role in blood transfusion and liver diseases. *Pediatric Infectious Disease Journal.* 2006; 25(5): 390–4.
24 Narayanan Menon KV. Non-A to E hepatitis. *Current Opinion in Infectious Diseases.* 2002; 15(5): 529–34.
25 Ghany M, Liang TJ. Drug targets and molecular mechanisms of drug resistance in chronic hepatitis B. *Gastroenterology.* 2007; 132(4): 1574–85.
26 Chang MH. Hepatitis B virus infection. *Seminars in Fetal and Neonatal Medicine.* 2007; 12(3): 160–7.
27 Pungpapong S, Kim WR, Poterucha JJ. Natural history of hepatitis B virus infection: an update for clinicians. *Mayo Clinic Proceedings.* 2007; 82(8): 967–75.
28 Chang MH. Hepatitis B virus infection. *Seminars in Fetal and Neonatal Medicine.* 2007; 12(3): 160–7.
29 Arbuthnot P, Longshaw V, Naidoo T et al. Opportunities for treating chronic hepatitis B and C virus infection using RNA interference. *Journal of Viral Hepatitis.* 2007; 14(7): 447–59.
30 Kew MC, Kramvis A, Yu MC et al. Increased hepatocarcinogenic potential of hepatitis B virus genotype A in Bantu-speaking sub-saharan Africans. *Journal of Medical Virology.* 2005; 75(4): 513–21.

31 Livingston SE, Simonetti JP, McMahon BJ et al. Hepatitis B virus genotypes in Alaska Native people with hepatocellular carcinoma: preponderance of genotype F. *Journal of Infectious Diseases.* 2007; 195(1): 5–11.
32 Toan NL, Song le H, Kremsner PG et al. Impact of the hepatitis B virus genotype and genotype mixtures on the course of liver disease in Vietnam. *Hepatology.* 2006; 43(6): 1375–84.
33 Mojiri A, Behzad-Behbahani A, Saberifirozi M et al. Hepatitis B virus genotypes in southwest Iran: molecular, serological and clinical outcomes. *World Journal of Gastroenterology.* 2008; 14(10): 1510–3.
34 Lin CL, Kao JH. Hepatitis B viral factors and clinical outcomes of chronic hepatitis B. *Journal of Biomedical Science.* 2008; 15(2): 137–45.
35 Chu CM, Liaw YF. Chronic hepatitis B virus infection acquired in childhood: special emphasis on prognostic and therapeutic implication of delayed HBeAg seroconversion. *Journal of Viral Hepatitis.* 2007; 14(3): 147–52.
36 Livingston SE, Simonetti JP, Bulkow LR et al. Clearance of hepatitis B e antigen in patients with chronic hepatitis B and genotypes A, B, C, D, and F. *Gastroenterology.* 2007; 133(5): 1452–7.
37 Fattovich G, Bortolotti F, Donato F. Natural history of chronic hepatitis B: special emphasis on disease progression and prognostic factors. *Journal of Hepatology.* 2008; 48(2): 335–52.
38 Tangkijvanich P, Mahachai V, Komolmit P et al. Hepatitis B virus genotypes and hepatocellular carcinoma in Thailand. *World Journal of Gastroenterology.* 2005; 11(15): 2238–43.
39 Chevaliez S, Pawlotsky JM. Hepatitis C virus: virology, diagnosis and management of antiviral therapy. *World Journal of Gastroenterology.* 2007; 13(17): 2461–6.
40 Fry DE. Occupational risks of blood exposure in the operating room. *American Surgeon.* 2007; 73(7): 637–46.
41 Chevaliez S, Pawlotsky JM. Hepatitis C virus: virology, diagnosis and management of antiviral therapy. *World Journal of Gastroenterology.* 2007; 13(17): 2461–6.
42 Arbuthnot P, Longshaw V, Naidoo T et al. Opportunities for treating chronic hepatitis B and C virus infection using RNA interference. *Journal of Viral Hepatitis.* 2007; 14(7): 447–59.
43 Koziel MJ, Peters MG. Viral hepatitis in HIV infection. *New England Journal of Medicine.* 2007; 356(14): 1445–54.
44 Arbuthnot P, Longshaw V, Naidoo T et al. Opportunities for treating chronic hepatitis B and C virus infection using RNA interference. *Journal of Viral Hepatitis.* 2007; 14(7): 447–59.
45 Castera L. Steatosis, insulin resistance and fibrosis progression in chronic hepatitis C. *Minerva Gastroenterologica e Dietologica.* 2006; 52(2): 125–34.
46 Hjelkrem MC, Torres DM, Harrison SA. Nonalcoholic fatty liver disease. *Minerva Medica.* 2008; 99(6): 583–93.
47 International Agency for Research on Cancer. *IARC Monographs on the Evaluation of Carcinogenic Risks to Humans.* Available at http://monographs.iarc.fr/ENG/Classification/crthgr01.php. Accessed October 2007.
48 McGlynn KA, London WT. Epidemiology and natural history of hepatocellular carcinoma. *Best Practice and Research Clinical Gastroenterology.* 2005; 19(1): 3–23.

49. International Agency for Research on Cancer. *Hepatitis Viruses. Summary Data eEported and Evaluation*. 1997. WHO. Available at http://monographs.iarc.fr/ENG/Monographs/vol59/volume59.pdf. Accessed October 2007.
50. Parkin DM. The global health burden of infection-associated cancers in the year 2002. *International Journal of Cancer*. 2006; 118(12): 3030–44.
51. Bosch FX, Ribes J, Cleries R et al. Epidemiology of hepatocellular carcinoma. *Clinics in Liver Disease*. 2005; 9(2): 191–211, v.
52. Erickson SK. Nonalcoholic fatty liver disease. *Journal of Lipid Research*. 2009; 50: S412–16.
53. Evans AA, O'Connell AP, Pugh JC et al. Geographic variation in viral load among hepatitis B carriers with differing risks of hepatocellular carcinoma. *Cancer Epidemiology, Biomarkers and Prevention*. 1998; 7(7): 559–65.
54. Hassan MM, Hwang LY, Hatten CJ et al. Risk factors for hepatocellular carcinoma: synergism of alcohol with viral hepatitis and diabetes mellitus. *Hepatology*. 2002; 36(5): 1206–13.
55. Davila JA, Morgan RO, Shaib Y et al. Hepatitis C infection and the increasing incidence of hepatocellular carcinoma: a population-based study. *Gastroenterology*. 2004; 127(5): 1372–80.
56. Raza SA, Clifford GM, Franceschi S. Worldwide variation in the relative importance of hepatitis B and hepatitis C viruses in hepatocellular carcinoma: a systematic review. *British Journal of Cancer*. 2007; 96(7): 1127–34.
57. Hislop TG, Teh C, Low A et al. Hepatitis B knowledge, testing and vaccination levels in Chinese immigrants to British Columbia, Canada. *Canadian Journal of Public Health*. 2007; 98(2): 125–9.
58. Fung SK, Wong FS, Wong DK et al. Hepatitis B virus genotypes, precore and core promoter variants among predominantly Asian patients with chronic HBV infection in a Canadian center. *Liver International*. 2006; 26(7): 796–804.
59. Lang K, Danchenko N, Gondek K et al. The burden of illness associated with hepatocellular carcinoma in the United States. *Journal of Hepatology*. 2009; 50(1): 89–99.
60. El-Serag HB, Mason AC. Risk factors for the rising rates of primary liver cancer in the United States. *Archives of Internal Medicine*. 2000; 160(21): 3227–30.
61. Patrick DM, Bigham M, Ng H et al. Elimination of acute hepatitis B among adolescents after one decade of an immunization program targeting Grade 6 students. *Pediatric Infectious Disease Journal*. 2003; 22(10): 874–7.
62. Bronowicki JP, Bineau C, Feugier P et al. Primary lymphoma of the liver: clinical-pathological features and relationship with HCV infection in French patients. *Hepatology*. 2003; 37(4): 781–7.
63. Salmon JS, Thompson MA, Arildsen RC et al. Non-Hodgkin's lymphoma involving the liver: clinical and therapeutic considerations. *Clinical Lymphoma and Myeloma*. 2006; 6(4): 273–80.
64. Chen CJ, Jeng LB, Huang SF. Lymphoepithelioma-like hepatocellular carcinoma. *Chang Gung Medical Journal*. 2007; 30(2): 172–7.
65. Chen TC, Ng KF, Kuo T. Intrahepatic cholangiocarcinoma with lymphoepithelioma-like component. *Modern Pathology*. 2001; 14(5): 527–32.
66. Shaib Y, El-Serag HB. The epidemiology of cholangiocarcinoma. *Seminars in Liver Disease*. 2004; 24(2): 115–25.
67. Yamamoto S, Kubo S, Hai S et al. Hepatitis C virus infection as a likely etiology of intrahepatic cholangiocarcinoma. *Cancer Science*. 2004; 95(7): 592–5.

68 Shaib YH, El-Serag HB, Nooka AK et al. Risk factors for intrahepatic and extrahepatic cholangiocarcinoma: a hospital-based case-control study. *American Journal of Gastroenterology*. 2007; 102(5): 1016–21.
69 Torbenson M, Yeh MM, Abraham SC. Bile duct dysplasia in the setting of chronic hepatitis C and alcohol cirrhosis. *American Journal of Surgical Pathology*. 2007; 31(9): 1410–3.
70 Donato F, Gelatti U, Tagger A et al. Intrahepatic cholangiocarcinoma and hepatitis C and B virus infection, alcohol intake, and hepatolithiasis: a case-control study in Italy. *Cancer Causes and Control*. 2001; 12(10): 959–64.
71 Lee TY, Lee SS, Jung SW et al. Hepatitis B virus infection and intrahepatic cholangiocarcinoma in Korea: a case-control study. *American Journal of Gastroenterology*. 2008; 103(7): 1716–20.
72 Zhou YM, Yin ZF, Yang JM et al. Risk factors for intrahepatic cholangiocarcinoma: a case-control study in China. *World Journal of Gastroenterology*. 2008; 14(4): 632–5.
73 Welzel TM, Graubard BI, El-Serag HB et al. Risk factors for intrahepatic and extrahepatic cholangiocarcinoma in the United States: a population-based case-control study. *Clinical Gastroenterology and Hepatology* 2007; 5(10): 1221–8.
74 El-Serag HB, Engels EA, Landgren O et al. Risk of hepatobiliary and pancreatic cancers after hepatitis C virus infection: a population-based study of U.S. veterans. *Hepatology*. 2009; 49(1): 116–23.
75 Bondini S, Kallman J, Wheeler A et al. Impact of non-alcoholic fatty liver disease on chronic hepatitis B. *Liver International*. 2007; 27(5): 607–11.
76 Koike K. Hepatitis C as a metabolic disease: implication for the pathogenesis of NASH. *Hepatology Research*. 2005; 33(2): 145–50.
77 Targher G, Bertolini L, Padovani R et al. Differences and similarities in early atherosclerosis between patients with non-alcoholic steatohepatitis and chronic hepatitis B and C. *Journal of Hepatology*. 2007; 46(6): 1126–32.
78 Pyrsopoulos NT, Reddy KR. Extrahepatic manifestations of chronic viral hepatitis. *Current Gastroenterology Reports*. 2001; 3(1): 71–8.
79 Muller AM, Ihorst G, Mertelsmann R et al. Epidemiology of non-Hodgkin's lymphoma (NHL): trends, geographic distribution, and etiology. *Annals of Hematology*. 2005; 84(1): 1–12.
80 Kuniyoshi M, Nakamuta M, Sakai H et al. Prevalence of hepatitis B or C virus infections in patients with non-Hodgkin's lymphoma. *Journal of Gastroenterology and Hepatology*. 2001; 16(2): 215–9.
81 Ulcickas Yood M, Quesenberry CP, Jr., Guo D et al. Incidence of non-Hodgkin's lymphoma among individuals with chronic hepatitis B virus infection. *Hepatology*. 2007; 46(1): 107–12.
82 Lim ST, Fei G, Quek R et al. The relationship of hepatitis B virus infection and non-Hodgkin's lymphoma and its impact on clinical characteristics and prognosis. *European Journal of Haematology*. 2007; 79(2): 132–7.
83 El-Sayed GM, Mohamed WS, Nouh MA et al. Viral genomes and antigen detection of hepatitis B and C viruses in involved lymph nodes of Egyptian non-Hodgkin's lymphoma patients. *Egyptian Journal of Immunology*. 2006; 13(1): 105–14.
84 Marcucci F, Mele A, Spada E et al. High prevalence of hepatitis B virus infection in B-cell non-Hodgkin's lymphoma. *Haematologica*. 2006; 91(4): 554–7.
85 Wang F, Xu RH, Han B et al. High incidence of hepatitis B virus infection in B-cell subtype non-Hodgkin lymphoma compared with other cancers. *Cancer*. 2007; 109(7): 1360–4.

86 Arcaini L, Burcheri S, Rossi A et al. Prevalence of HCV infection in nongastric marginal zone B-cell lymphoma of MALT. *Annals of Oncology.* 2007; 18(2): 346–50.
87 Ferreri AJ, Zucca E. Marginal-zone lymphoma. *Critical Reviews in Oncology/Hematology.* 2007; 63(3): 245–56.
88 Giordano TP, Henderson L, Landgren O et al. Risk of non-Hodgkin lymphoma and lymphoproliferative precursor diseases in US veterans with hepatitis C virus. *Journal of the American Medical Association.* 2007; 297(18): 2010–7.
89 Nieters A, Kallinowski B, Brennan P et al. Hepatitis C and risk of lymphoma: results of the European multicenter case-control study EPILYMPH. *Gastroenterology.* 2006; 131(6): 1879–86.
90 Bianco E, Marcucci F, Mele A et al. Prevalence of hepatitis C virus infection in lymphoproliferative diseases other than B-cell non-Hodgkin's lymphoma, and in myeloproliferative diseases: an Italian Multi-Center case-control study. *Haematologica.* 2004; 89(1): 70–6.
91 Spinelli JJ, Lai AS, Krajden M et al. Hepatitis C virus and risk of non-Hodgkin lymphoma in British Columbia, Canada. *International Journal of Cancer.* 2008; 122(3): 630–3.
92 Mazzaro C, Tirelli U, Pozzato G. Hepatitis C virus and non-Hodgkin's lymphoma 10 years later. *Digestive and Liver Disease.* 2005; 37(4): 219–26.
93 Chi ZC, Ma SZ. Rheumatologic manifestations of hepatic diseases. *Hepatobiliary and Pancreatic Diseases International.* 2003; 2(1): 32–7.
94 Han SH. Extrahepatic manifestations of chronic hepatitis B. *Clinics in Liver Disease.* 2004; 8(2): 403–18.
95 Mason A, Theal J, Bain V et al. Hepatitis B virus replication in damaged endothelial tissues of patients with extrahepatic disease. *American Journal of Gastroenterology.* 2005; 100(4): 972–6.
96 Rong Q, Huang J, Su E et al. Infection of hepatitis B virus in extrahepatic endothelial tissues mediated by endothelial progenitor cells. *Virology Journal.* 2007; 4: 36.
97 Umeda M, Marusawa H, Seno H et al. Hepatitis B virus infection in lymphatic tissues in inactive hepatitis B carriers. *Journal of Hepatology.* 2005; 42(6): 806–12.
98 Zignego AL, Giannini C, Ferri C. Hepatitis C virus-related lymphoproliferative disorders: an overview. *World Journal of Gastroenterology.* 2007; 13(17): 2467–78.
99 Zignego AL, Ferri C, Pileri SA et al. Extrahepatic manifestations of Hepatitis C Virus infection: a general overview and guidelines for a clinical approach. *Digestive and Liver Disease.* 2007; 39(1): 2–17.
100 Galossi A, Guarisco R, Bellis L et al. Extrahepatic manifestations of chronic HCV infection. *Journal of Gastrointestinal and Liver Diseases.* 2007; 16(1): 65–73.
101 Lizardi-Cervera J, Poo JL, Romero-Mora K et al. Hepatitis C virus infection and non-Hodgkin's lymphoma: a review and case report of nine patient. *Annals of Hepatology.* 2006; 5(4): 257–62.
102 Shintani Y, Fujie H, Miyoshi H et al. Hepatitis C virus infection and diabetes: direct involvement of the virus in the development of insulin resistance. *Gastroenterology.* 2004; 126(3): 840–8.

103 Lormeau C, Falgarone G, Roulot D et al. Rheumatologic manifestations of chronic hepatitis C infection. *Joint Bone Spine*. 2006; 73(6): 633–8.
104 Sanzone AM, Begue RE. Hepatitis C and arthritis: an update. *Infectious Disease Clinics of North America*. 2006; 20(4): 877–89.
105 Antonelli A, Ferri C, Fallahi P et al. Thyroid cancer in HCV-related chronic hepatitis patients: a case-control study. *Thyroid*. 2007; 17(5): 447–51.
106 Ali A, Zein NN. Hepatitis C infection. *Cleveland Clinic Journal of Medicine*. 2005; 72(11): 1005–8.
107 Bianchi FB, Muratori P, Granito A et al. Hepatitis C and autoreactivity. *Digestive and Liver Disease*. 2007; 39(suppl 1): S22–4.
108 Saadoun D, Landau DA, Calabrese LH et al. Hepatitis C-associated mixed cryoglobulinaemia: a crossroad between autoimmunity and lymphoproliferation. *Rheumatology*. 2007; 46(8): 1234–42.
109 Muratori L, Bogdanos DP, Muratori P et al. Susceptibility to thyroid disorders in hepatitis C. *Clinical Gastroenterology and Hepatology*. 2005; 3(6): 595–603.
110 Craxi A, Laffi G, Zignego AL. Hepatitis C virus (HCV) infection: a systemic disease. *Molecular Aspects of Medicine*. 2008; 29(1–2): 85–95.
111 Okuse C, Yotsuyanagi H, Koike K. Hepatitis C as a systemic disease: virus and host immunologic responses underlie hepatic and extrahepatic manifestations. *Journal of Gastroenterology*. 2007; 42(11): 857–65.
112 Ferri C, Antonelli A, Mascia MT et al. B-cells and mixed cryoglobulinemia. *Autoimmunity Reviews*. 2007; 7(2): 114–20.
113 Berk DR, Mallory SB, Keeffe EB et al. Dermatologic disorders associated with chronic hepatitis C: effect of interferon therapy. *Clinical Gastroenterology and Hepatology*. 2007; 5(2): 142–51.
114 Viguier M, Rivet J, Agbalika F et al. B-cell lymphomas involving the skin associated with hepatitis C virus infection. *International Journal of Dermatology*. 2002; 41(9): 577–82.
115 Nagao Y, Sata M. Hepatitis C virus and lichen planus. *Journal of Gastroenterology and Hepatology*. 2004; 19(10): 1101–13.
116 Sansonno D, Carbone A, De Re V et al. Hepatitis C virus infection, cryoglobulinaemia, and beyond. *Rheumatology*. 2007; 46(4): 572–8.
117 Ferri C, Antonelli A, Mascia MT et al. B-cells and mixed cryoglobulinemia. *Autoimmunity Reviews*. 2007; 7(2): 114–20.
118 Sansonno D, Carbone A, De Re V et al. Hepatitis C virus infection, cryoglobulinaemia, and beyond. *Rheumatology*. 2007; 46(4): 572–8.
119 Trejo O, Ramos-Casals M, Lopez-Guillermo A et al. Hematologic malignancies in patients with cryoglobulinemia: association with autoimmune and chronic viral diseases. *Seminars in Arthritis and Rheumatism*. 2003; 33(1): 19–28.
120 Ramos-Casals M, Garcia-Carrasco M, Brito Zeron MP et al. Viral etiopathogenesis of Sjogren's syndrome: role of the hepatitis C virus. *Autoimmunity Reviews*. 2002; 1(4): 238–43.
121 Ramos-Casals M, Loustaud-Ratti V, De Vita S et al. Sjogren syndrome associated with hepatitis C virus: a multicenter analysis of 137 cases. *Medicine*. 2005; 84(2): 81–9.
122 Ramos-Casals M, Trejo O, Garcia-Carrasco M et al. Triple association between hepatitis C virus infection, systemic autoimmune diseases, and B cell lymphoma. *Journal of Rheumatology*. 2004; 31(3): 495–9.

123 Ramos-Casals M, De Vita S, Tzioufas AG. Hepatitis C virus, Sjogren's syndrome and B-cell lymphoma: linking infection, autoimmunity and cancer. *Autoimmunity Reviews*. 2005; 4(1): 8–15.
124 Malek SN, Hatfield AJ, Flinn IW. MALT Lymphomas. *Current Treatment Options in Oncology*. 2003; 4(4): 269–79.
125 Zinzani PL, Magagnoli M, Galieni P et al. Nongastrointestinal low-grade mucosa-associated lymphoid tissue lymphoma: analysis of 75 patients. *Journal of Clinical Oncology*. 1999; 17(4): 1254.
126 Ramos-Casals M, la Civita L, de Vita S et al. Characterization of B cell lymphoma in patients with Sjogren's syndrome and hepatitis C virus infection. *Arthritis and Rheumatism*. 2007; 57(1): 161–70.
127 Ortiz-Movilla N, Lazaro P, Rodriguez-Inigo E et al. Hepatitis C virus replicates in sweat glands and is released into sweat in patients with chronic hepatitis C. *Journal of Medical Virology*. 2002; 68(4): 529–36.
128 Ohoka S, Tanaka Y, Amako Y et al. Sialadenitis in patients with chronic hepatitis C is not directly related to hepatitis C virus. *Hepatology Research*. 2003; 27(1): 23–9.
129 De Re V, De Vita S, Gasparotto D et al. Salivary gland B cell lymphoproliferative disorders in Sjogren's syndrome present a restricted use of antigen receptor gene segments similar to those used by hepatitis C virus-associated non-Hodgkins's lymphomas. *European Journal of Immunology*. 2002; 32(3): 903–10.
130 De Vita S, De Re V, Sansonno D et al. Lack of HCV infection in malignant cells refutes the hypothesis of a direct transforming action of the virus in the pathogenesis of HCV-associated B-cell NHLs. *Tumori*. 2002; 88(5): 400–6.
131 Suarez F, Lortholary O, Hermine O et al. Infection-associated lymphomas derived from marginal zone B cells: a model of antigen-driven lymphoproliferation. *Blood*. 2006; 107(8): 3034–44.
132 Ambrosetti A, Zanotti R, Pattaro C et al. Most cases of primary salivary mucosa-associated lymphoid tissue lymphoma are associated either with Sjoegren syndrome or hepatitis C virus infection. *British Journal of Haematology*. 2004; 126(1): 43–9.
133 Sene D, Limal N, Cacoub P. Hepatitis C virus-associated extrahepatic manifestations: a review. *Metabolic Brain Disease*. 2004; 19(3–4): 357–81.
134 De Vita S, De Re V, Sansonno D et al. Gastric mucosa as an additional extrahepatic localization of hepatitis C virus: viral detection in gastric low-grade lymphoma associated with autoimmune disease and in chronic gastritis. *Hepatology*. 2000; 31(1): 182–9.
135 Besson C, Canioni D, Lepage E et al. Characteristics and outcome of diffuse large B-cell lymphoma in hepatitis C virus-positive patients in LNH 93 and LNH 98 Groupe d'Etude des Lymphomes de l'Adulte programs. *Journal of Clinical Oncology*. 2006; 24(6): 953–60.
136 Takeshita M, Sakai H, Okamura S et al. Splenic large B-cell lymphoma in patients with hepatitis C virus infection. *Human Pathology*. 2005; 36(8): 878–85.
137 Arcaini L, Paulli M, Boveri E et al. Splenic and nodal marginal zone lymphomas are indolent disorders at high hepatitis C virus seroprevalence with distinct presenting features but similar morphologic and phenotypic profiles. *Cancer*. 2004; 100(1): 107–15.

138 Antonelli A, Ferri C, Fallahi P et al. Thyroid cancer in HCV-related chronic hepatitis patients: a case-control study. *Thyroid.* 2007; 17(5): 447–51.
139 Krueger H, McLean D, Williams D. *The Prevention of Second Primary Cancers.* Basel: Karger, 2008.
140 Brennan P, Scelo G, Hemminki K et al. Second primary cancers among 109 000 cases of non-Hodgkin's lymphoma. *British Journal of Cancer.* 2005; 93(1): 159–66.
141 Antonelli A, Ferri C, Fallahi P et al. Thyroid disorders in chronic hepatitis C virus infection. *Thyroid.* 2006; 16(6): 563–72.
142 Landau DA, Saadoun D, Calabrese LH et al. The pathophysiology of HCV induced B-cell clonal disorders. *Autoimmunity Reviews.* 2007; 6(8): 581–7.
143 Kelaidi C, Rollot F, Park S et al. Response to antiviral treatment in hepatitis C virus-associated marginal zone lymphomas. *Leukemia.* 2004; 18(10): 1711–6.
144 Ferri C, Antonelli A, Mascia MT et al. B-cells and mixed cryoglobulinemia. *Autoimmunity Reviews.* 2007; 7(2): 114–20.
145 Atkins M, Nolan M. Sexual transmission of hepatitis B. *Current Opinions in Infectious Diseases.* 2005; 18(1): 67–72.
146 Zuckerman JN. Review: hepatitis B immune globulin for prevention of hepatitis B infection. *Journal of Medical Virology.* 2007; 79(7): 919–21.
147 Health Protection Agency. *Hepatitis B - General Information.* 2005. Available at http://www.hpa.org.uk/infections/topics_az/hepatitis_b/gen_info.htm. Accessed October 2007.
148 Alter MJ. Epidemiology of hepatitis B in Europe and worldwide. *Journal of Hepatology.* 2003; 39(suppl 1): S64–9.
149 Benhamou Y. Hepatitis B in the HIV-coinfected patient. *Journal of Acquired Immune Deficiency Syndromes.* 2007; 45(suppl 2): S57–65.
150 Centers for Disease Control and Prevention. Incidence of acute hepatitis B--United States, 1990–2002. *Morbidity and Mortality Weekly Report.* 2004; 52(51–52): 1252–4.
151 Benhamou Y. Hepatitis B in the HIV-coinfected patient. *Journal of Acquired Immune Deficiency Syndromes.* 2007; 45(suppl 2): S57–65.
152 Hoffmann CJ, Thio CL. Clinical implications of HIV and hepatitis B co-infection in Asia and Africa. *Lancet Infectious Diseases.* 2007; 7(6): 402–9.
153 Chang MH. Hepatitis B virus infection. *Seminars in Fetal and Neonatal Medicine.* 2007; 12(3): 160–7.
154 Tajiri H, Tanaka Y, Kagimoto S et al. Molecular evidence of father-to-child transmission of hepatitis B virus. *Journal of Medical Virology.* 2007; 79(7): 922–6.
155 Hoffmann CJ, Thio CL. Clinical implications of HIV and hepatitis B co-infection in Asia and Africa. *Lancet Infectious Diseases.* 2007; 7(6): 402–9.
156 Chang MH. Impact of hepatitis B vaccination on hepatitis B disease and nucleic acid testing in high-prevalence populations. *Journal of Clinical Virology.* 2006; 36(suppl 1): S45–50.
157 Fry DE. Occupational risks of blood exposure in the operating room. *American Surgeon.* 2007; 73(7): 637–46.
158 Alter MJ. Epidemiology of hepatitis B in Europe and worldwide. *Journal of Hepatology.* 2003; 39(suppl 1): S64–9.
159 Fry DE. Occupational risks of blood exposure in the operating room. *American Surgeon.* 2007; 73(7): 637–46.

160 Stramer SL. Current risks of transfusion-transmitted agents: a review. *Archives of Pathology and Laboratory Medicine.* 2007; 131(5): 702–7.
161 Dodd RY, Notari EPt, Stramer SL. Current prevalence and incidence of infectious disease markers and estimated window-period risk in the American Red Cross blood donor population. *Transfusion.* 2002; 42(8): 975–9.
162 Allain JP, Candotti D, Soldan K et al. The risk of hepatitis B virus infection by transfusion in Kumasi, Ghana. *Blood.* 2003; 101(6): 2419–25.
163 Slowik MK, Jhaveri R. Hepatitis B and C viruses in infants and young children. *Seminars in Pediatric Infectious Diseases.* 2005; 16(4): 296–305.
164 Li XM, Shi MF, Yang YB et al. Effect of hepatitis B immunoglobulin on interruption of HBV intrauterine infection. *World Journal of Gastroenterology.* 2004; 10(21): 3215–7.
165 Li XM, Yang YB, Hou HY et al. Interruption of HBV intrauterine transmission: a clinical study. *World Journal of Gastroenterology.* 2003; 9(7): 1501–3.
166 Chang MH. Hepatitis B virus infection. *Seminars in Fetal and Neonatal Medicine.* 2007; 12(3): 160–7.
167 Benhamou Y. Hepatitis B in the HIV-coinfected patient. *Journal of Acquired Immune Deficiency Syndromes.* 2007; 45(suppl 2): S57–65.
168 Pungpapong S, Kim WR, Poterucha JJ. Natural history of hepatitis B virus infection: an update for clinicians. *Mayo Clinic Proceedings.* 2007; 82(8): 967–75.
169 Alter MJ. Epidemiology of hepatitis B in Europe and worldwide. *Journal of Hepatology.* 2003; 39(suppl 1): S64–9.
170 Matthews GV, Nelson MR. The management of chronic hepatitis B infection. *International Journal of STD and AIDS.* 2001; 12(6): 353–7.
171 Chang MH. Hepatitis B virus infection. *Seminars in Fetal and Neonatal Medicine.* 2007; 12(3): 160–7.
172 Michielsen PP, Van Damme P. Viral hepatitis and pregnancy. *Acta Gastro-Enterologica Belgica.* 1999; 62(1): 21–9.
173 Gambarin-Gelwan M. Hepatitis B in pregnancy. *Clinics in Liver Disease.* 2007; 11(4): 945–63, x.
174 Zuckerman J, van Hattum J, Cafferkey M et al. Should hepatitis B vaccination be introduced into childhood immunisation programmes in northern Europe? *Lancet Infectious Diseases.* 2007; 7(6): 410–9.
175 Pungpapong S, Kim WR, Poterucha JJ. Natural history of hepatitis B virus infection: an update for clinicians. *Mayo Clinic Proceedings.* 2007; 82(8): 967–75.
176 Zuckerman J, van Hattum J, Cafferkey M et al. Should hepatitis B vaccination be introduced into childhood immunisation programmes in northern Europe? *Lancet Infectious Diseases.* 2007; 7(6): 410–9.
177 Brabin B, Beeching NJ, Bunn JE et al. Hepatitis B prevalence among Somali households in Liverpool. *Archives of Disease in Childhood.* 2002; 86(1): 67–8.
178 Kretzschmar M, de Wit GA, Smits LJ et al. Vaccination against hepatitis B in low endemic countries. *Epidemiology and Infection.* 2002; 128(2): 229–44.
179 Zuckerman J, van Hattum J, Cafferkey M et al. Should hepatitis B vaccination be introduced into childhood immunisation programmes in northern Europe? *Lancet Infectious Diseases.* 2007; 7(6): 410–9.

180 See the Health Canada webpage at hc-sc.gc.ca/sr-sr/pubs/hpr-rpms/wp-dt/2001-0105-immigration/ method_e.html. Accessed November 2007.
181 Patrick DM, Bigham M, Ng H et al. Elimination of acute hepatitis B among adolescents after one decade of an immunization program targeting Grade 6 students. *Pediatric Infectious Disease Journal.* 2003; 22(10): 874–7.
182 Sherman M. Department of Medicine, University of Toronto. Personal communication (January, 2008).
183 Gish RG, Gadano AC. Chronic hepatitis B: current epidemiology in the Americas and implications for management. *Journal of Viral Hepatitis.* 2006; 13(12): 787–98.
184 Sherman KE, Peters M, Koziel MJ. HIV and liver disease forum: conference proceedings. *Hepatology.* 2007; 45(6): 1566–77.
185 Alter MJ. Epidemiology of hepatitis C. *Hepatology.* 1997; 26(3 suppl 1): 62S–5S.
186 Perez CM, Suarez E, Torres EA et al. Seroprevalence of hepatitis C virus and associated risk behaviours: a population-based study in San Juan, Puerto Rico. *International Journal of Epidemiology.* 2005; 34(3): 593–9.
187 Sherman M. Department of Medicine, University of Toronto. Personal communication (January, 2008).
188 Data available at http://www.cdc.gov/ncidod/diseases/hepatitis/c_training/edu/1/default.htm. Accessed May 2005.
189 Scheinmann R, Hagan H, Lelutiu-Weinberger C et al. Non-injection drug use and hepatitis C virus: A systematic review. *Drug and Alcohol Dependence.* 2007; 89(1): 1–12.
190 Shannon K, Ishida T, Morgan R et al. Potential community and public health impacts of medically supervised safer smoking facilities for crack cocaine users. *Harm Reduction Journal.* 2006; 3: 1.
191 McGovern BH. Hepatitis C in the HIV-infected patient. *Journal of Acquired Immune Deficiency Syndromes.* 2007; 45(suppl 2): S47–56.
192 Gotz HM, van Doornum G, Niesters HG et al. A cluster of acute hepatitis C virus infection among men who have sex with men--results from contact tracing and public health implications. *AIDS.* 2005; 19(9): 969–74.
193 McGovern BH. Hepatitis C in the HIV-infected patient. *Journal of Acquired Immune Deficiency Syndromes.* 2007; 45(suppl 2): S47–56.
194 Sulkowski MS. The HIV-coinfected patient: managing viral hepatitis. *Journal of Acquired Immune Deficiency Syndromes.* 2007; 45(suppl 2): S36–7.
195 Koziel MJ, Peters MG. Viral hepatitis in HIV infection. *New England Journal of Medicine.* 2007; 356(14): 1445–54.
196 Fischer B, Rehm J, Kim G et al. Safer injection facilities (SIFs) for injection drug users (IDUs) in Canada. A review and call for an evidence-focused pilot trial. *Canadian Journal of Public Health.* 2002; 93(5): 336–8.
197 Roy E, Alary M, Morissette C et al. High hepatitis C virus prevalence and incidence among Canadian intravenous drug users. *International Journal of STD and AIDS.* 2007; 18(1): 23–7.
198 Sherman KE, Peters M, Koziel MJ. HIV and liver disease forum: conference proceedings. *Hepatology.* 2007; 45(6): 1566–77.
199 Shepard CW, Finelli L, Alter MJ. Global epidemiology of hepatitis C virus infection. *Lancet Infectious Diseases.* 2005; 5(9): 558–67.
200 Fischler B. Hepatitis C virus infection. *Seminars in Fetal and Neonatal Medicine.* 2007; 12(3): 168–73.

201 Sherman KE, Peters M, Koziel MJ. HIV and liver disease forum: conference proceedings. *Hepatology*. 2007; 45(6): 1566–77.
202 Mok J, Pembrey L, Tovo PA et al. When does mother to child transmission of hepatitis C virus occur? Archives of Disease in Childhood. *Fetal and Neonatal Edition*. 2005; 90(2): F156–60.
203 Slowik MK, Jhaveri R. Hepatitis B and C viruses in infants and young children. *Seminars in Pediatric Infectious Diseases*. 2005; 16(4): 296–305.
204 Kumar RM, Shahul S. Role of breast-feeding in transmission of hepatitis C virus to infants of HCV-infected mothers. *Journal of Hepatology*. 1998; 29(2): 191–7.
205 Lin HH, Kao JH, Hsu HY et al. Absence of infection in breast-fed infants born to hepatitis C virus-infected mothers. *Journal of Pediatrics*. 1995; 126(4): 589–91.
206 Polywka S, Schroter M, Feucht HH et al. Low risk of vertical transmission of hepatitis C virus by breast milk. *Clinical Infectious Diseases*. 1999; 29(5): 1327–9.
207 Fischler B. Hepatitis C virus infection. *Seminars in Fetal and Neonatal Medicine*. 2007; 12(3): 168–73.
208 Stramer SL. Current risks of transfusion-transmitted agents: a review. *Archives of Pathology and Laboratory Medicine*. 2007; 131(5): 702–7.
209 Dodd RY, Notari EPt, Stramer SL. Current prevalence and incidence of infectious disease markers and estimated window-period risk in the American Red Cross blood donor population. *Transfusion*. 2002; 42(8): 975–9.
210 Fry DE. Occupational risks of blood exposure in the operating room. *American Surgeon*. 2007; 73(7): 637–46.
211 Fischler B. Hepatitis C virus infection. *Seminars in Fetal and Neonatal Medicine*. 2007; 12(3): 168–73.
212 Alter MJ. Epidemiology of hepatitis C virus infection. *World Journal of Gastroenterology*. 2007; 13(17): 2436–41.
213 Yen T, Keeffe EB, Ahmed A. The epidemiology of hepatitis C virus infection. *Journal of Clinical Gastroenterology*. 2003; 36(1): 47–53.
214 Rose VL. CDC issues new recommendations for the prevention and control of hepatitis C virus infection. *American Family Physician*. 1999; 59(5): 1321–3.
215 Wong T, Lee SS. Hepatitis C: a review for primary care physicians. *Canadian Medical Association Journal*. 2006; 174(5): 649–59.
216 Zahariadis G, Plitt SS, O'Brien S et al. Prevalence and estimated incidence of blood-borne viral pathogen infection in organ and tissue donors from northern Alberta. *American Journal of Transplantation*. 2007; 7(1): 226–34.
217 Wu HX, Wu J, Wong T et al. Incidence and risk factors for newly acquired hepatitis C virus infection among Aboriginal versus non-Aboriginal Canadians in six regions, 1999–2004. *European Journal of Clinical Microbiology and Infectious Diseases*. 2007; 26(3): 167–74.
218 Sherman M. Department of Medicine, University of Toronto. Personal communication (January, 2008).
219 Armstrong GL, Wasley A, Simard EP et al. The prevalence of hepatitis C virus infection in the United States, 1999 through 2002. *Annals of Internal Medicine*. 2006; 144(10): 705–14.
220 Hsieh TH, Liu CJ, Chen DS et al. Natural course and treatment of hepatitis D virus infection. *Journal of the Formosan Medical Association*. 2006; 105(11): 869–81.

221 Fiedler M, Roggendorf M. Immunology of HDV infection. *Current Topics in Microbiology and Immunology.* 2006; 307: 187–209.
222 Herzer K, Sprinzl MF, Galle PR. Hepatitis viruses:Live and let die. *Liver International.* 2007; 27(3): 293–301.
223 Tan J, Lok AS. Update on viral hepatitis: 2006. *Current Opinion in Gastroenterology.* 2007; 23(3): 263–7.
224 Rivkin A. Entecavir: a new nucleoside analogue for the treatment of chronic hepatitis B. *Drugs of Today.* 2007; 43(4): 201–20.
225 Schwartz M, Roayaie S, Konstadoulakis M. Strategies for the management of hepatocellular carcinoma. *Nature Clinical Practice Oncology.* 2007; 4(7): 424–32.
226 Liu CJ, Kao JH. Hepatitis B virus-related hepatocellular carcinoma: epidemiology and pathogenic role of viral factors. *Journal of the Chinese Medical Association.* 2007; 70(4): 141–5.
227 Hoofnagle JH, Doo E, Liang TJ et al. Management of hepatitis B: summary of a clinical research workshop. *Hepatology.* 2007; 45(4): 1056–75.
228 Slowik MK, Jhaveri R. Hepatitis B and C viruses in infants and young children. *Seminars in Pediatric Infectious Diseases.* 2005; 16(4): 296–305.
229 Chen SL, Morgan TR. The natural history of hepatitis C virus (HCV) infection. *International Journal of Medical Sciences.* 2006; 3(2): 47–52.
230 Hoofnagle JH, Doo E, Liang TJ et al. Management of hepatitis B: summary of a clinical research workshop. *Hepatology.* 2007; 45(4): 1056–75.
231 Hoffmann CJ, Thio CL. Clinical implications of HIV and hepatitis B co-infection in Asia and Africa. *Lancet Infectious Diseases.* 2007; 7(6): 402–9.
232 Kew MC, Kramvis A, Yu MC et al. Increased hepatocarcinogenic potential of hepatitis B virus genotype A in Bantu-speaking sub-saharan Africans. *Journal of Medical Virology.* 2005; 75(4): 513–21.
233 Chan HL, Hui AY, Wong ML et al. Genotype C hepatitis B virus infection is associated with an increased risk of hepatocellular carcinoma. *Gut.* 2004; 53(10): 1494–8.
234 Chen CJ, Yang HI, Su J et al. Risk of hepatocellular carcinoma across a biological gradient of serum hepatitis B virus DNA level. *Journal of the American Medical Association.* 2006; 295(1): 65–73.
235 Iloeje UH, Yang HI, Su J et al. Predicting cirrhosis risk based on the level of circulating hepatitis B viral load. *Gastroenterology.* 2006; 130(3): 678–86.
236 Fattovich G. Natural history and prognosis of hepatitis B. *Seminars in Liver Disease.* 2003; 23(1): 47–58.
237 Yim HJ, Lok AS. Natural history of chronic hepatitis B virus infection: what we knew in 1981 and what we know in 2005. *Hepatology.* 2006; 43(2 suppl 1): S173–81.
238 Information adapted from Pungpapong S, Kim WR, Poterucha JJ. Natural history of hepatitis B virus infection: an update for clinicians. *Mayo Clinic Proceedings.* 2007; 82(8): 967–75.
239 Sarin K, Kumar MJ, Tyagi P. HBV carrier or chronic HBV infection: need for change in terminology. *Journal of Gastroenterology and Hepatology.* 2004; 19: S103–7.
240 Pungpapong S, Kim WR, Poterucha JJ. Natural history of hepatitis B virus infection: an update for clinicians. *Mayo Clinic Proceedings.* 2007; 82(8): 967–75.

241 Ahmed F, Perz JF, Kwong S et al. National trends and disparities in the incidence of hepatocellular carcinoma, 1998–2003. *Preventing Chronic Disease.* 2008; 5(3): A74.

242 Dyer Z, Peltekian K, van Zanten SV. Review article: the changing epidemiology of hepatocellular carcinoma in Canada. *Alimentary Pharmacology and Therapeutics.* 2005; 22(1): 17–22.

243 Souvignet C, Lejeune O, Trepo C. Interferon-based treatment of chronic hepatitis C. *Biochimie.* 2007; 89(6–7): 894–8.

244 Tan J, Lok AS. Update on viral hepatitis: 2006. *Current Opinion in Gastroenterology.* 2007; 23(3): 263–7.

245 Weigand K, Stremmel W, Encke J. Treatment of hepatitis C virus infection. *World Journal of Gastroenterology.* 2007; 13(13): 1897–905.

246 Arbuthnot P, Longshaw V, Naidoo T et al. Opportunities for treating chronic hepatitis B and C virus infection using RNA interference. *Journal of Viral Hepatitis.* 2007; 14(7): 447–59.

247 Szabo E, Paska C, Kaposi Novak P et al. Similarities and differences in hepatitis B and C virus induced hepatocarcinogenesis. *Pathology Oncology Research.* 2004; 10(1): 5–11.

248 Anzola M. Hepatocellular carcinoma: role of hepatitis B and hepatitis C viruses proteins in hepatocarcinogenesis. *Journal of Viral Hepatitis.* 2004; 11(5): 383–93.

249 Lee CM, Hung CH, Lu SN et al. Viral etiology of hepatocellular carcinoma and HCV genotypes in Taiwan. *Intervirology.* 2006; 49(1–2): 76–81.

250 Arbuthnot P, Longshaw V, Naidoo T et al. Opportunities for treating chronic hepatitis B and C virus infection using RNA interference. *Journal of Viral Hepatitis.* 2007; 14(7): 447–59.

251 Trinchet JC, Ganne-Carrie N, Nahon P et al. Hepatocellular carcinoma in patients with hepatitis C virus-related chronic liver disease. *World Journal of Gastroenterology.* 2007; 13(17): 2455–60.

252 McGlynn KA, London WT. Epidemiology and natural history of hepatocellular carcinoma. *Best Practice and Research Clinical Gastroenterology.* 2005; 19(1): 3–23.

253 Chuang SC, Vecchia CL, Boffetta P. Liver cancer: descriptive epidemiology and risk factors other than HBV and HCV infection. *Cancer Letters.* 2008: Epublished ahead of print.

254 Dragani TA, Zocchetti C. Occupational exposure to vinyl chloride and risk of hepatocellular carcinoma. *Cancer Causes and Control.* 2008; 19(10): 1193–200.

255 Yosry A. Schistosomiasis and neoplasia. *Contributions to Microbiology.* 2006; 13: 81–100.

256 Gomaa AI, Khan SA, Toledano MB et al. Hepatocellular carcinoma: epidemiology, risk factors and pathogenesis. *World Journal of Gastroenterology.* 2008; 14(27): 4300–8.

257 Anwar WA, Khaled HM, Amra HA et al. Changing pattern of hepatocellular carcinoma (HCC) and its risk factors in Egypt: possibilities for prevention. *Mutation Research.* 2008; 659(1–2): 176–84.

258 Strickland GT. Liver disease in Egypt: hepatitis C superseded schistosomiasis as a result of iatrogenic and biological factors. *Hepatology.* 2006; 43(5): 915–22.

259 Anwar WA, Khaled HM, Amra HA et al. Changing pattern of hepatocellular carcinoma (HCC) and its risk factors in Egypt: possibilities for prevention. *Mutation Research.* 2008; 659(1-2): 176-84.

260 Shiha G, Zalata KR. Does schistosomiasis interfere with application of the Knodell score for assessment of chronic hepatitis C? *Medical Science Monitor.* 2002; 8(2): CR72-7.

261 Yu MC, Yuan JM. Environmental factors and risk for hepatocellular carcinoma. *Gastroenterology.* 2004; 127(5 suppl 1): S72-8.

262 McGlynn KA, London WT. Epidemiology and natural history of hepatocellular carcinoma. *Best Practice and Research Clinical Gastroenterology.* 2005; 19(1): 3-23.

263 Raoul JL. Natural history of hepatocellular carcinoma and current treatment options. *Seminars in Nuclear Medicine.* 2008; 38(2): S13-8.

264 Chuang SC, Vecchia CL, Boffetta P. Liver cancer: descriptive epidemiology and risk factors other than HBV and HCV infection. *Cancer Letters.* 2008: Epublished ahead of print.

265 Yuan JM, Govindarajan S, Arakawa K et al. Synergism of alcohol, diabetes, and viral hepatitis on the risk of hepatocellular carcinoma in blacks and whites in the U.S. *Cancer.* 2004; 101(5): 1009-17.

266 Hassan MM, Hwang LY, Hatten CJ et al. Risk factors for hepatocellular carcinoma: synergism of alcohol with viral hepatitis and diabetes mellitus. *Hepatology.* 2002; 36(5): 1206-13.

267 Chung RT, Andersen J, Volberding P et al. Peginterferon Alfa-2a plus ribavirin versus interferon alfa-2a plus ribavirin for chronic hepatitis C in HIV-coinfected persons. *New England Journal of Medicine.* 2004; 351(5): 451-9.

268 Carrat F, Bani-Sadr F, Pol S et al. Pegylated interferon alfa-2b vs standard interferon alfa-2b, plus ribavirin, for chronic hepatitis C in HIV-infected patients: a randomized controlled trial. *Journal of the American Medical Association.* 2004; 292(23): 2839-48.

269 Petrovic LM. HIV/HCV co-infection: histopathologic findings, natural history, fibrosis, and impact of antiretroviral treatment: a review article. *Liver International.* 2007; 27(5): 598-606.

270 Rockstroh JK. Influence of viral hepatitis on HIV infection. *Journal of Hepatology.* 2006; 44(1 suppl): S25-7.

271 Garcia-Samaniego J, Rodriguez M, Berenguer J et al. Hepatocellular carcinoma in HIV-infected patients with chronic hepatitis C. *American Journal of Gastroenterology.* 2001; 96(1): 179-83.

272 Overton ET, Sungkanuparph S, Powderly WG et al. Undetectable plasma HIV RNA load predicts success after hepatitis B vaccination in HIV-infected persons. *Clinical Infectious Diseases.* 2005; 41(7): 1045-8.

273 Cooper CL, Davis HL, Angel JB et al. CPG 7909 adjuvant improves hepatitis B virus vaccine seroprotection in antiretroviral-treated HIV-infected adults. *AIDS.* 2005; 19(14): 1473-9.

274 Teoh NC, Farrell GC. Management of chronic hepatitis C virus infection: a new era of disease control. *Internal Medicine Journal.* 2004; 34(6): 324-37.

275 U.S Preventive Services Task Force. Screening for hepatitis C virus infection in adults: recommendation statement. *Annals of Internal Medicine.* 2004; 140(6): 462-4.

276 Valsamakis A. Molecular testing in the diagnosis and management of chronic hepatitis B. *Clinical Microbiology Reviews.* 2007; 20(3): 426–39.

277 Adler M, Goubau P, Leroux-Roels G et al. Practical use of hepatitis C and B molecular tools: Belgian guidelines. *Acta Gastro-enterologica Belgica.* 2005; 68(3): 308–13.

278 Zoulim F. New nucleic acid diagnostic tests in viral hepatitis. *Seminars in Liver Disease.* 2006; 26(4): 309–17.

279 Chevaliez S, Pawlotsky JM. Hepatitis C virus: virology, diagnosis and management of antiviral therapy. *World Journal of Gastroenterology.* 2007; 13(17): 2461–6.

280 Jerome KR, Gretch DR. Laboratory approaches to the diagnosis of hepatitis C virus infection. Minerva *Gastroenterologica e Dietologica.* 2004; 50(1): 9–20.

281 Fischler B. Hepatitis C virus infection. *Seminars in Fetal and Neonatal Medicine.* 2007; 12(3): 168–73.

282 Lisker-Melman M, Sayuk GS. Defining optimal therapeutic outcomes in chronic hepatitis. *Archives of Medical Research.* 2007; 38(6): 652–60.

283 Herrine SK. Approach to the patient with chronic hepatitis C virus infection. *Annals of Internal Medicine.* 2002; 136(10): 747–57.

284 Podzorski RP. Molecular testing in the diagnosis and management of hepatitis C virus infection. *Archives of Pathology and Laboratory Medicine.* 2002; 126(3): 285–90.

285 Pungpapong S, Kim WR, Poterucha JJ. Natural history of hepatitis B virus infection: an update for clinicians. *Mayo Clinic Proceedings.* 2007; 82(8): 967–75.

286 Monto A, Wright TL. The epidemiology and prevention of hepatocellular carcinoma. *Seminars in Oncology.* 2001; 28(5): 441–9.

287 Sherman M. Department of Medicine, University of Toronto. Personal communication (January, 2008).

288 Moriwaki H. Prevention of liver cancer: basic and clinical aspects. *Experimental & Molecular Medicine.* 2002; 34(5): 319–25.

289 Mast EE, Alter MJ, Margolis HS. Strategies to prevent and control hepatitis B and C virus infections: a global perspective. *Vaccine.* 1999; 17(13–14): 1730–3.

290 Law MG, Batey RG. Injecting drug use in Australia: needle/syringe programs prove their worth, but hepatitis C still on the increase. *Medical Journal of Australia.* 2003; 178(5): 197–8.

291 Hope VD, Judd A, Hickman M et al. Prevalence of hepatitis C among injection drug users in England and Wales: is harm reduction working? *American Journal of Public Health.* 2001; 91(1): 38–42.

292 Judd A, Hickman M, Jones S et al. Incidence of hepatitis C virus and HIV among new injecting drug users in London: prospective cohort study. *British Medical Journal.* 2005; 330(7481): 24–5.

293 Birkhead GS, Klein SJ, Candelas AR et al. Integrating multiple programme and policy approaches to hepatitis C prevention and care for injection drug users: a comprehensive approach. *International Journal on Drug Policy.* 2007; 18(5): 417–25.

294 Fry DE. Occupational risks of blood exposure in the operating room. *American Surgeon.* 2007; 73(7): 637–46.

295 Note that the idea of post-exposure does not mean that the intervention is necessarily initiated after exposure. Clearly, prophylactic vaccination happens beforehand, and even some co-factor strategies (e.g., smoking cessation) may happen before any exposure to a virus. However, the point is that these types of prevention only become relevant once exposure has occurred.

296 Banatvala JE, Van Damme P. Hepatitis B vaccine -- do we need boosters? *Journal of Viral Hepatitis.* 2003; 10(1): 1–6.

297 Van Damme P, Van Herck K. A review of the long-term protection after hepatitis A and B vaccination. *Travel Medicine and Infectious Disease.* 2007; 5(2): 79–84.

298 Sjogren MH. Prevention of hepatitis B in nonresponders to initial hepatitis B virus vaccination. *American Journal of Medicine.* 2005; 118(suppl 10A): 34S–9S.

299 *Health Authority Redesign Accomplishments. A Four Year Picture.* 2005. BC Ministry of Health. Available at https://www.healthservices.gov.bc.ca/socsec/pdf/phsa_redesign.pdf. Accessed September 2007.

300 Centers for Disease Control and Prevention. Global progress toward universal childhood hepatitis B vaccination, 2003. *Morbidity and Mortality Weekly Report.* 2003; 52(36): 868–70.

301 Chien YC, Jan CF, Kuo HS et al. Nationwide hepatitis B vaccination program in Taiwan: effectiveness in the 20 years after it was launched. *Epidemiologic Reviews.* 2006; 28: 126–35.

302 Chang MH. Impact of hepatitis B vaccination on hepatitis B disease and nucleic acid testing in high-prevalence populations. *Journal of Clinical Virology.* 2006; 36(suppl 1): S45–50.

303 Peny JM, Gleizes O, Covilard JP. Financial requirements of immunisation programmes in developing countries: a 2004–2014 perspective. *Vaccine.* 2005; 23(37): 4610–8.

304 Shepard CW, Simard EP, Finelli L et al. Hepatitis B virus infection: epidemiology and vaccination. *Epidemiologic Reviews.* 2006; 28: 112–25.

305 World Health Organization. *WHO vaccine-preventable diseases: monitoring system.* 2007. Available at http://whqlibdoc.who.int/hq/2007/WHO_IVB_2007_eng.pdf. Accessed April 2007.

306 Jacobson VJ, Szilagyi P. Patient reminder and recall systems to improve immunization rates. *Cochrane Database of Systematic Reviews.* 2005.

307 Gaudino JA, deHart MP, Cheadle A et al. Childhood immunization registries: gaps between knowledge and action among family practice physicians and pediatricians in Washington state, 1998. *Archives of Pediatrics and Adolescent Medicine.* 2002; 156(10): 978–85.

308 LeBaron CW, Starnes DM, Rask KJ. The impact of reminder-recall interventions on low vaccination coverage in an inner-city population. *Archives of Pediatrics and Adolescent Medicine.* 2004; 158(3): 255–61.

309 Shefer A, Santoli J, Wortley P et al. Status of quality improvement activities to improve immunization practices and delivery: findings from the immunization quality improvement symposium, October 2003. *Journal of Public Health Management and Practice.* 2006; 12(1): 77–89.

310 Minkovitz CS, Belote AD, Higman SM et al. Effectiveness of a practice-based intervention to increase vaccination rates and reduce missed opportunities. *Archives of Pediatrics and Adolescent Medicine.* 2001; 155(3): 382–6.

311 Gyorkos TW, Tannenbaum TN, Abrahamowicz M et al. Evaluation of the effectiveness of immunization delivery methods. *Canadian Journal of Public Health*. 1994; 85(suppl 1): S14–30.
312 World Health Organization. Hepatitis B vaccines. *Weekly Epidemiological Record*. 2004; 79(28): 255–63.
313 Francois G, Hallauer J, Van Damme P. Hepatitis B vaccination: how to reach risk groups. *Vaccine*. 2002; 21(1–2): 1–4.
314 Gjorup IE, Smith E, Borgwardt L et al. Twenty-year survey of the epidemiology of hepatitis B in Denmark: effect of immigration. *Scandanavian Journal of Infectious Diseases*. 2003; 35(4): 260–4.
315 Zuckerman J, van Hattum J, Cafferkey M et al. Should hepatitis B vaccination be introduced into childhood immunisation programmes in northern Europe? *Lancet Infectious Diseases*. 2007; 7(6): 410–9.
316 Minuk GY, Uhanova J. Viral hepatitis in the Canadian Inuit and First Nations populations. *Canadian Journal of Gastroenterology*. 2003; 17(12): 707–12.
317 World Health Organization. Hepatitis B vaccines. *Weekly Epidemiological Record*. 2004; 79(28): 255–63.
318 Schwarz KB, Balistreri W. Viral hepatitis. *Journal of Pediatric Gastroenterology and Nutrition*. 2002; 35(suppl 1): S29–32.
319 Jonas MM. Treatment of chronic hepatitis B in children. *Journal of Pediatric Gastroenterology and Nutrition*. 2006; 43(suppl 1): S56–60.
320 Kerkar N. Hepatitis B in children: complexities in management. *Pediatric Transplantation*. 2005; 9(5): 685–91.
321 Forns X, Payette PJ, Ma X et al. Vaccination of chimpanzees with plasmid DNA encoding the hepatitis C virus (HCV) envelope E2 protein modified the infection after challenge with homologous monoclonal HCV. *Hepatology*. 2000; 32(3): 618–25.
322 Slowik MK, Jhaveri R. Hepatitis B and C viruses in infants and young children. *Seminars in Pediatric Infectious Diseases*. 2005; 16(4): 296–305.
323 Schwarz KB, Balistreri W. Viral hepatitis. *Journal of Pediatric Gastroenterology and Nutrition*. 2002; 35(suppl 1): S29–32.
324 See recommendation webpage at www.ahrq.gov/clinic/3rduspstf/hepbscr/hepbrs.pdf. Accessed November 2007.
325 U.S. Preventive Services Task Force. Screening for hepatitis C virus infection in adults: recommendation statement. *Annals of Internal Medicine*. 2004; 140(6): 462–4.
326 Herrine SK. Approach to the patient with chronic hepatitis C virus infection. *Annals of Internal Medicine*. 2002; 136(10): 747–57.
327 See recommendation webpage at www.ahrq.gov/clinic/3rduspstf/hepbscr/hepbrs.pdf. Accessed November 2007.
328 Shepard CW, Simard EP, Finelli L et al. Hepatitis B virus infection: epidemiology and vaccination. *Epidemiologic Reviews*. 2006; 28: 112–25.
329 Hoffmann CJ, Thio CL. Clinical implications of HIV and hepatitis B co-infection in Asia and Africa. *Lancet Infectious Diseases*. 2007; 7(6): 402–9.
330 Chang MH. Hepatitis B virus infection. *Seminars in Fetal and Neonatal Medicine*. 2007; 12(3): 160–7.
331 See the webpage summary at www.bchealthguide.org/healthfiles/hfile25b.stm. Accessed November 2007.

332 See the drug label webpage at www.talecris-pi.info/inserts/hyperhepb.pdf. Accessed November 2007.
333 Zuckerman JN. Protective efficacy, immunotherapeutic potential, and safety of hepatitis B vaccines. *Journal of Medical Virology.* 2006; 78(2): 169–77.
334 Zuckerman JN. Review: hepatitis B immune globulin for prevention of hepatitis B infection. *Journal of Medical Virology.* 2007; 79(7): 919–21.
335 Pungpapong S, Kim WR, Poterucha JJ. Natural history of hepatitis B virus infection: an update for clinicians. *Mayo Clinic Proceedings.* 2007; 82(8): 967–75.
336 Caruntu FA, Benea L. Acute hepatitis C virus infection: diagnosis, pathogenesis, treatment. *Journal of Gastrointestinal and Liver Diseases.* 2006; 15(3): 249–56.
337 Isaguliants MG, Ozeretskovskaya NN. Host background factors contributing to hepatitis C virus clearance. *Current Pharmaceutical Biotechnology.* 2003; 4(3): 185–93.
338 See the webpage at www.liverfoundation.org/about/advocacy/hcvscreening. Accessed November 2007.
339 Hill L, Henry B, Schweikert S. Screening for chronic hepatitis C: American College of Preventive Medicine practice policy statement. *American Journal of Preventive Medicine.* 2005; 28(3): 327–30.
340 Adapted from the 1998 U.S. prevention recommendations available at www.cdc.gov/mmwr/preview/ mmwrhtml/00055154.htm. Accessed November 2007.
341 Franceschi S, Montella M, Polesel J et al. Hepatitis viruses, alcohol, and tobacco in the etiology of hepatocellular carcinoma in Italy. *Cancer Epidemiology, Biomarkers and Prevention.* 2006; 15(4): 683–9.
342 Chen CC, Yang SY, Liu CJ et al. Association of cytokine and DNA repair gene polymorphisms with hepatitis B-related hepatocellular carcinoma. *International Journal of Epidemiology.* 2005; 34(6): 1310–8.
343 Donato F, Gelatti U, Limina RM et al. Southern Europe as an example of interaction between various environmental factors: a systematic review of the epidemiologic evidence. *Oncogene.* 2006; 25(27): 3756–70.
344 Seitz HK, Stickel F. Risk factors and mechanisms of hepatocarcinogenesis with special emphasis on alcohol and oxidative stress. *Biological Chemistry.* 2006; 387(4): 349–60.
345 Wang LY, You SL, Lu SN et al. Risk of hepatocellular carcinoma and habits of alcohol drinking, betel quid chewing and cigarette smoking: a cohort of 2416 HBsAg-seropositive and 9421 HBsAg-seronegative male residents in Taiwan. *Cancer Causes and Control.* 2003; 14(3): 241–50.
346 Lisker-Melman M, Sayuk GS. Defining optimal therapeutic outcomes in chronic hepatitis. *Archives of Medical Research.* 2007; 38(6): 652–60.
347 Souvignet C, Lejeune O, Trepo C. Interferon-based treatment of chronic hepatitis C. *Biochimie.* 2007; 89(6–7): 894–8.
348 Keeffe EB, Dieterich DT, Han SH et al. A treatment algorithm for the management of chronic hepatitis B virus infection in the United States: 2008 update. *Clinical Gastroenterology and Hepatology.* 2008; 6(12): 1315–41.
349 Lisker-Melman M, Sayuk GS. Defining optimal therapeutic outcomes in chronic hepatitis. *Archives of Medical Research.* 2007; 38(6): 652–60.
350 Papatheodoridis GV, Manolakopoulos S, Archimandritis AJ. Current treatment indications and strategies in chronic hepatitis B virus infection. *World Journal of Gastroenterology.* 2008; 14(45): 6902–10.

351 Delaney WEt, Borroto-Esoda K. Therapy of chronic hepatitis B: trends and developments. *Current Opinion in Pharmacology.* 2008; 8(5): 532–40.
352 Maylin S, Martinot-Peignoux M, Ripault MP et al. Sustained virological response is associated with clearance of hepatitis C virus RNA and a decrease in hepatitis C virus antibody. *Liver International.* 2009; 29(4): 511–7.
353 Maylin S, Martinot-Peignoux M, Moucari R et al. Eradication of hepatitis C virus in patients successfully treated for chronic hepatitis C. *Gastroenterology.* 2008; 135(3): 821–9.
354 Pegylation is the process of attaching polyethylene glycol to interferon, improving efficacy and achieving a more feasible dosing regimen by allowing a reduced frequency of administration.
355 Weigand K, Stremmel W, Encke J. Treatment of hepatitis C virus infection. *World Journal of Gastroenterology.* 2007; 13(13): 1897–905.
356 Feld JJ, Hoofnagle JH. Mechanism of action of interferon and ribavirin in treatment of hepatitis C. *Nature.* 2005; 436(7053): 967–72.
357 Deutsch M, Hadziyannis SJ. Old and emerging therapies in chronic hepatitis C: an update. *Journal of Viral Hepatitis.* 2008; 15(1): 2–11.
358 Souvignet C, Lejeune O, Trepo C. Interferon-based treatment of chronic hepatitis C. *Biochimie.* 2007; 89(6–7): 894–8.
359 Arbuthnot P, Longshaw V, Naidoo T et al. Opportunities for treating chronic hepatitis B and C virus infection using RNA interference. *Journal of Viral Hepatitis.* 2007; 14(7): 447–59.
360 Fischler B. Hepatitis C virus infection. *Seminars in Fetal and Neonatal Medicine.* 2007; 12(3): 168–73.
361 Pawlotsky JM, Chevaliez S, McHutchison JG. The hepatitis C virus life cycle as a target for new antiviral therapies. *Gastroenterology.* 2007; 132: 1979–98.
362 Rodis J. Chronic hepatitis C virus infection: a review for pharmacists. *Journal of the American Pharmaceutical Association.* 2007; 47(4): 508–20.
363 Fischler B. Hepatitis C virus infection. *Seminars in Fetal and Neonatal Medicine.* 2007; 12(3): 168–73.
364 Bacon BR, McHutchison JG. Into the light: strategies for battling hepatitis C. *American Journal of Managed Care.* 2007; 13(suppl 12): S319–26.
365 Okanoue T, Minami M, Makiyama A et al. Natural course of asymptomatic hepatitis C virus-infected patients and hepatocellular carcinoma after interferon therapy. *Clinical Gastroenterology and Hepatology.* 2005; 3(10 suppl 2): S89–91.
366 Yu ML, Huang CF, Dai CY et al. Long-term effects of interferon-based therapy for chronic hepatitis C. *Oncology.* 2007; 72(suppl 1): 16–23.
367 Hirakawa M, Ikeda K, Arase Y et al. Hepatocarcinogenesis following HCV RNA eradication by interferon in chronic hepatitis patients. *Internal Medicine.* 2008; 47(19): 1637–43.
368 Tanaka A, Uegaki S, Kurihara H et al. Hepatic steatosis as a possible risk factor for the development of hepatocellular carcinoma after eradication of hepatitis C virus with antiviral therapy in patients with chronic hepatitis C. *World Journal of Gastroenterology.* 2007; 13(39): 5180–7.
369 Hofmann WP, Soriano V, Zeuzem S. Antiviral combination therapy for treatment of chronic hepatitis B, hepatitis C, and human immunodeficiency virus infection. *Handbook for Experimental Pharmacology.* 2009; 189: 321–46.

370 Zeuzem S, Nelson DR, Marcellin P. Dynamic evolution of therapy for chronic hepatitis C: how will novel agents be incorporated into the standard of care? *Antiviral Therapy.* 2008; 13(6): 747–60.
371 Hoofnagle JH, Doo E, Liang TJ et al. Management of hepatitis B: summary of a clinical research workshop. *Hepatology.* 2007; 45(4): 1056–75.
372 Lok AS. Navigating the maze of hepatitis B treatments. *Gastroenterology.* 2007; 132(4): 1586–94.
373 Tan J, Lok AS. Update on viral hepatitis: 2006. *Current Opinion in Gastroenterology.* 2007; 23(3): 263–7.
374 Chang MH. Hepatitis B virus infection. *Seminars in Fetal and Neonatal Medicine.* 2007; 12(3): 160–7.
375 Ghany M, Liang TJ. Drug targets and molecular mechanisms of drug resistance in chronic hepatitis B. *Gastroenterology.* 2007; 132(4): 1574–85.
376 Lok AS. Navigating the maze of hepatitis B treatments. *Gastroenterology.* 2007; 132(4): 1586–94.
377 Schwarz KB. Pediatric issues in new therapies for hepatitis B and C. *Current Gastroenterology Reports.* 2003; 5(3): 233–9.
378 Jonas MM, Mizerski J, Badia IB et al. Clinical trial of lamivudine in children with chronic hepatitis B. *New England Journal of Medicine.* 2002; 346(22): 1706–13.
379 Slowik MK, Jhaveri R. Hepatitis B and C viruses in infants and young children. *Seminars in Pediatric Infectious Diseases.* 2005; 16(4): 296–305.
380 Jonas MM. Treatment of chronic hepatitis B in children. *Journal of Pediatric Gastroenterology and Nutrition.* 2006; 43(suppl 1): S56–60.
381 Hsu HY, Tsai HY, Wu TC et al. Interferon-alpha treatment in children and young adults with chronic hepatitis B: a long-term follow-up study in Taiwan. *Liver International.* 2008; (Apr 5):
382 Emerick K. Treatment of hepatitis C in children. *Pediatric Infectious Disease Journal.* 2004; 23(3): 257–8.
383 Schwarz KB. Pediatric issues in new therapies for hepatitis B and C. *Current Gastroenterology Reports.* 2003; 5(3): 233–9.
384 Schwarz KB, Balistreri W. Viral hepatitis. *Journal of Pediatric Gastroenterology and Nutrition.* 2002; 35(suppl 1): S29–32.
385 Emerick K. Treatment of hepatitis C in children. *Pediatric Infectious Disease Journal.* 2004; 23(3): 257–8.
386 Sherman M, Shafran S, Burak K et al. Management of chronic hepatitis C: consensus guidelines. *Canadian Journal of Gastroenterology.* 2007; 21(suppl C): 25C–34C.
387 Ramos-Casals M, Jara LJ, Medina F et al. Systemic autoimmune diseases co-existing with chronic hepatitis C virus infection (the HISPAMEC Registry): patterns of clinical and immunological expression in 180 cases. *Journal of Internal Medicine.* 2005; 257(6): 549–57.
388 Zoulim F, Chevallier M, Maynard M et al. Clinical consequences of hepatitis C virus infection. *Reviews in Medical Virology.* 2003; 13(1): 57–68.
389 Ramos-Casals M, Garcia-Carrasco M, Brito Zeron MP et al. Viral etiopathogenesis of Sjogren's syndrome: role of the hepatitis C virus. *Autoimmunity Reviews.* 2002; 1(4): 238–43.

390 Zignego AL, Giannini C, Monti M et al. Hepatitis C virus lymphotropism: lessons from a decade of studies. *Digestive and Liver Disease.* 2007; 39(suppl 1): S38–45.
391 Pal S, Sullivan DG, Kim S et al. Productive replication of hepatitis C virus in perihepatic lymph nodes in vivo: implications of HCV lymphotropism. *Gastroenterology.* 2006; 130(4): 1107–16.
392 Sherman M, Shafran S, Burak K et al. Management of chronic hepatitis B: consensus guidelines. *Canadian Journal of Gastroenterology.* 2007; 21(suppl C): 5C–24C.
393 Kottilil S, Jackson JO, Polis MA. Hepatitis B & hepatitis C in HIV-infection. *Indian Journal of Medical Research.* 2005; 121(4): 424–50.

9

HELICOBACTER PYLORI

Gastric carcinogenesis is a complex, multistep and multifactorial event in which the role of *Helicobacter pylori* infection has been established by numerous epidemiological investigations.[1]

INTRODUCTION

Helicobacter pylori bacterium represents one of the most common organisms existing in humans, colonizing the stomachs of over half of the people in the world.[2,3] The gastritis that occurs in infected individuals is mostly asymptomatic. About 20% of those infected will eventually experience a clinical outcome, including peptic ulcers or a type of gastric cancer, specifically adenocarcinoma or mucosa-associated lymphoid tissue (MALT) lymphoma.[4-7] An estimated 1–3% of people infected with *H. pylori* develop adenocarcinoma, compared to less than 0.1% for MALT lymphoma.[8,9] The role of *H. pylori* in extragastric disease, including some other cancers, is also being investigated. Benign conditions of interest include hepatobiliary, cardiovascular, hematologic, and urologic disorders.[10-14] However, gastric cancer continues to dominate the research agenda with respect to *H. pylori*.

Despite a global decline in gastric cancer incidence rates, particularly in developed countries, this malignancy remains the fourth most common cancer worldwide, and the second leading cause of cancer-related mortality, with over 400,000 deaths each year.[15-17] Regions with high gastric cancer incidence include Eastern Asia, Eastern Europe, and South America.[18,19]

Even though there was a formal confirmation of carcinogenicity in 1994 by the WHO's International Agency for Research on Cancer (IARC),[20] the public health perspective on *H. pylori* has been marked by ambivalence.[21] This is because *H. pylori* colonization of the stomach is sometimes classified not as a disease per se but rather a phenomenon akin to the routine presence of α-hemolytic streptococci in the upper respiratory tract and of certain *Escherichia coli* strains in the colon.[22] All multicellular organisms are colonized with other organisms, where there is benefit to both invader and host (i.e., mutualistic colonization) or at least the host is unaffected (i.e., colonization that is commensal). The difference between colonization and infection can be circumstantial; thus even a (mostly) nonpathogenic invader can produce significant disease under certain conditions. Unless otherwise specified, moving from colonization to true infection with *H. pylori* (i.e., being *H. pylori*-positive) is equivalent to having a certain concentration of antibody in the blood and/or signs of active disease (as indicated through enzyme assays or histologic examination).

H. pylori may qualify for the classification of "partially mutualistic" when present in human hosts. The caution concerning universal, population-wide eradication stems in part from the evidence that the presence of *H. pylori* may in fact reduce the risk of certain benign conditions, such as gastroesophageal reflux disease (GERD), and perhaps even exert a protective effect against adenocarcinoma in the esophagus and the adjacent region of the stomach (the so-called gastric cardia).[23-25] For this reason, eradication of the bacterium has typically been restricted to those with symptomatic disease; in other words, while therapeutic eradication has been pursued, universal eradication has not.

Given the high cost of detection and eradication of *H. pylori* colonization, and the fact that countries such as the United States and Canada already enjoy low and declining incidence of gastric cancer, the need for prevention efforts targeting cancer per se remains uncertain. For example, the timing of interventions is controversial. Thus, though standard antibiotic treatment is in fact efficacious in eliminating infection, it is generally agreed that such therapy may be too late after the patient reaches a certain stage of premalignant disease.[26] As already suggested, prophylactic approaches have been even more controversial. Even if population-wide measures can be defended, researchers are still investigating whether or not they would reduce the risk of gastric cancer development.[27-29] Despite the misgivings, the emergence of antibiotic-resistant strains of *H. pylori* and the high rate of infection recurrence have intensified the drive to develop a prophylactic vaccine.[30–32] The proponents of more aggressive public health responses to *H. pylori* (including attempts to universally eradicate it from humans through prophylactic vaccination) point out that the "dire consequences" of eliminating the bacterium from the human biological system have been exaggerated.[33]

Having introduced some of the key themes and issues related to *H. pylori* and cancer, more detailed information about the bacterium itself will now be provided, followed by the subtopics previously laid out in this book, namely, evidence of associated cancers, disease mechanism and process (including cofactors), transmission and occurrence of the agent, detection methods, and prevention approaches.

THE BACTERIUM

H. pylori is a spiral-shaped and flagellated Gram-negative bacterium that colonizes the gastric mucosa of humans.[34,35] It was first isolated in 1982. Traces of *H. pylori* found in mummified human remains, however, suggest that the bacterium has existed as an infectious agent for at least 3,000 years, and other evidence indicates the possibility of an even earlier origin.[36–39]

Samples of *H. pylori* harvested from the stomachs of different individuals are highly polymorphic; strain variation also has been observed within a single host.[40] Analysis has suggested that there is a functional core of 1,100–1,300 genes common to all *H. pylori* strains. These genes govern metabolism, transcription, and biosynthesis of amino acids, as well as other cellular processes that are essential to the maintenance and expansion of the bacterial colony.[41] Several hundred other genes are potentially variable from strain to strain; among other functions, these genes code for cell-surface proteins that in turn may account for a particular strain's adaptation to a genetically diverse host.[42]

H. pylori bacteria may have the capacity to lose and possibly acquire exogenous DNA. Research has indicated that this phenomenon is consistent with "a model of continuous microevolution within its cognate host."[43] However, recent studies have called into question the extent to which genetic exchange occurs and influences transmission and host adaptation.[44,45]

It seems evident that only certain strains of *H. pylori* are pathogenic.[46–48] Furthermore, identified pathogenic types have also been variably associated with disease outcomes.[49] It has been difficult to tie specific virulence factors[50] to disease manifestations; in fact, strains containing the same factors have been identified in both symptomatic and asymptomatic persons.[51] At least one fundamental distinction, however, is well supported by research. It seems that *H. pylori* may be divided into two subgroups based on cytotoxin-associated gene A (*CagA*), specifically whether it is expressed (type 1) or not (type 2).[52] The *CagA* gene has been identified as a marker of virulence[53]; it is associated with a so-called "genomic island" in the DNA of *H. pylori* that is responsible for injecting the CagA protein into gastric epithelial cells, with a subsequent impact on cellular mechanisms.[54,55] Other pathogenicity islands in the *H. pylori* genome are also being intensively studied. Variations in *H. pylori* strains based on the role of CagA (and other virulence factors) have been posited as a possible explanation of geographic differences in gastric cancer incidence.[56]

Moving beyond the strain and pathogenicity variations of *H. pylori* itself, it is important to note that different Helicobacter species (e.g., *H. bilis*, *H. heilmannii*) have been implicated in both animal and human diseases.[57] The first case report of *H. heilmannii* associated with gastric adenocarcinoma was published in 2008.[58]

Given the important public health implications of *H. pylori* and its demonstrated involvement in stomach diseases, the bacterium's two discoverers, B Marshall and R Warren, were recognized with the Nobel Prize in 2005.[59] Although many research questions about *H. pylori* remain unanswered, a review by Clyne and colleagues in 2007 revealed that over 20,000 academic reports related to this bacterium have already been published.[60] Indeed, it is one of only a few infectious agents with its own dedicated journal, launched over a decade ago.[61]

EVIDENCE OF ASSOCIATED CANCERS

While other bacteria may play a role in carcinogenesis at different body sites, *H. pylori* is certainly the most studied bacterial cause of malignancy.[62] According to IARC, infection with *H. pylori* causes a substantial proportion of gastric cancers.[63-65] Compared to the uninfected population, the risk of developing gastric cancer in infected individuals appears to be two to six times higher.[66-68] This association will be further explored, followed by a brief overview of other potential cancer connections that have been investigated.

As noted earlier, when gastric cancer occurs, it usually appears in the form of adenocarcinoma.[69] The other main malignancy linked to *H. pylori*, MALT lymphoma, is a form of non-Hodgkin's lymphoma that usually affects the gastrointestinal (GI) tract, though it can also occur in other organs. With the link to MALT lymphoma confirmed,

H. pylori joins the list of infectious agents implicated in cancers of the lymphatic system.[70] Hepatitis B and C are also members of this list, an inventory that will be expanded in chapters to follow. It should be noted that, since MALT lymphoma is relatively rare, any discussion of gastric cancer in the remainder of this chapter will generally be in reference to adenocarcinoma.

A Necessary Cause of Gastric Cancer?

The task of determining the level of risk attribution of *H. pylori* is complicated by the fact that loss of infection occurs in some cases of gastric cancer, which may result in a decline in serum antibodies for the bacterium; the resulting negative seroprevalence test is equivalent to a missed disease association.[71-73] Of course, positive seroprevalence is also ambiguous in association studies, as the presence of antibodies is not proof of current infection.[74] Despite these methodological challenges, good evidence has been developed suggesting that *H. pylori* infection is a very important, though not sufficient, cause of gastric cancer.[75-77] However, even being confirmed as a necessary causal factor would be a dramatic result in oncology, catapulting the association into the same rare category as human papillomavirus (HPV) and cervical cancer. This consideration leads naturally to the following questions: What is the strength of disease association? And is "necessary" a legitimate qualifier of the causal role of *H. pylori*?

Indirect evidence for an etiologic link between *H. pylori* and gastric cancer has been observed in developed countries, where a decrease in *H. pylori* infection rates has matched a substantial decline in gastric cancer incidence in recent decades.[78] Communities with very low gastric cancer incidence have been marked by an *H. pylori* infection rate as low as 2%.[79,80]

Direct evidence has also been compelling. A study based on subjects drawn from 17 developed countries (United States, Japan, and 11 European states) was published just prior to the IARC classification of *H. pylori* as a carcinogen. It revealed that infected subjects had a sixfold higher risk of developing gastric cancer compared to those who were uninfected.[81] By comparison, a large Japanese study in 2006 pegged the infection-related relative risk of gastric cancer between 5 and 10 (depending on assumptions about what could be construed as *H. pylori* positivity).[82] The strongest corroborating evidence, based on a 2001 study in Japan, showed that gastric cancer occurred only in infected patients, that is, those with a specified level of antibodies for the bacterium or signs of gastric disease indicated by histologic examination or a rapid urease test (see the section "Bacterial Detection Methods").[83] The results of this study suggest that *H. pylori* infection is a necessary cause of cancer in the majority of gastric subsites.

Site-Specific Impacts

But how does one reconcile the idea of infection as a necessary cause with the proportion of gastric cancer usually attributed to the bacterium, namely, 60–70%?[84,85] One would instead expect a figure approaching 100%. The explanation might be found in the complexities of stomach anatomy, and especially the distinction between cardia and noncardia regions of the stomach. The cardia is the small zone of the stomach near the esophageal junction; noncardia refers to the rest of the stomach. A 2001 analysis of 12 case-control studies again found a sixfold increase of gastric cancer in *H. pylori*-positive individuals, but only for persistent infection in the *noncardia* region.[86]

The complexities of diagnosis and localizing the site of cancer development has sometimes created subsite misclassification within studies.[87,88] Despite the obstacles, researchers have been able to propose that cancer of the gastric cardia has two main origins, one involving *H. pylori* infection (and thus with an etiology similar to distal or noncardia gastric cancer) and one related to gastric reflux disease (and thus aligned with distal esophageal adenocarcinoma).[89,90] This dual etiology accounts for bacteria-related gastric cancer being less than 100% of total cases, and also helps to explain why it is possible to have an increase in adenocarcinoma of the gastric cardia even though gastric cancer has generally been declining in developed countries.[91,92]

The anatomic distinctions may drive a potentially important etiologic pattern with respect to gastric cancer. While *H. pylori* appears to be strongly associated with noncardia gastric cancer (i.e., with adenocarcinoma across the majority of the stomach mucosa), the link with cancer in the cardia zone is weaker, and perhaps null. One study group even noted a *protective* effect in developed, western countries as opposed to those in Asia.[93,94] Whatever other factors may be in play, there is evidence that cancers of the cardia should be distinguished from distal regions of the stomach in terms of their genetic pathway and, furthermore, it appears that the cardia-localized tumors are more aggressive.[95] The proposal that *H. pylori* infection can be protective against such tumors is controversial.[96]

Restricting the focus to noncardia or distal gastric cancer indicates that the association with *H. pylori* could be very strong indeed. In fact, a 2004 German study suggested that *H. pylori* infection may be "close to" being a necessary condition for the development of noncardia gastric cancer. Applying strict exclusion criteria to their cases, the research team reported a relative risk of noncardia gastric cancer of 18.3 for any *H. pylori* infection, and 28.4 for CagA-positive bacteria.[97]

However, a recent study based in multiple European settings suggested a relative risk for noncardia cancer of 6.5 (95% CI 3.3–12.6) in individuals with CagA seropositivity.[98] This figure is closer to the result of earlier meta-analyses. The discrepancy with the German study may be explained by the fact mentioned at the beginning of this section, namely, that *H. pylori* density drops when gastric mucosa is affected by metaplasia or neoplasia. One implication of this phenomenon is the possibility that "the magnitude of the noncardia association may be underestimated."[99] Evidence of this complexity was offered in a 2004 Japanese study that tracked the cancer risk level attached to a progression of disease, from *H. pylori* infection with no chronic atrophic gastritis (AG) through to substantial and persistent AG expression and extensive metaplasia but no longer any direct sign of *H. pylori* infection.[100]

The data in Table 9.1 show that it is possible for gastric cancer to develop as a sequela to AG that itself is known to be caused by *H. pylori* but where bacterial infection per se is no longer detectable by serologic means. While this study offers one compelling explanation for ongoing confusion about the relative risks of gastric cancer caused by infection, the fact that recent evaluations of *H. pylori* involvement in carcinogenesis vary widely (from "very substantial" to "still under investigation") confirms that this research area will remain active for some time to come.[101]

Finally, attributable burden must be distinguished from the individual risk of getting cancer when infected. While evidence seems to support the conclusion that a very large percentage of cancer in certain gastric sites can be attributed to *H. pylori* infection, the actual risk of carcinogenesis in a particular case of infection is much more difficult to evaluate. The involvement of endogenous cofactors such as host genetics, as well as environmental cofactors related to tobacco use and diet, certainly contributes great complexity to the discussion.[102-104] The etiologic evidence related to smoking is particularly compelling.[105-108] The topic of cofactors will be further explored in the following section.

Table 9.1. Risk Factors in Progression of Gastric Cancer

Disease Stage	Relative Risk	95% CI
H. pylori + / chronic AG −	7.13	0.95–53.33
H. pylori + / chronic AG +	14.85	1.96–107.7
H. pylori − / severe AG	61.85	5.6–682.64

Source: Ohata et al., *International Journal of Cancer*, 2004.

Investigative Cancer Associations

Interest in a potential role for *H. pylori* in cancers beyond the stomach has recently intensified. As might be expected, the focus has been primarily on the digestive system, including the esophagus and liver, though cancer associations are being evaluated in diverse anatomic areas, including urological and oropharyngeal sites.[109,110]

While not consistent across all studies,[111] recent meta-analyses and new research have confirmed a protective role for *H. pylori* with respect to esophageal adenocarcinoma (but not squamous cell carcinoma).[112-114] Site variation in gastric atrophy mechanisms related to the bacteria has been suggested as part of the explanation for the protective effect.[115,116] According to one 2008 study, the inverse association seems to be weaker in women than men.[117] Overall, however, the manifest decline of *H. pylori* colonization in Western countries may be contributing to the recent increase in esophageal adenocarcinoma.[118]

The question of whether *H. pylori* plays a role in the development of liver cancer (specifically hepatocellular carcinoma, or HCC) remains controversial. The fact that DNA of *H. pylori* and other *Helicobacter* species has been found in the liver tissues of HCC patients is certainly suggestive, as is the ability of experimental infection with *H. hepaticus* to cause chronic hepatitis and liver cancer in mice.[119,120] A 2008 study even showed that *H. pylori* could adhere to and invade hepatocytes in vitro.[121] However, results continue to be conflicting. A recent meta-analysis, though acknowledging the potential for bias, confirmed an association between *H. pylori* infection and the risk of HCC; on the other hand, a 2008 U.S. study could not locate *Helicobacter* DNA in actual liver tumors.[122]

The research related to other parts of the digestive system has been limited. Studies seem to support a role for *Helicobacter* species in the development of biliary tract cancer but not for *H. pylori* in pancreatic carcinogenesis.[123-126] *H. pylori* may be one of a number of microbes involved with colorectal cancer.[127,128] Support for this conclusion was offered through two recent reviews of the literature.[129,130] However, other recent studies have produced contrary results or adopted a more cautious approach on the question of causation.[131-134] Research related to the respiratory system has generated a similar ambiguous pattern. For example, two studies from 2008 on laryngeal cancer risk and *H. pylori* involvement offered opposing conclusions.[135,136]

In sum, no cancer rivals gastric adenocarincoma in terms of evidence for *H. pylori*-associated causation. Mixed results appear to be the norm for studies of malignancies at most other sites.

TRANSMISSION AND OCCURRENCE OF THE BACTERIUM

The fact that H. pylori is a pandemic infection suggests multiple transmission pathways, but little is known for certain about this topic.[137] Uncontroversial concepts include the observation that the natural acquisition of H. pylori occurs mostly in early childhood and, once established, colonization typically persists throughout life unless treated.[138–141] However, no matter what the age of acquisition, the exact mode of transmission of H. pylori has not been clearly defined.[142–144]

The prevailing understanding is that the bacterium is transmitted from person to person, with oral–oral and fecal–oral routes commonly suggested.[145–147] Several recent studies have in fact called into question the fecal–oral route, at least among children, thus distinguishing H. pylori from hepatitis A in terms of the main mode of pediatric transmission.[148–150] A 2009 systematic review of the literature concluded that maternal transmission is the main source for pediatric H. pylori infection in low-prevalence populations.[151]

Oral–anal and oral–vaginal pathways (e.g., through adult sexual contact) have also been posited, but not conclusively demonstrated.[152] If the vagina is ever confirmed as a reservoir of H. pylori, there will be increased interest in the potential for vertical transmission to babies in the birth canal.[153] One 2004 study of stool samples from 3-day-old infants ($n = 50$) found H. pylori DNA in 30% of cases, which points to the potential for a vertical pathway.[154]

Final transmission routes of interest relate to the health care system itself. Iatrogenic spread of H. pylori during endoscopies has been demonstrated.[155] Hospital workers with direct patient contact may also be at increased risk for H. pylori infection, though some recent research has not supported this conclusion.[156,157]

Potential "vehicles" of infection operating on various pathways include saliva, vomit, feces, dental plaque, and contaminated food or water.[158–160] The role of breastfeeding remains controversial.[161] Whatever the specific contribution of breast milk and other sources, a generally increased rate of transmission among family members is well-established.[162–164] Consistent with suspected transmission modes, indirect risk factors for infection include overcrowding, poor sanitation, and inadequate hygiene. A positive association with measures of low socioeconomic status has also been demonstrated.[165–168]

There have been suggestions that the dosage of H. pylori required for primary infection may be difficult to acquire from classic reservoirs in the environment. It is possible, however, that infections acquired through contaminated drinking water or food that are easily fought off by the host may still exert an influence on population prevalence through intraspecies recombination during transient passage of *H. pylori* through the GI tract. Genetic diversity in fact is seen as an influence on the ability of the bacterium to colonize the human body.[169] This may be one explanation for the role of sanitation and other public health controls in slowing the spread of *H. pylori* in industrialized countries.[170]

There are substantial variations in the prevalence of *H. pylori* infection between different geographical regions.[171] Infection rates are relatively high in many developing countries, with prevalence in some jurisdictions approaching 80–90%; this compares with rates of only 20–65% in cohorts over age 30 years in developed countries.[172–174] One oft-cited analysis estimated the average prevalence of *H. pylori* to be 35% in developed countries and 85% in developing countries.[175] The regional differences seem to be established early; children in developing countries can demonstrate an infection prevalence of 70% by age 15, compared to only 5–15% in developed countries.[176,177]

Prevalence tends to increase with age, at the rate of about 1% per year.[178] While some researchers have attempted to draw a connection between this pattern and the natural history features noted earlier (i.e., acquisition starting in childhood and a lack of clearance without therapy), the mechanisms are not immediately clear.[179] Other authorities have simply ascribed the increasing prevalence with age to a birth cohort effect related to diminished acquisition in more recent pediatric populations as socioeconomic conditions have improved over time in some countries.[180]

In contrast to the clear age association, there does not appear to be any significant gender influence on *H. pylori* infection rates.[181,182]

The inverse relationship between socioeconomic status and *H. pylori* prevalence has already been noted. Indeed, the lifetime infection rate in the most affluent countries is dropping toward 10% or even lower.[183] This trend has been particularly noted in the United States, where "markedly improved sanitation in the second half of the 19th century greatly reduced *H. pylori* transmission, initiating a decline in *H. pylori* infection that will ultimately lead to its elimination from the U.S. population."[184]

On the other hand, several population-based studies have confirmed the importance of low socioeconomic conditions in elevated acquisition of *H. pylori* infection.[185] The clearest example of this dynamic in the Canadian context is seen in Aboriginal populations living in situations marked by poverty. For instance, research in one Aboriginal community reported a remarkable 95% rate of *H. pylori* infection among adults.[186] A follow-up study in the same community detected a 16%

H. *pylori* acquisition rate among children in just 1 year.[187] By contrast, a recent study of Canadian children who underwent endoscopic examination showed an average *H. pylori* prevalence of only 5%, despite the fact that the particular cohort was deemed medically at-risk.[188] The latter figure represented a significant decline over the last decade, a trend that apparently has not been matched among some Aboriginal populations. Similarly, research among Alaskan Inuit showed that 72% of individuals had acquired *H. pylori* antibodies by age 24 years.[189] Similar concerns about *H. pylori* prevalence has arisen in northern Aboriginal populations in other countries.[190]

The impact of moving from lower to higher socioeconomic conditions has also been demonstrated among immigrant populations in the United States. One study showed that the prevalence of *H. pylori* in immigrant, first-, and second-generation Hispanics was 31%, 9%, and 3%, respectively.[191] Even more dramatically, prevalence rates among New York City residents born in east Asia have been found to be as high as 70%.[192]

Earlier, a trend of decreasing *H. pylori* infection was described among a specific cohort of Canadian children undergoing a diagnostic examination. In fact, *H. pylori* prevalence in the general population of the United States, Europe, and other developed settings has declined considerably in recent years.[193,194] An example of this trend across one decade of age-stratified data in Japan is offered in Figure 9.1.[195]

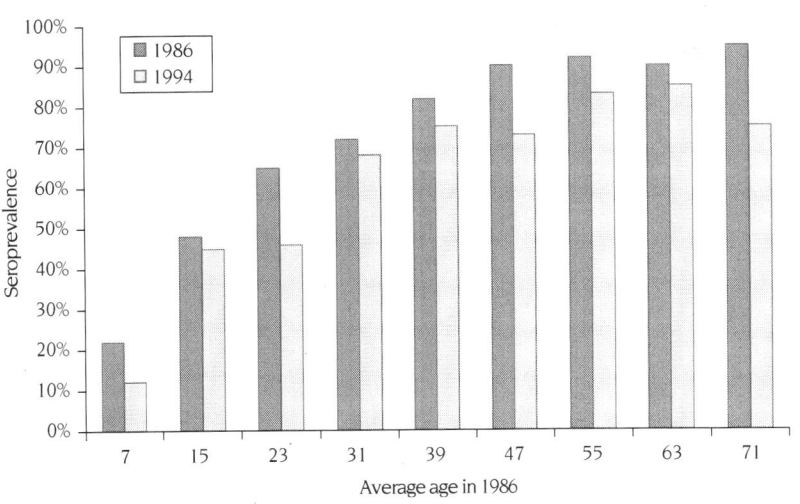

Figure 9.1. Prevalence of *Helicobacter pylori* infection, Japan, 1986–1994. *Source*: Kumagai et al., *Journal of Infectious Diseases*, 1998. Used by permission.

DISEASE MECHANISM AND PROCESSES

The general pattern involved with microbe-related cancer was introduced in the beginning of the book. Infection with *H. pylori* appears to follow distinct pathogenic pathways, resulting in unique disease outcomes in different individuals.[196,197] In this section, the various elements involved with the development of *H. pylori*-related cancer will be elucidated.

First, there is the important requirement of persistent infection, similar to that seen with HPV and cervical cancer.[198,199] The main difference with the bacterium is that it exhibits a much higher degree of persistence. Indeed, *H. pylori* has been recognized as a "paradigm for a bacterium that causes chronic infections."[200] Generally, its mode of action as a pathogen has been characterized by terms such as *slow* or *stealth*. Left untreated, *H. pylori* is able to continuously evade the immune system; in fact, it can persist in the stomach throughout the life of the host.[201-205]

How *H. pylori* is able to survive in the stomach despite the host's immune response is not completely understood.[206,207] It was already noted in the description of the bacterium that genomic diversity may play a role in immune evasion.[208] Another explanation for the lack of bacterial clearance may be the existence of *H. pylori* in the extracellular environment of the gastric mucosa.[209] A recent Japanese study detailed the ability of the bacterium to overcome host self-renewal processes within the gastric epithelium and thus help sustain infection.[210]

A number of other virulence mechanisms have been posited to be part of the process of evading host defenses and eventual colonization.[211,212] The factors include the bacterial enzyme urease, which is involved in neutralizing gastric acid; flagella, which provide the motility to approach and invade the gastric mucosa; and bacterial enzymes, which facilitate acquisition of nutritional elements from the host.[213,214]

The fundamental hallmarks of *H. pylori*-related disease are an inflammatory response, increased levels of stomach acid, and damage to surrounding tissues.[215-217] On a microscopic level, an accumulation of immune cells in the gastric mucosa has been detected.[218,219] The intensity of the resulting gastritis varies, but symptoms are typically minimal-to-nonexistent.[220]

An infection causes gastric cancer both through the direct impact of the organism (and its products) on the mucosa and by indirect effects related to alteration of the mucosal environment that is created by *H. pylori*-induced gastritis.[221,222] Thus, the bacterium's CagA protein is known to have a direct oncogenic potential. On the other hand, the severity and site of the body's inflammatory response to *H. pylori* infection are known to affect the risk of carcinogenesis.[223,224] Chronic inflammation can lead to a series of premalignant changes in the stomach lining, which may result in the development of gastric cancer.[225-227]

Disease Risk Factors

In addition to bacterial characteristics, environmental and host genetic factors are also believed to contribute to gastric cancer development.[228-232] Environmental factors that have been associated with disease progression include tobacco use, excessive alcohol use, and high levels of salt intake.[233-237] There is evidence that increased consumption of fruits and vegetables may lower the risk of developing gastric cancer; this has been particularly linked to the impact of dietary vitamin C on reducing the harmful effects of inflammation and the formation of carcinogenic N-nitroso compounds.[238-240]

Only a small minority of patients with premalignant lesions ultimately develop a full malignancy, again suggesting the importance of risk factors beyond *H. pylori* infection.[241] There is typically a long latency period between acquisition of infection and any cancer progression.[242] For example, peptic ulcers tend to appear in patients in their 20s and 30s, whereas less than 10% of gastric cancers appear before age 45.[243] Because gastric cancer is usually not diagnosed until it reaches an advanced stage, patients generally have a poor prognosis—the 5-year survival rate of less than 20%.[244,245] In cases where early diagnosis is achieved, a 5-year survival rate of over 90% has been reported.[246]

BACTERIAL DETECTION METHODS

There is ongoing concern about the warrant for a systematic, universal eradication program (see the following discussion, and also the section "Prevention Approaches"). This has sharpened the focus on prevention in groups at higher risk for gastric cancer. Screening based on the presence of actual epithelial changes may be perceived as impractical; worse, a positive result may be too late for effective prevention related to *H. pylori*. Thus, there has been a clear emphasis on appropriate means to detect or confirm chronic infection with the bacterium before disease development, and certainly prior to manifest symptoms. Indeed, initial versions of any systematic eradication program would almost certainly depend on just such a detect-and-treat strategy.

H. pylori infection can be detected or diagnosed either by noninvasive or invasive methods. Noninvasive approaches include the urea breath test (UBT), fecal or stool antigen test, and an immunological assay of *H. pylori*-specific antibodies in body fluids such as sera, urine, saliva, or gastric juice.[247–251] As with many areas of medicine, the availability of DNA-testing (in this case, for specific *H. pylori* types) has begun to offer great promise for researchers and clinicians alike.[252,253]

While the UBT and stool antigen test detect active infection, antibodies are markers of both past and present exposure to *H. pylori*; therefore, they cannot be used to prove that the patient is currently infected.[254,255] Serum assays can, however, provide additional information about the strain of *H. pylori* involved and the status of the gastric mucosa; this is accomplished through the identification of virulence factors such as CagA and/or disease progression markers.[256–261]

The various noninvasive detection methods are continually being refined and evaluated against one another in terms of both effectiveness and cost-effectiveness.[262–266]

Invasive detection methods for *H. pylori* and related disease involve endoscopy, sometimes combined with a biopsy in order to facilitate more accurate histological examination, bacterial culture, or a rapid urease test.[267–270]

The many detection methods noted earlier, generating a multiplicity of management protocols, make navigation through the options very complex.[271] It is useful at this point only to briefly introduce the main clinical or public health settings where detection of *H. pylori* might apply.

The detection of *H. pylori* with respect to gastric cancer control may be pursued in four broad contexts: mass screening in an average-risk population, targeted screening in moderate-risk to high-risk populations, diagnostic testing in the event of gastric symptoms, and surveillance following therapy for *H. pylori* infection and/or related disease. It is axiomatic that screening programs are not pursued unless beneficial follow-up of a positive test is feasible and available; specifically, the capacity to interrupt or reverse disease progression must exist. Although there is some recent qualified support for the cost-effectiveness of population screening for *H. pylori*,[272–274] mass eradication does not seem to have a strong evidence base, particularly in regions of low endemicity.[275] Thus, it is relatively safe to eliminate mass or population screening for *H. pylori* (or related disease) as a compelling option in the majority of developed countries.[276,277]

The next category, targeted screening, has received greater attention in the literature, though the applications are still quite limited. Consensus guidelines support the detection and eradication of *H. pylori* in first degree relatives of patients with gastric cancer. Although not directly related to cancer, *H. pylori* detection and eradication may also prevent peptic ulcer development in individuals taking nonsteroidal anti-inflammatory drugs (NSAIDs).[278]

Opportunistic testing for (and diagnosis of) *H. pylori* infection in the case of upper GI symptoms remains the area of greatest clinical interest. Endoscopy is the accepted reference test for diagnosing ulcers and upper GI malignancies, with a sensitivity and specificity of >95%.[279] However, since a high proportion of the population experiences dyspepsia at some point in a 6-month period, it is impractical to employ an expensive and invasive method such as endoscopy as the primary diagnostic approach. Thus, a test-and-treat strategy is recommended in adult patients less than 45 years old with persistent dyspepsia, based on one or other of the noninvasive *H. pylori* detection methods described earlier.[280] It should be noted that older studies questioned whether this approach to managing dyspepsia would be cost-saving to a health care system; newer trials have been more encouraging in this regard.[281-285]

The strongest arguments for general endoscopic screening for gastric cancer precursors (such as AG) apply to countries with endemic infection.[286] When AG is known to be present, noninvasive tests for *H. pylori* infection may become very relevant to understanding the risk level and appropriate follow-up of a patient.[287,288] Importantly, once certain factors (i.e., so-called "alarm" symptoms, older age, and/or *H. pylori*-positivity) have been used to demark a cohort at high risk for malignancy, then biennial screening by endoscopy for gastric cancer *does* demonstrate clear effectiveness and even cost-effectiveness.[289,290]

Surveillance after *H. pylori* eradication is also of clinical importance. At least 4 weeks following treatment, a test to verify eradication of infection should be conducted.[291] Often, the UBT is employed for this purpose, though certain configurations of the fecal antigen test have been promoted as an alternative.[292,293]

PREVENTION APPROACHES

As noted in an earlier section, the research trend appears to be oriented toward confirming *H. pylori* as a strong causal factor for gastric cancer, and possibly even as necessary for the development of noncardia gastric adenocarcinoma.[294] This fact naturally establishes the bacterium as a very appropriate, and even urgent, target for primary prevention of disease. Each of these now-familiar prevention categories will be reviewed in this last major section.

| Avoiding Exposure | Preventing Infection | Prophylactic Eradication | Preventing Cofactor | Therapeutic Eradication | Interrupting Transformation |

1. Avoiding Exposure to the Agent

The primary prevention of disease related to *H. pylori*, particularly by avoiding exposure to the bacterium, is hampered by the poor understanding of transmission routes.[295] Realistic options include limiting possible fecal–oral transfer between persons through hygiene practices in the home, health care settings, etc. Raising living standards or conditions has sometimes been perceived as an indirect means of such protection; for example, less crowding in home and other settings may simply reduce the opportunities for transferring the bacteria. In the absence of very specific strategies to interrupt transmission to individuals, public health efforts have usually focused on improving general sanitation in a community. Given the uncertainty around water-borne transmission of *H. pylori*, the rationale for the effectiveness of such measures remains speculative.[296] The importance of drinking water in the spread of infection is currently much better understood for a long list of other microbial pathogens.[297]

| Avoiding Exposure | Preventing Infection | Prophylactic Eradication | Preventing Cofactor | Therapeutic Eradication | Interrupting Transformation |

2. Preventing Infection after Exposure to the Agent

When it is available, a vaccine often becomes the "gold standard" approach to neutralizing adverse effects of exposure to a microbe. The emergence of antibiotic resistance has increased the interest in vaccination for *H. pylori*. If anything, motivation is even higher in developing countries, where effective antibiotic therapies are not very accessible due to their high cost.[298,299]

As *H. pylori* infections are generally acquired during childhood, prophylactic vaccination programs will likely be most effective if targeted at young children.[300,301] Research pursued in a developed setting has suggested that a vaccination program implemented for at least 10 years would significantly reduce *H. pylori* infection rates.[302] The same U.S. study group calculated that the development of a prophylactic vaccine, even with an efficacy as low as 55%, would be cost-effective.[303]

Despite extensive investigation, including some success with animal models, there are currently no approved vaccines for *H. pylori*.[304–306]

| Avoiding Exposure | Preventing Infection | **Prophylactic Eradication** | Preventing Cofactor | Therapeutic Eradication | Interrupting Transformation |

3. Prophylactic Eradication or Suppression

Population-wide eradication of *H. pylori* is not recommended as a strategy for gastric cancer prevention, at least not in developed countries with low and/or declining prevalence of *H. pylori*.[307] There are four main arguments against such a practice:

1. As noted earlier, a person may have intragastric *H. pylori* but be asymptomatic. When "benign" symptoms such as dyspepsia occur, and an infection is confirmed, the condition is then easily treatable. While not a proof of the value of prophylactic eradication per se, it is of interest that therapeutic eradication is a potential approach to benign conditions associated with *H. pylori*. Thus, a recent Cochrane review noted that *H. pylori* eradication therapy has a small but statistically significant effect on non-ulcer dyspepsia in study groups with detected infection; furthermore, economic modeling suggests that the benefit, albeit modest, may still be cost-effective, though more research is clearly needed.[308]
2. Although still controversial, there is evidence that *H. pylori* infection may protect against the development of certain diseases in the gastric cardia and the esophagus, including adenocarcinoma.[309–311] However, given the low absolute incidence of cancer in the esophagus, the potential protective benefits of infection are likely outweighed by the risks related to gastric cancer development.[312,313] Indeed, there is evidence that the *combined* risk of gastric and esophageal cancer is actually increased in the population infected with *H. pylori*.[314]
3. Perhaps most importantly, formal proof of the impact of eradication on the incidence of gastric cancer is still being developed. Even if its effectiveness was fully established, systematic eradication of the bacteria would represent an expensive and perhaps excessive application of antibiotics, which could ultimately promote the emergence of resistant strains.[315]
4. In many developed countries, both *H. pylori* infection and (especially distal) gastric adenocarcinoma have already declined to very low levels.[316] In such contexts, the most substantial preventive effect of eradication in terms of gastric cancer seems to be achieved among groups clearly at risk, such as those infected with CagA-positive

H. pylori strains or possibly those having certain genetic polymorphisms that in turn are associated with inflammation markers.[317]

There may be a more compelling rationale for population-wide eradication in developing countries or settings that are prone to endemic infection with *H. pylori*.[318] However, even in such countries there is a continued debate about the appropriateness of systematic eradication of the bacterium.[319,320]

| Avoiding Exposure | Preventing Infection | Prophylactic Eradication | **Preventing Cofactor** | Therapeutic Eradication | Interrupting Transformation |

4. Cofactor Prevention

H. pylori infection may be approaching "necessary" status as a causative agent for specific gastric cancers in specific subsites, but it does not appear to be a sufficient condition to initiate a tumor. The suspected cofactors were listed earlier in this chapter. Of these, the intake of salt, including via salt-preserved foods, has been of particular interest.[321] A potential mechanism elucidated in animal studies points to the impact of salt on the mucous microenvironment of the gastric lining.[322] As an example of the extensive epidemiologic evidence, 2,476 Japanese men over 40 years were stratified according to their daily salt intake in a prospective study. A significant salt–cancer association was observed, but only in subjects who had both *H. pylori* infection and AG; the age- and sex-adjusted odds ratio was 2.87 (95% CI 1.14–7.24).[323] This suggests that salt intake is a true cofactor, and thus a plausible target for gastric cancer prevention in individuals who are infected with *H. pylori*.

Smoking cessation is another potentially strong candidate for reducing gastric cancer in the event of *H. pylori* infection.[324] In one German study among subjects positive for the bacteria, the relative risk of noncardia gastric cancer was 6.1 among nonsmokers compared to 16.6 for smokers.[325]

On the protective side, there is evidence that increased consumption of fruits and vegetables may lower the risk of developing gastric cancer.[326,327] Although some studies have suggested that antioxidants and other dietary supplements such as vitamin C, beta-carotene, and folic acid may also reduce the risk, a Cochrane review did not support this conclusion.[328]

Moderate intake of alcohol consistently demonstrates a protective association with respect to *H. pylori* infection.[329,330] There has been a debate about whether moderate alcohol intake can prevent or eradicate infection.[331]

Because of prevalent conditions such as arthritis, GERD, and ulcers, effective treatments such as NSAIDs and gastric acid controls (e.g., proton pump inhibitors) are widely prescribed by clinicians. NSAIDs may actually reduce the risk of gastric carcinogenesis, though more research is needed to clarify the precise benefits and disadvantages.[332-335] Some of the complexities involved include the fact that the use of NSAIDs actually *promotes* the development of GI ulcers, whereas employing acid inhibitors (i.e., gastric protectants) may be a risk factor for gastric carcinogenesis.[336-339] This suggests the potential importance of finding some "middle ground" of disease control by applying the least damaging combination of antibiotics, gastric protectants, and NSAIDs.[340,341] The topic of NSAIDs will be discussed further in a subsequent section.

Avoiding Exposure	Preventing Infection	Prophylactic Eradication	Preventing Cofactor	**Therapeutic Eradication**	Interrupting Transformation

5. Therapeutic Eradication or Suppression

Therapeutic vaccines against *H. pylori* and gastric cancer continue to be intensively investigated in tandem with the quest for a prophylactic intervention, but serious scientific and clinical challenges must be overcome.[342] In the meantime, a variety of other antibacterial approaches have been extensively studied, with the end-point of interest often being the eradication of *H. pylori* in individual patients.

The use of antibiotics in combination with a proton pump inhibitor (targeting gastric acid secretion) is very effective at clearing the infection, a conclusion that has been confirmed in many countries, including Canada.[343] Although patients with premalignant gastric lesions and confirmed *H. pylori* positivity are often prescribed eradication treatment, results from clinical trials are in conflict as to whether the risk of gastric cancer development is actually reduced.[344,345] More specifically, the question lingers about whether there is a "point of no return" during disease progression after which eradication would be too late.[346-349] Despite the uncertainties, many researchers and reviewers have concluded that eradication prior to atrophy of the gastric mucosa may be the best chance of reducing cancer risk.[350-353]

The classic study in this regard was conducted by Wong et al. in China in 2004.[354] The researchers randomized 1,630 healthy carriers of *H. pylori*. Half of them received triple therapy consisting of omeprazole, amoxicillin, and metronidazole, and the other half a placebo. The main outcome measure of interest was the incidence of gastric cancer. While there was no significant difference between the intervention and placebo groups when they were considered as a whole, looking more closely at a subset of the treatment arm did provide some encouragement. Thus, in patients who had no precancerous lesions at the start of the study, the triple therapy appeared to prevent any gastric cancer from developing.

In addition to ongoing concerns about the prevention efficacy of eradication, there are other challenges in terms of a real-world application of this approach. For instance, while a low rate of reinfection has been observed following eradication treatment in the United States and Europe, studies in *H. pylori* prevalent areas have revealed higher rates of reinfection.[355,356] One recent theory about recolonization after eradication suggests that, contrary to earlier conclusions, *H. pylori* can exist within human cells.[357]

The emergence of antibiotic-resistant strains of *H. pylori* is another growing concern related to eradication efficacy.[358,359] It has been estimated that 10% of *H. pylori* strains are resistant to clarithromycin in developed countries, compared to 25–50% in developing countries.[360] By comparison, research in Canada found that resistance is consistently around 20% for metronidazole but less than 4% for clarithromycin.[361] A Canadian study also found that antibiotic resistance varies geographically.[362] Finally, inadequate patient compliance is another cause of treatment failure.[363] Reasons for noncompliance include side effects and the fact that alleviation of symptoms may not be immediate.[364] One study of 2,751 patients demonstrated a side effects rate of about 23%.[365] Typical side effects seen with *H. pylori* therapy include diarrhea, abdominal pain, and nausea.

One exception to the modest results seen in eradication studies involves the type of gastric cancer seen more rarely, namely MALT lymphoma. Interestingly, MALT lymphoma is the "only known malignancy whose course can be directly changed by the removal of a pathogen."[366] In fact, eradication of *H. pylori* can lead to complete remission of the cancer, as well as exercising a preventive effect.[367,368] Some provisos should be raised in this regard. First, though histological remission may be achieved in up to 90% of patients following antibiotic therapy, molecular disease has been known to persist and possibly account for late relapses.[369,370] This raises a categorical question about whether such intervention should be considered "eradication" at all. Finally, it seems that *H. pylori* treatment does not have any effect on extragastric lymphomas.[371]

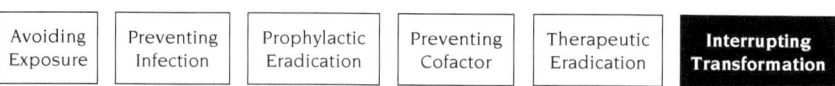

6. Interrupting Transformation Related to Infection

As noted in the section on detection, neither screening nor diagnostic approaches to *H. pylori* are very relevant if a suitable intervention does not exist that could reduce the incidence of gastric cancer in a population positive for infection. Several treatments other than eradication have been investigated, with no overwhelming success story so far in terms of cancer prevention.[372]

The interventions of this sort generally fall under the heading of chemoprevention, or the use of medications to suppress or reverse carcinogenesis.[373,374] Candidate therapies include supplementation with vitamin C and/or beta-carotene and the use of NSAIDs. Unfortunately, antioxidant supplementation has only demonstrated borderline effects on premalignant gastric lesions.[375] The preventive application of NSAIDs (such as aspirin) is complicated by the fact that these substances, while reducing gastric cancer incidence, are also known to cause peptic ulcers.[376] For this reason, purportedly safer medications of this type have increasingly gained attention, although some of these agents have also come under fire (and even been withdrawn from the market) due to reports of cardiac side effects.[377,378]

Other chemoprevention approaches have been applied at various stages of disease progression. Generally, the strategies remain unproven. For example, calcium intake has been employed to counteract the effect of excessive dietary salt, but data are mixed.[379,380] Likewise, while probiotic products (based, for the most part, on bacteria producing lactic acid) have been widely used in Japan and Europe for years, their various health claims are controversial. With respect to gastric cancer, there is some evidence for several beneficial effects of probiotics, including normalization of the intestinal microflora, modulation of immune function, and inhibition of *H. pylori* colonization.[381] It seems that standard antibiotic treatment may be enhanced with combined administration of probiotics, including the reduction of side effects.[382,383]

CONCLUSION

H. pylori represents a microbe of great scientific complexity and interest. The clinical implications and applications drive the research agenda, especially those involving cancer prevention. The bacterium bears an intriguing resemblance in aspects of its activity to that of HPV in the context of malignant disease. First, the bacterium is ubiquitous among human populations (though it is currently better controlled than HPV in developed nations).

Second, both pathogens are involved with a combination of benign and malignant diseases, making the health economics of prevention or treatment especially complicated. One immediate implication of any cancer prevention efforts is the possibility of some collateral benefits in terms of benign conditions. In fact, the investigation of the disease associations of both agents is still very active, suggesting that prevention synergies may increase in the future.

Third, the most notable cancers associated with each agent share an important common cofactor, namely, smoking. This may allow for some prevention synergies linking HPV and *H. pylori.*

Fourth, both pathogens demonstrate forms of tissue tropism combined with some degree of site specificity. In the latter regard, there is in each case one site (i.e., uterine cervix, noncardia gastric lining) where the microbe appears to be a necessary (but not sufficient) cause of malignancy. This is a rare phenomenon in oncology, one that holds great promise for cancer prevention. In this regard, there are many avenues of prevention, detection, and treatment for both pathogens, either currently available or being actively explored. The sense of urgency is partly driven by the fact that HPV and *H. pylori* are the agents that cause the highest number of cancer cases in most developed countries and globally.[384]

The most pertinent difference between *H. pylori* and HPV is in the proven effectiveness of primary and secondary prevention strategies related to cancer. Prevention strategies for HPV are considerably further advanced, especially with respect to the vital arena of vaccination. Any advantage *H. pylori* may enjoy because of the availability of nonsurgical approaches to treatment is tempered by the modest impact demonstrated to date on gastric cancer prevention. The impetus to pursue an effective set of prevention strategies will likely continue to be strong given the public health impact of *H. pylori* in general and its specific role in carcinogenesis. Indeed, by some global assessments, infection with the bacterium is the most common exogenous cause of cancer after smoking.[385] In keeping with the theme of this book, approaches to prevent infection should be a primary goal of a "multi-pronged effort to curtail suffering and death from *H. pylori* infection-associated cancers."[386]

NOTES

1 Farinati F, Cardin R, Cassaro M et al. Helicobacter pylori, inflammation, oxidative damage and gastric cancer: a morphological, biological and molecular pathway. *European Journal of Cancer Prevention.* 2008; 17(3): 195–200.
2 Clyne M, Dolan B, Reeves EP. Bacterial factors that mediate colonization of the stomach and virulence of Helicobacter pylori. *FEMS Microbiology Letters.* 2007; 268(2): 135–43.
3 Das JC, Paul N. Epidemiology and pathophysiology of Helicobacter pylori infection in children. *Indian Journal of Pediatrics.* 2007; 74(3): 287–90.

4 Graham DY, Yamaoka Y, Malaty HM. Contemplating the future without Helicobacter pylori and the dire consequences hypothesis. *Helicobacter.* 2007; 12 (suppl 2): 64–8.
5 Lesbros-Pantoflickova D, Corthesy-Theulaz I, Blum AL. Helicobacter pylori and probiotics. *Journal of Nutrition.* 2007; 137(3 suppl 2): 812S–8S.
6 Kinoshita Y. 2. Lifestyle-related diseases and Helicobacter pylori infection. *Internal Medicine.* 2007; 46(2): 105–6.
7 Cianci R, Montalto M, Pandolfi F et al. Third-line rescue therapy for Helicobacter pylori infection. *World Journal of Gastroenterology.* 2006; 12(15): 2313–9.
8 Fox JG, Wang TC. Inflammation, atrophy, and gastric cancer. *Journal of Clinical Investigation.* 2007; 117(1): 60–9.
9 Suzuki H, Hibi T, Marshall BJ. Helicobacter pylori: present status and future prospects in Japan. *Journal of Gastroenterology.* 2007; 42(1): 1–15.
10 Nilsson HO, Pietroiusti A, Gabrielli M et al. Helicobacter pylori and extragastric diseases—other Helicobacters. *Helicobacter.* 2005; 10(suppl 1): 54–65.
11 Singh RK, McMahon AD, Patel H et al. Prospective analysis of the association of infection with CagA bearing strains of Helicobacter pylori and coronary heart disease. *Heart.* 2002; 88(1): 43–6.
12 Bohr UR, Annibale B, Franceschi F et al. Extragastric manifestations of Helicobacter pylori infection—other Helicobacters. *Helicobacter.* 2007; 12(suppl 1): 45–53.
13 Pellicano R, Peyre S, Astegiano M et al. Updated review (2006) on Helicobacter pylori as a potential target for the therapy of ischemic heart disease. *Panminerva Medica.* 2006; 48(4): 241–6.
14 Al-Marhoon MS. Is there a role for Helicobacter pylori infection in urological diseases? *Urology Journal.* 2008; 5(3): 139–43.
15 Romano M, Ricci V, Zarrilli R. Mechanisms of disease: Helicobacter pylori-related gastric carcinogenesis—implications for chemoprevention. *Nature Clinical Practice.* 2006; 3(11): 622–32.
16 Matysiak-Budnik T, Megraud F. Helicobacter pylori infection and gastric cancer. *European Journal of Cancer.* 2006; 42(6): 708–16.
17 Hatakeyama M. Oncogenic mechanisms of the Helicobacter pylori CagA protein. Nature Reviews. *Cancer.* 2004; 4(9): 688–94.
18 Smith MG, Hold GL, Tahara E et al. Cellular and molecular aspects of gastric cancer. *World Journal of Gastroenterology.* 2006; 12(19): 2979–90.
19 de Vries AC, Haringsma J, Kuipers EJ. The detection, surveillance and treatment of premalignant gastric lesions related to Helicobacter pylori infection. *Helicobacter.* 2007; 12(1): 1–15.
20 *IARC Monographs on the Evaluation of Carcinogenic Risks to Humans.* 1994. Volume 61: schistosomes, Liver Flukes and *Helicobacter pylori.* Available at: monographs.iarc.fr/ENG/Classification/crthgr01.php. Accessed May, 2008. (http://monographs.iarc.fr/ENG/Monographs/vol61/volume61.pdf).
21 Axon A. How to influence health providers. *Helicobacter.* 2007; 12(suppl 2): 80–4.
22 Kuipers EJ, Janssen MJ, de Boer WA. Good bugs and bad bugs: indications and therapies for Helicobacter pylori eradication. *Current Opinion in Pharmacology.* 2003; 3(5): 480–5.
23 Shahabi S, Rasmi Y, Jazani NH et al. Protective effects of Helicobacter pylori against gastroesophageal reflux disease may be due to a neuroimmunological anti-inflammatory mechanism. *Immunology and Cell Biology.* 2008; 86(2): 175–8.

24 Lai LH, Sung JJ. Helicobacter pylori and benign upper digestive disease. *Best Practice and Research. Clinical Gastroenterology.* 2007; 21(2): 261–79.
25 Islami F, Kamangar F. Helicobacter pylori and esophageal cancer risk: a meta-analysis. *Cancer Prevention Research* 2008; 1(5): 329–38.
26 Malfertheiner P, Megraud F, O'Morain C et al. Current concepts in the management of Helicobacter pylori infection: the Maastricht III Consensus Report. *Gut.* 2007; 56(6): 772–81.
27 Kato M, Asaka M, Ono S et al. Eradication of Helicobacter pylori for primary gastric cancer and secondary gastric cancer after endoscopic mucosal resection. *Journal of Gastroenterology.* 2007; 42(suppl 17): 16–20.
28 Rocco A, Nardone G. Diet, H pylori infection and gastric cancer: evidence and controversies. *World Journal of Gastroenterology.* 2007; 13(21): 2901–12.
29 Ables AZ, Simon I, Melton ER. Update on Helicobacter pylori treatment. *American Family Physician.* 2007; 75(3): 351–8.
30 Wilson KT, Crabtree JE. Immunology of Helicobacter pylori: insights into the failure of the immune response and perspectives on vaccine studies. *Gastroenterology.* 2007; 133(1): 288–308.
31 D'Elios MM, Andersen LP. Helicobacter pylori inflammation, immunity, and vaccines. *Helicobacter.* 2007; 12(suppl 1): 15–9.
32 Vorobjova T, Watanabe T, Chiba T. Helicobacter pylori immunology and vaccines. *Helicobacter.* 2008; 13 (suppl 1): 18–22.
33 Graham DY, Yamaoka Y, Malaty HM. Contemplating the future without Helicobacter pylori and the dire consequences hypothesis. *Helicobacter.* 2007; 12(suppl 2): 64–8.
34 Clyne M, Dolan B, Reeves EP. Bacterial factors that mediate colonization of the stomach and virulence of Helicobacter pylori. *FEMS Microbiology Letters.* 2007; 268(2): 135–43.
35 Kabir S. The current status of Helicobacter pylori vaccines: a review. *Helicobacter.* 2007; 12(2): 89–102.
36 Egan BJ, O'Morain CA. A historical perspective of Helicobacter gastroduodenitis and its complications. *Best Practice and Research. Clinical Gastroenterology.* 2007; 21(2): 335–46.
37 Suerbaum S, Josenhans C. Helicobacter pylori evolution and phenotypic diversification in a changing host. *Nature Reviews. Microbiology.* 2007; 5(6): 441–52.
38 Linz B, Balloux F, Moodley Y et al. An African origin for the intimate association between humans and Helicobacter pylori. *Nature.* 2007; 445(7130): 915–8.
39 Ghose C, Perez-Perez GI, Dominguez-Bello MG et al. East Asian genotypes of Helicobacter pylori strains in Amerindians provide evidence for its ancient human carriage. *Proceedings of the National Academy of Sciences of the United States of America.* 2002; 99(23): 15107–11.
40 Israel DA, Salama N, Krishna U et al. Helicobacter pylori genetic diversity within the gastric niche of a single human host. *Proceedings of the National Academy of Sciences of the United States of America.* 2001; 98(25): 14625–30.
41 Han YH, Liu WZ, Shi YZ et al. Comparative genomics profiling of clinical isolates of Helicobacter pylori in Chinese populations using DNA microarray. *Journal of Microbiology.* 2007; 45(1): 21–8.

42 Salama N, Guillemin K, McDaniel TK et al. A whole-genome microarray reveals genetic diversity among Helicobacter pylori strains. *Proceedings of the National Academy of Sciences of the United States of America*. 2000; 97(26): 14668–73.
43 Israel DA, Salama N, Krishna U et al. Helicobacter pylori genetic diversity within the gastric niche of a single human host. *Proceedings of the National Academy of Sciences of the United States of America*. 2001; 98(25): 14625–30.
44 Kivi M, Rodin S, Kupershmidt I et al. Helicobacter pylori genome variability in a framework of familial transmission. *BioMed Central Microbiology*. 2007; 7: 54.
45 Salama NR, Gonzalez-Valencia G, Deatherage B et al. Genetic analysis of Helicobacter pylori strain populations colonizing the stomach at different times postinfection. *Journal of Bacteriology*. 2007; 189(10): 3834–45.
46 Hatakeyama M, Brzozowski T. Pathogenesis of Helicobacter pylori infection. *Helicobacter*. 2006; 11 (suppl 1): 14–20.
47 Prinz C, Schwendy S, Voland P. H pylori and gastric cancer: shifting the global burden. *World Journal of Gastroenterology*. 2006; 12(34): 5458–64.
48 Matysiak-Budnik T, Megraud F. Helicobacter pylori infection and gastric cancer. *European Journal of Cancer*. 2006; 42(6): 708–16.
49 Svennerholm AM, Lundgren A. Progress in vaccine development against Helicobacter pylori. *FEMS Immunology and Medical Microbiology*. 2007; 50(2): 146–56.
50 Virulence factors are molecules that influence host function to allow the pathogen to thrive. Basic cellular processes, such as metabolism or cell structural components, may be vital to existence and growth, but are not considered virulence factors since they do not directly influence the host.
51 Clyne M, Dolan B, Reeves EP. Bacterial factors that mediate colonization of the stomach and virulence of Helicobacter pylori. *FEMS Microbiology Letters*. 2007; 268(2): 135–43.
52 Jafarzadeh A, Rezayati MT, Nemati M. Specific serum immunoglobulin G to H pylori and CagA in healthy children and adults (south-east of Iran). *World Journal of Gastroenterology*. 2007; 13(22): 3117–21.
53 Siman JH, Engstrand L, Berglund G et al. Helicobacter pylori and CagA seropositivity and its association with gastric and oesophageal carcinoma. *Scandinavian Journal of Gastroenterology*. 2007; 42(8): 933–40.
54 Perez-Perez GI, Salomaa A, Kosunen TU et al. Evidence that cagA(+) Helicobacter pylori strains are disappearing more rapidly than cagA(-) strains. *Gut*. 2002; 50(3): 295–8.
55 Kwok T, Zabler D, Urman S et al. Helicobacter exploits integrin for type IV secretion and kinase activation. *Nature*. 2007; 449(7164): 862–6.
56 Yamaoka Y, Kato M, Asaka M. Geographic differences in gastric cancer incidence can be explained by differences between Helicobacter pylori strains. *Internal Medicine*. 2008; 47(12): 1077–83.
57 Jergens AE, Wilson-Welder JH, Dorn A et al. Helicobacter bilis triggers persistent immune reactivity to antigens derived from the commensal bacteria in gnotobiotic C3H/HeN mice. *Gut*. 2007; 56(7): 934–40.
58 Duttala SV, Majumdar AP, Parikh RK et al. H. heilmannii infection and gastric carcinogenesis. *Indian Journal of Gastroenterology*. 2008; 27(3): 131–2.

59 Megraud F, Lehours P. Helicobacter pylori detection and antimicrobial susceptibility testing. *Clinical Microbiology Reviews.* 2007; 20(2): 280–322.
60 Clyne M, Dolan B, Reeves EP. Bacterial factors that mediate colonization of the stomach and virulence of Helicobacter pylori. *FEMS Microbiology Letters.* 2007; 268(2): 135–43.
61 Graham DY. Helicobacter: a new scientific journal. *Helicobacter.* 1996; 1(1): 1–3.
62 Vogelmann R, Amieva MR. The role of bacterial pathogens in cancer. *Current Opinion in Microbiology.* 2007; 10(1): 76–81.
63 IARC Monographs on the Evaluation of Carcinogenic Risks to Humans. 1994. Volume 61: schistosomes, Liver Flukes and *Helicobacter pylori.* Available at: monographs.iarc.fr/ENG/Classification/crthgr01.php.
64 Fox JG, Wang TC. Inflammation, atrophy, and gastric cancer. *Journal of Clinical Investigation.* 2007; 117(1): 60–9.
65 Dubois A, Boren T. Helicobacter pylori is invasive and it may be a facultative intracellular organism. *Cellular Microbiology.* 2007; 9(5): 1108–16.
66 Tsuji S, Tsujii M, Murata H et al. Helicobacter pylori eradication to prevent gastric cancer: underlying molecular and cellular mechanisms. *World Journal of Gastroenterology.* 2006; 12(11): 1671–80.
67 Ables AZ, Simon I, Melton ER. Update on Helicobacter pylori treatment. *American Family Physician.* 2007; 75(3): 351–8.
68 Kuipers EJ, Sipponen P. Helicobacter pylori eradication for the prevention of gastric cancer. *Helicobacter.* 2006; 11(suppl 1): 52–7.
69 de Vries AC, Haringsma J, Kuipers EJ. The detection, surveillance and treatment of premalignant gastric lesions related to Helicobacter pylori infection. *Helicobacter.* 2007; 12(1): 1–15.
70 Hjalgrim H, Engels EA. Infectious aetiology of Hodgkin and non-Hodgkin lymphomas: a review of the epidemiological evidence. *Journal of Internal Medicine.* 2008; 264(6): 537–48.
71 Malaty HM. Epidemiology of Helicobacter pylori infection. *Best Practice and Research. Clinical Gastroenterology.* 2007; 21(2): 205–14.
72 Rocco A, Nardone G. Diet, H pylori infection and gastric cancer: evidence and controversies. *World Journal of Gastroenterology.* 2007; 13(21): 2901–12.
73 Dubois A, Boren T. Helicobacter pylori is invasive and it may be a facultative intracellular organism. *Cellular Microbiology.* 2007; 9(5): 1108–16.
74 McLoughlin RM, Sebastian SS, O'Connor HJ et al. Review article: test and treat or test and scope for Helicobacter pylori infection. Any change in gastric cancer prevention? *Alimentary Pharmacology and Therapeutics.* 2003; 17(suppl 2): 82–8.
75 Fox JG, Wang TC. Inflammation, atrophy, and gastric cancer. *Journal of Clinical Investigation.* 2007; 117(1): 60–9.
76 Dubois A, Boren T. Helicobacter pylori is invasive and it may be a facultative intracellular organism. *Cellular Microbiology.* 2007; 9(5): 1108–16.
77 Tsugane S, Sasazuki S. Diet and the risk of gastric cancer: review of epidemiological evidence. *Gastric Cancer.* 2007; 10(2): 75–83.
78 Egan BJ, O'Morain CA. A historical perspective of Helicobacter gastroduodenitis and its complications. *Best Practice and Research. Clinical Gastroenterology.* 2007; 21(2): 335–46.
79 Tokudome S, Samsuria Soeripto WD, Triningsih FX et al. Helicobacter pylori infection appears essential for stomach carcinogenesis: observations in Semarang, Indonesia. *Cancer Science.* 2005; 96(12): 873–5.

80 Tokudome S, Soeripto, Triningsih FX et al. Rare Helicobacter pylori infection as a factor for the very low stomach cancer incidence in Yogyakarta, Indonesia. *Cancer Letters.* 2005; 219(1): 57–61.
81 An international association between Helicobacter pylori infection and gastric cancer. The EUROGAST Study Group. *The Lancet.* 1993; 341(8857): 1359–62.
82 Sasazuki S, Inoue M, Iwasaki M et al. Effect of Helicobacter pylori infection combined with CagA and pepsinogen status on gastric cancer development among Japanese men and women: a nested case-control study. *Cancer Epidemiology, Biomarkers and Prevention.* 2006; 15(7): 1341–7.
83 Uemura N, Okamoto S, Yamamoto S et al. Helicobacter pylori infection and the development of gastric cancer. *New England Journal of Medicine.* 2001; 345(11): 784–9.
84 Parkin DM. The global health burden of infection-associated cancers in the year 2002. *International Journal of Cancer.* 2006; 118(12): 3030–44.
85 Mc Loughlin RM, Sebastian SS, O'Connor HJ et al. Review article: test and treat or test and scope for Helicobacter pylori infection. Any change in gastric cancer prevention? *Alimentary Pharmacology and Therapeutics.* 2003; 17(suppl 2): 82–8.
86 Helicobacter and Cancer Collaborative Group. Gastric cancer and Helicobacter pylori: a combined analysis of 12 case control studies nested within prospective cohorts. *Gut.* 2001; 49(3): 347–53.
87 Ekstrom AM, Signorello LB, Hansson LE et al. Evaluating gastric cancer misclassification: a potential explanation for the rise in cardia cancer incidence. *Journal of the National Cancer Institute.* 1999; 91(9): 786–90.
88 Blaser MJ, Saito D. Trends in reported adenocarcinomas of the oesophagus and gastric cardia in Japan. *European Journal of Gastroenterology and Hepatology.* 2002; 14(2): 107–13.
89 Hansen S, Vollset SE, Derakhshan MH et al. Two distinct aetiologies of cardia cancer; evidence from premorbid serological markers of gastric atrophy and Helicobacter pylori status. *Gut.* 2007; 56(7): 918–25.
90 McColl KE. Cancer of the gastric cardia. *Best Practice and Research. Clinical Gastroenterology.* 2006; 20(4): 687–96.
91 Maeda H, Okabayashi T, Nishimori I et al. Clinicopathologic features of adenocarcinoma at the gastric cardia: is it different from distal cancer of the stomach? *Journal of the American College of Surgeons.* 2008; 206(2): 306–10.
92 Lee JY, Kim HY, Kim KH et al. No changing trends in incidence of gastric cardia cancer in Korea. *Journal of Korean Medical Science.* 2003; 18(1): 53–7.
93 Kamangar F, Dawsey SM, Blaser MJ et al. Opposing risks of gastric cardia and noncardia gastric adenocarcinomas associated with Helicobacter pylori seropositivity. *Journal of the National Cancer Institute.* 2006; 98(20): 1445–52.
94 Kamangar F, Qiao YL, Blaser MJ et al. Helicobacter pylori and oesophageal and gastric cancers in a prospective study in China. *British Journal of Cancer.* 2007; 96(1): 172–6.
95 Tajima Y, Yamazaki K, Makino R et al. Differences in the histological findings, phenotypic marker expressions and genetic alterations between adenocarcinoma of the gastric cardia and distal stomach. *British Journal of Cancer.* 2007; 96(4): 631–8.
96 Xia HH, Yang Y, Wong BC. Relationship between Helicobacter pylori infection and gastroesophageal reflux disease. *Chinese Journal of Digestive Diseases.* 2004; 5(1): 1–6.

97 Brenner H, Arndt V, Stegmaier C et al. Is Helicobacter pylori infection a necessary condition for noncardia gastric cancer? *American Journal of Epidemiology.* 2004; 159(3): 252–8.

98 Palli D, Masala G, Del Giudice G et al. CagA+ Helicobacter pylori infection and gastric cancer risk in the EPIC-EURGAST study. *International Journal of Cancer.* 2007; 120(4): 859–67.

99 Helicobacter and Cancer Collaborative Group. Gastric cancer and Helicobacter pylori: a combined analysis of 12 case control studies nested within prospective cohorts. *Gut.* 2001; 49(3): 347–53.

100 Ohata H, Kitauchi S, Yoshimura N et al. Progression of chronic atrophic gastritis associated with Helicobacter pylori infection increases risk of gastric cancer. *International Journal of Cancer.* 2004; 109(1): 138–43.

101 Eslick GD. Helicobacter pylori infection causes gastric cancer? A review of the epidemiological, meta-analytic, and experimental evidence. *World Journal of Gastroenterology.* 2006; 12(19): 2991–9.

102 Perez-Perez GI, Garza-Gonzalez E, Portal C et al. Role of cytokine polymorphisms in the risk of distal gastric cancer development. *Cancer Epidemiology, Biomarkers and Prevention.* 2005; 14(8): 1869–73.

103 Gylling A, Abdel-Rahman WM, Juhola M et al. Is gastric cancer part of the tumour spectrum of hereditary non-polyposis colorectal cancer? A molecular genetic study. *Gut.* 2007; 56(7): 926–33.

104 Rocco A, Nardone G. Diet, H pylori infection and gastric cancer: evidence and controversies. *World Journal of Gastroenterology.* 2007; 13(21): 2901–12.

105 Freedman ND, Abnet CC, Leitzmann MF et al. A prospective study of tobacco, alcohol, and the risk of esophageal and gastric cancer subtypes. *American Journal of Epidemiology.* 2007; 165(12): 1424–33.

106 Sjodahl K, Lu Y, Nilsen TI et al. Smoking and alcohol drinking in relation to risk of gastric cancer: a population-based, prospective cohort study. *International Journal of Cancer.* 2007; 120(1): 128–32.

107 Lindblad M, Rodriguez LA, Lagergren J. Body mass, tobacco and alcohol and risk of esophageal, gastric cardia, and gastric non-cardia adenocarcinoma among men and women in a nested case-control study. *Cancer Causes and Control.* 2005; 16(3): 285–94.

108 Engel LS, Chow WH, Vaughan TL et al. Population attributable risks of esophageal and gastric cancers. *Journal of the National Cancer Institute.* 2003; 95(18): 1404–13.

109 Al-Marhoon MS. Is there a role for Helicobacter pylori infection in urological diseases? *Urology Journal.* 2008; 5(3): 139–43.

110 Lukes P, Astl J, Pavlik E et al. Helicobacter pylori in tonsillar and adenoid tissue and its possible role in oropharyngeal carcinogenesis. *Folia Biologica.* 2008; 54(2): 33–9.

111 Siman JH, Engstrand L, Berglund G et al. Helicobacter pylori and CagA seropositivity and its association with gastric and oesophageal carcinoma. *Scandinavian Journal of Gastroenterology.* 2007; 42(8): 933–40.

112 Rokkas T, Pistiolas D, Sechopoulos P et al. Relationship between Helicobacter pylori infection and esophageal neoplasia: a meta-analysis. *Clinical Gastroenterology and Hepatology.* 2007; 5(12): 1413–7, 7 e1–2.

113 Zhuo X, Zhang Y, Wang Y et al. Helicobacter pylori infection and oesophageal cancer risk: association studies via evidence-based meta-analyses. *Clinical Oncology.* 2008; 20(10): 757–62.

114 Robins G, Crabtree JE, Bailey A et al. International variation in Helicobacter pylori infection and rates of oesophageal cancer. *European Journal of Cancer.* 2008; 44(5): 726–32.

115 Anderson LA, Murphy SJ, Johnston BT et al. Relationship between Helicobacter pylori infection and gastric atrophy and the stages of the oesophageal inflammation, metaplasia, adenocarcinoma sequence: results from the FINBAR case-control study. *Gut.* 2008; 57(6): 734–9.

116 Fruh M, Zhou W, Zhai R et al. Polymorphisms of inflammatory and metalloproteinase genes, Helicobacter pylori infection and the risk of oesophageal adenocarcinoma. *British Journal of Cancer.* 2008; 98(4): 689–92.

117 Lofdahl HE, Lu Y, Lagergren J. Sex-specific risk factor profile in oesophageal adenocarcinoma. *British Journal of Cancer.* 2008; 99(9): 1506–10.

118 Islami F, Kamangar F. Helicobacter pylori and esophageal cancer risk: a meta-analysis. *Cancer Prevention Research.* 2008; 1(5): 329–38.

119 Xuan SY, Xin YN, Chen AJ et al. Association between the presence of H pylori in the liver and hepatocellular carcinoma: a meta-analysis. *World Journal of Gastroenterology.* 2008; 14(2): 307–12.

120 Abu Al-Soud W, Stenram U, Ljungh A et al. DNA of Helicobacter spp. and common gut bacteria in primary liver carcinoma. *Digestive and Liver Disease.* 2008; 40(2): 126–31.

121 Ito K, Yamaoka Y, Ota H et al. Adherence, internalization, and persistence of Helicobacter pylori in hepatocytes. *Digestive Diseases and Sciences.* 2008; 53(9): 2541–9.

122 Vivekanandan P, Torbenson M. Low frequency of Helicobacter DNA in benign and malignant liver tissues from Baltimore, United States. *Human Pathology.* 2008; 39(2): 213–6.

123 Pandey M, Shukla M. Helicobacter species are associated with possible increase in risk of hepatobiliary tract cancers. *Surgical Oncology.* 2009; 18(1): 51–6.

124 de Martel C, Plummer M, Parsonnet J et al. Helicobacter species in cancers of the gallbladder and extrahepatic biliary tract. *British Journal of Cancer.* 2009; 100(1): 194–9.

125 Lindkvist B, Johansen D, Borgstrom A et al. A prospective study of Helicobacter pylori in relation to the risk for pancreatic cancer. *BMC Cancer.* 2008; 8: 321.

126 de Martel C, Llosa AE, Friedman GD et al. Helicobacter pylori infection and development of pancreatic cancer. *Cancer Epidemiology, Biomarkers and Prevention.* 2008; 17(5): 1188–94.

127 Burnett-Hartman AN, Newcomb PA, Potter JD. Infectious agents and colorectal cancer: a review of Helicobacter pylori, Streptococcus bovis, JC virus, and human papillomavirus. *Cancer Epidemiology, Biomarkers and Prevention.* 2008; 17(11): 2970–9.

128 Hecht G. In the beginning was Helicobacter pylori: roles for microbes in other intestinal disorders. *Gastroenterology.* 2007; 132(2): 481–3.

129 Zumkeller N, Brenner H, Zwahlen M et al. Helicobacter pylori infection and colorectal cancer risk: a meta-analysis. *Helicobacter.* 2006; 11(2): 75–80.

130 Zhao YS, Wang F, Chang D et al. Meta-analysis of different test indicators: Helicobacter pylori infection and the risk of colorectal cancer. *International Journal of Colorectal Disease*. 2008; 23(9): 875–82.

131 Bulajic M, Stimec B, Ille T et al. PCR detection of helicobacter pylori genome in colonic mucosa: normal and malignant. *Contributions / Macedonian Academy of Sciences and Arts, Section of Biological and Medical Sciences*. 2007; 28(2): 25–38.

132 Machida-Montani A, Sasazuki S, Inoue M et al. Atrophic gastritis, Helicobacter pylori, and colorectal cancer risk: A case-control study. *Helicobacter*. 2007; 12(4): 328–32.

133 Bulajic M, Stimec B, Jesenofsky R et al. Helicobacter pylori in colorectal carcinoma tissue. *Cancer Epidemiology, Biomarkers and Prevention*. 2007; 16(3): 631–3.

134 Jones M, Helliwell P, Pritchard C et al. Helicobacter pylori in colorectal neoplasms: is there an aetiological relationship? *World Journal of Surgical Oncology*. 2007; 5: 51.

135 Zhuo XL, Wang Y, Zhuo WL et al. Possible association of Helicobacter pylori infection with laryngeal cancer risk: an evidence-based meta-analysis. *Archives of Medical Research*. 2008; 39(6): 625–8.

136 Masoud N, Manouchehr K, Najmeh D et al. Lack of association between Helicobacter pylori and laryngeal carcinoma. *Asian Pacific Journal of Cancer Prevention*. 2008; 9(1): 81–2.

137 Delport W, van der Merwe SW. The transmission of Helicobacter pylori: the effects of analysis method and study population on inference. *Best Practice and Research. Clinical Gastroenterology*. 2007; 21(2): 215–36.

138 Weyermann M, Adler G, Brenner H et al. The mother as source of Helicobacter pylori infection. *Epidemiology*. 2006; 17(3): 332–4.

139 Malaty HM, El-Kasabany A, Graham DY et al. Age at acquisition of Helicobacter pylori infection: a follow-up study from infancy to adulthood. *The Lancet*. 2002; 359(9310): 931–5.

140 Kivi M, Tindberg Y. Helicobacter pylori occurrence and transmission: a family affair? *Scandinavian Journal of Infectious Diseases*. 2006; 38(6–7): 407–17.

141 Rowland M, Daly L, Vaughan M et al. Age-specific incidence of Helicobacter pylori. *Gastroenterology*. 2006; 130(1): 65–72.

142 Clyne M, Dolan B, Reeves EP. Bacterial factors that mediate colonization of the stomach and virulence of Helicobacter pylori. *FEMS Microbiology Letters*. 2007; 268(2): 135–43.

143 Delport W, van der Merwe SW. The transmission of Helicobacter pylori: the effects of analysis method and study population on inference. *Best Practice and Research. Clinical Gastroenterology*. 2007; 21(2): 215–36.

144 Kusters JG, van Vliet AH, Kuipers EJ. Pathogenesis of Helicobacter pylori infection. *Clinical Microbiology Reviews*. 2006; 19(3): 449–90.

145 Das JC, Paul N. Epidemiology and pathophysiology of Helicobacter pylori infection in children. *Indian Journal of Pediatrics*. 2007; 74(3): 287–90.

146 Mourad-Baars P, Chong S. Helicobacter pylori infection in pediatrics. *Helicobacter*. 2006; 11(suppl 1): 40–5.

147 Bittencourt PF, Rocha GA, Penna FJ et al. Gastroduodenal peptic ulcer and Helicobacter pylori infection in children and adolescents. *Jornal de Pediatria*. 2006; 82(5): 325–34.

148 Egemen A, Yilmaz O, Akil I et al. Evaluation of association between hepatitis A and Helicobacter pylori infections and routes of transmission. *Turkish Journal of Pediatrics*. 2006; 48(2): 135–9.
149 Yang YJ, Wang SM, Chen CT et al. Lack of evidence for fecal-oral transmission of Helicobacter pylori infection in Taiwanese. *Journal of the Formosan Medical Association*. 2003; 102(6): 375–8.
150 Malaty HM, Tanaka E, Kumagai T et al. Seroepidemiology of Helicobacter pylori and hepatitis A virus and the mode of transmission of infection: a 9-year cohort study in rural Japan. *Clinical Infectious Diseases*. 2003; 37(8): 1067–72.
151 Weyermann M, Rothenbacher D, Brenner H. Acquisition of helicobacter pylori infection in early childhood: independent contributions of infected mothers, fathers, and siblings. *American Journal of Gastroenterology*. 2009; 104(1): 182–9.
152 Eslick GD. Sexual transmission of Helicobacter pylori via oral-anal intercourse. *International Journal of STD and AIDS*. 2002; 13(1): 7–11.
153 Eslick GD. Helicobacter pylori infection transmitted sexually via oral-genital contact: a hypothetical model. *Sexually Transmitted Infections*. 2000; 76(6): 489–92.
154 Fujimura S, Kato S, Nagai K et al. Detection of Helicobacter pylori in the stools of newborn infants. *Pediatric Infectious Disease Journal*. 2004; 23(11): 1055–6.
155 Brown LM. Helicobacter pylori: epidemiology and routes of transmission. *Epidemiologic Reviews*. 2000; 22(2): 283–97.
156 Mastromarino P, Conti C, Donato K et al. Does hospital work constitute a risk factor for Helicobacter pylori infection? *Journal of Hospital Infection*. 2005; 60(3): 261–8.
157 Noone PA, Waclawski ER, Watt AD. Are endoscopy nurses at risk of infection with Helicobacter pylori from their work? *Occupational Medicine*. 2006; 56(2): 122–8.
158 Suzuki H, Hibi T, Marshall BJ. Helicobacter pylori: present status and future prospects in Japan. *Journal of Gastroenterology*. 2007; 42(1): 1–15.
159 Malaty HM. Epidemiology of Helicobacter pylori infection. *Best Practice and Research. Clinical Gastroenterology*. 2007; 21(2): 205–14.
160 Kusters JG, van Vliet AH, Kuipers EJ. Pathogenesis of Helicobacter pylori infection. *Clinical Microbiology Reviews*. 2006; 19(3): 449–90.
161 Magalhaes Queiroz DM, Luzza F. Epidemiology of Helicobacter pylori infection. *Helicobacter*. 2006; 11 (suppl 1): 1–5.
162 Bittencourt PF, Rocha GA, Penna FJ et al. Gastroduodenal peptic ulcer and Helicobacter pylori infection in children and adolescents. *Jornal de Pediatria*. 2006; 82(5): 325–34.
163 Kivi M, Johansson AL, Reilly M et al. Helicobacter pylori status in family members as risk factors for infection in children. *Epidemiology and Infection*. 2005; 133(4): 645–52.
164 Farrell S, Doherty GM, Milliken I et al. Risk factors for Helicobacter pylori infection in children: an examination of the role played by intrafamilial bed sharing. *Pediatric Infectious Disease Journal*. 2005; 24(2): 149–52.
165 Ables AZ, Simon I, Melton ER. Update on Helicobacter pylori treatment. *American Family Physician*. 2007; 75(3): 351–8.

166 Delport W, van der Merwe SW. The transmission of Helicobacter pylori: the effects of analysis method and study population on inference. *Best Practice and Research. Clinical Gastroenterology.* 2007; 21(2): 215–36.
167 Singh K, Ghoshal UC. Causal role of Helicobacter pylori infection in gastric cancer: an Asian enigma. *World Journal of Gastroenterology.* 2006; 12(9): 1346–51.
168 Nagel G, Linseisen J, Boshuizen HC et al. Socioeconomic position and the risk of gastric and oesophageal cancer in the European Prospective Investigation into Cancer and Nutrition (EPIC-EURGAST). *International Journal of Epidemiology.* 2007; 36(1): 66–76.
169 Suerbaum S, Josenhans C. Helicobacter pylori evolution and phenotypic diversification in a changing host. *Nature Reviews. Microbiology.* 2007; 5(6): 441–52.
170 Azevedo NF, Guimaraes N, Figueiredo C et al. A new model for the transmission of Helicobacter pylori: role of environmental reservoirs as gene pools to increase strain diversity. *Critical Reviews in Microbiology.* 2007; 33(3): 157–69.
171 Malaty HM. Epidemiology of Helicobacter pylori infection. *Best Practice and Research. Clinical Gastroenterology.* 2007; 21(2): 205–14.
172 Svennerholm AM, Lundgren A. Progress in vaccine development against Helicobacter pylori. *FEMS Immunology and Medical Microbiology.* 2007; 50(2): 146–56.
173 Delport W, van der Merwe SW. The transmission of Helicobacter pylori: the effects of analysis method and study population on inference. *Best Practice and Research. Clinical Gastroenterology.* 2007; 21(2): 215–36.
174 Horvitz G, Gold BD. Gastroduodenal diseases of childhood. *Current Opinion in Gastroenterology.* 2006; 22(6): 632–40.
175 Helicobacter and Cancer Collaborative Group. Gastric cancer and Helicobacter pylori: a combined analysis of 12 case control studies nested within prospective cohorts. *Gut.* 2001; 49(3): 347–53.
176 Khuroo MS. Helicobacter pylori: the unique organism. *Annals of Saudi Medicine.* 2002; 22(3–4): 192–201.
177 Delport W, van der Merwe SW. The transmission of Helicobacter pylori: the effects of analysis method and study population on inference. *Best Practice and Research. Clinical Gastroenterology.* 2007; 21(2): 215–36.
178 Graham DY, Malaty HM, Evans DG et al. Epidemiology of Helicobacter pylori in an asymptomatic population in the United States: effect of age, race and socioeconomic status. *Gastroenterology.* 1991;100: 1495–1501.
179 Weyermann M, Adler G, Brenner H et al. The mother as source of Helicobacter pylori infection. *Epidemiology.* 2006; 17(3): 332–4.
180 Perez-Perez GI, Salomaa A, Kosunen TU et al. Evidence that cagA(+) Helicobacter pylori strains are disappearing more rapidly than cagA(−) strains. *Gut.* 2002; 50(3): 295–8.
181 Delport W, van der Merwe SW. The transmission of Helicobacter pylori: the effects of analysis method and study population on inference. *Best Practice and Research. Clinical Gastroenterology.* 2007; 21(2): 215–36.
182 Das JC, Paul N. Epidemiology and pathophysiology of Helicobacter pylori infection in children. *Indian Journal of Pediatrics.* 2007; 74(3): 287–90.
183 Suzuki H, Hibi T, Marshall BJ. Helicobacter pylori: present status and future prospects in Japan. *Journal of Gastroenterology.* 2007; 42(1): 1–15.

184 Suerbaum S, Michetti P. Helicobacter pylori infection. *New England Journal of Medicine.* 2002; 347(15): 1175–86.
185 Magalhaes Queiroz DM, Luzza F. Epidemiology of Helicobacter pylori infection. *Helicobacter.* 2006; 11(suppl 1): 1–5.
186 Bernstein CN, McKeown I, Embil JM et al. Seroprevalence of Helicobacter pylori, incidence of gastric cancer, and peptic ulcer-associated hospitalizations in a Canadian Indian population. *Digestive Diseases and Sciences.* 1999; 44(4): 668–74.
187 Sinha SK, Martin B, Gold BD et al. The incidence of Helicobacter pylori acquisition in children of a Canadian First Nations community and the potential for parent-to-child transmission. *Helicobacter.* 2004; 9(1): 59–68.
188 Mourad-Baars P, Chong S. Helicobacter pylori infection in pediatrics. *Helicobacter.* 2006; 11(suppl 1): 40–5.
189 Zhu J, Davidson M, Leinonen M et al. Prevalence and persistence of antibodies to herpes viruses, Chlamydia pneumoniae and Helicobacter pylori in Alaskan Eskimos: the GOCADAN Study. *Clinical Microbiology and Infection.* 2006; 12(2): 118–22.
190 Goodman KJ, Jacobson K, Veldhuyzen van Zanten S. Helicobacter pylori infection in Canadian and related Arctic Aboriginal populations. *Canadian Journal of Gastroenterology.* 2008; 22(3): 289–95.
191 Tsai CJ, Perry S, Sanchez L et al. Helicobacter pylori infection in different generations of Hispanics in the San Francisco Bay Area. *American Journal of Epidemiology.* 2005; 162(4): 351–7.
192 Perez-Perez GI, Olivares AZ, Foo FY et al. Seroprevalence of Helicobacter pylori in New York City populations originating in East Asia. *Journal of Urban Health.* 2005; 82(3): 510–6.
193 Horvitz G, Gold BD. Gastroduodenal diseases of childhood. *Current Opinion in Gastroenterology.* 2006; 22(6): 632–40.
194 Collins J, Ali-Ibrahim A, Smoot DT. Antibiotic therapy for Helicobacter pylori. *Medical Clinics of North America.* 2006; 90(6): 1125–40.
195 Kumagai T, Malaty HM, Graham DY et al. Acquisition versus loss of Helicobacter pylori infection in Japan: results from an 8-year birth cohort study. *Journal of Infectious Diseases.* 1998; 178(3): 717–21.
196 Fox JG, Wang TC. Inflammation, atrophy, and gastric cancer. *Journal of Clinical Investigation.* 2007; 117(1): 60–9.
197 Lochhead P, El-Omar EM. Helicobacter pylori infection and gastric cancer. *Best Practice and Research. Clinical Gastroenterology.* 2007; 21(2): 281–97.
198 Israel DA, Peek RM, Jr. The role of persistence in Helicobacter pylori pathogenesis. *Current Opinion in Gastroenterology.* 2006; 22(1): 3–7.
199 Buret AG, Fedwick JP, Flynn AN. Host epithelial interactions with Helicobacter pylori: a role for disrupted gastric barrier function in the clinical outcome of infection? *Canadian Journal of Gastroenterology.* 2005; 19(9): 543–52.
200 Suerbaum S, Josenhans C. Helicobacter pylori evolution and phenotypic diversification in a changing host. *Nature Reviews. Microbiology.* 2007; 5(6): 441–52.
201 Algood HM, Cover TL. Helicobacter pylori persistence: an overview of interactions between H. pylori and host immune defenses. *Clinical Microbiology Reviews.* 2006; 19(4): 597–613.

202 Beswick EJ, Suarez G, Reyes VE. H pylori and host interactions that influence pathogenesis. *World Journal of Gastroenterology.* 2006; 12(35): 5599–605.
203 Suarez G, Reyes VE, Beswick EJ. Immune response to H. pylori. *World Journal of Gastroenterology.* 2006; 12(35): 5593–8.
204 Correa P, Houghton J. Carcinogenesis of Helicobacter pylori. *Gastroenterology.* 2007; 133(2): 659–72.
205 Velin D, Michetti P. Immunology of Helicobacter pylori infection. *Digestion.* 2006; 73(2-3): 116–23.
206 Clyne M, Dolan B, Reeves EP. Bacterial factors that mediate colonization of the stomach and virulence of Helicobacter pylori. *FEMS Microbiology Letters.* 2007; 268(2): 135–43.
207 Portal-Celhay C, Perez-Perez GI. Immune responses to Helicobacter pylori colonization: mechanisms and clinical outcomes. *Clinical Science.* 2006; 110(3): 305–14.
208 Cooke CL, Huff JL, Solnick JV. The role of genome diversity and immune evasion in persistent infection with Helicobacter pylori. *FEMS Immunology and Medical Microbiology.* 2005; 45(1): 11–23.
209 Fox JG, Wang TC. Inflammation, atrophy, and gastric cancer. *Journal of Clinical Investigation.* 2007; 117(1): 60–9.
210 Mimuro H, Suzuki T, Nagai S et al. Helicobacter pylori dampens gut epithelial self-renewal by inhibiting apoptosis, a bacterial strategy to enhance colonization of the stomach. *Cell Host and Microbe.* 2007; 2(4): 250–63.
211 Allen LA. Phagocytosis and persistence of Helicobacter pylori. *Cellular Microbiology.* 2007; 9(4): 817–28.
212 Sgouros SN, Bergele C. Clinical outcome of patients with Helicobacter pylori infection: the bug, the host, or the environment? *Postgraduate Medical Journal.* 2006; 82(967): 338–42.
213 Sagaert X, De Wolf-Peeters C, Noels H et al. The pathogenesis of MALT lymphomas: where do we stand? *Leukemia.* 2007; 21(3): 389–96.
214 Fox JG, Wang TC. Inflammation, atrophy, and gastric cancer. *Journal of Clinical Investigation.* 2007; 117(1): 60–9.
215 Suarez G, Reyes VE, Beswick EJ. Immune response to H. pylori. *World Journal of Gastroenterology.* 2006; 12(35): 5593–8.
216 Beswick EJ, Suarez G, Reyes VE. H pylori and host interactions that influence pathogenesis. *World Journal of Gastroenterology.* 2006; 12(35): 5599–605.
217 Peek RM, Jr., Crabtree JE. Helicobacter infection and gastric neoplasia. *Journal of Pathology.* 2006; 208(2): 233–48.
218 Suarez G, Reyes VE, Beswick EJ. Immune response to H. pylori. *World Journal of Gastroenterology.* 2006; 12(35): 5593–8.
219 Allen LA. Phagocytosis and persistence of Helicobacter pylori. *Cellular Microbiology.* 2007; 9(4): 817–28.
220 Fox JG, Wang TC. Inflammation, atrophy, and gastric cancer. *Journal of Clinical Investigation.* 2007; 117(1): 60–9.
221 Lochhead P, El-Omar EM. Helicobacter pylori infection and gastric cancer. *Best Practice and Research. Clinical Gastroenterology.* 2007; 21(2): 281–97.
222 Das JC, Paul N. Epidemiology and pathophysiology of Helicobacter pylori infection in children. *Indian Journal of Pediatrics.* 2007; 74(3): 287–90.
223 Fox JG, Wang TC. Inflammation, atrophy, and gastric cancer. *Journal of Clinical Investigation.* 2007; 117(1): 60–9.

224 Wilson KT, Crabtree JE. Immunology of Helicobacter pylori: insights into the failure of the immune response and perspectives on vaccine studies. *Gastroenterology.* 2007; 133(1): 288–308.
225 Malfertheiner P, Megraud F, O'Morain C et al. Current concepts in the management of Helicobacter pylori infection: the Maastricht III Consensus Report. *Gut.* 2007; 56(6): 772–81.
226 Holmes RS, Vaughan TL. Epidemiology and pathogenesis of esophageal cancer. *Seminars in Radiation Oncology.* 2007; 17(1): 2–9.
227 Matysiak-Budnik T, Megraud F. Helicobacter pylori infection and gastric cancer. *European Journal of Cancer.* 2006; 42(6): 708–16.
228 Sgouros SN, Bergele C. Clinical outcome of patients with Helicobacter pylori infection: the bug, the host, or the environment? *Postgraduate Medical Journal.* 2006; 82(967): 338–42.
229 Ando T, Goto Y, Ishiguro K et al. The interaction of host genetic factors and Helicobacter pylori infection. *Inflammopharmacology.* 2007; 15(1): 10–4.
230 Kato M, Asaka M, Ono S et al. Eradication of Helicobacter pylori for primary gastric cancer and secondary gastric cancer after endoscopic mucosal resection. *Journal of Gastroenterology.* 2007; 42(suppl 17): 16–20.
231 Trautmann K, Stolte M, Miehlke S. Eradication of H pylori for the prevention of gastric cancer. *World Journal of Gastroenterology.* 2006; 12(32): 5101–7.
232 Correa P, Houghton J. Carcinogenesis of Helicobacter pylori. *Gastroenterology.* 2007; 133(2): 659–72.
233 Lochhead P, El-Omar EM. Helicobacter pylori infection and gastric cancer. *Best Practice and Research. Clinical Gastroenterology.* 2007; 21(2): 281–97.
234 de Vries AC, Haringsma J, Kuipers EJ. The detection, surveillance and treatment of premalignant gastric lesions related to Helicobacter pylori infection. *Helicobacter.* 2007; 12(1): 1–15.
235 Tatematsu M, Tsukamoto T, Toyoda T. Effects of eradication of Helicobacter pylori on gastric carcinogenesis in experimental models. *Journal of Gastroenterology.* 2007; 42(suppl 17): 7–9.
236 Pritchard DM, Crabtree JE. Helicobacter pylori and gastric cancer. *Current Opinion in Gastroenterology.* 2006; 22(6): 620–5.
237 Singh K, Ghoshal UC. Causal role of Helicobacter pylori infection in gastric cancer: an Asian enigma. *World Journal of Gastroenterology.* 2006; 12(9): 1346–51.
238 Lochhead P, El-Omar EM. Helicobacter pylori infection and gastric cancer. *Best Practice and Research. Clinical Gastroenterology.* 2007; 21(2): 281–97.
239 Matsuzaka M, Fukuda S, Takahashi I et al. The decreasing burden of gastric cancer in Japan. *Tohoku Journal of Experimental Medicine.* 2007; 212(3): 207–19.
240 Leung WK, Sung JJ. Chemoprevention of gastric cancer. *European Journal of Gastroenterology and Hepatology.* 2006; 18(8): 867–71.
241 Chmiela M, Michetti P. Inflammation, immunity, vaccines for Helicobacter infection. *Helicobacter.* 2006; 11(suppl 1): 21–6.
242 Malaty HM. Epidemiology of Helicobacter pylori infection. *Best Practice and Research. Clinical Gastroenterology.* 2007; 21(2): 205–14.

243 Milne AN, Sitarz R, Carvalho R et al. Early onset gastric cancer: on the road to unraveling gastric carcinogenesis. *Current Molecular Medicine*. 2007; 7(1): 15–28.
244 Smith MG, Hold GL, Tahara E et al. Cellular and molecular aspects of gastric cancer. *World Journal of Gastroenterology*. 2006; 12(19): 2979–90.
245 Matysiak-Budnik T, Megraud F. Helicobacter pylori infection and gastric cancer. *European Journal of Cancer*. 2006; 42(6): 708–16.
246 Tan YK, Fielding JW. Early diagnosis of early gastric cancer. *European Journal of Gastroenterology and Hepatology*. 2006; 18: 821–9.
247 Ricci C, Holton J, Vaira D. Diagnosis of Helicobacter pylori: invasive and non-invasive tests. *Best Practice and Research. Clinical Gastroenterology*. 2007; 21(2): 299–313.
248 Dzierzanowska-Fangrat K, Lehours P, Megraud F et al. Diagnosis of Helicobacter pylori infection. *Helicobacter*. 2006; 11(suppl 1): 6–13.
249 Gisbert JP, Pajares JM. Review article: C-urea breath test in the diagnosis of Helicobacter pylori infection—a critical review. *Alimentary Pharmacology and Therapeutics*. 2004; 20(10): 1001–17.
250 Ren Z, Borody T, Pang G et al. Evaluation of anti-Helicobacter pylori IgG2 antibody for the diagnosis of Helicobacter pylori infection in western and Chinese populations. *Alimentary Pharmacology and Therapeutics*. 2005; 21(1): 83–9.
251 Tucci A, Tucci P, Bisceglia M et al. Real-time detection of Helicobacter Pylori infection and atrophic gastritis: comparison between conventional methods and a novel device for gastric juice analysis during endoscopy. *Endoscopy*. 2005; 37(10): 966–76.
252 Nyan DC, Welch AR, Dubois A et al. Development of a noninvasive method for detecting and monitoring the time course of Helicobacter pylori infection. *Infection and Immunity*. 2004; 72(9): 5358–64.
253 Kabir S. Detection of Helicobacter pylori DNA in feces and saliva by polymerase chain reaction: a review. *Helicobacter*. 2004; 9(2): 115–23.
254 Ricci C, Holton J, Vaira D. Diagnosis of Helicobacter pylori: invasive and non-invasive tests. *Best Practice and Research. Clinical Gastroenterology*. 2007; 21(2): 299–313.
255 Malfertheiner P, Megraud F, O'Morain C et al. Current concepts in the management of Helicobacter pylori infection: the Maastricht III Consensus Report. *Gut*. 2007; 56(6): 772–81.
256 Yan J, Mao YF, Shao ZX. Frequencies of the expression of main protein antigens from Helicobacter pylori isolates and production of specific serum antibodies in infected patients. *World Journal of Gastroenterology*. 2005; 11(3): 421–5.
257 Han FC, Li XJ, Jiang H et al. Detection of H. pylori antibody profile in serum by protein array. *World Journal of Gastroenterology*. 2006; 12(25): 4044–8.
258 Simala-Grant JL, Taylor DE. Molecular biology methods for the characterization of Helicobacter pylori infections and their diagnosis. *Acta Pathologica, Microbiologica, et Immunologica Scandinavica*. 2004; 112(11–12): 886–97.
259 Sipponen P, Graham DY. Importance of atrophic gastritis in diagnostics and prevention of gastric cancer: application of plasma biomarkers. *Scandinavian Journal of Gastroenterology*. 2007; 42(1): 2–10.
260 Plebani M, Basso D. Non-invasive assessment of chronic liver and gastric diseases. *Clinica Chimica Acta*. 2007; 381(1): 39–49.

261 Miki K. Gastric cancer screening using the serum pepsinogen test method. *Gastric Cancer.* 2006; 9(4): 245–53.
262 Gatta L, Ricci C, Tampieri A et al. Accuracy of breath tests using low doses of 13C-urea to diagnose Helicobacter pylori infection: a randomised controlled trial. *Gut.* 2006; 55(4): 457–62.
263 Hooton C, Keohane J, Clair J et al. Comparison of three stool antigen assays with the 13C- urea breath test for the primary diagnosis of Helicobacter pylori infection and monitoring treatment outcome. *European Journal of Gastroenterology and Hepatology.* 2006; 18(6): 595–9.
264 Cirak MY, Akyon Y, Megraud F. Diagnosis of Helicobacter pylori. *Helicobacter.* 2007; 12(suppl 1): 4–9.
265 Elwyn G, Taubert M, Davies S et al. Which test is best for Helicobacter pylori? A cost-effectiveness model using decision analysis. *British Journal of General Practice.* 2007; 57(538): 401–3.
266 Rasool S, Abid S, Jafri W. Validity and cost comparison of 14carbon urea breath test for diagnosis of H Pylori in dyspeptic patients. *World Journal of Gastroenterology.* 2007; 13(6): 925–9.
267 Ricci C, Holton J, Vaira D. Diagnosis of Helicobacter pylori: invasive and non-invasive tests. *Best Practice and Research. Clinical Gastroenterology.* 2007; 21(2): 299–313.
268 Gisbert JP, Abraira V. Accuracy of Helicobacter pylori diagnostic tests in patients with bleeding peptic ulcer: a systematic review and meta-analysis. *American Journal of Gastroenterology.* 2006; 101(4): 848–63.
269 Tseng CA, Wang WM, Wu DC. Comparison of the clinical feasibility of three rapid urease tests in the diagnosis of Helicobacter pylori infection. *Digestive Diseases and Sciences.* 2005; 50(3): 449–52.
270 Yakoob J, Abid S, Jafri W et al. Comparison of biopsy-based methods for the detection of Helicobacter pylori infection. *British Journal of Biomedical Science.* 2006; 63(4): 159–62.
271 Garcia-Altes A, Rota R, Barenys M et al. Cost-effectiveness of a 'score and scope' strategy for the management of dyspepsia. *European Journal of Gastroenterology and Hepatology.* 2005; 17(7): 709–19.
272 Roderick P, Davies R, Raftery J et al. Cost-effectiveness of population screening for Helicobacter pylori in preventing gastric cancer and peptic ulcer disease, using simulation. *Journal of Medical Screening.* 2003; 10(3): 148–56.
273 Davies R, Crabbe D, Roderick P et al. A simulation to evaluate screening for Helicobacter pylori infection in the prevention of peptic ulcers and gastric cancers. *Health Care Management Science.* 2002; 5(4): 249–58.
274 Lane JA, Murray LJ, Noble S et al. Impact of Helicobacter pylori eradication on dyspepsia, health resource use, and quality of life in the Bristol helicobacter project: randomised controlled trial. *British Medical Journal.* 2006; 332(7535): 199–204.
275 Tan YK, Fielding JW. Early diagnosis of early gastric cancer. *European Journal of Gastroenterology and Hepatology.* 2006; 18(8): 821–9.
276 Mason JM, Moayyedi P, Young PJ et al. Population-based and opportunistic screening and eradication of Helicobacter pylori. An analysis using trial baseline data. Leeds H. pylori Study Group. *International Journal of Technology Assessment in Health Care.* 1999; 15(4): 649–60.
277 Leja M, Dumitrascu DL. Should we screen for Helicobacter pylori to prevent gastric cancer? *Digestive Diseases.* 2007; 25(3): 218–21.

278 Malfertheiner P, Megraud F, O'Morain C et al. Current concepts in the management of Helicobacter pylori infection: the Maastricht III Consensus Report. *Gut.* 2007; 56(6): 772–81.
279 Plebani M, Basso D. Non-invasive assessment of chronic liver and gastric diseases. *Clinica Chimica Acta.* 2007; 381(1): 39–49.
280 Malfertheiner P, Megraud F, O'Morain C et al. Current concepts in the management of Helicobacter pylori infection: the Maastricht III Consensus Report. *Gut.* 2007; 56(6): 772–81.
281 Briggs AH, Sculpher MJ, Logan RP et al. Cost effectiveness of screening for and eradication of Helicobacter pylori in management of dyspeptic patients under 45 years of age. *British Medical Journal.* 1996; 312(7042): 1321–5.
282 Mason JM, Moayyedi P, Young PJ et al. Population-based and opportunistic screening and eradication of Helicobacter pylori. An analysis using trial baseline data. Leeds H. pylori Study Group. *International Journal of Technology Assessment in Health Care.* 1999; 15(4): 649–60.
283 Ford AC, Forman D, Nathan J et al. Clinical trial: knowledge of negative Helicobacter pylori status reduces subsequent dyspepsia-related resource use. *Alimentary Pharmacology and Therapeutics.* 2007; 26(9): 1267–75.
284 Hu WH, Lam SK, Lam CL et al. Comparison between empirical prokinetics, Helicobacter test-and-treat and empirical endoscopy in primary-care patients presenting with dyspepsia: a one-year study. *World Journal of Gastroenterology.* 2006; 12(31): 5010–6.
285 Klok RM, Arents NL, de Vries R et al. Economic evaluation of a randomized trial comparing Helicobacter pylori test-and-treat and prompt endoscopy strategies for managing dyspepsia in a primary-care setting. *Clinical Therapeutics.* 2005; 27(10): 1647–57.
286 Nardone G, Rocco A, Compare D et al. Is screening for and surveillance of atrophic gastritis advisable? *Digestive Diseases.* 2007; 25(3): 214–7.
287 Lahner E, Vaira D, Figura N et al. Role of noninvasive tests (C-urea breath test and stool antigen test) as additional tools in diagnosis of Helicobacter pylori infection in patients with atrophic body gastritis. *Helicobacter.* 2004; 9(5): 436–42.
288 Korstanje A, van Eeden S, Offerhaus GJ et al. The 13carbon urea breath test for the diagnosis of Helicobacter pylori infection in subjects with atrophic gastritis: evaluation in a primary care setting. *Alimentary Pharmacology and Therapeutics.* 2006; 24(4): 643–50.
289 Dan YY, So JB, Yeoh KG. Endoscopic screening for gastric cancer. *Clinical Gastroenterology and Hepatology.* 2006; 4(6): 709–16.
290 Plebani M, Basso D. Non-invasive assessment of chronic liver and gastric diseases. *Clinica Chimica Acta.* 2007; 381(1): 39–49.
291 Malfertheiner P, Megraud F, O'Morain C et al. Current concepts in the management of Helicobacter pylori infection: the Maastricht III Consensus Report. *Gut.* 2007; 56(6): 772–81.
292 Hooton C, Keohane J, Clair J et al. Comparison of three stool antigen assays with the 13C- urea breath test for the primary diagnosis of Helicobacter pylori infection and monitoring treatment outcome. *European Journal of Gastroenterology and Hepatology.* 2006; 18(6): 595–9.
293 Paimela HM, Oksala NK, Kaariainen IP et al. Faecal antigen tests in the confirmation of the effect of Helicobacter eradication therapy. *Annals of Medicine.* 2006; 38(5): 352–6.

294 Tokudome S, Hosono A, Suzuki S. Population-attributable fractions in gastric cancer risk factors: the necessity to focus on Helicobacter pylori infection. *Gastric Cancer.* 2006; 9(3): 240–1.
295 Brown LM. Helicobacter pylori: epidemiology and routes of transmission. *Epidemiologic Reviews.* 2000; 22(2): 283–97.
296 Bellack NR, Koehoorn MW, MacNab YC et al. A conceptual model of water's role as a reservoir in Helicobacter pylori transmission: a review of the evidence. *Epidemiology and Infection.* 2006; 134(3): 439–49.
297 Ashbolt NJ. Microbial contamination of drinking water and disease outcomes in developing regions. *Toxicology.* 2004; 198(1–3): 229–38.
298 Svennerholm AM, Lundgren A. Progress in vaccine development against Helicobacter pylori. *FEMS Immunology and Medical Microbiology.* 2007; 50(2): 146–56.
299 Wilson KT, Crabtree JE. Immunology of Helicobacter pylori: insights into the failure of the immune response and perspectives on vaccine studies. *Gastroenterology.* 2007; 133(1): 288–308.
300 Svennerholm AM, Lundgren A. Progress in vaccine development against Helicobacter pylori. *FEMS Immunology and Medical Microbiology.* 2007; 50(2): 146–56.
301 Kabir S. The current status of Helicobacter pylori vaccines: a review. *Helicobacter.* 2007; 12(2): 89–102.
302 Rupnow MF, Shachter RD, Owens DK et al. Quantifying the population impact of a prophylactic Helicobacter pylori vaccine. *Vaccine.* 2001; 20(5–6): 879–85.
303 Rupnow MF, Owens DK, Shachter R et al. Helicobacter pylori vaccine development and use: a cost-effectiveness analysis using the Institute of Medicine Methodology. *Helicobacter.* 1999; 4(4): 272–80.
304 Chmiela M, Michetti P. Inflammation, immunity, vaccines for Helicobacter infection. *Helicobacter.* 2006; 11(suppl 1): 21–6.
305 Wilson KT, Crabtree JE. Immunology of Helicobacter pylori: insights into the failure of the immune response and perspectives on vaccine studies. *Gastroenterology.* 2007; 133(1): 288–308.
306 Aebischer T, Schmitt A, Walduck AK et al. Helicobacter pylori vaccine development: facing the challenge. *International Journal of Medical Microbiology.* 2005; 295(5): 343–53.
307 Prinz C, Schwendy S, Voland P. H pylori and gastric cancer: shifting the global burden. *World Journal of Gastroenterology.* 2006; 12(34): 5458–64.
308 Moayyedi P, Soo S, Deeks J et al. Eradication of Helicobacter pylori for non-ulcer dyspepsia. *Cochrane Database of Systematic Reviews.* 2006.
309 Pera M, Manterola C, Vidal O et al. Epidemiology of esophageal adenocarcinoma. *Journal of Surgical Oncology.* 2005; 92(3): 151–9.
310 Holmes RS, Vaughan TL. Epidemiology and pathogenesis of esophageal cancer. *Seminars in Radiation Oncology.* 2007; 17(1): 2–9.
311 Kuipers EJ. Proton pump inhibitors and Helicobacter pylori gastritis: friends or foes? *Basic and Clinical Pharmacology and Toxicology.* 2006; 99(3): 187–94.
312 Megraud F, Lehours P. Helicobacter pylori and gastric cancer prevention is possible. *Cancer Detection and Prevention.* 2004; 28(6): 392–8.
313 Prinz C, Schwendy S, Voland P. H pylori and gastric cancer: shifting the global burden. *World Journal of Gastroenterology.* 2006; 12(34): 5458–64.

314 Henrik Siman J, Forsgren A, Berglund G et al. Helicobacter pylori infection is associated with a decreased risk of developing oesophageal neoplasms. *Helicobacter.* 2001; 6(4): 310–6.
315 Megraud F, Lehours P. Helicobacter pylori and gastric cancer prevention is possible. *Cancer Detection and Prevention.* 2004; 28(6): 392–8.
316 Suzuki H, Hibi T, Marshall BJ. Helicobacter pylori: present status and future prospects in Japan. *Journal of Gastroenterology.* 2007; 42(1): 1–15.
317 Prinz C, Schwendy S, Voland P. H pylori and gastric cancer: shifting the global burden. *World Journal of Gastroenterology.* 2006; 12(34): 5458–64.
318 Sugano K. Prevention of gastric cancer: urgent need to implement Helicobacter pylori eradication therapy as a primary preventive measure in Japan. *Journal of Gastroenterology.* 2007; 42(suppl 17): 1–2.
319 Ahuja V. The case for Helicobacter pylori eradication in India: sensationalism, skepticism and scientific salesmanship. *Indian Journal of Gastroenterology.* 2006; 25(1): 20–4.
320 Ramakrishna BS. Helicobacter pylori infection in India: the case against eradication. *Indian Journal of Gastroenterology.* 2006; 25(1): 25–8.
321 Tsugane S, Sasazuki S. Diet and the risk of gastric cancer: review of epidemiological evidence. *Gastric Cancer.* 2007; 10(2): 75–83.
322 Kato S, Tsukamoto T, Mizoshita T et al. High salt diets dose-dependently promote gastric chemical carcinogenesis in Helicobacter pylori-infected Mongolian gerbils associated with a shift in mucin production from glandular to surface mucous cells. *International Journal of Cancer.* 2006; 119(7): 1558–66.
323 Shikata K, Kiyohara Y, Kubo M et al. A prospective study of dietary salt intake and gastric cancer incidence in a defined Japanese population: the Hisayama study. *International Journal of Cancer.* 2006; 119(1): 196–201.
324 Machida-Montani A, Sasazuki S, Inoue M et al. Association of Helicobacter pylori infection and environmental factors in non-cardia gastric cancer in Japan. *Gastric Cancer.* 2004; 7(1): 46–53.
325 Brenner H, Arndt V, Bode G et al. Risk of gastric cancer among smokers infected with Helicobacter pylori. *International Journal of Cancer.* 2002; 98(3): 446–9.
326 Matsuzaka M, Fukuda S, Takahashi I et al. The decreasing burden of gastric cancer in Japan. *Tohoku Journal of Experimental Medicine.* 2007; 212(3): 207–19.
327 Romano M, Ricci V, Zarrilli R. Mechanisms of disease: Helicobacter pylori-related gastric carcinogenesis—implications for chemoprevention. *Nature Clinical Practice.* 2006; 3(11): 622–32.
328 Bjelakovic G, Nikolova D, Simonetti RG et al. Antioxidant supplements for preventing gastrointestinal cancers. *Cochrane Database of Systematic Reviews.* 2007.
329 Murray LJ, Lane AJ, Harvey IM et al. Inverse relationship between alcohol consumption and active Helicobacter pylori infection: the Bristol Helicobacter project. *American Journal of Gastroenterology.* 2002; 97(11): 2750–5.
330 Gikas A, Triantafillidis JK, Apostolidis N et al. Relationship of smoking and coffee and alcohol consumption with seroconversion to Helicobacter pylori: a longitudinal study in hospital workers. *Journal of Gastroenterology and Hepatology.* 2004; 19(8): 927–33.

331 Luzza F, Imeneo M, Maletta M et al. Smoking, alcohol and coffee consumption, and H pylori infection. Alcohol consumption eliminates rather than prevents infection with H pylori. *British Medical Journal.* 1998; 316(7136): 1019.
332 Ables AZ, Simon I, Melton ER. Update on Helicobacter pylori treatment. *American Family Physician.* 2007; 75(3): 351–8.
333 Leung WK, Sung JJ. Chemoprevention of gastric cancer. *European Journal of Gastroenterology and Hepatology.* 2006; 18(8): 867–71.
334 Dai Y, Wang WH. Non-steroidal anti-inflammatory drugs in prevention of gastric cancer. *World Journal of Gastroenterology.* 2006; 12(18): 2884–9.
335 Hwang HJ, Youn YH, Kim JH et al. Low-dose aspirin affects the clinicopathological features of gastric cancer. *Digestion.* 2006; 73(1): 54–9.
336 Lanas A, Hunt R. Prevention of anti-inflammatory drug-induced gastrointestinal damage: benefits and risks of therapeutic strategies. *Annals of Medicine.* 2006; 38(6): 415–28.
337 Lanas A, Scheiman J. Low-dose aspirin and upper gastrointestinal damage: epidemiology, prevention and treatment. *Current Medical Research and Opinion.* 2007; 23(1): 163–73.
338 Vonkeman HE, Klok RM, Postma MJ et al. Direct medical costs of serious gastrointestinal ulcers among users of NSAIDs. *Drugs and Aging.* 2007; 24(8): 681–90.
339 Kuipers EJ. Proton pump inhibitors and Helicobacter pylori gastritis: friends or foes? *Basic and Clinical Pharmacology and Toxicology.* 2006; 99(3): 187–94.
340 Futagami S, Suzuki K, Hiratsuka T et al. Chemopreventive effect of celecoxib in gastric cancer. *Inflammopharmacology.* 2007; 15(1): 1–4.
341 Fischbach LA, Correa P, Ramirez H et al. Anti-inflammatory and tissue-protectant drug effects: results from a randomized placebo-controlled trial of gastritis patients at high risk for gastric cancer. *Alimentary Pharmacology and Therapeutics.* 2001; 15(6): 831–41.
342 Chui SY, Clay TM, Lyerly HK et al. The development of therapeutic and preventive vaccines for gastric cancer and Helicobacter pylori. *Cancer Epidemiology, Biomarkers and Prevention.* 2005; 14(8): 1883–9.
343 Rodgers C, van Zanten SV. A meta-analysis of the success rate of Helicobacter pylori therapy in Canada. *Canadian Journal of Gastroenterology.* 2007; 21(5): 295–300.
344 Kato M, Asaka M, Ono S et al. Eradication of Helicobacter pylori for primary gastric cancer and secondary gastric cancer after endoscopic mucosal resection. *Journal of Gastroenterology.* 2007; 42(suppl 17): 16–20.
345 Ables AZ, Simon I, Melton ER. Update on Helicobacter pylori treatment. *American Family Physician.* 2007; 75(3): 351–8.
346 Lochhead P, El-Omar EM. Helicobacter pylori infection and gastric cancer. *Best Practice and Research. Clinical Gastroenterology.* 2007; 21(2): 281–97.
347 Kuipers EJ, Sipponen P. Helicobacter pylori eradication for the prevention of gastric cancer. *Helicobacter.* 2006; 11(suppl 1): 52–7.
348 Tan YK, Fielding JW. Early diagnosis of early gastric cancer. *European Journal of Gastroenterology and Hepatology.* 2006; 18(8): 821–9.
349 Murakami K, Kodama M, Fujioka T. Latest insights into the effects of Helicobacter pylori infection on gastric carcinogenesis. *World Journal of Gastroenterology.* 2006; 12(17): 2713–20.

350 Lochhead P, El-Omar EM. Helicobacter pylori infection and gastric cancer. *Best Practice and Research. Clinical Gastroenterology.* 2007; 21(2): 281–97.
351 Leemans WF, Janssen HL, de Man RA. Future prospectives for the management of chronic hepatitis B. *World Journal of Gastroenterology.* 2007; 13(18): 2554–67.
352 Malfertheiner P, Megraud F, O'Morain C et al. Current concepts in the management of Helicobacter pylori infection: the Maastricht III Consensus Report. *Gut.* 2007; 56(6): 772–81.
353 Prinz C, Schwendy S, Voland P. H pylori and gastric cancer: shifting the global burden. *World Journal of Gastroenterology.* 2006; 12(34): 5458–64.
354 Wong BC, Lam SK, Wong WM et al. Helicobacter pylori eradication to prevent gastric cancer in a high-risk region of China: a randomized controlled trial. *Journal of the American Medical Association.* 2004; 291(2): 187–94.
355 Svennerholm AM, Lundgren A. Progress in vaccine development against Helicobacter pylori. *FEMS Immunology and Medical Microbiology.* 2007; 50(2): 146–56.
356 Magalhaes Queiroz DM, Luzza F. Epidemiology of Helicobacter pylori infection. *Helicobacter.* 2006; 11(suppl 1): 1–5.
357 Dubois A, Boren T. Helicobacter pylori is invasive and it may be a facultative intracellular organism. *Cellular Microbiology.* 2007; 9(5): 1108–16.
358 Gerrits MM, van Vliet AH, Kuipers EJ et al. Helicobacter pylori and antimicrobial resistance: molecular mechanisms and clinical implications. *Lancet Infectious Diseases.* 2006; 6(11): 699–709.
359 Hunt RH, Smaill FM, Fallone CA et al. Implications of antibiotic resistance in the management of Helicobacter pylori infection: Canadian Helicobacter Study Group. *Canadian Journal of Gastroenterology.* 2000; 14(10): 862–8.
360 Yilmaz O, Demiray E. Clinical role and importance of fluorescence in situ hybridization method in diagnosis of H pylori infection and determination of clarithromycin resistance in H pylori eradication therapy. *World Journal of Gastroenterology.* 2007; 13(5): 671–5.
361 Fallone CA. Epidemiology of the antibiotic resistance of Helicobacter pylori in Canada. *Canadian Journal of Gastroenterology.* 2000; 14(10): 879–82.
362 Hunt RH, Smaill FM, Fallone CA et al. Implications of antibiotic resistance in the management of Helicobacter pylori infection: Canadian Helicobacter Study Group. *Canadian Journal of Gastroenterology.* 2000; 14(10): 862–8.
363 McLoughlin RM, O'Morain CA, O'Connor HJ. Eradication of Helicobacter pylori: recent advances in treatment. *Fundamental and Clinical Pharmacology.* 2005; 19(4): 421–7.
364 Wolle K, Malfertheiner P. Treatment of Helicobacter pylori. *Best Practice and Research. Clinical Gastroenterology.* 2007; 21(2): 315–24.
365 Broutet N, Tchamgoue S, Pereira E et al. Risk factors for failure of Helicobacter pylori therapy—results of an individual data analysis of 2751 patients. *Alimentary Pharmacology and Therapeutics.* 2003; 17(1): 99–109.
366 Beswick EJ, Suarez G, Reyes VE. H pylori and host interactions that influence pathogenesis. *World Journal of Gastroenterology.* 2006; 12(35): 5599–605.
367 Sagaert X, De Wolf-Peeters C, Noels H et al. The pathogenesis of MALT lymphomas: where do we stand? *Leukemia.* 2007; 21(3): 389–96.
368 Stolte M, Bayerdorffer E, Morgner A et al. Helicobacter and gastric MALT lymphoma. *Gut.* 2002; 50(suppl 3): III19–24.

369 Montalban C, Santon A, Redondo C et al. Long-term persistence of molecular disease after histological remission in low-grade gastric MALT lymphoma treated with H. pylori eradication. Lack of association with translocation t(11;18): a 10-year updated follow-up of a prospective study. *Annals of Oncology*. 2005; 16(9): 1539–44.

370 Zucca E, Cavalli F. Are antibiotics the treatment of choice for gastric lymphoma? *Current Hematology Reports*. 2004; 3(1): 11–6.

371 Grunberger B, Wohrer S, Streubel B et al. Antibiotic treatment is not effective in patients infected with Helicobacter pylori suffering from extragastric MALT lymphoma. *Journal of Clinical Oncology*. 2006; 24(9): 1370–5.

372 Leung WK, Sung JJ. Chemoprevention of gastric cancer. *European Journal of Gastroenterology and Hepatology*. 2006; 18(8): 867–71.

373 Nardone G, Rocco A. Chemoprevention of gastric cancer: role of COX-2 inhibitors and other agents. *Digestive Diseases*. 2004; 22(4): 320–6.

374 Romano M, Ricci V, Zarrilli R. Mechanisms of disease: Helicobacter pylori-related gastric carcinogenesis—implications for chemoprevention. *Nature Clinical Practice*. 2006; 3(11): 622–32.

375 Leung WK, Sung JJ. Chemoprevention of gastric cancer. *European Journal of Gastroenterology and Hepatology*. 2006; 18(8): 867–71.

376 Grau MV, Rees JR, Baron JA. Chemoprevention in gastrointestinal cancers: current status. *Basic and Clinical Pharmacology and Toxicology*. 2006; 98(3): 281–7.

377 Nardone G, Rocco A. Chemoprevention of gastric cancer: role of COX-2 inhibitors and other agents. *Digestive Diseases*. 2004; 22(4): 320–6.

378 Brownstein JS, Sordo M, Kohane IS et al. The tell-tale heart: population-based surveillance reveals an association of rofecoxib and celecoxib with myocardial infarction. *PLoS ONE*. 2007; 2(9): e840.

379 You WC, Li JY, Zhang L et al. Etiology and prevention of gastric cancer: a population study in a high risk area of China. *Chinese Journal of Digestive Diseases*. 2005; 6(4): 149–54.

380 Fischbach LA, Correa P, Ramirez H et al. Anti-inflammatory and tissue-protectant drug effects: results from a randomized placebo-controlled trial of gastritis patients at high risk for gastric cancer. *Alimentary Pharmacology and Therapeutics*. 2001; 15(6): 831–41.

381 Lin DC. Probiotics as functional foods. *Nutrition in Clinical Practice*. 2003; 18(6): 497–506.

382 Lesbros-Pantoflickova D, Corthesy-Theulaz I, Blum AL. Helicobacter pylori and probiotics. *Journal of Nutrition*. 2007; 137(3 suppl 2): 812S–8S.

383 Gotteland M, Brunser O, Cruchet S. Systematic review: are probiotics useful in controlling gastric colonization by Helicobacter pylori? *Alimentary Pharmacology and Therapeutics*. 2006; 23(8): 1077–86.

384 van Lier EA, van Kranen HJ, van Vliet JA et al. Estimated number of new cancer cases attributable to infection in the Netherlands in 2003. *Cancer Letters*. 2008; 272(2): 226–31.

385 Axon A. How to influence health providers. *Helicobacter*. 2007; 12(suppl 2): 80–4.

386 Mbulaiteye SM, Hisada M, El-Omar EM. Helicobacter Pylori associated global gastric cancer burden. *Frontiers in Bioscience*. 2009; 14: 1490–504.

10

EPSTEIN-BARR VIRUS

Epstein-Barr virus is a ubiquitous human pathogen that usually maintains a harmonious relationship with its host. Rarely, this host–virus balance is perturbed, causing a diverse group of malignancies in both immunocompetent and immunosuppressed patients.[1]

INTRODUCTION

Epstein-Barr virus is also known by the more "taxonomically transparent" label of human herpesvirus type 4 (HHV-4). The better known, eponymous name can be traced to two of the researchers who first investigated the virus, MA Epstein and YM Barr.[2] Epstein-Barr virus (EBV) is the label used consistently in this book.

EBV is often recognized as the human tumor virus first identified (with only the discovery of hepatitis B competing to be of the same vintage). EBV was isolated in 1964 from a lymphoma that commonly afflicts children in sub-Saharan Africa.[3] This cancer was described by the surgeon Denis Burkitt (after whom it is named), though several other researchers were also involved.[4] Since that time, EBV has been implicated in a wide variety of cancers, most of which emerge years after the primary infection.[5]

About 100 herpesviruses have been isolated, but it appears that only 8 types infect humans. The best known of these are the herpes simplex viruses, types 1 and 2. As noted in the "Introduction" to this book, all the human herpesviruses have been investigated for a cancer connection, but so far only one other, HHV-8, has been strongly confirmed as a carcinogenic agent. More information on HHV-8, and the human herpesviruses as a whole, may be found in Chapter 11.

EBV is a ubiquitous virus that infects the majority of people in the world by the time they reach adulthood.[6] Some studies suggest that over 95% of adults in the world are EBV-positive.[7] This means that it is unusual not to be infected with EBV. The very high prevalence rate is driven by two main factors: relative ease of transmission and lifelong persistence of infection.[8,9]

Fortunately, most EBV carriers are asymptomatic. The virus is best known for prompting an immune response in infected adolescents that is marked by acute infectious mononucleosis (IM), colloquially referred to as "mono" or sometimes "kissing disease" (because of the presumed behavior leading to transmission). The triggering mechanisms that cause a small proportion of infected individuals to develop one of a wide spectrum of malignancies remain unclear. Driven by the hope of discovering preventive and therapeutic strategies, untangling EBV cancer pathways remains an intense research focus.[10,11]

THE VIRUS

EBV, a linear double-stranded DNA virus, has been known to exist in the human population in two main genetic forms, usually referred to as A and B, with the first type (or EBV-A) predominating.[12] Other genetic variations have been identified, an area of research that has only accelerated with the advent of new molecular investigation techniques.[13,14] There is evidence that EBV subtypes and variants exhibit different geographic distributions, preferential disease associations, and/or variable influences on the clinical behavior of specific malignancies.[15-21] For example, EBV-A seems to be prevalent in Burkitt lymphoma (BL) in some jurisdictions.[22,23] Furthermore, there have long been suggestions that EBV-B exhibits a tropism for nasopharyngeal epithelial cells (and related cancer), although other studies have questioned this conclusion.[24,25] More recently, EBV-B has been connected to oral squamous cell carcinoma in an isolated geographic setting, namely, Japan's island of Okinawa.[26] EBV genetic variants continue to be refined, both in terms of transforming potential (based on experimental cell lines) and epidemiologic linkages—especially in the context of nasopharyngeal carcinoma (NPC).[27,28]

Despite the volume of emerging evidence, the characterization of disease-specific associations with EBV subtypes and variants remains incomplete. Some researchers remain unconvinced that there are any connections among EBV genetic variation, preferred cellular targets, and disease development. A recent review noted that "there is a lack of large, well-designed epidemiologic studies of risk associations with EBV variants."[29] This means, for example, that the dramatic differences found in the rate of NPC across geographical regions[30] may be attributable to differences in host genetics or environmental cofactors rather than EBV type variation. In other words, the geographic distribution of EBV genetic variants may be ultimately confirmed as having little bearing on disease susceptibility.[31]

The herpesviruses as a group will be further outlined in the next chapter on human herpesvirus type 8 (HHV-8). For now, it will suffice to note that herpesviruses such as EBV, herpes simplex virus, and HHV-6 have a marked tropism for cells of the immune system.[32] Furthermore, unlike the categories known as alpha- and beta-herpesviruses, the gamma-herpesvirus (which includes EBV and HHV-8) are geared toward B lymphocyte infection.[33] It will become clear that this is only the beginning of what is known about EBV natural history and biology.

EVIDENCE OF ASSOCIATED CANCERS

After more than 40 years of research, the information that has emerged concerning EBV and carcinogenesis is very complex.[34,35] One conclusion at least is clear: as indicated in Table 10.4 at the end of this chapter, the list of candidate cancer associations has greatly expanded beyond the two classic connections discovered in the 1960s, that is, endemic BL and NPC.[36,37] According to the oft-quoted analysis of infection and cancer produced by Parkin in 2006, about one out of every 100 cancers in the world may be attributed to EBV.[38] The range of cancers making up this complement is remarkable.

Consistent with the discussion about disease processes to follow, one review suggested that since "the complexity and duration of EBV-host interaction provides numerous possibilities for a malignant outcome, the heterogeneity of the cancers associated with EBV is not surprising."[39] Determining the full range of the EBV-carcinogenesis connection has required painstaking research. The nature of EBV infection—which involves "strategies to minimize or eliminate its pathogenic potential, in the interest of maintaining infection and the survival of the host"[40]—means that causal associations between the virus and disease have been difficult to prove. One intriguing challenge in the identification of EBV in cancerous tissues involves ensuring that the virus has not simply "come along for the ride" as a latent infection within immune cells that are contributing to an inflammatory response.[41,42] The presence of EBV as a passenger in cancerous tissue has been especially raised in the context of controversial disease associations, such as breast cancer.[43]

The malignancies where an EBV etiologic linkage has been best established will be reviewed first, starting with the origin of the EBV disease story, the lymphoma first identified among African children by Burkitt.

Burkitt Lymphoma

Burkitt lymphoma[44] is a B-cell non-Hodgkin's lymphoma (NHL) usually classified under three headings; each category represents different geographic distribution and viral involvement (Table 10.1).[45,46]

Nonendemic BL is the version of the disorder seen most often in Western countries. It is still rare in such settings, although incidence has recently increased. The escalating rates have been attributed to expanding cases of immunosuppression associated with HIV/AIDS. Compared to the endemic type of BL found in Africa, the HIV-associated form is not as closely related to EBV; less than 40% of cases are positive for the virus, whereas African children with the disease demonstrate essentially 100% EBV involvement.[47,48]

In light of this book's focus on the infectious causes of cancer, the apparent association of endemic BL with malaria is of particular interest. In fact, in an effort to understand the epidemiology of BL in a region such as equatorial Africa, a number of cofactors have been investigated. While malaria is the most well-established candidate, researchers are realizing that other factors are probably required to explain why BL is

Table 10.1. Characteristics of Burkitt Lymphoma Types

	Endemic	*Sporadic*	*HIV-associated*
Geography	Equatorial Africa, Papua New Guinea	Worldwide	Worldwide
Prevalence (per 100,000)	1–20	0.01	Variable (related to HIV prevalence)
Age range	2–14 years	All ages	All ages
EBV association	98%	5–10%	30–40%
Cofactor	Malaria coinfection		HIV infection
Tissue site	Extranodal	Lymph node	Lymph node
Most common body site(s)	Jaw	Abdomen	Abdomen, bone marrow

Source: Brady et al., *Journal of Clinical Pathology*, 2007.

not much more common than it is. This has led to the remarkable suggestion that at least one of the other cofactors for BL is also an infection, specifically involving certain arboviruses[49] that share the same insect vector that carries the protozoan parasite causing malaria.[50] If true, this would position BL as a unique instance of cancer with a polymicrobial origin comprising at least three infections.

Hodgkin's Disease and Non-Hodgkin's Lymphomas

Suspicion of an infectious cause for Hodgkin's disease (HD) is "almost as old as the recognition of the disease as such."[51] EBV has been implicated in HD, though positivity for the virus varies from 10% to 95% depending on the specific disease subtype. About half of the Hodgkin's cases in the United States demonstrate the presence of EBV. However, the rate goes up to 95% in HIV-associated cases.[52] Although technically not considered an AIDS-defining condition, in the developed world HD competes with Kaposi sarcoma as the cancer most often diagnosed in HIV-positive individuals.[53] While being immunocompromised appears to be an important factor in HD caused by EBV, coinfection with HIV does not explain the entire presentation of disease. Indeed, EBV-positive HD seems to result from an "intricate interplay of early- and later-life environmental, hormonal, and genetic factors."[54]

A subset of HD appears to not be caused by EBV; this group constitutes 30–50% of cases in the developed world, and over 90% in developing countries.[55] The search for another infectious cause for this type of HD has proven to be elusive. Proposed agents include the measles virus, where the evidence has been mixed,[56,57] and (more recently) the Torque teno virus.[58]

EBV has been implicated in a bewildering array of NHLs beyond BL. For example, there are several AIDS-related lymphomas that have been linked to EBV, including the most common category of NHL, diffuse large cell lymphoma, and its subtypes.[59,60] Generally, AIDS-related NHLs are either systemic (e.g., a certain subset of BL) or more localized (notably, targeting the central nervous system). As a class, these malignancies tend to be aggressive. The systemic types typically demonstrate EBV positivity in 30–90% of cases.[61]

EBV sometimes seems to work alongside HIV as an enhancer of disease susceptibility. This is especially seen in EBV-positive individuals coinfected with HHV-8.[62] The two viruses interact in such a way that HHV-8-induced lysis is inhibited, promoting viral latency and the eventual development of primary effusion lymphoma (PEL).[63] The disease pathways of PEL are complex. For instance, EBV may cause a type of disease similar to PEL that does not involve HHV-8 (see Chapter 11).[64]

Researchers have also found that coinfection with the two types of herpesviruses can lead to simultaneous cancers that are unrelated.[65] In sum, EBV and HHV-8 have many overlapping features and disease involvements, including increased cancer risk in the face of HIV coinfection.[66] One review suggested that 50% of AIDS-related lymphomas can be traced to one and/or the other of the human gammaherpesviruses.[67]

Pathways of immune-incompetence other than HIV infection (e.g., inherited disorders, conditioning drugs used in transplantation) can lead to lymphoproliferative conditions that manifest an EBV connection. For example, EBV infection is linked to approximately 90% of the B-cell lymphomas associated with post-transplant lymphoproliferative disorder (PTLD); as a whole, these conditions represent a serious complication for transplant recipients.[68]

Although mainly infecting B-cells, EBV can infect other immune system cells.[69,70] In particular, certain T-cell NHLs have been associated with the virus.[71,72] There is some indication that an immunocompromised state (especially related to HIV coinfection) can create a prolonged, active EBV infection, which in turn exacerbates the movement of EBV beyond its natural home in B-cells to involvement in T-cell malignancies.[73,74] One example is a lymphoma involving both T-cells and natural killer cells that demonstrates a remarkable 90% EBV-positivity when localized in the nasal area[75,76]; this rivals the degree of association observed in NPC (see the following discussion).

Nasopharyngeal Carcinoma

Nasopharyngeal carcinoma is strongly associated with EBV.[77,78] It is a highly metastatic malignancy without effective cure; furthermore, while many NPC risk factors are well-established, the details of the underlying disease mechanism remain largely unknown.[79,80]

NPC is infrequent in the West, with the exception of some Inuit groups.[81] The disease is more common in the Canton province of China, in Hong Kong, and, to a lesser degree, in other locations in southeast Asia.[82,83] This geographic localization has often been explained in terms of the risk of NPC associated with the consumption of salted fish.[84,85] As incidence is generally high in people of Chinese descent regardless of where they live, the possibility of host genetic factors cannot be ignored. To the extent that host or lifestyle factors are involved, immigration from endemic areas may increase the burden of NPC in Western countries.[86] On a final note, intermediate rates of NPC have been observed in the Middle East, North Africa, and southern European regions situated on the Mediterranean basin.[87]

Other Disease Associations

In addition to the preceding conditions, EBV-related malignancy has also been investigated in the context of different epithelial sites and a number of other tissue types.[88] This includes certain gastric cancers, salivary gland tumors, hepatocellular carcinomas, and (in immunosuppressed patients) smooth muscle tumors known as leiomyosarcomas.[89–92] A potential role in bladder and cervical cancer has also recently been reported.[93,94] Whatever the theoretical interest in the various potential disease associations, it must be admitted that the detection of EBV in any such cases does not yet have prognostic or therapeutic significance.[95] However, given the disease burden attached to some of the cancers potentially influenced by EBV, investigating the role of the virus will undoubtedly continue as a research focus. A case in point is gastric cancer, where the proportion caused by EBV may be as high as 10%.[96,97] Moreover, the potential role of EBV in lymphoepithelioma-like carcinomas of the stomach approaches 100%; these rare tumors are thought to have a pathogenic mechanism similar to NPC.[98]

While most attention has naturally focused on confirming positive associations with cancer, any research concluding that there is not a causal relationship is also very useful in shaping priorities. An example is a 2004 study suggesting that EBV does not have a role in small-cell carcinoma of the lung.[99] Likewise, there have been negative reports concerning EBV involvement in breast cancer, though this area of research remains controversial. Other studies have demonstrated the presence of EBV genetic material in breast tumor cells, but rarely in control tissue; this suggests that the virus may be involved in some instances of breast carcinogenesis.[100]

Although already an extensive inventory, it has barely scratched the surface. To provide a window on the full range of malignancies where an EBV connection has been established or investigated, the key literature is summarized in Table 10.4 at the end of this chapter. While intriguing at the level of basic research, from a public health perspective it is important to not become too distracted by the long list of diseases. In order to draw attention to the most important prevention targets, an overview of the substantial EBV–cancer associations is provided in Table 10.2. The EBV-attributable proportion of other cancers, even common ones such as oral squamous cell carcinoma, that are not included in Table 10.2 is either very small or still controversial.

Even when there is a high proportion of cases attributable to EBV, it must be acknowledged that many of the cancers are rare in absolute terms in developed countries such as the United States and Canada; the same reality likely applies on a worldwide basis.

Table 10.2. EBV Association in Selected Cancers

Disease	EBV Positivity (%)
Burkitt lymphoma (endemic)	>95
Hodgkin's disease (subtype)	>95
Nasal NK/T cell lymphoma	>90
Gastric lymphoepithelioma-like carcinoma	>90
Gastric adenocarcinoma	5–25
Posttransplantation lymphoproliferative disorders	>90
Nasopharyngeal carcinoma	>95
AIDS-associated lymphoma, CNS	>95
AIDS-associated lymphoma, other	30–90

Source: Thompson et al., Clinical Cancer Research, 2004.

On the other hand, much of the epidemiology, including attributable proportions, is still being clarified. For example, the fraction of the total NHL burden in Canada attributable to EBV has not been ascertained. As a starting point of discussion, one estimate suggested that some 10% of T-cell lymphomas in the world are caused by the virus.[102]

The EBV-disease connection does not end with cancer. The virus appears to have a causative role in a spectrum of nonmalignant diseases, starting of course with IM. Some of the identified diseases may in fact be cancer precursors; for example, "chronic active EBV infection" appears to be a true premalignant condition.[103,104]

One of the most intriguing pathogenic mechanisms linked to EBV is autoimmunity.[105,106] The autoimmune diseases that have been proposed as falling in some way within the orbit of EBV infection include systemic lupus erythematosus, rheumatoid arthritis, and multiple sclerosis.[107–110]

TRANSMISSION AND OCCURRENCE OF THE AGENT

The primary means of EBV transmission involves saliva; this is because EBV preferentially infects lymphoid tissues (specifically, B-cells) and squamous epithelium in the oropharynx. The virus can continue to be shed into the mouth and thence into saliva for years after the primary infection occurs.[111]

Vertical transmission of EBV may be an important factor in the development of acute lymphoblastic leukemia (ALL)[112] in children. Some researchers have found that reactivated EBV in infected mothers seems to be passed to the offspring in utero, which then leads to virally induced leukemia.[113,114] However, the evidence is inconsistent, and thus the proposed linkage between vertically transmitted virus and ALL remains controversial.[115,116]

There has been an interesting inversion in the developing pictures of EBV and HHV-8 transmission. In short, HHV-8, first considered to be mainly a sexually transmitted infection (especially among homosexual males), is now also seen to be transmissible by saliva (see Chapter 11); whereas EBV, traditionally considered to be spread by saliva, may also be transmitted by sexual contact (as well as blood transfusion and transplantation).[117,118] In terms of supporting evidence, there have been reports of EBV detected in genital secretions, indicating that sexual transmission of the virus is possible. In one study, the degree to which IM patients, their sexual partners, and nonsexual personal contacts shared the same viral isolates was tested by genital analysis.[119] There was significantly more overlap of EBV isolates among the sexual partners. However, the levels of EBV detected in the cervical, male urethral, and semen samples were so low relative to typical salivary complements, sexual transmission was still deemed to be a minor pathway compared with oral-to-oral contact.

DISEASE MECHANISM AND PROCESSES

Given what is arguably the most prevalent human infection in the world, and the cancer-causing agent that has been studied for the longest period of time, it is surprising to discover how much of the EBV disease process remains to be elucidated. The explanation relates to complexities in the interaction between EBV and its human host.

Multiple Targets and Processes

As already suggested in the section on disease associations, there are many "benign" and malignant conditions that appear to be directly caused by the virus. This phenomenon has its roots in multiple cellular tropisms. EBV has been shown to infect and affect the following cell types:[120-122]

- B lymphocytes
- Oral squamous cells (keratinocytes)

- Gastric epithelial cells
- T-cells (multiple phenotypes)
- Natural killer cells
- Monocytes and granulocytes
- Hodgkin-Reed-Sternberg cells

The complexity of the range of host cells is only increased when one considers the multiple body sites where infected cells and tissue may be found. It all adds up to a wide spectrum of diseases caused by EBV. Precisely how do these diseases develop, especially the various cancers?

The disease processes of EBV exhibit both familiar and unique features. For instance, some aspects of the EBV disease mechanism overlap with other viral infections where persistence within the host plays a role in the eventual emergence of cancer. Taken together, the elements of disease development comprise the following:

1. Where the virus becomes established in the host (i.e., the cell or cells of primary infection) and how it gains entry to cells
2. How it transfers between different cell types
3. The manner in which the virus escapes host immune responses and persists as a latent infection
4. The dynamics of reactivation, viral replication, and host cell lysis prior to transmission
5. The specific factors that influence carcinogenesis

As already suggested, many questions about these areas are still being explored. Ultimately, better understanding the natural history of EBV infection and disease development provides the foundation for prevention modalities.

Pathways of Infection and Latency

The cells where EBV infection may be found, though many and varied, can be categorized as belonging either to the immune system or to one of the mucosal epithelia in the host. While B-cells in lymphoid tissue (especially the tonsils) or circulating in the blood seem to be a dominant locus of EBV persistence,[123] there continues to be a debate about whether lymphoid or epithelial tissue represents the key site of viral passage into the human biological system.[124,125] More specifically, researchers have investigated whether viral transmission via saliva leads to a primary oropharyngeal infection centered on squamous epithelial cells or on B-cells.[126,127]

The two main theories about primary infection indicate that either the virus directly accesses B-cells in the oral mucosa, or it spends time in epithelial cells (where it undergoes amplification) before transferring to B-cells.[128] Other ideas have been recently advanced, including the possible movement of EBV from B-cells in lymphoid tissue to circulating monocytes and finally to keratinocytes in the oral epithelium.[129,130] The latter cells then allow for viral reactivation, proliferation, shedding, and transmission to new hosts—though admittedly the evidence for this version of events has been strongest in the context of immunocompromised individuals. Other research has recently suggested that involvement of memory B-cells is not necessary for EBV to ultimately persist in (and be shed from) the oropharynx.[131–133] Clearly, the biological pathways of EBV infection continue to be a fluid area of investigation.

Although the broad themes are still emerging, studies have elucidated some of the molecular aspects of primary infection. For instance, researchers have identified that the process of EBV binding to cells, and subsequently gaining entry, involves a number of host envelope proteins.[134] This binding "profligacy" is actually common to the herpesvirus as a group. Whatever its origin, the variety of ways these viruses can attach to the surface of a cell is one of the reasons that EBV is able to affect so many cell types.[135] The specific manner of binding may shed light on some of the unanswered questions about primary infection. It seems that EBV first binds to B-cells, but remains on the cellular surface (known as an ectopic infection) before transferring to epithelial cells of the oropharynx.[136]

The mechanism by which EBV transfers between different cell types (especially in the absence of cellular lysis) has been investigated in some detail. There is evidence of a very efficient system allowing EBV to move from B-cells to epithelial cells, and vice versa.[137] This involves intimate contact between the envelopes of the two cell types (which researchers have referred to, rather poetically, as "kissing"); the tight attachment allows for intercellular transfer of the virus, a process which has been shown to occur in as little as 10 minutes.[138,139]

One of the main reasons for the ongoing interest in confirming a role for epithelial cells in the EBV lifecycle is the evidence that infection of B-cells appears to be generally unproductive. In other words, while EBV may favor memory B-cells as the site of persistence/latency, viral proliferation does not occur predominantly in such cells.[140] This has led one reviewer to conclude that "infection of B cells...can hardly explain the successful spread of the virus in the human population."[141]

Although the precise pathways and timing of primary EBV infection are still being worked out, it is clear that the virus ultimately creates a latent, growth-transforming infection in mucosal B-cells that leads to the expansion of affected cells in the tonsils, and probably in other lymphoid tissues. The number of infected B-cells in the blood also rises dramatically, constituting 1–10% of the B-cell complement in cases of IM.[142]

While many of the infected cells are removed by the host's immune system, some persist by downregulating latent antigen expression and entering a resting state in the memory B-cell pool. A remarkable phenomenon that has been uncovered is the variety of viral gene expressions seen in different host cells. Thus, it seems that EBV employs a different latency (and transformation) strategy in BL, NPC, gastric adenocarcinoma, etc.[143–146] This creates great challenges for prevention and treatment research; in short, the various immunotherapies under development must be tested in terms of efficacy against the different EBV latency mechanisms.[147,148]

Each of the latency strategies employs only a small subset of the 85 proteins known to be coded by the virus.[149] Beyond this basic mechanism of persistence, EBV viral products are known to affect a wide range of host cell molecules while on the pathway to B-cell growth, immortalization, and ultimately tumor development.[150–152] However, it is outside the scope of this book to review in detail the growing body of data related to molecular processes.

Reactivation, Replication, and Lysis

Movement to the lytic phase of EBV infection is counteracted by specific and potent immune responses.[153,154] In fact, it is the hyperactivation of the host T-cells that is the fundamental basis of the immunopathology known as IM, which is of course the paradigmatic "benign" EBV disease.

The most substantial viral proliferation (and thus risk of transmission) may be traced to oropharyngeal epithelial cells during active, primary infections. However, movement out of a latent state occasionally seems to occur in B-cells as well; these reactivated cells are able to pass virus to epithelial cells (mainly in the oropharynx), which then leads to new instances of viral replication and cellular lysis. This phenomenon might explain the "low-level virus shedding found in the throat of long-term virus carriers."[155]

Different mechanisms for inducing reactivation out of a latent state have been proposed. One of the best understood triggers is coinfection, especially involving other herpesviruses, such as cytomegalovirus.[156] The molecular aspects of reactivation are still being elucidated, but already there is evidence that the process in EBV is different than that seen in other herpesviruses.[157] A fascinating and important instance of

EBV reactivation and replication involves coinfection with the protozoa *Plasmodium falciparum*, one of the causes of malaria; as seen earlier, malaria may combine with EBV and other factors to create a "class of sufficient causation" leading to BL.[158]

Carcinogenesis

Replication and lysis, as described earlier, are prerequisites for infecting new, locally resident B-cell populations in the same host, for transmission to new hosts, and for the onset of IM. However, it is the phenomenon of latency that is most problematic in terms of malignant transformation.[159]

The factors and conditions that help to propel cells with latent EBV infection into a full carcinogenic mode are not yet well understood.[160] However, it is not surprising that one risk factor proposed for EBV-related carcinogenesis is the immunocompromised state created as a byproduct of pretransplant conditioning, HIV infection, and other instigators.

While it is true that BL, as well as EBV-related HD, are elevated in HIV-positive cohorts, the connection between immune competence and the rate of EBV-related malignancies is still not entirely clear. For example, some research has suggested that those who are positive for both HIV and EBV do not have an elevated risk for NHL.[161] In fact, the strongest evidence of an association between a compromised immune system and EBV-related disease has been observed for the rare lesions known as leiomyosarcoma.[162] A recent study added plasmablastic lymphoma of the oral cavity to the list of HIV-related malignancies caused by EBV.[163] Prior to this point, the inventory of EBV-associated oral disease in HIV patients has been essentially restricted to the nonmalignant condition known as oral hairy leukoplakia.[164,165]

Prevention Opportunities

The chief value of this general review of EBV disease mechanism is anticipating how the various biological strategies employed by the virus may be exploited by interventions that will prevent disease. Thus, as will be described in a later section of the chapter, the complex immunologic response to EBV offers doorways for intervention.[166] One of the key quests has revolved around "therapeutic approaches aimed at preventing EBV latency in B-cells [to] thwart the development of virus-associated tumors."[167] The fact that the lytic phase of EBV infection is more susceptible to immune surveillance and response in the human body offers an intriguing possibility. In short, it would be useful to find ways to reactivate the virus latent in early cancer cells into the early part of the lytic cycle, and then direct chemotherapeutic agents or a boosted immune system against the now more immunologically "visible" target.[168] Another example more pertinent to the main theme of this book is the apparent ability of EBV to gain entry to oropharyngeal epithelial cells via multiple routes, including cell-to-cell transfers and (in the case of cell-free virions) via the basolateral membrane of polarized cells. As one recent review noted, this indicates that "multiple approaches to prevention of epithelial infection with EBV will be necessary."[169]

Naturally, much more could be said about the detailed processes involved with each of the EBV-related malignancies, but this would extend the chapter inordinately. A brief note on one cancer, NPC, at least provides a glimpse into the known complexity, as well as suggesting the information that remains to be discovered. Among several mechanisms mediating the oncogenic evolution of NPC cells, EBV infection induces the activation of telomerase, an enzyme implicated in cell immortalization. Researchers have begun to unravel the complex intracellular signaling pathways employed in the modulation of telomerase levels in infected cells, thereby shedding light on potential therapeutic interventions for this disease.[170]

VIRAL DETECTION METHODS

Since 90% or more of most adult populations are infected with EBV, universal screening is not very relevant. As suggested earlier, the unusual situation is when a person does not test positive for the virus.

Table 10.3. EBV Detection Methods

Method	Features
Serological	
Immunofluorescence assay (IFA)	Classical method; gold standard; highly specific
Enzyme-linked immunosorbent assay (ELISA)	Rapid and highly sensitive
Blot techniques	Highly specific; mainly confirmatory
Heterophile antibody agglutination	Less sensitive, less specific; 10–50% of children <4 years of age do not produce heterophile antibodies
Molecular	
Polymerase chain reaction (PCR)	Used to detect virus load and reactivation
In situ hybridization, *in situ* PCR	Used to detect EBV-associated tumors
Virus antigens, immunohistochemistry, and immunocytology	Used to detect EBV-associated tumors

Source: Hess, *Journal of Clinical Microbiology*, 2004.

In some geographic areas, targeted screening is carried out in high-risk populations, such as family members of NPC patients in southern China.[171] Viral detection localized to a tissue and site is also used to confirm a diagnosis of EBV-associated disease. The methods of detection that are employed can be classified as either serological or molecular. The most common techniques are outlined in the Table 10.3.

Despite the increasing accuracy of polymerase chain reaction (PCR) and other molecular methods in recent years, serological testing is still preferred for primary detection in immunocompetent individuals. Even with technological improvements,[172] immunoassay results are sometimes indeterminate, in which case further diagnostic approaches such as PCR would be employed. Conversely, in immunocompromised patients missing the usual serological markers, molecular methods are more appropriate. This especially entails the quantification of viral load by a standardized PCR assay system.[173,174]

PREVENTION APPROACHES

The pattern established in previous chapters will again be followed, organizing prevention approaches to EBV and related diseases in categories that relate to the overall disease pathway. With the exception of cofactor control, all of the interventions described later have some direct connection to EBV infection or its related disease processes.

Avoiding Exposure	Preventing Infection	Prophylactic Eradication	Preventing Cofactor	Therapeutic Eradication	Interrupting Transformation

1. Avoiding Exposure to the Agent

Given the very high prevalence of the virus, and the fact that the type of casual contact associated with transmission is so ubiquitous, avoiding EBV exposure does not seem to be a feasible strategy. An area of interest, however, is the geographic variation observed for age of infection in children. In developing countries, most children are infected before 1 year of age, whereas only 50% of children aged 5–9 years are infected in developed nations.[175] Given that the primary medium for EBV transmission is saliva, the earlier age of infection observed in the developing world may be partly due to crowded and/or unsanitary living conditions. Sharing beds and eating utensils could easily enhance opportunities for EBV transfer. Low socioeconomic status may also lead to malnutrition, resulting in impaired immunity, and thus a greater likelihood of developing EBV-associated disease.[176] It is possible that, at

| Avoiding Exposure | **Preventing Infection** | Prophylactic Eradication | Preventing Cofactor | Therapeutic Eradication | Interrupting Transformation |

2. Preventing Infection after Exposure to the Agent

There are no vaccines for preventing EBV infection currently in use. Development of a vaccine has been very slow due to lack of an appropriate animal model, and also because of uncertainty about the purpose of such an intervention.[177] Nonetheless, efforts are still being made to develop an EBV vaccine that prevents initial infection.[178–180] At least two candidate vaccines have been brought to the trial stage.[181]

Results for a vaccine to prevent IM in healthy young adults were recently published.[182] It was determined that the vaccine significantly reduced the incidence of IM relative to the placebo group, though it was not effective in preventing asymptomatic EBV infection (i.e., colonization).

| Avoiding Exposure | Preventing Infection | **Prophylactic Eradication** | Preventing Cofactor | Therapeutic Eradication | Interrupting Transformation |

3. Prophylactic Eradication or Suppression

The ubiquity of the virus in human populations has also meant that there is little motivation to investigate eradication strategies in asymptomatic individuals. However, approaches that could be applied to such a task are being investigated. Recalling the role that immunosuppression plays in the development of certain EBV-associated malignancies, some of the most promising research involves therapies aimed at reestablishing immunocompetence.[183,184] This strategy can theoretically be used prophylactically in at-risk populations, but mostly the focus has been on the treatment and reversal of incipient disease (see section "Therapeutic Eradication or Suppression").

| Avoiding Exposure | Preventing Infection | Prophylactic Eradication | **Preventing Cofactor** | Therapeutic Eradication | Interrupting Transformation |

4. Cofactor Prevention

Given its importance in specific populations in both the developed and developing world, NPC has received a substantial amount of attention in the literature. Environmental and genetic factors that contribute to NPC risk were recently reviewed by Chang and Adami.[185] The most dominant cofactor was the consumption of salt-preserved fish, a traditional staple of the diet in southern China and several other NPC-endemic areas. Consuming other salt-preserved foods, such as seal meat among the Inuit, also seems to elevate risk; in fact, all NPC-endemic populations have salt-preserved foods as a dietary staple.[186,187] Of particular concern is the use of salted fish for weaning infants, especially in families of lower socioeconomic status. According to one study among Malaysian Chinese adults, those who reported daily consumption of salted fish during childhood have an NPC relative risk of 17.4 (95% CI 2.7–111.1) compared to groups characterized by nonconsumption.[188]

Although more moderately associated, another dietary risk factor for NPC is lack of consumption of fruits and vegetables. A study in Guangzhou, China, found that NPC patients had eaten significantly less fresh fruits and vegetables, especially during early childhood, compared with a control group.[189]

Other environmental risk factors for NPC that have been investigated include smoking, alcohol consumption, malaria, herbal medicines, and occupational exposures such as wood dust and formaldehyde. There are many conflicting reports regarding these exposures, making definitive conclusions about NPC association challenging.[190-192] Consistent with the present state of the research, a recent review suggested that, "other than dietary modifications, no concrete preventive measures for NPC exist."[193]

In other malignancies, a number of coinfections have been postulated as factors interacting with EBV. Of these, the best-researched is the link between malaria and BL. A study in Uganda, focusing on children with BL, measured antibodies for both EBV and malaria; BL cases were five times more likely than controls to demonstrate both infections.[194] This may indicate that EBV and malaria act synergistically in the pathogenesis of BL, and that malaria prevention measures may have the collateral benefit of preventing this EBV-associated lymphoma.

Another infection that is a potential cofactor in EBV-associated conditions is HIV, specifically with respect to BL, B-lymphoproliferative disease (BLPD), and a variety of T-cell malignancies.[195] Thus, prevention and treatment of HIV infection might have an effect on associated EBV disease. Reducing the incidence of a certain class of tumors could be achieved by adjustments to sexual behavior or, eventually, through HIV vaccination.[196]

Immunosuppression in transplant patients is also suggested to be a cofactor in BLPD, as well as the various T-cell lymphomas related to EBV infection; as noted earlier in the chapter, the specific name for

BLPD in such cases is PTLD.[197] As is usual in this area of medical care, the search for safer transplant conditioning regimes could have direct preventive implications. Sometimes protective remedial action is also possible. For example, bone marrow transplant (BMT) recipients are at especially high risk of developing EBV-associated PTLD. Studies have shown that administration of EBV-specific cytotoxic T-lymphocytes (CTLs) in BMT patients resulted in decreased EBV load, conferring protection against the emergence of PTLD.[198–200]

| Avoiding Exposure | Preventing Infection | Prophylactic Eradication | Preventing Cofactor | **Therapeutic Eradication** | Interrupting Transformation |

5. Therapeutic Eradication or Suppression

There are currently no drugs licensed for treatment of EBV infection in clinical settings. Although a number of pharmaceuticals are known to inhibit EBV replication, they have had limited success in clinical trials. Because these drugs impact the viral lytic cycle, they are not effective against latent EBV infections per se. To fill this gap, novel antivirals are being sought that target nonreplicative viral proteins, with the intention of interrupting carcinogenesis (see section "Interrupting Transformation Related to Infection").[201]

The possibility of actually eradicating the virus from individuals with latent infection continues to be investigated. Latent membrane protein 2A (LMP-2A), which is consistently expressed by infected B-cells, is a particular area of interest. One study has identified several proteins influenced by LMP-2A that may be potential targets for therapeutic agents.[202] Such strategies are ultimately aimed at disrupting latency mechanisms, exposing the virus to host immunity, and thus increasing the probability of clearance.[203]

Immunotherapies have perhaps generated the greatest interest, especially in the context of NPC. There are two categories under investigation—adoptive and active immunotherapy.[204] One research focus with respect to adoptive immunotherapy involves the infusion of donor CTLs, though this treatment carries with it the danger of graft-versus-host disease.[205–207] CTL therapy appears to hold some promise,[208] although this has been seen more for the autologous rather than allogenic variety of transplantation. Active EBV immunotherapy, or the application of therapeutic vaccines, is also being investigated, but progress has been modest to date.[209] Ultimately, a true preventive role for immunotherapies will depend on both safety evaluations and a record of proven efficacy with EBV-related cancer precursors.

| Avoiding Exposure | Preventing Infection | Prophylactic Eradication | Preventing Cofactor | Therapeutic Eradication | **Interrupting Transformation** |

6. Interrupting Transformation Related to Infection

Therapies that target virally induced transformation mechanisms are being pursued in the context of EBV infection and a variety of related diseases.[210,211] For example, it was noted earlier that EBV can infect T-lymphocytes. One condition that results from such infection is a version of the nonmalignant condition known as hemophagocytic syndrome (HPS); a proportion of people with this disease progress to T-cell lymphoma.[212] The EBV-encoded LMP-1 is considered to be the driving force behind neoplastic transformation in such situations. One of the functions of LMP-1 is the activation of a transcription pathway that confers resistance to programmed cell death (and possibly to anticancer drugs).[213] Inhibition of the transcription pathway has, therefore, been identified as a potential target for therapeutic strategies aimed at HPS and/or T-cell lymphoma arising from EBV infection.

CONCLUSION

With the massive global prevalence of EBV infection, and given its routine oral transmission, it is difficult to hold out much hope for the classic primary prevention objective of eliminating exposure to the infection. As well, in light of limited understanding of the oncogenic mechanisms for the many types of cancer associated with EBV, comprehensive prevention methods later in the disease process also remain elusive. Notwithstanding the promise of immunotherapies and antivirals, it must be acknowledged that the prevention and management of EBV-related morbidity remain in the "nascent stages."[214]

As the oldest known oncogenic virus, EBV has contributed greatly to many aspects of basic cancer knowledge.[215] EBV, along with HHV-8, offers a unique opportunity to compare the cancer mechanisms of two viruses from the same family, namely, the gamma-herpesviruses. In fact, the two viruses demonstrate clear similarities, including lymphotropism (specifically of a B-cell variety) and a repertoire of very effective immune evasion strategies.[216] As well, biological interaction between the two viral types (similar to that found between closely related retroviruses, HIV and HTLV) is an area of keen interest for researchers.[217]

The involvement of polymicrobial infections in the development of cancer is a growing focus in oncology. This topic raises important questions about how to define a carcinogenic agent. If all cofactors were included, from those contributing to persistent infection to initiators of neoplasia to promoters of tumor progression, then the list of cancer-causing agents would be many times longer than the existing table of contents for this book. For instance, HIV undoubtedly would occupy a full chapter. EBV is central to such a discussion. In fact, EBV promises to extend the investigation in intriguing ways by moving beyond dual infection to carcinogenesis involving at least three agents, even ones drawn from different categories of microbes. In view here is the proposed linkage between two viruses (EBV and an arbovirus) and one protozoa (the malaria-causing parasite *P. falciparum*) in the development of BL.[218]

EBV exhibits some interesting parallels with other agents examined in this book. The virus seems to occupy a sort of middle ground in terms of disease associations. On the one hand, its remarkable specificity as the carcinogen in BL and NPC is reminiscent of HPV-related tumors in the female cervix and in other mucosal tissues with direct access to the exterior of the body. On the other hand, similar to a virus such as hepatitis C, EBV manifests tropism for multiple cellular types and, as a consequence, seems to have connections with a growing and varied inventory of malignancies. As is true with other agents reviewed in this book, the story concerning EBV and cancer, although already decades old, is far from finished.

Table 10.4. Epstein-Barr Virus-associated Cancers

Cancer	Characteristics	Occurrence	Prognosis	Studies (by Lead Author and Date)
B-cell malignancies				
Burkitt lymphoma	EBV association >95% (endemic type); also associated with malaria, HIV	Most frequent in equatorial Africa, especially in children; more common in males	Cure rate above 50% with chemotherapy	Carpenter (2008); Orem (2008); Rainey (2008); Kamranvar (2007)
Hodgkin's disease	EBV association >95% (lymphocyte depleted type); immunocompromised individuals at higher risk	891 new cases in Canada in 2004; more common in males	5-year survival rate of 80–95%	Canadian Cancer Society (2008); Ambinder (2007); Cickusic (2007); Kapatai (2007); Andersson (2006); Khan (2006)
AIDS-associated B-cell lymphomas	EBV association for CNS lymphoma: >95%; EBV association for other lymphomas: 30–90% (includes primary effusion and diffuse large cell lymphomas)			Angeletti (2008); Ferrazzo (2007); Rezk (2007); Epeldegui (2006)
Post-transplantation lymphoproliferative disorders	EBV association >90%; a group of B-cell lymphomas; affect individuals immunocompromised due to conditioning before transplants	Occur in 1 in 500 patients within a year of transplant; higher risk in children and heart transplant patients	5-year survival rate of about 60%	Cohen (2007); Dolcetti (2007); Johnson (2006)

(Continued)

Table 10.4. (Continued)

Cancer	Characteristics	Occurrence	Prognosis	Studies (by Lead Author and Date)
Lymphomatoid granulomatosis	Affects immunocompromised individuals; involves lungs, skin, and central nervous system	Rare; more than twice as common in males	No known cure, often leads to death within a year	Nishihara (2007); Rezk (2007)
Pyothorax-associated lymphoma	Associated with previous artificial pneumothorax	Most common among Japanese patients		Takakuwa (2008); Aozasa (2006)
Senile EBV-associated B-cell lymphoproliferative disorders		Only affects elderly patients, median age 76		Shiozawa (2007); Shimoyama (2006); Oyama (2003)
Methotrexate-associated B-cell lymphoma	Affects immunocompromised individuals			Said (2007)
Wiskott-Aldrich syndrome-associated B-cell lymphoma	Affects immunocompromised individuals			Sebire (2003); Sasahara (2001)
X-linked lymphoproliferative disorder-associated B-cell lymphoma	Affects immunocompromised individuals	Rare condition; only in males		Coffey (1998)

T-cell malignancies

Extranodal NK/T-cell lymphoma, nasal type	EBV association >90%; can also occur in the skin; affects immunocompromised individuals	Associated with East Asian populations; two or three times more common in males	Median survival varies from 6 to 25 months	Liang (2008); Hsieh (2007); Rezk (2007)
Peripheral T-cell lymphoma, unspecified	Disease course often aggressive	Accounts for <10% of non-Hodgkin's lymphomas worldwide; uncommon in North America	5-year survival rate of 30–35%	Prochazka (2007); Tan (2006)
Angioimmunoblastic T-cell lymphoma	Involves the skin in 40–50% of cases; a type of peripheral T-cell lymphoma	Comprises 1–2% of all non-Hodgkin's lymphomas; median patient age 65 years; more common in males	25% of patients achieve complete remission with chemotherapy	Dunleavy (2007); Rezk (2007)
Enteropathy-type T-cell lymphoma	A type of peripheral T-cell lymphoma; aggressive; associated with celiac disease; investigational for EBV connection		1- and 5-year survival rates of 40% and 20%, respectively	Rezk (2007); Quintanilla-Martinez (1997); de Bruin (1995)
Subcutaneous panniculitis-like lymphoma	A type of peripheral T-cell lymphoma; EBV association found in some Japanese cases	Rare; accounts for <1% of all non-Hodgkin's lymphomas	50% mortality rate	Takeshita (2004); Liu (2002); Harada (1994)
Hepatosplenic T-cell lymphoma	A type of peripheral T-cell lymphoma; aggressive; investigational for EBV connection	Rare; more common among males	Most patients die within 2 years	Rezk (2007); Ohshima (2000)

(Continued)

Table 10.4. (Continued)

Cancer	Characteristics	Occurrence	Prognosis	Studies (by Lead Author and Date)
Nonhepatosplenic γδ T-cell lymphoma	Can occur in skin, intestine, nose, lymph nodes, lung, and thyroid	Rare		Rezk (2007); Arnulf (1998); Kagami (1997)
Sinonasal angiocentric T-cell lymphoma		Rare in United States and Europe; clusters in Japan, Hong Kong, and Central America	Not well known	Rodriguez (2000); O'Leary (1995)
Virus-associated hemophagocytic syndrome T-cell lymphomas	Affects immunocompromised individuals			Chuang (2007)
Other hematological malignancies				
Acute lymphoblastic leukemia	Investigational for EBV connection; associated with maternal infection	Most common in childhood, more common in males	85% cure rate in children	O'Connor (2007); Tedeschi (2007); Kim (2006)
Multiple myeloma	Cancer of plasma cells	1892 new cases in Canada in 2004; more common in males	Considered incurable	Canadian Cancer Society (2008); Csire (2007)
Epithelial cell malignancies				
Nasopharyngeal carcinoma	EBV association >95%; sometimes referred to as nonglandular NPC	Most common in regions of East Asia and Africa; 231 new cases in Canada in 2004	65% five-year survival rate	Canadian Cancer Society (2008); Tao (2007); Mirzamani (2006); Zhong (2006)

Lymphoepithelioma-like carcinomas	EBV association for gastric type >90%; other varieties include salivary, sinonasal, thymus, and lungs	Generally rare; some sites more common among Asian populations		Herath (2008); Herbst (2006); Hsu (2006); Larbcharoensub (2006); Papalambros (2003); Castro (2001); Zong (2001); Chapel (2000)
Gastric adenocarcinoma	EBV association 5–25%; adenocarcinoma constitutes 90% of stomach tumors, the second leading cause of cancer-related death worldwide	Two-thirds of stomach cancers occur in developing countries; more common in males	5-year survival rate less than 20% in United States	Deyrup (2008); Akiba (2008); Crew (2006); Hsieh (1998)
Oral squamous cell carcinoma	Strongly associated with smoking and heavy alcohol consumption	More common in males; most cases occur after age 50	5-year survival rates range from 17% to 90%, depending on specific malignancy	Bagan (2008); Gonzalez-Moles (2002)
Oropharyngeal squamous cell carcinoma	EBV association controversial	114 new cases in Canada in 2004		Canadian Cancer Society (2008); Szkaradkiewicz (2002); Khabie (2001)
Esophageal squamous cell carcinoma	Strongly associated with smoking and heavy alcohol consumption	More common in males; median patient age is 67	5-year survival rate of 20–25%	Awerkiew (2003)
Breast carcinoma	Investigational for EBV connection	Most common cancer among females; incidence increases with age	5-year survival rate of 80%	Fawzy (2008); Bonnet (1999)

(Continued)

Table 10.4. (Continued)

Cancer	Characteristics	Occurrence	Prognosis	Studies (by Lead Author and Date)
Primary sinonasal nasopharyngeal-type undifferentiated carcinoma	Most often occurs in nasal cavity	Rare; more common in males		Jeng (2002)
Cervical carcinoma		Second most common cancer in females worldwide		Kim (2005); Szkaradkiewicz (2004); Sasagawa (2000)
Hepatocellular carcinoma	Accounts for 80–90% of all liver cancers	More common in males	Usually leads to death within 3–6 months	Li (2004)
Mesenchymal malignancies				
Follicular dendritic cell sarcoma	Occurs in liver and lymph nodes	Rare; more common in females		Bai (2006)
Leiomyosarcoma	Affects immunocompromised individuals		No known cure	Sprangers (2008)

BIBLIOGRAPHY FOR TABLE 10.4

Akiba S, Koriyama C, Herrera-Goepfert R et al. Epstein-Barr virus associated gastric carcinoma: epidemiological and clinicopathological features. *Cancer Science*. 2008; 99: 195–201.

Ambinder RF. Epstein-barr virus and Hodgkin lymphoma. *Hematology / the Education Program of the American Society of Hematology*. 2007; 2007: 204–9.

Andersson J. Epstein-Barr virus and Hodgkin's lymphoma. *Herpes*. 2006; 13: 12–6.

Angeletti PC, Zhang L, Wood C. The viral etiology of AIDS-associated malignancies. *Advances in Pharmacology*. 2008; 56: 509–57.

Aozasa K. Pyothorax-associated lymphoma. *Journal of Clinical and Experimental Hematopathology*. 2006; 46: 5–10.

Arnulf B, Copie-Bergman C, Delfau-Larue MH et al. Nonhepatosplenic gammadelta T-cell lymphoma: a subset of cytotoxic lymphomas with mucosal or skin localization. *Blood*. 1998; 91: 1723–31.

Awerkiew S, Bollschweiler E, Metzger R et al. Esophageal cancer in Germany is associated with Epstein-Barr-virus but not with papillomaviruses. *Medical Microbiology and Immunology*. 2003; 192: 137–40.

Bagan JV, Jimenez Y, Murillo J et al. Epstein-Barr virus in oral proliferative verrucous leukoplakia and squamous cell carcinoma: a preliminary study. *Medicina Oral, Patologia Oral y Cirugia Bucal*. 2008; 13: E110–3.

Bai LY, Kwang WK, Chiang IP et al. Follicular dendritic cell tumor of the liver associated with Epstein-Barr virus. *Japanese Journal of Clinical Oncology*. 2006; 36: 249–53.

Bonnet M, Guinebretiere JM, Kremmer E et al. Detection of Epstein-Barr virus in invasive breast cancers. *Journal of the National Cancer Institute*. 1999; 91: 1376–81.

Canadian Cancer Society. *Canadian Cancer Statistics 2008*. 2008.

Carpenter LM, Newton R, Casabonne D et al. Antibodies against malaria and Epstein-Barr virus in childhood Burkitt lymphoma: a case-control study in Uganda. *International Journal of Cancer*. 2008; 122: 1319–23.

Castro CY, Ostrowski ML, Barrios R et al. Relationship between Epstein-Barr virus and lymphoepithelioma-like carcinoma of the lung: a clinicopathologic study of 6 cases and review of the literature. *Human Pathology*. 2001; 32: 863–72.

Chapel F, Fabiani B, Davi F et al. Epstein-Barr virus and gastric carcinoma in Western patients: comparison of pathological parameters and p53 expression in EBV-positive and negative tumours. *Histopathology*. 2000; 36: 252–61.

Chuang HC, Lay JD, Hsieh WC et al. Pathogenesis and mechanism of disease progression from hemophagocytic lymphohistiocytosis to Epstein-Barr virus-associated T-cell lymphoma: nuclear factor-kappa B pathway as a potential therapeutic target. Cancer Science. 2007; 98: 1281–7.

Cickusic E, Mustedanagic-Mujanovic J, Iljazovic E et al. Association of Hodgkin's lymphoma with Epstein Barr virus infection. *Bosnian Journal of Basic Medical Sciences*. 2007; 7: 58–65.

Coffey AJ, Brooksbank RA, Brandau O et al. Host response to EBV infection in X-linked lymphoproliferative disease results from mutations in an SH2-domain encoding gene. *Nature Genetics*. 1998; 20: 129–35.

Cohen JM, Cooper N, Chakrabarti S et al. EBV-related disease following haematopoietic stem cell transplantation with reduced intensity conditioning. *Leukemia & Lymphoma.* 2007; 48: 256-69.

Crew KD, Neugut AI. Epidemiology of Gastric Cancer. *World Journal of Gastroenterology.* 2006; 12: 354-62.

Csire M, Mikala G, Peto M et al. Detection of four lymphotropic herpesviruses in Hungarian patients with multiple myeloma and lymphoma. *Federation of European Microbiological Societies Immunology and Medical Microbiology.* 2007; 49: 62-7.

de Bruin PC, Jiwa NM, Oudejans JJ et al. Epstein-Barr virus in primary gastrointestinal T cell lymphomas. Association with gluten-sensitive enteropathy, pathological features, and immunophenotype. *American Journal of Pathology.* 1995; 146: 861-7.

Deyrup AT. Epstein-Barr virus-associated epithelial and mesenchymal neoplasms. *Human Pathology.* 2008; 39(4): 473-83.

Dolcetti R. B lymphocytes and Epstein-Barr virus: the lesson of post-transplant lymphoproliferative disorders. *Autoimmunity Reviews.* 2007; 7: 96-101.

Dunleavy K, Wilson WH, Jaffe ES. Angioimmunoblastic T cell lymphoma: pathobiological insights and clinical implications. *Current Opinion in Hematology.* 2007; 14: 348-53.

Epeldegui M, Widney DP, Martinez-Maza O. Pathogenesis of AIDS lymphoma: role of oncogenic viruses and B cell activation-associated molecular lesions. *Current Opinion in Oncology.* 2006; 18: 444-8.

Fawzy S, Sallam M, Mohammad Awad N. Detection of Epstein-Barr virus in breast carcinoma in Egyptian women. *Clinical Biochemistry.* 2008; 41: 486-92.

Ferrazzo KL, Mesquita RA, Aburad AT et al. EBV detection in HIV-related oral plasmablastic lymphoma. *Oral Diseases.* 2007; 13: 564-9.

Gonzalez-Moles MA, Gutierrez J, Rodriguez MJ et al. Epstein-Barr virus latent membrane protein-1 (LMP-1) expression in oral squamous cell carcinoma. *Laryngoscope.* 2002; 112: 482-7.

Harada H, Iwatsuki K, Kaneko F. Detection of Epstein-Barr virus genes in malignant lymphoma with clinical and histologic features of cytophagic histiocytic panniculitis. *Journal of the American Academy of Dermatology.* 1994; 31: 379-83.

Herath CH, Chetty R. Epstein-Barr virus-associated lymphoepithelioma-like gastric carcinoma. *Archives of Pathology & Laboratory Medicine.* 2008; 132: 706-9.

Herbst H, Niedobitek G. Sporadic EBV-associated lymphoepithelial salivary gland carcinoma with EBV-positive low-grade myoepithelial component. *Virchows Archiv.* 2006; 448: 648-54.

Hsieh LL, Lin PJ, Chen TC et al. Frequency of Epstein-Barr virus-associated gastric adenocarcinoma in Taiwan. *Cancer Letters.* 1998; 129: 125-9.

Hsieh PP, Tung CL, Chan AB et al. EBV viral load in tumor tissue is an important prognostic indicator for nasal NK/T-cell lymphoma. *American Journal of Clinical Pathology.* 2007; 128: 579-84.

Hsu YC, Lu HF, Huang CC et al. Malignant lymphoepithelial lesions of the salivary gland. *Otolaryngology - Head and Neck Surgery.* 2006; 134: 661-6.

Jeng YM, Sung MT, Fang CL et al. Sinonasal undifferentiated carcinoma and nasopharyngeal-type undifferentiated carcinoma: two clinically, biologi-

cally, and histopathologically distinct entities. *American Journal of Surgical Pathology.* 2002; 26: 371–6.
Johnson LR, Nalesnik MA, Swerdlow SH. Impact of Epstein-Barr virus in monomorphic B-cell posttransplant lymphoproliferative disorders: a histogenetic study. *American Journal of Surgical Pathology.* 2006; 30: 1604–12.
Kagami Y, Nakamura S, Suzuki R et al. A nodal gamma/delta T-cell lymphoma with an association of Epstein-Barr virus. *American Journal of Surgical Pathology.* 1997; 21: 729–36.
Kamranvar SA, Gruhne B, Szeles A et al. Epstein-Barr virus promotes genomic instability in Burkitt's lymphoma. *Oncogene.* 2007; 26: 5115–23.
Kapatai G, Murray P. Contribution of the Epstein Barr virus to the molecular pathogenesis of Hodgkin lymphoma. *Journal of Clinical Pathology.* 2007; 60: 1342–9.
Khabie N, Savva A, Kasperbauer JL et al. Epstein-Barr virus DNA is not increased in tonsillar carcinoma. *Laryngoscope.* 2001; 111: 811–4.
Khan G. Epstein-Barr virus, cytokines, and inflammation: a cocktail for the pathogenesis of Hodgkin's lymphoma? *Experimental Hematology.* 2006; 34: 399–406.
Kim AS, Eastmond DA, Preston RJ. Childhood acute lymphocytic leukemia and perspectives on risk assessment of early-life stage exposures. *Mutation Research.* 2006; 613: 138–60.
Kim NR, Lin Z, Kim KR et al. Epstein-Barr virus and p16INK4A methylation in squamous cell carcinoma and precancerous lesions of the cervix uteri. *Journal of Korean Medical Science.* 2005; 20: 636–42.
Larbcharoensub N, Tubtong N, Praneetvatakul V et al. Epstein-Barr virus associated lymphoepithelial carcinoma of the parotid gland; a clinicopathological report of three cases. *Journal of the Medical Association of Thailand.* 2006; 89: 1536–41.
Li W, Wu BA, Zeng YM et al. Epstein-Barr virus in hepatocellular carcinogenesis. *World Journal of Gastroenterology.* 2004; 10: 3409–13.
Liang X, Graham DK. Natural killer cell neoplasms. *Cancer.* 2008; 112: 1425–36.
Liu V, McKee PH. Cutaneous T-cell lymphoproliferative disorders: approach for the surgical pathologist: recent advances and clarification of confused issues. *Advances in Anatomic Pathology.* 2002; 9: 79–100.
Mirzamani N, Salehian P, Farhadi M et al. Detection of EBV and HPV in nasopharyngeal carcinoma by in situ hybridization. *Experimental and Molecular Pathology.* 2006; 81: 231–4.
Nishihara H, Tateishi U, Itoh T et al. Immunohistochemical and gene rearrangement studies of central nervous system lymphomatoid granulomatosis. *Neuropathology.* 2007; 27: 413–8.
O'Connor SM, Boneva RS. Infectious etiologies of childhood leukemia: plausibility and challenges to proof. *Environmental Health Perspectives.* 2007; 115: 146–50.
O'Leary G, Kennedy SM. Association of Epstein-Barr virus with sinonasal angiocentric T cell lymphoma. *Journal of Clinical Pathology.* 1995; 48: 946–9.
Ohshima K, Haraoka S, Harada N et al. Hepatosplenic gammadelta T-cell lymphoma: relation to Epstein-Barr virus and activated cytotoxic molecules. *Histopathology.* 2000; 36: 127–35.

Orem J, Mbidde EK, Weiderpass E. Current investigations and treatment of Burkitt's lymphoma in Africa. *Tropical Doctor.* 2008; 38: 7–11.

Oyama T, Ichimura K, Suzuki R et al. Senile EBV+ B-cell lymphoproliferative disorders: a clinicopathologic study of 22 patients. *American Journal of Surgical Pathology.* 2003; 27: 16–26.

Papalambros E, Felekouras E, Pikoulis E et al. Epstein-Barr virus - associated adenocarcinoma of the stomach: a rare entity with distinct characteristics. *Journal of the Balkan Union of Oncology.* 2003; 8: 329–31.

Prochazka V, Trneny M, Pytlik R et al. Peripheral T-cell lymphoma, unspecified— the analysis of the data from the Czech Lymphoma Study Group (CLSG) registry. *Biomedical papers of the Medical Faculty of the University Palacky, Olomouc, Czechoslovakia.* 2007; 151: 103–7.

Quintanilla-Martinez L, Lome-Maldonado C, Ott G et al. Primary non-Hodgkin's lymphoma of the intestine: high prevalence of Epstein-Barr virus in Mexican lymphomas as compared with European cases. *Blood.* 1997; 89: 644–51.

Rainey JJ, Rochford R, Sumba PO et al. Family environment is associated with endemic Burkitt lymphoma: a population-based case-control study. *American Journal of Tropical Medicine and Hygiene.* 2008; 78: 338–43.

Rezk SA, Weiss LM. Epstein-Barr virus-associated lymphoproliferative disorders. *Human Pathology.* 2007; 38: 1293–304.

Rodriguez J, Romaguera JE, Manning J et al. Nasal-type T/NK lymphomas: a clinicopathologic study of 13 cases. *Leukemia & Lymphoma.* 2000; 39: 139–44.

Said JW. Immunodeficiency-related Hodgkin lymphoma and its mimics. *Advances in Anatomic Pathology.* 2007; 14: 189–94.

Sasagawa T, Shimakage M, Nakamura M et al. Epstein-Barr virus (EBV) genes expression in cervical intraepithelial neoplasia and invasive cervical cancer: a comparative study with human papillomavirus (HPV) infection. *Human Pathology.* 2000; 31: 318–26.

Sasahara Y, Fujie H, Kumaki S et al. Epstein-Barr virus-associated hodgkin's disease in a patient with Wiskott-Aldrich syndrome. *Acta Paediatrica.* 2001; 90: 1348–51.

Sebire NJ, Haselden S, Malone M et al. Isolated EBV lymphoproliferative disease in a child with Wiskott-Aldrich syndrome manifesting as cutaneous lymphomatoid granulomatosis and responsive to anti-CD20 immunotherapy. *Journal of Clinical Pathology.* 2003; 56: 555–7.

Shimoyama Y, Oyama T, Asano N et al. Senile Epstein-Barr virus-associated B-cell lymphoproliferative disorders: a mini review. *Journal of Clinical and Experimental Hematopathology.* 2006; 46: 1–4.

Shiozawa E, Saito B, Yamochi-Onizuka T et al. Senile EBV-associated B-cell lymphoproliferative disorder of indolent clinical phenotype with recurrence as aggressive lymphoma. *Pathology International.* 2007; 57: 688–93.

Sprangers B, Smets S, Sagaert X et al. Posttransplant Epstein-Barr virus-associated myogenic tumors: case report and review of the literature. *American Journal of Transplantation.* 2008; 8: 253–8.

Statistics Canada. Cancer Incidence in Canada 2004 to 2005. 2007. Available at http://www.statcan.ca/english/freepub/82-231-XIE/82-231-XIE2007001.pdf. Accessed April 2008.

Szkaradkiewicz A, Kruk-Zagajewska A, Wal M et al. Epstein-Barr virus and human papillomavirus infections and oropharyngeal squamous cell carcinomas. *Clinical and Experimental Medicine.* 2002; 2: 137–41.

Szkaradkiewicz A, Wal M, Kuch A et al. Human papillomavirus (HPV) and Epstein-Barr virus (EBV) cervical infections in women with normal and abnormal cytology. *Polish Journal of Microbiology*. 2004; 53: 95–9.

Takakuwa T, Tresnasari K, Rahadiani N et al. Cell origin of pyothorax-associated lymphoma: a lymphoma strongly associated with Epstein-Barr virus infection. *Leukemia*. 2008; 22: 620–7.

Takeshita M, Okamura S, Oshiro Y et al. Clinicopathologic differences between 22 cases of CD56-negative and CD56-positive subcutaneous panniculitis-like lymphoma in Japan. *Human Pathology*. 2004; 35: 231–9.

Tan BT, Warnke RA, Arber DA. The frequency of B- and T-cell gene rearrangements and epstein-barr virus in T-cell lymphomas: a comparison between angio-immunoblastic T-cell lymphoma and peripheral T-cell lymphoma, unspecified with and without associated B-cell proliferations. *Journal of Molecular Diagnostics*. 2006; 8: 466–75.

Tao Q, Chan AT. Nasopharyngeal carcinoma: molecular pathogenesis and therapeutic developments. *Expert Reviews in Molecular Medicine*. 2007; 9: 1–24.

Tedeschi R, Bloigu A, Ogmundsdottir HM et al. Activation of maternal Epstein-Barr virus infection and risk of acute leukemia in the offspring. *American Journal of Epidemiology*. 2007; 165: 134–7.

Zhong BL, Zong YS, Lin SX et al. Epstein-Barr virus infection in precursor lesions of nasopharyngeal carcinoma. *Chinese Journal of Cancer*. 2006; 25: 136–42.

Zong Y, Liu K, Zhong B et al. Epstein-Barr virus infection of sinonasal lymphoepithelial carcinoma in Guangzhou. *Chinese Medical Journal*. 2001; 114: 132–6.

NOTES

1 Deyrup AT. Epstein-Barr virus-associated epithelial and mesenchymal neoplasms. *Human Pathology*. 2008; 39(4): 473–83.

2 Epstein MA, Achong BG, Barr YM. Virus particles in cultured lymphoblasts from Burkitt's lymphoma. *The Lancet*. 1964; 1(7335): 702–3.

3 Thorley-Lawson DA, Allday MJ. The curious case of the tumour virus: 50 years of Burkitt's lymphoma. *Nature Reviews. Microbiology*. 2008; 6(12): 913–24.

4 Coakley D. Denis Burkitt and his contribution to haematology/oncology. *British Journal of Haematology*. 2006; 135(1): 17–25.

5 Thompson MP, Kurzrock R. Epstein-Barr virus and cancer. *Clinical Cancer Research*. 2004; 10(3): 803–21.

6 Yachie A, Kanegane H, Kasahara Y. Epstein-Barr virus-associated T-/natural killer cell lymphoproliferative diseases. *Seminars in Hematology*. 2003; 40(2): 124–32.

7 Brady G, MacArthur GJ, Farrell PJ. Epstein-Barr virus and Burkitt lymphoma. *Journal of Clinical Pathology*. 2007; 60(12): 1397–402.

8 Thompson MP, Kurzrock R. Epstein-Barr virus and cancer. *Clinical Cancer Research*. 2004; 10(3): 803–21.

9 Schmidt CW, Misko IS. The ecology and pathology of Epstein-Barr virus. *Immunology and Cell Biology*. 1995; 73(6): 489–504.

10 Niller HH, Salamon D, Ilg K et al. EBV-associated neoplasms: alternative pathogenetic pathways. *Medical Hypotheses*. 2004; 62(3): 387–91.

11 Ambinder RF. Epstein-Barr virus-associated lymphoproliferative disorders. *Reviews in Clinical & Experimental Hematology.* 2003; 7(4): 362–74.
12 The labels type 1 and type 2 have also been also used for the classic strains of the virus. See Abdel-Hamid M, Chen JJ, Constantine N et al. EBV strain variation: geographical distribution and relation to disease state. *Virology.* 1992; 190(1): 168–75. Note that this usage creates some ambiguity since the alternate name for EBV is already human herpesvirus type 4.
13 Triantos D, Leao JC, Porter SR et al. Tissue distribution of Epstein-Barr virus genotypes in hosts coinfected by HIV. *AIDS* 1998; 12(16): 2141–6.
14 Gorzer I, Niesters HG, Cornelissen JJ et al. Characterization of Epstein-Barr virus Type I variants based on linked polymorphism among EBNA3A, -3B, and -3C genes. *Virus Research.* 2006; 118(1–2): 105–14.
15 Saechan V, Mori A, Mitarnun W et al. Analysis of LMP1 variants of EBV in Southern Thailand: evidence for strain-associated T-cell tropism and pathogenicity. *Journal of Clinical Virology.* 2006; 36(2): 119–25.
16 Kim JE, Kim YA, Jeon YK et al. Comparative analysis of NK/T-cell lymphoma and peripheral T-cell lymphoma in Korea: clinicopathological correlations and analysis of EBV strain type and 30-bp deletion variant LMP1. *Pathology International.* 2003; 53(11): 735–43.
17 Wang JT, Sheeng TS, Su IJ et al. EBNA-1 sequence variations reflect active EBV replication and disease status or quiescent latency in lymphocytes. *Journal of Medical Virology.* 2003; 69(3): 417–25.
18 Sandvej K, Zhou XG, Hamilton-Dutoit S. EBNA-1 sequence variation in Danish and Chinese EBV-associated tumours: evidence for geographical polymorphism but not for tumour-specific subtype restriction. *Journal of Pathology.* 2000; 191(2): 127–31.
19 Tiwawech D, Srivatanakul P, Karalak A et al. Association between EBNA2 and LMP1 subtypes of Epstein-Barr virus and nasopharyngeal carcinoma in Thais. *Journal of Clinical Virology.* 2008; 42(1): 1–6.
20 See HS, Yap YY, Yip WK et al. Epstein-Barr virus latent membrane protein-1 (LMP-1) 30-bp deletion and Xho I-loss is associated with type III nasopharyngeal carcinoma in Malaysia. *World Journal of Surgical Oncology.* 2008; 6: 18.
21 Zhang XS, Wang HH, Hu LF et al. V-val subtype of Epstein-Barr virus nuclear antigen 1 preferentially exists in biopsies of nasopharyngeal carcinoma. *Cancer Letters.* 2004; 211(1): 11–8.
22 Queiroga EM, Gualco G, Weiss LM et al. Burkitt lymphoma in Brazil is characterized by geographically distinct clinicopathologic features. *American Journal of Clinical Pathology.* 2008; 130(6): 946–56.
23 Queiroga EM, Gualco G, Chioato L et al. Viral studies in Burkitt lymphoma: association with Epstein-Barr virus but not HHV-8. *American Journal of Clinical Pathology.* 2008; 130(2): 186–92.
24 Chen XY, Pepper SD, Arrand JR. Prevalence of the A and B types of Epstein-Barr virus DNA in nasopharyngeal carcinoma biopsies from southern China. *Journal of General Virology.* 1992; 73(Pt 2): 463–6.
25 Shu CH, Chang YS, Liang CL et al. Distribution of type A and type B EBV in normal individuals and patients with head and neck carcinomas in Taiwan. *Journal of Virological Methods.* 1992; 38(1): 123–30.
26 Higa M, Kinjo T, Kamiyama K et al. Epstein-Barr virus (EBV)-related oral squamous cell carcinoma in Okinawa, a subtropical island, in southern

Japan—simultaneously infected with human papillomavirus (HPV). *Oral Oncology.* 2003; 39(4): 405–14.
27 Diduk SV, Smirnova KV, Pavlish OA et al. Functionally significant mutations in the Epstein-Barr virus LMP1 gene and their role in activation of cell signaling pathways. *Biochemistry. Biokhimiia.* 2008; 73(10): 1134–9.
28 Tiwawech D, Srivatanakul P, Karalak A et al. Association between EBNA2 and LMP1 subtypes of Epstein-Barr virus and nasopharyngeal carcinoma in Thais. *Journal of Clinical Virology.* 2008; 42(1): 1–6.
29 Chang ET, Adami HO. The enigmatic epidemiology of nasopharyngeal carcinoma. *Cancer Epidemiology, Biomarkers and Prevention.* 2006; 15(10): 1765–77.
30 Zhou Y, Nabeshima K, Koga K et al. Comparison of Epstein-Barr virus genotypes and clinicohistopathological features of nasopharyngeal carcinoma between Guilin, China and Fukuoka, Japan. *Oncology Reports.* 2008; 19(6): 1413–20.
31 Ayadi W, Feki L, Khabir A et al. Polymorphism analysis of Epstein-Barr virus isolates of nasopharyngeal carcinoma biopsies from Tunisian patients. *Virus Genes.* 2007; 34(2): 137–45.
32 Gosselin J, Flamand L, D'Addario M et al. Modulatory effects of Epstein-Barr, herpes simplex, and human herpes-6 viral infections and coinfections on cytokine synthesis. A comparative study. *Journal of Immunology.* 1992; 149(1): 181–7.
33 Barozzi P, Potenza L, Riva G et al. B cells and Herpesviruses: a model of lymphoproliferation. *Autoimmunity Reviews.* 2007; 7(2): 132–6.
34 Niedobitek G, Meru N, Delecluse HJ. Epstein-Barr virus infection and human malignancies. *International Journal of Experimental Pathology.* 2001; 82(3): 149–70.
35 Young LS, Rickinson AB. Epstein-Barr virus: 40 years on. *Nature Reviews Cancer.* 2004; 4(10): 757–68.
36 Kutok JL, Wang F. Spectrum of Epstein-Barr virus-associated diseases. *Annual Review of Pathology.* 2006; 1: 375–404.
37 Pattle SB, Farrell PJ. The role of Epstein-Barr virus in cancer. *Expert Opinion on Biological Therapy.* 2006; 6(11): 1193–205.
38 Parkin DM. The global health burden of infection-associated cancers in the year 2002. *International Journal of Cancer.* 2006; 118(12): 3030–44.
39 Hsu JL, Glaser SL. Epstein-barr virus-associated malignancies: epidemiologic patterns and etiologic implications. *Critical Reviews of Oncology/Hematology.* 2000; 34(1): 27–53.
40 Thorley-Lawson DA, Gross A. Persistence of the Epstein-Barr virus and the origins of associated lymphomas. *New England Journal of Medicine.* 2004; 350(13): 1328–37.
41 Thorley-Lawson DA. EBV the prototypical human tumor virus—just how bad is it? *Journal of Allergy and Clinical Immunology.* 2005; 116(2): 251–61.
42 Horiuchi K, Mishima K, Ichijima K et al. Epstein-Barr virus in the proliferative diseases of squamous epithelium in the oral cavity. *Oral Surgery, Oral Medicine, Oral Pathology, Oral Radiology, and Endodontics.* 1995; 79(1): 57–63.
43 Xue SA, Lampert IA, Haldane JS et al. Epstein-Barr virus gene expression in human breast cancer: protagonist or passenger? *British Journal of Cancer.* 2003; 89(1): 113–9.

44 Also known as Burkitt's lymphoma.
45 Brady G, MacArthur GJ, Farrell PJ. Epstein-Barr virus and Burkitt lymphoma. *Journal of Clinical Pathology.* 2007; 60(12): 1397–402. With additional information from Rochford R, Cannon MJ, Moormann AM. Endemic Burkitt's lymphoma: a polymicrobial disease? *Nature Reviews Microbiology.* 2005; 3(2): 182–7.
46 Brady G, Macarthur GJ, Farrell PJ. Epstein-Barr virus and Burkitt lymphoma. *Postgraduate Medical Journal.* 2008; 84(993): 372–7.
47 Dolcetti R, Guidoboni M, Gloghini A et al. EBV-associated tumors: pathogenetic insights for improved disease monitoring and treatment. *Current Cancer Therapy Reviews.* 2005; 1: 27–44.
48 Subar M, Neri A, Inghirami G et al. Frequent c-myc oncogene activation and infrequent presence of Epstein-Barr virus genome in AIDS-associated lymphoma. *Blood.* 1988; 72(2): 667–71.
49 Arbovirus is shorthand for arthropod-borne virus, the arthropod in question often being a mosquito. Viruses included in this category include chikungunya, West Nile virus, and Rift Valley fever.
50 van den Bosch CA. Is endemic Burkitt's lymphoma an alliance between three infections and a tumour promoter? *Lancet Oncology.* 2004; 5(12): 738–46.
51 Hjalgrim H, Engels EA. Infectious aetiology of Hodgkin and non-Hodgkin lymphomas: a review of the epidemiological evidence. *Journal of Internal Medicine.* 2008; 264(6): 537–48.
52 Gandhi MK, Tellam JT, Khanna R. Epstein-Barr virus-associated Hodgkin's lymphoma. *British Journal of Haematology.* 2004; 125(3): 267–81.
53 Dolcetti R, Boiocchi M, Gloghini A et al. Pathogenetic and histogenetic features of HIV-associated Hodgkin's disease. *European Journal of Cancer.* 2001; 37(10): 1276–87.
54 Glaser SL, Gulley ML, Clarke CA et al. Racial/ethnic variation in EBV-positive classical Hodgkin lymphoma in California populations. *International Journal of Cancer.* 2008; 123(7): 1499–507.
55 Paltiel O. The elusive search for a viral culprit in non-EBV-associated Hodgkin lymphoma. *Leukemia and Lymphoma.* 2007; 48(4): 647–8.
56 Benharroch D, Shemer-Avni Y, Myint YY et al. Measles virus: evidence of an association with Hodgkin's disease. *British Journal of Cancer.* 2004; 91(3): 572–9.
57 Wilson KS, Freeland JM, Gallagher A et al. Measles virus and classical Hodgkin lymphoma: no evidence for a direct association. *International Journal of Cancer.* 2007; 121(2): 442–7.
58 Figueiredo CP, Franz-Vasconcelos HC, Giunta G et al. Detection of Torque teno virus in Epstein-Barr virus positive and negative lymph nodes of patients with Hodgkin lymphoma. *Leukemia and Lymphoma.* 2007; 48(4): 731–5.
59 Hjalgrim H, Engels EA. Infectious aetiology of Hodgkin and non-Hodgkin lymphomas: a review of the epidemiological evidence. *Journal of Internal Medicine.* 2008; 264(6): 537–48.
60 Riedel DJ, Gonzalez-Cuyar LF, Zhao XF et al. Plasmablastic lymphoma of the oral cavity: a rapidly progressive lymphoma associated with HIV infection. *Lancet Infectious Diseases.* 2008; 8(4): 261–7.
61 Cesarman E. Epstein-Barr virus (EBV) and lymphomagenesis. *Frontiers in Bioscience.* 2002; 7: e58–65.
62 Mack AA, Sugden B. EBV is necessary for proliferation of dually infected primary effusion lymphoma cells. *Cancer Research.* 2008; 68(17): 6963–8.

63 Xu D, Coleman T, Zhang J et al. Epstein-Barr virus inhibits Kaposi's sarcoma-associated herpesvirus lytic replication in primary effusion lymphomas. *Journal of Virology.* 2007; 81(11): 6068–78.
64 Ascoli V, Lo-Coco F. Body cavity lymphoma. *Current Opinion in Pulmonary Medicine.* 2002; 8(4): 317–22.
65 Carbone A. KSHV/HHV-8 associated Kaposi's sarcoma in lymph nodes concurrent with Epstein-Barr virus associated Hodgkin lymphoma. *Journal of Clinical Pathology.* 2005; 58(6): 626–8.
66 Tran H, Nourse J, Hall S et al. Immunodeficiency-associated lymphomas. *Blood Reviews.* 2008; 22(5): 261–81.
67 Wood C, Harrington W, Jr. AIDS and associated malignancies. *Cell Research.* 2005; 15(11–12): 947–52.
68 Snow AL, Martinez OM. Epstein-Barr virus: evasive maneuvers in the development of PTLD. *American Journal of Transplantation.* 2007; 7(2): 271–7.
69 Jones JF, Shurin S, Abramowsky C et al. T-cell lymphomas containing Epstein-Barr viral DNA in patients with chronic Epstein-Barr virus infections. *New England Journal of Medicine.* 1988; 318(12): 733–41.
70 Aozasa K, Takakuwa T, Hongyo T et al. Nasal NK/T-cell lymphoma: epidemiology and pathogenesis. *International Journal of Hematology.* 2008; 87(2): 110–7.
71 Ueda S, Maeda Y, Yamaguchi T et al. Influence of Epstein-Barr virus infection in adult T-cell leukemia. *Hematology.* 2008; 13(3): 154–62.
72 Carbone A, Gloghini A, Dotti G. EBV-associated lymphoproliferative disorders: classification and treatment. *Oncologist.* 2008; 13(5): 577–85.
73 Bekker V, Scherpbier H, Beld M et al. Epstein-Barr virus infects B and non-B lymphocytes in HIV-1-infected children and adolescents. *Journal of Infectious Diseases.* 2006; 194(9): 1323–30.
74 Yachie A, Kanegane H, Kasahara Y. Epstein-Barr virus-associated T-/natural killer cell lymphoproliferative diseases. *Seminars in Hematology.* 2003; 40(2): 124–32.
75 Suzuki R, Takeuchi K, Ohshima K et al. Extranodal NK/T-cell lymphoma: diagnosis and treatment cues. *Hematological Oncology.* 2008; 26(2): 66–72.
76 Aozasa K, Takakuwa T, Hongyo T et al. Nasal NK/T-cell lymphoma: epidemiology and pathogenesis. *International Journal of Hematology.* 2008; 87(2): 110–7.
77 Niedobitek G, Agathanggelou A, Nicholls JM. Epstein-Barr virus infection and the pathogenesis of nasopharyngeal carcinoma: viral gene expression, tumour cell phenotype, and the role of the lymphoid stroma. *Seminars in Cancer Biology.* 1996; 7(4): 165–74.
78 Dolcetti R, Menezes J. Epstein-Barr virus and undifferentiated nasopharyngeal carcinoma: new immunobiological and molecular insights on a long-standing etiopathogenic association. *Advanced Cancer Research.* 2003; 87: 127–57.
79 Abdulamir AS, Hafidh RR, Abdulmuhaimen N et al. The distinctive profile of risk factors of nasopharyngeal carcinoma in comparison with other head and neck cancer types. *BMC Public Health.* 2008; 8: 400.
80 Liu JP, Cassar L, Pinto A et al. Mechanisms of cell immortalization mediated by EB viral activation of telomerase in nasopharyngeal carcinoma. *Cell Research.* 2006; 16(10): 809–17.
81 Boysen T, Friborg J, Andersen A et al. The Inuit cancer pattern—the influence of migration. *International Journal of Cancer.* 2008; 122(11): 2568–72.

82 Thompson MP, Kurzrock R. Epstein-Barr virus and cancer. *Clinical Cancer Research.* 2004; 10(3): 803–21.
83 Busson P, Keryer C, Ooka T et al. EBV-associated nasopharyngeal carcinomas: from epidemiology to virus-targeting strategies. *Trends in Microbiology.* 2004; 12(8): 356–60.
84 Chang ET, Adami HO. The enigmatic epidemiology of nasopharyngeal carcinoma. *Cancer Epidemiology, Biomarkers and Prevention.* 2006; 15(10): 1765–77.
85 Hsu JL, Glaser SL. Epstein-barr virus-associated malignancies: epidemiologic patterns and etiologic implications. *Critical Reviews of Oncology/Hematology.* 2000; 34(1): 27–53.
86 Young LS, Murray PG. Epstein-Barr virus and oncogenesis: from latent genes to tumours. *Oncogene.* 2003; 22(33): 5108–21.
87 Chang ET, Adami HO. The enigmatic epidemiology of nasopharyngeal carcinoma. *Cancer Epidemiology, Biomarkers and Prevention.* 2006; 15(10): 1765–77.
88 Deyrup AT. Epstein-Barr virus-associated epithelial and mesenchymal neoplasms. *Human Pathology.* 2008; 39(4): 473–83.
89 Wu MS, Shun CT, Wu CC et al. Epstein-Barr virus-associated gastric carcinomas: relation to H. pylori infection and genetic alterations. *Gastroenterology.* 2000; 118(6): 1031–8.
90 Wang CP, Chang YL, Ko JY et al. Lymphoepithelial carcinoma versus large cell undifferentiated carcinoma of the major salivary glands. *Cancer.* 2004; 101(9): 2020–7.
91 McClain KL, Leach CT, Jenson HB et al. Association of Epstein-Barr virus with leiomyosarcomas in children with AIDS. *New England Journal of Medicine.* 1995; 332(1): 12–8.
92 Macsween KF, Crawford DH. Epstein-Barr virus-recent advances. *Lancet Infectious Diseases.* 2003; 3(3): 131–40.
93 Abe T, Shinohara N, Tada M et al. Infiltration of Epstein-Barr virus-harboring lymphocytes occurs in a large subset of bladder cancers. *International Journal of Urology.* 2008; 15(5): 429–34.
94 Santos NB, Villanova FE, Andrade PM et al. Epstein-Barr virus detection in invasive and pre-invasive lesions of the uterine cervix. *Oncology Reports.* 2009; 21(2): 403–5.
95 Herrmann K, Niedobitek G. Epstein-Barr virus-associated carcinomas: facts and fiction. *Journal of Pathology.* 2003; 199(2): 140–5.
96 Ryan JL, Morgan DR, Dominguez RL et al. High levels of Epstein-Barr virus DNA in latently infected gastric adenocarcinoma. *Laboratory Investigation.* 2009; 89(1): 80–90.
97 Fukayama M, Hino R, Uozaki H. Epstein-Barr virus and gastric carcinoma: virus-host interactions leading to carcinoma. *Cancer Science.* 2008; 99(9): 1726–33.
98 Sousa H, Pinto-Correia AL, Medeiros R et al. Epstein-Barr virus is associated with gastric carcinoma: the question is what is the significance? *World Journal of Gastroenterology.* 2008; 14(27): 4347–51.
99 Chu PG, Cerilli L, Chen YY et al. Epstein-Barr virus plays no role in the tumorigenesis of small-cell carcinoma of the lung. *Modern Pathology.* 2004; 17(2): 158–64.

100 Lawson JS, Gunzburg WH, Whitaker NJ. Viruses and human breast cancer. *Future Microbiology*. 2006; 1: 33–51.
101 Canadian Cancer Society, National Cancer Institute of Canada. *Canadian Cancer Statistics 2008*.
102 Crawford DH. Biology and disease associations of Epstein-Barr virus. *Philosophical Transactions of the Royal Society of London*. 2001; 356(1408): 461–73.
103 Yachie A, Kanegane H, Kasahara Y. Epstein-Barr virus-associated T-/natural killer cell lymphoproliferative diseases. *Seminars in Hematology*. 2003; 40(2): 124–32.
104 Ohshima K, Kimura H, Yoshino T et al. Proposed categorization of pathological states of EBV-associated T/natural killer-cell lymphoproliferative disorder (LPD) in children and young adults: overlap with chronic active EBV infection and infantile fulminant EBV T-LPD. *Pathology International*. 2008; 58(4): 209–17.
105 Barzilai O, Sherer Y, Ram M et al. Epstein-Barr virus and cytomegalovirus in autoimmune diseases: are they truly notorious? A preliminary report. *Annals of the New York Academy of Sciences*. 2007; 1108: 567–77.
106 Lunemann JD, Kamradt T, Martin R et al. Epstein-barr virus: environmental trigger of multiple sclerosis? *Journal of Virology*. 2007; 81(13): 6777–84.
107 James JA, Harley JB, Scofield RH. Epstein-Barr virus and systemic lupus erythematosus. *Current Opinion in Rheumatology*. 2006; 18(5): 462–7.
108 Balandraud N, Roudier J, Roudier C. Epstein-Barr virus and rheumatoid arthritis. *Autoimmunity Reviews*. 2004; 3(5): 362–7.
109 DeLorenze GN, Munger KL, Lennette ET et al. Epstein-Barr virus and multiple sclerosis: evidence of association from a prospective study with long-term follow-up. *Archives of Neurology*. 2006; 63(6): 839–44.
110 Niller HH, Wolf H, Minarovits J. Regulation and dysregulation of Epstein-Barr virus latency: implications for the development of autoimmune diseases. *Autoimmunity*. 2008; 41(4): 298–328.
111 Murray PG, Young LS. The Role of the Epstein-Barr virus in human disease. *Frontiers in Bioscience*. 2002; 7: d519–40.
112 Other names for this disease are acute lymphocytic leukemia, acute lymphoid leukemia, and acute lymphoblastic leukemia/lymphoma.
113 Tedeschi R, Bloigu A, Ogmundsdottir HM et al. Activation of maternal Epstein-Barr virus infection and risk of acute leukemia in the offspring. *American Journal of Epidemiology*. 2007; 165(2): 134–7.
114 Lehtinen M, Koskela P, Ogmundsdottir HM et al. Maternal herpesvirus infections and risk of acute lymphoblastic leukemia in the offspring. *American Journal of Epidemiology*. 2003; 158(3): 207–13.
115 Belson M, Kingsley B, Holmes A. Risk factors for acute leukemia in children: a review. *Environmental Health Perspectives*. 2007; 115(1): 138–45.
116 McNally RJ, Eden TO. An infectious aetiology for childhood acute leukaemia: A review of the evidence. *British Journal of Haematology*. 2004; 127(3): 243–63.
117 Chagas CA, Endo LH, Dos-Santos WL et al. Is there a relationship between the detection of human herpesvirus 8 and Epstein-Barr virus in Waldeyer's ring tissues? *International Journal of Pediatric Otorhinolaryngology*. 2006; 70(11): 1923–7.

118 Macsween KF, Crawford DH. Epstein-Barr virus-recent advances. *Lancet Infectious Diseases.* 2003; 3(3): 131–40.
119 Thomas R, Macsween KF, McAulay K et al. Evidence of shared Epstein-Barr viral isolates between sexual partners, and low level EBV in genital secretions. *Journal of Medical Virology.* 2006; 78(9): 1204–9.
120 Kasahara Y, Yachie A. Cell type specific infection of Epstein-Barr virus (EBV) in EBV-associated hemophagocytic lymphohistiocytosis and chronic active EBV infection. *Critical Reviews in Oncology/Hematology.* 2002; 44(3): 283–94.
121 Hutt-Fletcher LM. Epstein-Barr virus entry. Journal of Virology. 2007; 81(15): 7825–32.
122 Knecht H, Berger C, Rothenberger S et al. The role of Epstein-Barr virus in neoplastic transformation. *Oncology.* 2001; 60(4): 289–302.
123 Laichalk LL, Hochberg D, Babcock GJ et al. The dispersal of mucosal memory B cells: evidence from persistent EBV infection. *Immunity.* 2002; 16(5): 745–54.
124 Faulkner GC, Krajewski AS, Crawford DH. The ins and outs of EBV infection. *Trends in Microbiology.* 2000; 8(4): 185–9.
125 Hoover SE, Kawada J, Wilson W et al. Oropharyngeal shedding of Epstein-Barr virus in the absence of circulating B cells. *Journal of Infectious Diseases.* 2008; 198(3): 318–23.
126 Feederle R, Neuhierl B, Bannert H et al. Epstein-Barr virus B95.8 produced in 293 cells shows marked tropism for differentiated primary epithelial cells and reveals interindividual variation in susceptibility to viral infection. *International Journal of Cancer.* 2007; 121(3): 588–94.
127 Niedobitek G, Agathanggelou A, Steven N et al. Epstein-Barr virus (EBV) in infectious mononucleosis: detection of the virus in tonsillar B lymphocytes but not in desquamated oropharyngeal epithelial cells. *Molecular Pathology.* 2000; 53(1): 37–42.
128 Hutt-Fletcher LM. Epstein-Barr virus entry. *Journal of Virology.* 2007; 81(15): 7825–32.
129 Tugizov S, Herrera R, Veluppillai P et al. Epstein-Barr virus (EBV)-infected monocytes facilitate dissemination of EBV within the oral mucosal epithelium. *Journal of Virology.* 2007; 81(11): 5484–96.
130 Walling DM, Ray AJ, Nichols JE et al. Epstein-Barr virus infection of Langerhans cell precursors as a mechanism of oral epithelial entry, persistence, and reactivation. *Journal of Virology.* 2007; 81(13): 7249–68.
131 Hoover SE, Kawada J, Wilson W et al. Oropharyngeal shedding of Epstein-Barr virus in the absence of circulating B cells. *Journal of Infectious Diseases.* 2008; 198(3): 318–23.
132 Conacher M, Callard R, McAulay K et al. Epstein-Barr virus can establish infection in the absence of a classical memory B-cell population. *Journal of Virology.* 2005; 79(17): 11128–34.
133 Chaganti S, Ma CS, Bell AI et al. Epstein-Barr virus persistence in the absence of conventional memory B cells: IgM+IgD+CD27+ B cells harbor the virus in X-linked lymphoproliferative disease patients. *Blood.* 2008; 112(3): 672–9.
134 Shannon-Lowe CD, Neuhierl B, Baldwin G et al. Resting B cells as a transfer vehicle for Epstein-Barr virus infection of epithelial cells. *Proceedings of the National Academy of Sciences of the United States of America.* 2006; 103(18): 7065–70.

135 Hutt-Fletcher LM. Epstein-Barr virus entry. *Journal of Virology.* 2007; 81(15): 7825–32.
136 Shannon-Lowe CD, Neuhierl B, Baldwin G et al. Resting B cells as a transfer vehicle for Epstein-Barr virus infection of epithelial cells. *Proceedings of the National Academy of Sciences of the United States of America.* 2006; 103(18): 7065–70.
137 Borza CM, Hutt-Fletcher LM. Alternate replication in B cells and epithelial cells switches tropism of Epstein-Barr virus. *Nature Medicine.* 2002; 8(6): 594–9.
138 Bornkamm GW, Behrends U, Mautner J. The infectious kiss: newly infected B cells deliver Epstein-Barr virus to epithelial cells. *Proceedings of the National Academy of Sciences of the United States of America.* 2006; 103(19): 7201–2.
139 Farrell PJ. Cell-switching and kissing. *Nature Medicine.* 2002; 8(6): 559–60.
140 Niller HH, Wolf H, Minarovits J. Regulation and dysregulation of Epstein-Barr virus latency: implications for the development of autoimmune diseases. *Autoimmunity.* 2008; 41(4): 298–328.
141 Bornkamm GW, Behrends U, Mautner J. The infectious kiss: newly infected B cells deliver Epstein-Barr virus to epithelial cells. *Proceedings of the National Academy of Sciences of the United States of America.* 2006; 103(19): 7201–2.
142 Hislop AD, Taylor GS, Sauce D et al. Cellular responses to viral infection in humans: lessons from Epstein-Barr virus. *Annual Review of Immunology.* 2007; 25: 587–617.
143 Minarovits J. Epigenotypes of latent herpesvirus genomes. *Current Topics in Microbiology and Immunology.* 2006; 310: 61–80.
144 Young LS, Murray PG. Epstein-Barr virus and oncogenesis: from latent genes to tumours. *Oncogene.* 2003; 22(33): 5108–21.
145 Kis LL, Takahara M, Nagy N et al. Cytokine mediated induction of the major Epstein-Barr virus (EBV)-encoded transforming protein, LMP-1. *Immunology Letters.* 2006; 104(1–2): 83–8.
146 Ogino T, Moriai S, Ishida Y et al. Association of immunoescape mechanisms with Epstein-Barr virus infection in nasopharyngeal carcinoma. *International Journal of Cancer.* 2007; 120(11): 2401–10.
147 Cohen JI, Bollard CM, Khanna R et al. Current understanding of the role of Epstein-Barr virus in lymphomagenesis and therapeutic approaches to EBV-associated lymphomas. *Leukemia and Lymphoma.* 2008; 49(suppl 1): 27–34.
148 Bollard CM, Cooper LJ, Heslop HE. Immunotherapy targeting EBV-expressing lymphoproliferative diseases. *Best Practice and Research Clinical Haematology.* 2008; 21(3): 405–20.
149 Bajaj BG, Murakami M, Robertson ES. Molecular biology of EBV in relationship to AIDS-associated oncogenesis. *Cancer Treatment and Research.* 2007; 133: 141–62.
150 Shore AM, White PC, Hui RC et al. Epstein-Barr virus represses the FoxO1 transcription factor through latent membrane protein 1 and latent membrane protein 2A. *Journal of Virology.* 2006; 80(22): 11191–9.
151 Lo AK, Lo KW, Tsao SW et al. Epstein-Barr virus infection alters cellular signal cascades in human nasopharyngeal epithelial cells. *Neoplasia.* 2006; 8(3): 173–80.

152 Klein E, Kis LL, Klein G. Epstein-Barr virus infection in humans: from harmless to life endangering virus-lymphocyte interactions. *Oncogene*. 2007; 26(9): 1297–305.
153 Paludan C, Munz C. CD4+ T cell responses in the immune control against latent infection by Epstein-Barr virus. *Current Molecular Medicine*. 2003; 3(4): 341–7.
154 Landais E, Saulquin X, Houssaint E. The human T cell immune response to Epstein-Barr virus. *International Journal of Developmental Biology*. 2005; 49(2–3): 285–92.
155 Hislop AD, Taylor GS, Sauce D et al. Cellular responses to viral infection in humans: lessons from Epstein-Barr virus. *Annual Review of Immunology*. 2007; 25: 587–617.
156 Aalto SM, Linnavuori K, Peltola H et al. Immunoreactivation of Epstein-Barr virus due to cytomegalovirus primary infection. *Journal of Medical Virology*. 1998; 56(3): 186–91.
157 Hayes RC, Leonfellner S, Pilgrim W et al. Incidence of nonmelanoma skin cancer in New Brunswick, Canada, 1992 to 2001. *Journal of Cutaneous Medicine and Surgery*. 2007; 11(2): 45–52.
158 Chene A, Donati D, Guerreiro-Cacais AO et al. A molecular link between malaria and Epstein-Barr virus reactivation. *Public Library of Science Pathogens*. 2007; 3(6): e80.
159 Ladell K, Dorner M, Zauner L et al. Immune activation suppresses initiation of lytic Epstein-Barr virus infection. *Cellular Microbiology*. 2007; 9(8): 2055–69.
160 Dolcetti R. B lymphocytes and Epstein-Barr virus: the lesson of post-transplant lymphoproliferative disorders. *Autoimmunity Reviews*. 2007; 7(2): 96–101.
161 Newton R, Carpenter L, Casabonne D et al. A prospective study of Kaposi's sarcoma-associated herpesvirus and Epstein-Barr virus in adults with human immunodeficiency virus-1. *British Journal of Cancer*. 2006; 94(10): 1504–9.
162 Hislop AD, Taylor GS, Sauce D et al. Cellular responses to viral infection in humans: lessons from Epstein-Barr virus. *Annual Review of Immunology*. 2007; 25: 587–617.
163 Ferrazzo KL, Mesquita RA, Aburad AT et al. EBV detection in HIV-related oral plasmablastic lymphoma. *Oral Diseases*. 2007; 13(6): 564–9.
164 Webster-Cyriaque J, Duus K, Cooper C et al. Oral EBV and KSHV infection in HIV. *Advances in Dental Research*. 2006; 19(1): 91–5.
165 Hille JJ, Webster-Cyriaque J, Palefski JM et al. Mechanisms of expression of HHV8, EBV and HPV in selected HIV-associated oral lesions. *Oral Diseases*. 2002; 8(suppl 2): 161–8.
166 Landais E, Saulquin X, Houssaint E. The human T cell immune response to Epstein-Barr virus. *International Journal of Developmental Biology*. 2005; 49(2–3): 285–92.
167 Young LS. Epstein-Barr-virus infection and persistence: a B-cell marriage in sickness and in health. *The Lancet*. 1999; 354(9185): 1141–2.
168 Amon W, Farrell PJ. Reactivation of Epstein-Barr virus from latency. *Reviews in Medical Virology*. 2005; 15(3): 149–56.
169 Tugizov SM, Berline JW, Palefsky JM. Epstein-Barr virus infection of polarized tongue and nasopharyngeal epithelial cells. *Nature Medicine*. 2003; 9(3): 307–14.

170 Liu JP, Cassar L, Pinto A et al. Mechanisms of cell immortalization mediated by EB viral activation of telomerase in nasopharyngeal carcinoma. *Cell Research.* 2006; 16(10): 809–17.
171 De Paoli P, Pratesi C, Bortolin MT. The Epstein Barr virus DNA levels as a tumor marker in EBV-associated cancers. *Journal of Cancer Research and Clinical Oncology.* 2007; 133(11): 809–15.
172 Binnicker MJ, Jespersen DJ, Harring JA et al. Evaluation of a multiplex flow immunoassay for detection of epstein-barr virus-specific antibodies. *Clinical and Vaccine Immunology.* 2008; 15(9): 1410–3.
173 Hess RD. Routine Epstein-Barr virus diagnostics from the laboratory perspective: Still challenging after 35 years. *Journal of Clinical Microbiology.* 2004; 42(8): 3381–7.
174 Kimura H, Ito Y, Suzuki R et al. Measuring Epstein-Barr virus (EBV) load: the significance and application for each EBV-associated disease. *Reviews in Medical Virology.* 2008; 18(5): 305–19.
175 Takeuchi K, Tanaka-Taya K, Kazuyama Y et al. Prevalence of Epstein-Barr virus in Japan: trends and future prediction. *Pathology International.* 2006; 56(3): 112–6.
176 Dinand V, Arya LS. Epidemiology of childhood Hodgkins disease: is it different in developing countries? *Indian Pediatrics.* 2006; 43(2): 141–7.
177 Balfour HH, Jr. Epstein-Barr virus vaccine for the prevention of infectious mononucleosis—and what else? *Journal of Infectious Diseases.* 2007; 196(12): 1724–6.
178 Moss DJ, Khanna R, Bharadwaj M. Will a vaccine to nasopharyngeal carcinoma retain orphan status? *Developments in Biologicals.* 2002; 110: 67–71.
179 Lopes V, Young LS, Murray PG. Epstein-Barr virus-associated cancers: A etiology and treatment. *Herpes.* 2003; 10(3): 78–82.
180 Lockey TD, Zhan X, Surman S et al. Epstein-Barr virus vaccine development: a lytic and latent protein cocktail. *Frontiers in Bioscience.* 2008; 13: 5916–27.
181 Macsween KF, Crawford DH. Epstein-Barr virus-recent advances. *Lancet Infectious Diseases.* 2003; 3(3): 131–40.
182 Sokal EM, Hoppenbrouwers K, Vandermeulen C et al. Recombinant gp350 vaccine for infectious mononucleosis: a phase 2, randomized, double-blind, placebo-controlled trial to evaluate the safety, immunogenicity, and efficacy of an Epstein-Barr virus vaccine in healthy young adults. *Journal of Infectious Diseases.* 2007; 196(12): 1749–53.
183 Khanna R, Tellam J, Duraiswamy J et al. Immunotherapeutic strategies for EBV-associated malignancies. *Trends in Molecular Medicine.* 2001; 7(6): 270–6.
184 Taylor GS. T cell-based therapies for EBV-associated malignancies. *Expert Opinion in Biological Therapy.* 2004; 4(1): 11–21.
185 Chang ET, Adami HO. The enigmatic epidemiology of nasopharyngeal carcinoma. *Cancer Epidemiology, Biomarkers and Prevention.* 2006; 15(10): 1765–77.
186 Poirier S, Hubert A, de-The G et al. Occurrence of volatile nitrosamines in food samples collected in three high-risk areas for nasopharyngeal carcinoma. *IARC Scientific Publications.* 1987; (84): 415–9.

187 Chang ET, Adami HO. The enigmatic epidemiology of nasopharyngeal carcinoma. *Cancer Epidemiology, Biomarkers and Prevention*. 2006; 15(10): 1765–77.
188 Armstrong RW, Armstrong MJ, Yu MC et al. Salted fish and inhalants as risk factors for nasopharyngeal carcinoma in Malaysian Chinese. *Cancer Research*. 1983; 43(6): 2967–70.
189 Yu MC, Huang TB, Henderson BE. Diet and nasopharyngeal carcinoma: a case-control study in Guangzhou, China. *International Journal of Cancer*. 1989; 43(6): 1077–82.
190 Chang ET, Adami HO. The enigmatic epidemiology of nasopharyngeal carcinoma. *Cancer Epidemiology, Biomarkers and Prevention*. 2006; 15(10): 1765–77.
191 Hildesheim A, Dosemeci M, Chan CC et al. Occupational exposure to wood, formaldehyde, and solvents and risk of nasopharyngeal carcinoma. *Cancer Epidemiology, Biomarkers and Prevention*. 2001; 10(11): 1145–53.
192 Chen CJ, Liang KY, Chang YS et al. Multiple risk factors of nasopharyngeal carcinoma: Epstein-Barr virus, malarial infection, cigarette smoking and familial tendency. *Anticancer Research*. 1990; 10(2B): 547–53.
193 Chang ET, Adami HO. The enigmatic epidemiology of nasopharyngeal carcinoma. *Cancer Epidemiology, Biomarkers and Prevention*. 2006; 15(10): 1765–77.
194 Carpenter LM, Newton R, Casabonne D et al. Antibodies against malaria and Epstein-Barr virus in childhood Burkitt lymphoma: a case-control study in Uganda. *International Journal of Cancer*. 2008; 122(6): 1319–23.
195 Crawford DH. Biology and disease associations of Epstein-Barr virus. *Philosophical Transactions of the Royal Society of London*. 2001; 356(1408): 461–73.
196 Mueller N. Overview: Viral agents and cancer. *Environmental Health Perspectives*. 1995; 103(suppl 8): 259–61.
197 Also known as post transplant lymphoproliferative disease.
198 Gustafsson A, Levitsky V, Zou JZ et al. Epstein-Barr virus (EBV) load in bone marrow transplant recipients at risk to develop posttransplant lymphoproliferative disease: prophylactic infusion of EBV-specific cytotoxic T cells. *Blood*. 2000; 95(3): 807–14.
199 Rooney CM, Smith CA, Ng CY et al. Infusion of cytotoxic T cells for the prevention and treatment of Epstein-Barr virus-induced lymphoma in allogeneic transplant recipients. *Blood*. 1998; 92(5): 1549–55.
200 Bollard CM, Cooper LJ, Heslop HE. Immunotherapy targeting EBV-expressing lymphoproliferative diseases. *Best Practice and Research Clinical Haematology*. 2008; 21(3): 405–20.
201 Gershburg E, Pagano JS. Epstein-Barr virus infections: prospects for treatment. *Journal of Antimicrobial Chemotherapy*. 2005; 56(2): 277–81.
202 Swanson-Mungerson M, Ikeda M, Lev L et al. Identification of latent membrane protein 2A (LMP2A) specific targets for treatment and eradication of Epstein-Barr virus (EBV)-associated diseases. *Journal of Antimicrobial Chemotherapy*. 2003; 52(2): 152–4.
203 Cohen JI, Bollard CM, Khanna R et al. Current understanding of the role of Epstein-Barr virus in lymphomagenesis and therapeutic approaches to EBV-associated lymphomas. *Leukemia and Lymphoma*. 2008; 49(suppl 1): 27–34.

204 Psyrri A, Burtness B. Viruses in head and neck cancers: prevention and therapy. *Expert Review of Anticancer Therapy.* 2008; 8(9): 1365–71.
205 Comito MA, Sun Q, Lucas KG. Immunotherapy for Epstein-Barr virus-associated tumors. *Leukemia and Lymphoma.* 2004; 45(10): 1981–7.
206 Murray PG, Young LS. Epstein-Barr virus infection: basis of malignancy and potential for therapy. *Expert Reviews in Molecular Medicine.* 2001; 2001: 1–20.
207 Gottschalk S, Heslop HE, Roon CM. Treatment of Epstein-Barr virus-associated malignancies with specific T cells. *Advanced Cancer Research.* 2002; 84: 175–201.
208 Merlo A, Turrini R, Dolcetti R et al. Adoptive cell therapy against EBV-related malignancies: a survey of clinical results. *Expert Opinion on Biological Therapy.* 2008; 8(9): 1265–94.
209 Psyrri A, Burtness B. Viruses in head and neck cancers: prevention and therapy. *Expert Review of Anticancer Therapy.* 2008; 8(9): 1365–71.
210 De Paoli P. Novel virally targeted therapies of EBV-associated tumors. *Current Cancer Drug Targets.* 2008; 8(7): 591–6.
211 Srimatkandada P, Loomis R, Carbone R et al. Combined proteasome and Bcl-2 inhibition stimulates apoptosis and inhibits growth in EBV-transformed lymphocytes: a potential therapeutic approach to EBV-associated lymphoproliferative diseases. *European Journal of Haematology.* 2008; 80(5): 407–18.
212 Chuang HC, Lay JD, Hsieh WC et al. Pathogenesis and mechanism of disease progression from hemophagocytic lymphohistiocytosis to Epstein-Barr virus-associated T-cell lymphoma: Nuclear factor-kappa B pathway as a potential therapeutic target. *Cancer Science.* 2007; 98(9): 1281–7.
213 Chuang HC, Lay JD, Hsieh WC et al. Pathogenesis and mechanism of disease progression from hemophagocytic lymphohistiocytosis to Epstein-Barr virus-associated T-cell lymphoma: nuclear factor-kappa B pathway as a potential therapeutic target. *Cancer Science.* 2007; 98(9): 1281–7.
214 Thompson MP, Kurzrock R. Epstein-Barr virus and cancer. *Clinical Cancer Research.* 2004; 10(3): 803–21.
215 Orem J, Mbidde EK, Lambert B et al. Burkitt's lymphoma in Africa, a review of the epidemiology and etiology. *African Health Sciences.* 2007; 7(3): 166–75.
216 Cesarman E, Mesri EA. Kaposi sarcoma-associated herpesvirus and other viruses in human lymphomagenesis. *Current Topics in Microbiology and Immunology.* 2007; 312: 263–87.
217 Jiang Y, Xu D, Zhao Y et al. Mutual Inhibition between Kaposi's Sarcoma-Associated Herpesvirus and Epstein-Barr Virus Lytic Replication Initiators in Dually-Infected Primary Effusion Lymphoma. *PLoS ONE.* 2008; 3(2): e1569.
218 van den Bosch CA. Is endemic Burkitt's lymphoma an alliance between three infections and a tumour promoter? *Lancet Oncology.* 2004; 5(12): 738–46.

11

HUMAN HERPESVIRUS TYPE 8

The link between human herpesvirus 8 (KSHV) and Kaposi's sarcoma has been proven, but many important aspects including risk factors, genetic predisposition to tumor development, transmission of KSHV, and the pathogenic potential of different genotypes remain to be elucidated.[1]

INTRODUCTION

Human herpesvirus type 8 (HHV-8), originally known as Kaposi sarcoma–associated herpesvirus (KSHV), was only isolated in 1994, making it one of the more recently identified oncogenic viruses.[2] By comparison, Epstein-Barr virus (EBV), a genetic relative of HHV-8, was isolated a full 30 years earlier.[3]

From the time of its discovery, HHV-8 has been linked with Kaposi sarcoma (KS), a tumor often presenting in the oral mucosa or skin; KS tumors are thought to arise in endothelial cells, specifically the lining of lymphatic vessels. KS is an important sequelae of human immunodeficiency virus (HIV) infection. Indeed, it is the hallmark malignancy in patients with acquired immune deficiency syndrome (AIDS). As such, the well-established causal association between KS and HHV-8 remains an ongoing clinical and public health concern.[4]

As will be outlined in this chapter, KS is not the only cancer connected with HHV-8. However, the other malignancies associated with the virus are even rarer than KS.[5] Thus, an argument can be made for the validity of the original qualifying term for the virus, "Kaposi-sarcoma–associated."

In fact, that name is still widely used, even when the discussion of disease expands beyond KS.[6] In the end, the more inclusive label HHV-8 was adopted within this book, in order to better represent the role of the virus in other cancers.

A 2003 review indicated that there were several outstanding issues surrounding HHV-8, including[7]:

- The evolution of the HHV-8 epidemic
- The distribution of HHV-8 with respect to KS
- Transmission modalities
- Natural history of infection
- The appropriate serological assays for detection and disease monitoring

Only partial progress has been made on these questions in recent years, suggesting that the subtitle from a 1999 editorial on the topic may still hold true today: some answers, more questions.[8] In this chapter, an update on what is currently known about HHV-8 and related cancers will be provided. As with other agents in this book, the basic science of the virus will be outlined, followed by sections on the evidence of associated cancers, disease mechanism and processes, transmission and occurrence of the agent, detection methods, and prevention approaches.

THE VIRUS AND ITS FAMILY

Herpesviridae is a family of DNA viruses that infect various animal species. The name comes from Greek *herpein*, which means "to creep," apparently a reference to the low disease activity during the often long latent phase of the infection. In fact, primary infection with herpesviruses typically results in lifelong persistence in the host.[9,10] A well-known example of this phenomenon is chickenpox (varicella), caused by HHV-3. While usually a pediatric disease, the latent virus may be reactivated in adulthood, resulting in herpes zoster (commonly known as shingles).

About 100 herpesvirus types have been isolated, with at least one found for most animal species examined to date; the spectrum of animal species involved is wide, from chickens to scallops, and mice to elephants.[11-14] A particular veterinary herpesvirus can further display a remarkable host range. For example, ovine herpesvirus type 2 has a natural reservoir in sheep, but can be transmitted to goats, cattle, bison, deer, and pigs.[15] The overall virus family is divided genetically into several subfamilies and genera; these are sometimes associated with characteristic host targets. For instance, the rhadinoviruses (also known as gamma-2-herpesvirinae), the subgroup that includes HHV-8, are associated with infection in primates.[16] In fact, HHV-8 represents the first human virus identified within the genus *Rhadinovirus*.[17]

The insights gained from herpesviruses that usually infect other animal species may enable researchers to better understand human infections and related diseases.[18,19] For instance, interspecies transmission can be revealing. Thus, the same mechanism that protects latently infected cells from being destroyed by the immune system in the normal animal hosts also creates a steady state where there is little or no expression of disease symptoms. On the other hand, viral transfer to a novel species produces a loss of "control over the amount of latently infected cells, which results in the development of lethal diseases."[20] By creating such transfers in experimental settings, researchers can mimic the functioning of the virus when its normal host experiences a compromised immune system. The hope is that by learning about the molecular pathways of herpesvirus disease, therapeutic and, possibly, preventive maneuvers related to HHV-8 in humans may be developed.[21]

Discovered in KS tissue in 1994, HHV-8 is the most recently identified of eight known human herpesviruses, each of which has a different clinical expression. In addition to EBV (discussed in Chapter 10), other human herpesviruses include cytomegalovirus (CMV) and herpes simplex virus (HSV). The basic classification and disease associations of the human herpesviruses are summarized in Table 11.1.[22] As indicated in the table, a link to cancer etiology has not been demonstrated for the types outside the gamma-herpesviruses.[23]

Table 11.1. Human Herpesviruses and Key Associated Diseases

Subfamily	Genus	HHV Type	Alternate Term	Malignant Disease	Nonmalignant Disease
Alpha-herpesvirinae	*Simplexvirus*	1	HSV-1		Oral herpes
		2	HSV-2		Genital herpes
	Varicellovirus	3	VZV		Chickenpox; shingles
Beta-herpesvirinae	*Cytomegalovirus*	5	CMV		Retinitis; hearing loss
	Roseolovirus	6, 7			Roseola
Gamma-herpesvirinae	*Lymphocryptovirus*	4	EBV	Lymphoma	Infectious mononucleosis
	Rhadinovirus	8	KSHV	Kaposi sarcoma	

Source: Moore, *Journal of Virology*, 1996.

Unlike other members of *Herpesviridae*, human herpesviruses appear to be species-specific in vivo.[24,25] That is, they are restricted to infecting humans. However, there is evidence that HHV-8 can infect a variety of animal cells in vitro.[26] The actual cellular tropisms of HHV-8 in the human host, though perhaps more limited than seen with EBV, are still wide-ranging.[27] Other human herpesviruses also infect different cell types; the precise niche range appears to be specific to each virus.[28] Returning to a previous example, HHV-3, also known as varicella-zoster virus (VZV), demonstrates multiple cellular tropisms before becoming latent in sensory neurons; the latter phenomenon is the key factor in the development of shingles, which can occur decades after the initial infection.

The herpesvirus particles are generally very complex. Like other viruses in this family, HHV-8 contains double-stranded DNA within a relatively large capsid that demonstrates icosahedral symmetry.[29]

Viral subtyping is generally marked by two phenomenon: stability over most of the viral genome, and variation in particular regions. The genotypes of HHV-8 have been traditionally based on *K1*, the most highly divergent gene in the viral genome. Analysis of *K1* variation in the past has suggested six subtypes, labeled A to E, plus Z. The existing subtypes may be refined (creating up to 24 evolutionary categories, each called a clade); research into other variations in the genome continues to extend subtyping in new directions.[30-33] If some of the genetic variants are proven to have different impacts in terms of carcinogenesis, then there may be implications for targeted screening. The indication that subtypes follow specific ethnic/geographic patterns (Table 11.2) may also be of relevance in prevention planning.[34]

In addition to the potential applications in pathology and prevention, HHV-8 genetic variation represents a tool (similar to other evolving pathogens) that can be used to investigate both ancient and recent

Table 11.2. Main Geographic Location of HHV-8 Subtypes

Subtype	Predominant Location and Ethnicity
A	United States, Europe, Northern Asia
A1	Israel (Ashkenazi Jews)
A5	Africa
B	Africa
C	United States, Europe, Northern Asia
C2, C6	North Africa (Sephardic Jews)
D	Pacific Islands
E	Brazil (Amerindians)
Z	Africa (Zambian children)

Source: Dourmishev et al., *Microbiology & Molecular Biology Reviews*, 2003.

human migration patterns.[35] One of the most dramatic examples of such developments is the evidence that a large cohort among HHV-8-positive individuals in the United States may have been derived from a single viral isolate that spread in concert with the AIDS epidemic.[36]

EVIDENCE OF ASSOCIATED CANCERS

HHV-8 is implicated in a narrower spectrum of cancers than found with EBV.[37] Three malignancies have a well-established association with HHV-8[38-40]:

- Kaposi sarcoma
- Primary effusion lymphoma (PEL) and related solid variants
- A subset of multicentric Castleman disease (MCD) that leads to plasmablastic lymphomas

While seemingly disparate in nature, the pathways of these three diseases all reflect some kind of immune system perturbation. In fact, the latter two conditions are both clearly lymphoproliferative disorders, a category of disease that is also associated with the other known gammaherpesvirus, EBV.[41] And, even more pertinent than the tangential connection of KS to lymphatic endothelium, cells central to the immune system are also thought to be involved in the progression of the disease.[42] Evidence for shared pathological elements among the three cancers was offered by a recent case report, where KS, PEL, and Castleman disease occurred over a 2-year period in the same HIV-positive patient.[43]

These three cancers will be further described in the following subsections.

Kaposi Sarcoma

Kaposi sarcoma[44] is a multifocal, highly vascular (and thus pigmented) lesion that most often occurs in mucosal and cutaneous areas. These include the oral and oropharyngeal mucosa, and the skin of the lower extremities, face, trunk, and genitalia. Lymph nodes can be involved, as well as organs of the respiratory and gastrointestinal tracts. Finally, KS has also been reported (rarely) in many other body sites, including the bones and the female breast.[45,46] Assuming that KS is a true cancer (see the following discussion), further classifying it as a sarcoma is appropriate given its apparent origin in endothelial cells.[47]

There is wide variety in the histological and clinical presentation of KS, which can make diagnosis difficult, especially during its proposed

Table 11.3. Clinicoepidemiologic Variants of Kaposi Sarcoma

KS Variant	Other Names	Risk Group	Geography	Lesion Location	Median Survival
Classic	Sporadic	Elderly people, particularly men; Ashkenazi Jewish or Middle Eastern origin	Southern and Eastern European countries; South America	Skin lesions confined to lower extremities; eventually progress to arms, mucosal tissues, and viscera	Years or decades
Endemic	African	Subvariants, including African cutaneous (adults) and lymphadenopathic (children)	Central and Eastern African countries	Differs with subvariant	Months or years
Post-transplant	Immunosuppression-associated; Iatrogenic	Organ-transplant recipients receiving immunosuppressive therapy (especially kidney recipients)	Worldwide; high rates in Classic and Endemic KS regions	Affects lymph nodes, mucosa, and visceral organs, sometimes in the absence of skin lesions	Months or years
Epidemic	AIDs-associated KS	HIV-positive individuals, especially men who have sex with men	Worldwide	Multifocal; frequently on the upper body, head and neck	Weeks or months

premalignant phase.[48] When first described by M. Kaposi (long before the advent of AIDS), KS was known as a rare, relatively indolent disease presenting in the skin on the legs of elderly European men.[49] The disease is now known to occur in four clinicoepidemiologic variants (Table 11.3): classic, endemic, iatrogenic or posttransplant, and epidemic.[50–56]

Classic KS, the form first reported by Dr. Kaposi in 1872, is usually benign and typically affects elderly men of Eastern European or Mediterranean descent.[57] Endemic KS, on the other hand, is one of the most common types of cancers in several African countries.[58] In North America and other developed regions, iatrogenic KS occurs mainly in organ transplant recipients that are subject to immunosuppression. The most aggressive variant of the disease, epidemic KS or AIDS-KS, is caused by an opportunistic or reactivated HHV-8 infection in AIDS patients, particularly among men who have sex with men (MSM).[59] For some of the clinical types of KS, further division into subvariants has been proposed.[60]

The advent of HIV infection has dramatically shifted the global pattern of KS; for instance, the substantial epidemic of HIV among the heterosexual population and MSM[61] in sub-Saharan Africa means that the endemic variant of KS is likely no longer the dominant concern. Indeed, driven by the effect of HIV coinfection, KS has become the most frequent cancer in many sub-Saharan African countries.[62] A particularly tragic aspect of this development pertains to the pediatric implications. While what is now known to be HHV-8-related disease has always occurred in children in endemic KS regions, the incidence of KS among children has dramatically increased in the era of AIDS.[63]

It was not until the rise of epidemic, or AIDS-related, KS that strong evidence emerged for an infectious etiology. In the same way that AIDS was once believed to be caused by the human T-cell lymphotropic virus, HIV was considered for a time to be the etiologic agent of KS. However, the implausibility of a direct causal role for HIV eventually became clear. For example, people infected with HIV by sexual routes had a much higher rate of KS than those who became HIV-positive through blood products or by vertical transmission; in other words, there was circumstantial evidence for the involvement of another infection that can be transmitted through sexual behaviors.[64,65]

Since the initial detection of HHV-8 in KS tissue, "overwhelming" molecular and serological evidence has accumulated that implicates HHV-8 as the viral agent for which researchers were searching.[66,67] In fact, it has been shown that HHV-8 infection is a necessary (though not sufficient) condition in the etiology of all four clinical forms of KS, not just the AIDS-related variety.[68]

The suggestion that HHV-8 is not a sufficient cause of KS is derived from the fact that every infected person does not develop the disease.[69] The assumption is that other causal mechanisms must be involved. Of course, HIV infection is the best known cofactor for the development of KS, though it is important to underline that, unlike HHV-8, HIV is not necessary for KS occurrence.[70,71] Other putative cofactors exist (and will be discussed later), but none rival the impact of HIV coinfection. In fact, it was the first cases of KS in the early 1980s among young MSM men in New York and San Francisco that heralded the beginning of the AIDS epidemic.[72] Results from several studies have shown that half of all MSM infected with HHV-8 and HIV develop KS within 5 to 10 years, making it the most common malignancy among this population.[73,74] The prognosis of AIDS-related KS is very poor, with patients often surviving for only a few months once symptoms appear.[75]

Controversies persist concerning KS. For instance, the exact origin of the characteristic KS tumor cell, called a spindle cell,[76] is still under debate. Although many source tissues have been proposed, current evidence suggests that spindle cells arise from the lymphatic endothelium, that is, the lining of lymphatic vessels.[77,78] Part of the confusion about the fundamental cellular makeup of KS may relate to the vascular spaces that are typically created within the lesions and that become filled with blood cells and a mixture of lymphoid cells; KS is also characterized by blood vessel proliferation, or angiogenesis. Despite the manifest vascularity, KS does not seem to be in essence a tumor of the linings of blood vessels. Support for the concept that HHV-8 is directly involved with lymph vessel cells rather than with blood vessel cells is provided by the fact that the virus has been found to not be associated with the development of angiosarcoma per se.[79]

As suggested earlier, there is also an ongoing discussion as to whether KS is actually a cancer. A distinction is often made between two sequelae of infection by different kinds of viruses: (1) inflammatory immune reactions and (2) "true" neoplasms or tumors that may or may not become malignant. Unfortunately, immune system reactivity and tumors are both marked by cellular proliferation, sometimes leading to misidentification. The basic difference between these two host responses to viral infection relates to the fundamental origins of neoplasia and hyperplasia. In short, the cells in a neoplastic lesion are marked by genetic clonality, which means they develop from a single cell, whereas hyperplastic immune responses can involve multiple cells with slight genetic variations.

In terms of KS, this is the precise focus of the complexity. In their early stages at least, KS lesions appear to be a polyclonal immune reaction to

HHV-8 infection rather than a true neoplasm.[80] KS can later evolve into a true clonal disease as part of its progression toward what are sometimes called late-nodular lesions.[81] At the same time, other research has suggested that even the advanced skin lesions in HIV-positive patients may be mostly a form of reactive, inflammatory proliferation.[82,83] Ultimately, whether or not a particular instance of KS accords with a technical definition of cancer may be a moot point; the most important clinical and public health reality is that it is a serious, sometimes deadly, disease with a clear viral etiology.

Other Lymphoproliferative Malignancies

The preceding discussion about types of cellular proliferation anticipates the broader picture that is emerging related to HHV-8 and cancer. Different disease conditions associated with the virus have quite complex presentations. For example, a true lymphoid neoplasia may be generated that resembles (and even physically overlaps with) benign lymphoproliferations that are normal reactions to infection. In short, distinguishing immune responses from true cancer seems to be an unavoidable part of understanding HHV-8 and its related diseases.

As noted earlier, there are two main lymphoproliferative disorders with demonstrated HHV-8 associations: MCD and PEL. The various clinical expressions of MCD are characterized by distinctive changes in lymph nodes. The two main histological variants are "hyaline vascular" and "plasma cell." The latter type is the one most often seen in the multicentric expression of the disease, which is frequently associated with HIV infection.[84] HIV-positive patients with MCD are consistently coinfected with HHV-8, confirming the virus as a necessary causal agent of at least this subset of the disease.[85] In the context of this book, it is critical to recognize that a portion of the MCD cases may progress to what is known as plasmablastic lymphoma, thus becoming a true part of the HHV-8 cancer spectrum. The majority of such cases occurs in the oral cavity, and usually are very aggressive.[86]

When found in HIV-positive patients, cancers such as KS and MCD are often marked by effusion.[87] This sort of presentation is also seen in PEL, a rare B-cell non-Hodgkin's lymphoma (NHL) that is again associated with HIV infection. At the same time, HIV, while an important cofactor, is not necessary for PEL development; in fact, several HIV-negative cases have been described.[88]

PEL often manifests as a malignancy with no contiguous tumor mass; instead, it exists within body cavities such as the pleural space and pericardium. The latter characteristic accounts for the former name of the disease, body cavity-based lymphoma. The prognosis for PEL is poor, with a median survival time of about 6 months.[89] This fact alone has increased the urgency around pursuing treatment and prevention options, including the identification of a direct etiologic agent. To this end, researchers have noted the regular detection of HHV-8 infection in PEL; in contrast, the virus is generally absent from the range of other NHLs found in humans.[90,91]

While the accumulating evidence has created wide acceptance of HHV-8 as the etiologic agent for PEL, the clinical studies are beset by complications. For instance, as noted in Chapter 10, EBV is a common coinfection in the B-lymphocytes involved with PEL. In fact, it seems that EBV may be responsible for a subset of disease similar to PEL but negative for HHV-8 infection. Multiplying the complexity, there are benign posttransplant lymphoproliferative effusions associated with both these viruses, as well as HHV-8-related effusions that apparently do not involve lymphocytes at all.[92] Finally, a few cases of PEL have been observed that are negative for HHV-8 and HIV, but which seem to be associated with hepatitis C virus (HCV).[93]

The preceding discussion raises a subtle point. In the bewildering world of lymphoma classification, there is a growing tendency to simply define a subset of disease based on its dominant etiologic agent. Applying this idea to viruses, a prerequisite for diagnosis may involve the demonstration of a particular viral genome within the tumor cells. So, it becomes possible to talk about, for example, "HHV-8-positive body cavity lymphoma" as a disease entity. In such instances, the attributable risk related to the virus would be, by definition, 100%.[94]

The history of HHV-8 research contains many unconfirmed and sometimes controversial links to other diseases.[95,96] These include prostate cancer and multiple myeloma, though both of these possibilities now seem to be discounted.[97-99] Other lymphomas have been considered, such as plasmablastic varieties unrelated to effusion or MCD, and a class of solid, extracavitary lymphomas that may be related to PEL and/or MCD.[100-102] As suggested earlier, case reports and patient series are regularly emerging that test the boundary between benign lymphoproliferations and true neoplasia, creating the potential in the future for an expanded spectrum of lymphoid cancers connected to HHV-8.[103-107]

TRANSMISSION AND OCCURRENCE OF THE AGENT

The question of how HHV-8 is transmitted has received substantial attention. Pica and Volpi noted in 2007 that, of the 600 papers published on HHV-8 over the preceding 3 years, more than 80 had focused on transmission.[108] Two main reasons can account for the research interest: (1) exposure prevention, an important subset of primary prevention, depends fundamentally on an awareness of transmission routes and their risk factors; and (2) there is still very little conclusively known about HHV-8 transmission.

The degree of challenge encountered in identifying transmission routes can be traced to several factors, ranging from the epidemiological to the biological. First, it is likely that there are multiple routes of HHV-8 infection. Second, the dominant path of viral transfer seems to vary according to geographic regions and the level of endemicity.[109] Third, there has been "political sensitivity" about the sometimes facile connections drawn between transmission data and sexual behaviors.[110] Fourth, though it is clear where HHV-8 ends up during disease development (e.g., in the case of KS, it is likely endothelial cells), there are still doubts about which cell types are the site of primary infection.[111] The candidate tropisms include B-lymphocytes, oral epithelial cells, and hematopoietic progenitor cells.[112,113] As a final research obstacle, Pica and Volpi stress the lack of gold standards for detecting HHV-8 antibodies and then making inferences about active infection.[114]

While detecting HHV-8 in cells and tissues presents its own challenges (see the pertinent section later in this chapter), progress has been made on identifying the viral reservoirs that facilitate transmission. But the actual process of transmission is at least as important as the potential media within which HHV-8 is transferred. In fact, there is much less clarity on the question of how the medium and/or virus are actually exchanged between hosts. This is a research gap that HHV-8 shares with other infectious agents described in this book.[115] Indeed, HHV-8 can serve as a paradigm to elucidate the general issues involved with untangling viral transmission.

Viral Transmission Variables

There are several factors to be considered when attempting to understand the transmission of a virus such as HHV-8. First, there is the question of viral reservoirs. Several candidates have been examined in the context of HHV-8 infection, the most notable being saliva, blood, and semen. The virus has been found in these three media throughout the world.[116–119] Indeed, it is possible that multiple body fluids are involved in the transmission of HHV-8.[120]

More precisely, HHV-8 DNA has been detected in oral epithelial cells shed in saliva, in B-lympocytes of the peripheral blood, and in both spermatozoa and mononuclear cells in the semen.[121] The virus also exists in a cell-free state in the blood during certain phases of its natural history.[122]

But it is oral shedding in HHV-8-positive individuals that offers the most accessible point for establishing the presence of the virus, a fact that has been confirmed in individuals with and without HIV coinfection.[123]

The intensity of the infection in a reservoir represents an important variable related to the risk of transmission. In this regard, saliva seems to dominate in the range of options. For example, one study showed (by a substantial margin) that oral secretions yielded both the highest frequency of HHV-8 detection and the highest number of DNA copies compared to all other body sites and fluids.[124] Not surprisingly, there is a trend toward even higher viral levels detected in saliva when the infected person has actually developed KS.[125]

Building on the fact that viremia (i.e., infection in the blood) seems to be intermittent, the comparison between saliva and plasma as reservoirs may help to explain why transmission by blood seems to be relatively inefficient.[126,127] In fact, though seroprevalence has been reported as high as 8% in developed countries, blood testing has sometimes detected zero virus, even in samples collected from HHV-8-positive individuals.[128-130] For this reason, universal screening of blood donors for HHV-8 generally has not been recommended in these jurisdictions.[131]

On the other hand, concerns continue to be raised about evidence of HHV-8 transmission by both transfusion and organ transplantation.[132,133] Here, it is important to distinguish a donated tissue contaminated by HHV-8 from the collateral effects of immunosuppressive conditioning that accompanies transplantation; a compromised immune system does not relate to transmission per se, but rather to the risk of chronic infection and disease progression after a primary infection has been acquired.[134]

Lingering issues around cell and tissue donation have been most noticeable in regions with relatively high viral seroprevalence (e.g., sub-Saharan Africa), especially with respect to patients requiring multiple donor units and/or regular transfusions.[135-137] Perspective on the different levels of public health concern is offered by the fact that transplantation-related KS is <0.1% in the United States and Northern European countries, but as high as 5% in the Middle East, a 50-fold variation.[138]

As a corollary to the issue of blood-based transmission, a modest body of literature has examined injection drug use as a risk factor for HHV-8 infection.[139-142] Although the evidence remains mixed, reports of infection among intravenous drug users seem to be infrequent, on a par with rate of transfusion-transmitted virus.[143] Certainly, the efficiency of the injection drug route appears to be much lower than seen with other parenterally transmitted viruses, such as HCV.

In terms of semen, the remaining candidate medium, one study concluded that HHV-8 is present "at concentrations that can be too low to allow its consistent detection."[144] Thus, semen appears to be of only marginal concern as a reservoir of HHV-8. On a related front, some studies have suggested that heterosexual activity, even of a high-risk variety, is an inefficient mode of HHV-8 transmission.[145]

In sum, saliva in the oral cavity generally seems to be the transfer medium demonstrating highest risk for HHV-8 transmission, exceeding both other body fluids and other mucosal sites. This growing consensus has gradually brought HHV-8 into line with other herpesviruses, where salivary transmission also appears to dominate over any other mode (including contact with genital mucosa).[146] This is why mononucleosis, associated with the herpesvirus EBV, is referred to as the "kissing disease." In the end, the key transmission medium in the known human gamma-herpesviruses seems to involve salivary exchange. However, it is important to recognize that HHV-8 is specifically marked by high risk of transmission through saliva exchanged in sexual activity, especially among men who have sex with men (see the later discussion).[147]

Researchers are pursuing more a detailed understanding of the host or viral factors that may affect oral shedding into the saliva. A recent study found that the presence of certain HLA alleles in the genome of African mothers promoted more intensive levels of HHV-8 in saliva, presumably generating a higher risk of transmission.[148] Another relevant molecular feature is the fact that the lytic genes of the virus (see section "Prevalence and Transmission") are specifically expressed during the differentiation of mucosal epithelium; the end point of differentiation is the sloughing off of cells from the outer layer of an epithelium, which helps to account for the notable presence of infectious virus in saliva.[149]

As noted earlier, another consideration in the area of transmission is the requirement that the medium and/or carrier cells come into contact with the receiving host, and specifically into proximity with cells susceptible to infection. Fulfillment of the latter criterion may be influenced by the ability of HHV-8 to infect a range of cells, including[150]:

- Typical KS spindle cells
- Endothelial cells lining the vascular spaces of KS lesions
- Monocytes in KS lesions
- B-lymphocytes in the peripheral blood, PEL, and MCD-related neoplasia
- Keratinocytes in epithelial linings

As for facilitating contact between infected saliva and one or more of these host cell types, a number of horizontal routes are possible, including:

- Nonsexual, oral–oral contact in domestic/family interactions
- Sexual activities, including oral–anal and oral–genital contact, as well as anal intercourse (where saliva may be used as a lubricant)

There is research evidence supporting each of these options.[151–154]

Additional risk categories for HHV-8 infection related to sexual practices include commercial sex workers, people who have multiple sex partners, MSM, and those engaging in sexual activities with HIV-positive individuals or other high-risk behaviors.[155–157]

The mechanisms of transmission and disease risk related to HIV/AIDS are especially complicated. An HIV-positive partner is at higher risk of being coinfected with HHV-8, and thus more likely to pass it on (see section "Prevalence and Transmission"); the new host also risks becoming infected with HIV, with the potential of immunosuppression and thus increased potential for a chronic HHV-8 infection that can lead to cancer. Compounding the health risks is the fact that the interaction between HIV and HHV-8 is definitely bilateral. In short, HHV-8 infection enhances HIV replication, the potential for transmission, and the risk of AIDS development.[158]

Prevalence and Transmission

A final major issue related to transmission involves the fact that the dominant route may be affected by the occurrence of the virus in a geographical region. In contrast to other herpesviruses, HHV-8 is not distributed evenly across the world. The average global seroprevalence of the virus is low,[159–161] but the range is extreme, from 5% or less in the United States and Northern Europe to as high as 58% among children in African countries.[162,163] HHV-8 seroprevalence in Canada has not been extensively studied. One project in the province of Quebec reported that, out of 150 renal transplant patients, none tested positive for anti-HHV-8 antibodies.[164]

It is important to note that high endemicity can also be attached to a particular subpopulation in a region. Thus, whereas Brazil's general HHV-8 seroprevalence is a modest 2.8–7.4%, Amerindian tribes within the country have been reported to have levels approaching 80%.[165,166]

The different prevalence rates influence transmission patterns. In areas of high endemicity, such as sub-Saharan Africa and southern European nations adjacent to the Mediterranean, HHV-8 transmission appears to occur primarily via domestic contact or nonsexual intimacy, probably involving saliva.[167] Transfer between siblings and from mother to child seem to be the main modalities.[168,169] The gradual increase in HHV-8 infection rates throughout childhood, with a leveling off by adolescence, supports this conclusion.[170] Some studies have identified a second increase in HHV-8 seroprevalence after the adolescent plateau; this may be explained by the onset and cumulative impact of other means of transmission, such as risky sexual activity throughout adulthood, or a periodic reactivation of latent virus that then leads to a replication phase.[171]

The fact that infection is so common in children in endemic countries points to the possibility of vertical transmission by one or more mechanisms. However, the low seroprevalence rates observed in infants born to infected mothers indicate that potential transfers during pregnancy, delivery, and breastfeeding are not a dominant concern.[172] This assessment seems to apply to nonendemic parts of the world as well. For example, one U.S. study revealed that HHV-8 DNA was detected in only 2 out of 89 babies born to mothers who were seropositive for the virus.[173]

By contrast with the geographical areas where risk related to domestic contact seems to dominate, sexual transmission is the most common route of transmission in low-endemic areas such as the United States and Northern Europe. The subgroup at highest risk is MSM, though the specific sexual activities involved are not completely elucidated.[174,175] As suggested earlier, some type of salivary involvement may be the operative route in a majority of cases.

Serious risk factors for transmission (and for chronic infection) found among MSM have created a modern pool of high HHV-8 prevalence. Among MSM, an estimated 25% of HIV-negative individuals and over 50% of HIV-positive individuals are infected with HHV-8.[176] The higher rate of infection among MSM, combined with frequent HIV coinfection, translates into KS incidence rates among men that are higher than found in women. This is illustrated in the U.S. setting by the information in Figure 11.1.[177] The observed decline in KS incidence among males since the 1990s is attributed to the success of highly active antiretroviral therapy (HAART).[178,179] This same positive pattern has been seen in Canada and many other jurisdictions.[180,181]

In sum, although various transmission routes continue to be investigated,[182] the emerging consensus is that horizontal transmission dominates, with nonsexual or sexual activities as the prevailing mode of HHV-8 transfer in different populations, albeit moderated by specific levels of endemicity. This raises the possibility of calibrating prevention strategies with the needs of the particular geographic region under consideration.

While variation in occurrence may help to explain current transmission patterns (i.e., the low rate of nonsexual, familial spread in

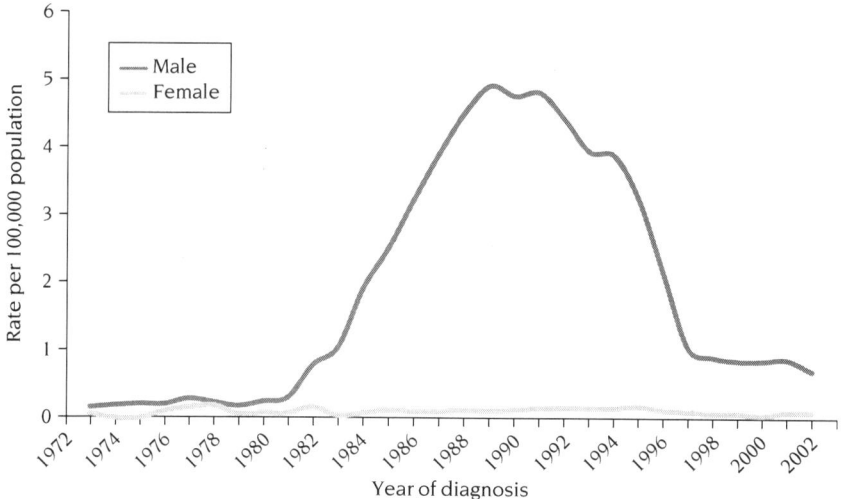

Figure 11.1. Incidence of Kaposi's sarcoma, United States, 1973–2002. *Source*: SEER Cancer Registry as cited by Casper, *Herpes*, 2006.

nonendemic areas), some researchers are still trying to understand environmental or even cultural factors that may have led to elevated HHV-8 prevalence in the first place.[183,184] The suggestions have included birth/residence near rivers, limited access to clean water, and exposure to iron or other substances.[185–187]

The proposal that bites from blood-sucking arthropods (such as mosquitoes) could act as a promoter of transmission has been pursued by an Italian research group since 2002. The suggestion is not that the mosquitoes carry the virus, but that HHV-8-positive mothers lick or otherwise apply saliva to their children's insect bites. As well, substances injected by the insect may play a role in establishing infection and/or inducing replication.[188,189] Supporting evidence was offered by a study that found an association between the distribution of mosquito species and rates of infection and KS development.[190] However, the so-called "promoter arthropod" hypothesis seems to have garnered only modest support among other researchers.

DISEASE MECHANISM AND PROCESSES

The various pathogenic elements involved with HHV-8-related cancer will be introduced in this section, particularly as they relate to KS. One reviewer has suggested that HHV-8 in fact possesses "a formidable repertoire of potent mechanisms that enable it to target and manipulate host cell pathways, leading to increased cell proliferation, increased cell survival, dysregulated angiogenesis, evasion of immunity, and malignant progression in the immunocompromised host."[191]

The HHV-8 lifecycle exhibits two distinct phases, a primary (and usually asymptomatic) infection that becomes latent, and a lytic period (marked by viral replication). This is actually a simplified scheme; there is evidence that expressions of latency and (low-grade) replication can exist simultaneously.[192]

The host immune response plays a crucial role at every stage: resisting persistent infection, controlling HHV-8 replication, and preventing tumors from developing in latently infected individuals.[193] When the immune system is suppressed (due to AIDS or as part of transplantation procedures), one or more phases of HHV-8-related disease (from latent infection to replication to carcinogenesis) may be promoted.[194] In short, the suppression of immune activity is crucial to some type of disease progression. Studies have shown, for instance, that AIDS-KS is specifically associated with a lack of HHV-8-specific T-cells in the host.[195]

As already noted, HHV-8 exhibits tropism for both lymphatic endothelial cells (the proposed origin point of KS) and lymphocytes (the basis of the other cancers associated with the virus). Peripheral blood mononuclear cells, which become infected by HHV-8 through poorly understood transmission pathways, are apparently able to transport the virus to different susceptible tissues.[196,197] In the case of KS, the likely target seems to be lymphatic endothelial cells (which eventually take on the spindle shape characteristic of the disease); this occurs predominantly in epithelial tissues, but possibly in lymph nodes or the lining of viscera.[198] As noted already, KS tumors are complex, highly vascular, and made up of many types of cells. The involvement of different tissues continues to raise questions about the ultimate target cell of HHV-8 in KS. For instance, a recent competing theory suggests that circulating blood progenitor cells harboring HHV-8 may be the precursors of KS spindle cells.[199]

Whatever the cell of origin may be, it is clear that HHV-8 programs infected tissues in multiple ways to achieve KS formation.[200,201] For example, even when the virus is latent in the recruited endothelial cells, it can express the lytic phase genes that may then promote features of tumor development (such as the proliferation of vascular tissue, also known as angiogenesis).[202–205] This usually initiates a long, multistep process, where the tumor seems to start out as a nonmalignant, polyclonal proliferation (which may even regress in certain variants of KS) before eventually becoming a true, uniclonal sarcoma.[206,207]

A fundamental question of pathology is this: how did the advent of HIV infections create an epidemic variant of KS? The answer seems to involve more than the indirect effects of immunosuppression. Indeed, the Tat protein characteristically expressed by HIV appears to also be directly involved in carcinogenesis. Research suggests that Tat may participate in KS development by inducing HHV-8 replication and increasing viral load.[208] It should be recalled that certain aspects of KS development depend precisely on unusual lytic protein expressions in the lesion; confirming a role for Tat in such processes would be of great theoretical (and possibly clinical) interest. Tat also has been shown to augment tissue growth factors, facilitate cell-to-cell viral transfer, and promote inflammatory cytokines (which in turn influence the emergence of spindle cells in KS).[209,210] As these functions become better understood, it may cause researchers to consider recategorizing HIV as at least a co-carcinogen in humans.

It is understood that HHV-8 is a necessary but not sufficient cause of KS.[211] As already suggested, HIV operates as a "super cofactor" in the initiation of KS, multiplying by thousands of times the risk of developing the tumor.[212] Although much less common today, the recreational use by MSM of inhalant nitrates as a vasodilator has been proposed as a behavioral cofactor in the development of KS.[213,214]

Other cofactors involved with KS, especially with the forms of the disease that are not related to HIV/AIDS, have not yet been well-defined. As already noted, the possibilities include encountering excess iron in the environment or exposure to chemical substances injected by mosquitoes. Dietary nitrosamines and aluminosilicates in volcanic soil have also been posited as cofactors that could explain the distribution of KS among HIV-negative populations; host-immune polymorphisms may also play a role.[215,216]

Once HHV-8 infection has become established, inducing lytic gene expression is likely a vital step in tumorogenesis. It seems that multiple cellular signals can reactivate the virus in spindle cells, shifting the infection from a latent to a replicating phase.[217] HIV apparently is not the only coinfection that can trigger such molecular events. Studies have shown that the presence of other human herpesviruses, such as HSV-1, can activate lytic cycle replication in HHV-8.[218-220] Considering the ubiquity of HSV-1, this sort of mechanism may in fact play a substantial role in KS development.

VIRAL DETECTION METHODS

Detecting HHV-8 infection may be accomplished indirectly, by means of the host response to the infection (i.e., the presence of antibodies), or directly (i.e., based on viral DNA or proteins). The methods employed include serological techniques, immunochemistry, in situ hybridization, and polymerase chain reaction (PCR).[221] Notwithstanding the variety of approaches available, more research is needed to determine the most effective way to diagnose infection and predict disease.[222-224] The simpler tests seem to produce conflicting results concerning which individuals are currently infected.[225,226] On the other hand, antibody assays may still be superior to more complex measurements of serum HHV-8 DNA load as a predictor of KS development.[227,228] There have been attempts to improve detection accuracy through the refinement of protocols, combining results from different types of testing, and basic technological improvements.[229-235] Interestingly, the advanced methodology of PCR has been recently enhanced by multiplex assays that enable testing for several herpesvirus types simultaneously.[236-238]

PREVENTION APPROACHES

Six prevention categories with a clear connection to infection per se have been consistently used in this book. Each of these six options will be reviewed with respect to HHV-8 in this last section of the chapter.

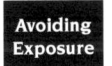

| **Avoiding Exposure** | Preventing Infection | Prophylactic Eradication | Preventing Cofactor | Therapeutic Eradication | Interrupting Transformation |

1. Avoiding Exposure to the Agent

The challenge related to classic exposure prevention is suggested by the results of one recent study, where only 6% of MSM were aware that KS is caused by a virus other than HIV.[239] Although the precise sexual behaviors related to HHV-8 transmission remain unclear, any safe sex practice could offer a first line of defense.[240] More specifically, it may be prudent to discourage any behaviors, especially among MSM, where saliva comes into contact with a partner's genitomucosal surfaces. One interventional approach in this regard involves the application of the antiherpes drug valacyclovir after dental treatment, though so far the impact on HHV-8 levels in saliva has been equivocal.[241]

While blood donor screening programs for HHV-8 antibodies or other biomarkers have generally not been implemented, this is likely not a great cause for concern in light of the low transmission rates that have been observed.[242] However, extra safety precautions may be warranted in the case of transfusion recipients who are immunocompromised; again, the issue is not higher transmission risk per se compared to other transfusion patients, but increased potential for any new infection to become chronic and lead to disease sequelae.[243] The extraordinary protective measures that can be adopted include testing of the relevant donors or their tissues for HHV-8-specific antibodies or viral nucleic acid, or both. Leukocyte reduction in blood units intended for immunocompromised transfusion recipients is also possible.[244] If deemed to be feasible, the eventual emergence of universal pathogen-inactivation programs applied to the blood supply would be a marked improvement over any sort of targeted strategies.[245]

Again, because of very low transmission risks in Asia, North America, and much of Europe, the need for pre- and posttransplantation strategies to counteract HHV-8 is hotly debated.[246,247] The threat level, and the ensuing response, may need to be considered more carefully in high-endemic regions.[248] In terms of exposure prevention per se, the issue is whether or not to screen for infection in tissues before transplantation. On the other hand, interventions to address the adverse effect of immunosuppression regimes fall under either the control of cofactors and disease progression or the detection and treatment of any infection that occurs (see the relevant sections later on).

Finally, whatever the ultimate determination of risk in the case of injection drug use and HHV-8 transmission, it is clear that there are many other compelling public health reasons to promote abstinence, treatment, and harm reduction measures related to this particular behavior.

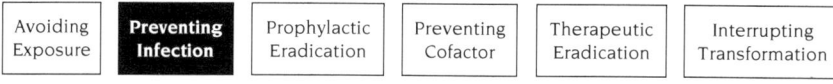

2. Preventing Infection after Exposure to the Agent

Although the intensive investigation of HHV-8 disease processes has certainly generated potential vaccine targets,[249] an immunization strategy for the virus has not yet been identified or initiated. It is not clear how quickly the relevant research will be pursued in light of the low global prevalence of the virus and the reality of more pressing vaccination priorities. However, the twin scourge of HIV and HHV-8 infection among some populations, and the fact that KS is still a major cause of mortality in patients with AIDS, may intensify vaccine research.

As with HIV and EBV, finding an efficient response to the genetic diversity of HHV-8 is a challenge to the development of both prophylactic and therapeutic measures. Ultimately, a full delineation of viral subtypes, their distribution, and any disease implications will determine whether population-specific vaccine strategies will eventually be required.[250]

| Avoiding Exposure | Preventing Infection | **Prophylactic Eradication** | Preventing Cofactor | Therapeutic Eradication | Interrupting Transformation |

3. Prophylactic Eradication or Suppression

Methods for prophylactically eradicating or suppressing HHV-8 infection are not available. The only suggested approach that approximates this category is the transfusion of virus-specific cytotoxic T-lymphocytes.[251] However, this arguably would only be applied in cases where immunosuppression is acting as a cofactor in disease development, and thus properly belongs to section "Cofactor Prevention."

| Avoiding Exposure | Preventing Infection | Prophylactic Eradication | **Preventing Cofactor** | Therapeutic Eradication | Interrupting Transformation |

4. Cofactor Prevention

The risk of developing KS among HHV-8-infected individuals is low unless the patient is coinfected with HIV or otherwise immunosuppressed (e.g., as part of a transplantation procedure). Properly evaluated, the relative risk of developing KS is extremely high in HIV-positive populations.[252] This makes preventing HIV infection an obvious priority in the drive to reduce malignancy related to HHV-8. In this context, it is important to recognize that the behavioral practices relevant to HIV prevention among MSM and other populations (e.g., condom use, limiting the number of sexual partners) would prevent a subset of HHV-8 transmission as well.[253] In short, reduced KS incidence may be multiplied through such sexual health efforts.

Of course, the most dramatic medical impact on HIV involves HAART; this is true in reference to both immune system reconstitution and possibly the reversal of other HIV-mediated pathogenetic processes that are still being elucidated.[254] The dramatic impact of HAART on KS rates was noted earlier in the context of the United States and Canada, and similar reports have emerged from many other jurisdictions. For instance, a large European study found that, among HIV-positive patients, the current incidence of KS is less than 10% of the rate seen in 1994.[255] The reduction is likely a result of effects on the immune system and certain unique HIV disease processes, rather than any direct cure of HHV-8 infection.[256]

Similar post-HAART improvements have also been seen in the occurrence of NHLs that are related to AIDS; the subset of these NHLs that are also associated with HHV-8 are presumably included in this pattern. In contrast, non-AIDS-related NHL incidence appears to be trending upward in the United States and other jurisdictions.[257]

Interrupting vertical transmission of HIV is certainly a priority in its own right, as well as being an important cofactor prevention measure for KS. Fortunately, herpesvirus management problems known to be caused by oral nucleoside therapy used with HIV-positive pregnant women are not that relevant to HHV-8 control, since vertical transmission has not been found to be a common route of HHV-8 infection in children.[258]

Preventing HHV-8-related disease in transplant patients is challenging. Adjusting proven immunosuppressant formulas can lead to reduced transplantation effectiveness. For example, data from a transplant tumor registry indicated that, among transplant patients with special protocols applied to control KS, 65% experienced graft failure or impaired graft function, compared to 21% of the total transplant population.[259] Nonetheless, innovative strategies continue to be pursued, for example, the incorporation of rapamycin, a new immunosuppressant that also generates antineoplastic effects.[260,261]

Two investigational cofactors have been a focus of prevention research in the past: mosquito bites and iron exposure. Thus, two regions of Italy that underwent mosquito suppression revealed a pattern of reduced HHV-8 seroprevalence; this was consistent with the involvement of blood-sucking insects in the transmission of the virus.[262] And, finally, one authority has suggested using chelators for iron withdrawal in animal models of KS to test its potency as a prevention mechanism.[263]

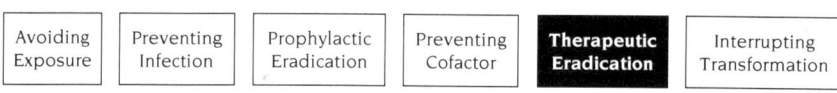

5. Therapeutic Eradication or Suppression

It is a matter of semantics whether being immunocompromised is considered a cofactor to be reversed (see section "Cofactor Prevention") or the target of a therapeutic intervention (such as HAART in AIDS patients). In either case, the effect on HHV-8 (and other coinfections) may be mostly characterized as indirect; this is notwithstanding the fact that immune reconstitution may eventually result in viral suppression through restored HHV-8-related cellular immunity.[264] In this section, however, the focus will be on interventions that are more specifically aimed at the virus.

Direct immunotherapies represent one option being investigated.[265] Similar to the scenario with respect to prophylactic eradication, a potentially effective intervention of this sort involves the introduction of

B-cells designed to stimulate virus-specific T-cells, especially in immunocompromised hosts.[266]

While research continues on a number of fronts, authorities have suggested that development of antiherpes measures to completely remove or neutralize a virus such as HHV-8 is unlikely.[267] Moderating viral load may prove to be a more feasible goal. Promising candidate drugs being pursued to suppress HHV-8 infection include ganciclovir, valganciclovir, and foscarnet. These agents have demonstrated the ability to inhibit HHV-8 replication in vitro and in a limited number of human trials.[268,269]

A prerequisite for this category of intervention is the detection of HHV-8. Some researchers have recommended applying one of the available viral detection modalities (see section "Viral Detection Methods") to the screening of individuals at risk for KS.[270] A robust screening program requires confidence about the effectiveness of a follow-up protocol, a criterion that has yet to be fulfilled for HHV-8 infection.

Avoiding Exposure	Preventing Infection	Prophylactic Eradication	Preventing Cofactor	Therapeutic Eradication	**Interrupting Transformation**

6. Interrupting Transformation Related to Infection

While relevant clinical trials are still small in number, there is a gradually expanding body of literature pointing to potential therapies targeting HHV-8-related carcinogenesis.[271-274] For example, there may be a role for strategies involving RNA interference or the interruption of angiogenesis.[275-277] Some studies are focusing specifically on molecular targets related to progression of the rarer HHV-8-related lymphoid cancers.[278]

As suggested in section "Therapeutic Eradication or Suppression," modifying disease in fact seems to be a more feasible goal than curing or eradicating infection. However, older therapies have not been shown to consistently counteract HHV-8-related disease processes; and none of the novel options are yet ready for the clinical setting.[279,280]

Finally, it is important to recall that qualifying for this prevention category requires some kind of impact on detected precursors of malignancy. It is unclear how relevant a "secondary prevention" approach might be in the context of KS management. It does seem likely, given that the initial histological presentation of KS can be quite minimal, that some type of premalignant screening would be an effective step preceding measures to control HHV-8-related disease processes. The most useful arena for such a program to be launched would probably be oral health checks, whether applied universally or among at-risk populations.[281]

CONCLUSION

HHV-8 bears some functional resemblance to other viruses described in this book. First, there is a clear overlap with EBV, an agent from the same herpesvirus subfamily. The shared features include suspected transmission mechanisms, specific target cells, and the complex dynamic between latent and lytic phases in the natural history of each virus. On another front, the pleiotropism of HHV-8 is reminiscent of HCV, an agent also known to infect a wide range of cells.

Like human papillomavirus (HPV) and human T-cell lymphotropic virus (see Chapter 12), HHV-8 represents 100% of the attributable risk for a specific cancer; in other words, each of these viruses operates as the necessary cause of the disease in question. There is also an obvious connection between HHV-8 and human T-cell lymphotropic virus in terms of their biological involvement with HIV coinfection.

HHV-8 may also be distinguished from viruses such as HPV and HCV in one very important respect: simply put, the virus will likely never occupy the same position on the clinical or public health agenda. Three factors have conspired to keep the urgency with respect to HHV-8 at a relatively low level, at least in developed countries:

- The seroprevalence of the virus in the population is generally modest
- Even when infection does become established, KS only develops in a subset of patients
- KS, which is the most burdensome consequence of HHV-8, has been dramatically reduced as a collateral benefit of HAART in AIDS patients

As a result of these considerations, though HHV-8 infection is still an important condition, it is not likely to become a public health priority in areas of low endemicity. In Canada, for instance, HHV-8 parallels HTLV-1 (see Chapter 12) in posing a very limited general health threat. Consequently, HHV-8 infection/KS does not appear in the Public Health Agency of Canada's most recent list of nationally notifiable diseases.[282]

Low urgency has perhaps contributed to the limited progress on prevention approaches. It is true that there has been a powerful indirect impact on KS from HAART; but vaccines and therapies directly targeting HHV-8 seem to only be at a conceptual or investigational stage. As for exposure prevention, the various potential strategies are hampered by uncertainty concerning transmission routes. Lack of compelling evidence for the risk of blood- and tissue-borne transmission has led to little concern in the arenas of transfusions, hemodialysis, and transplantation. Sometimes the problem involves knowing how to respond. For instance, planners in regions of high HHV-8 endemicity openly question whether prevention of casual, familial transmission is even feasible.

The obstacles described earlier do not mean that complacency should rule. Despite the reduced health burden it represents, epidemic KS remains "one of the tragic hallmarks of AIDS in Western countries."[283] Given the substantially increased risk of developing KS when a patient is coinfected with HHV-8 and HIV, the greatest advances in terms of exposure prevention may involve the promotion of safe sex practices that simultaneously address the transmission of both viruses. This approach of course would offer a myriad of other public health benefits.[284]

NOTES

1. Mancuso R, Biffi R, Valli M et al. HHV8 a subtype is associated with rapidly evolving classic Kaposi's sarcoma. *Journal of Medical Virology*. 2008; 80(12): 2153–60.
2. Chang Y, Cesarman E, Pessin MS et al. Identification of herpesvirus-like DNA sequences in AIDS-associated Kaposi's sarcoma. *Science*. 1994; 266(5192): 1865–9.
3. Rezk SA, Weiss LM. Epstein-Barr virus-associated lymphoproliferative disorders. *Human Pathology*. 2007; 38(9): 1293–304.
4. Greene W, Kuhne K, Ye F et al. Molecular biology of KSHV in relation to AIDS-associated oncogenesis. *Cancer Treatment and Research*. 2007; 133: 69–127.
5. Albrecht D, Meyer T, Lorenzen T et al. Epidemiology of HHV-8 infection in HIV-positive patients with and without Kaposi sarcoma: diagnostic relevance of serology and PCR. *Journal of Clinical Virology*. 2004; 30(2): 145–9.
6. For example, Du MQ, Bacon CM, Isaacson PG. Kaposi sarcoma-associated herpesvirus/human herpesvirus 8 and lymphoproliferative disorders. *Journal of Clinical Pathology*. 2007; 60(12): 1350–7.
7. Dukers NH, Rezza G. Human herpesvirus 8 epidemiology: what we do and do not know. *AIDS*. 2003; 17(12): 1717–30.
8. Jaffe HW, Pellett PE. Human herpesvirus 8 and Kaposi's sarcoma—some answers, more questions. *New England Journal of Medicine*. 1999; 340(24): 1912–3.
9. Gershburg E, Pagano JS. Conserved herpesvirus protein kinases. *Biochimica et Biophysica Acta*. 2008; 1784(1): 203–12.
10. Chen T, Hudnall SD. Anatomical mapping of human herpesvirus reservoirs of infection. *Modern Pathology*. 2006; 19(5): 726–37.
11. Jarosinski KW, Tischer BK, Trapp S et al. Marek's disease virus: lytic replication, oncogenesis and control. *Expert Review of Vaccines*. 2006; 5(6): 761–72.
12. Arzul I, Nicolas JL, Davison AJ et al. French scallops: a new host for ostreid herpesvirus-1. *Virology*. 2001; 290(2): 342–9.

13 Rajcani J, Kudelova M. Murine herpesvirus pathogenesis: a model for the analysis of molecular mechanisms of human gamma herpesvirus infections. *Acta Microbiologica et Immunologica Hungarica.* 2005; 52(1): 41–71.
14 Ehlers B, Dural G, Marschall M et al. Endotheliotropic elephant herpesvirus, the first betaherpesvirus with a thymidine kinase gene. *Journal of General Virology.* 2006; 87(Pt 10): 2781–9.
15 Ackermann M. Pathogenesis of gammaherpesvirus infections. *Veterinary Microbiology.* 2006; 113(3–4): 211–22.
16 Damania B, Desrosiers RC. Simian homologues of human herpesvirus 8. *Philosophical Transactions of the Royal Society of London. Series B, Biological Sciences.* 2001; 356(1408): 535–43.
17 Neipel F, Albrecht JC, Fleckenstein B. Human herpesvirus 8—the first human Rhadinovirus. *Journal of the National Cancer Institute. Monographs.* 1998; (23): 73–7.
18 O'Connor CM, Kedes DH. Rhesus monkey rhadinovirus: a model for the study of KSHV. *Current Topics in Microbiology and Immunology.* 2007; 312: 43–69.
19 Wang F, Rivailler P, Rao P et al. Simian homologues of Epstein-Barr virus. *Philosophical Transactions of the Royal Society of London. Series B, Biological Sciences.* 2001; 356(1408): 489–97.
20 Ackermann M. Pathogenesis of gammaherpesvirus infections. *Veterinary Microbiology.* 2006; 113(3–4): 211–22.
21 Sullivan RJ, Pantanowitz L, Casper C et al. Epidemiology, pathophysiology, and treatment of Kaposi sarcoma-associated herpesvirus disease: Kaposi sarcoma, primary effusion lymphoma, and multicentric Castleman disease. *Clinical Infectious Diseases.* 2008; 47(9): 1209–15.
22 Adapted from Moore PS, Gao SJ, Dominguez G et al. Primary characterization of a herpesvirus agent associated with Kaposi's sarcomae. *Journal of Virology.* 1996; 70(1): 549–58.
23 Berrington de Gonzalez A, Urban MI, Sitas F et al. Antibodies against six human herpesviruses in relation to seven cancers in black South Africans: a case control study. *Infectious Agents and Cancer.* 2006; 1: 2.
24 Garcia-Ramirez JJ, Ruchti F, Huang H et al. Dominance of virus over host factors in cross-species activation of human cytomegalovirus early gene expression. *Journal of Virology.* 2001; 75(1): 26–35.
25 Quinlivan M, Breuer J. Molecular and therapeutic aspects of varicella-zoster virus infection. *Expert Reviews in Molecular Medicine.* 2005; 7(15): 1–24.
26 Bechtel JT, Liang Y, Hvidding J et al. Host range of Kaposi's sarcoma-associated herpesvirus in cultured cells. *Journal of Virology.* 2003; 77(11): 6474–81.
27 Blackbourn DJ, Lennette E, Klencke B et al. The restricted cellular host range of human herpesvirus 8. *AIDS.* 2000; 14(9): 1123–33.
28 Krug LT, Teo CG, Tanaka-Taya K et al. Newly Identified Human Herpesviruses: HHV-6, HHV-7, and HHV-8. In: Fong IW and Alibeck K., eds. *New and Evolving Infections of the 21st Century.* New York: Springer New York; 2007.
29 Ablashi DV, Chatlynne LG, Whitman JE, Jr. et al. Spectrum of Kaposi's sarcoma-associated herpesvirus, or human herpesvirus 8, diseases. *Clinical Microbiology Reviews.* 2002; 15(3): 439–64.

30 Zhang D, Pu X, Wu W et al. Genotypic analysis on the ORF-K1 gene of human herpesvirus 8 from patients with Kaposi's sarcoma in Xinjiang, China. *Journal of Genetics and Genomics.* 2008; 35(11): 657–63.

31 Kasolo FC, Spinks J, Bima H et al. Diverse genotypes of Kaposi's sarcoma associated herpesvirus (KSHV) identified in infant blood infections in African childhood-KS and HIV/AIDS endemic region. *Journal of Medical Virology.* 2007; 79(10): 1555–61.

32 Zong JC, Kajumbula H, Boto W et al. Evaluation of global clustering patterns and strain variation over an extended ORF26 gene locus from Kaposi's sarcoma herpesvirus. *Journal of Clinical Virology.* 2007; 40(1): 19–25.

33 Whitby D, Marshall VA, Bagni RK et al. Genotypic characterization of Kaposi's sarcoma-associated herpesvirus in asymptomatic infected subjects from isolated populations. *Journal of General Virology.* 2004; 85(Pt 1): 155–63.

34 Dourmishev LA, Dourmishev AL, Palmeri D et al. Molecular genetics of Kaposi's sarcoma-associated herpesvirus (human herpesvirus-8) epidemiology and pathogenesis. *Microbiology and Molecular Biology Reviews.* 2003; 67(2): 175–212.

35 Hayward GS. KSHV strains: the origins and global spread of the virus. *Seminars in Cancer Biology.* 1999; 9(3): 187–99.

36 Zong JC, Metroka C, Reitz MS et al. Strain variability among Kaposi sarcoma-associated herpesvirus (human herpesvirus 8) genomes: evidence that a large cohort of United States AIDS patients may have been infected by a single common isolate. *Journal of Virology.* 1997; 71(3): 2505–11.

37 Laurent C, Meggetto F, Brousset P. Human herpesvirus 8 infections in patients with immunodeficiencies. *Human Pathology.* 2008; 39(7): 983–93.

38 Cesarman E, Mesri EA. Kaposi sarcoma-associated herpesvirus and other viruses in human lymphomagenesis. *Current Topics in Microbiology and Immunology.* 2007; 312: 263–87.

39 Schulz TF. The pleiotropic effects of Kaposi's sarcoma herpesvirus. *Journal of Pathology.* 2006; 208(2): 187–98.

40 Sullivan RJ, Pantanowitz L, Casper C et al. Epidemiology, pathophysiology, and treatment of Kaposi sarcoma-associated herpesvirus disease: Kaposi sarcoma, primary effusion lymphoma, and multicentric Castleman disease. *Clinical Infectious Diseases.* 2008; 47(9): 1209–15.

41 Barozzi P, Potenza L, Riva G et al. B cells and herpesviruses: a model of lymphoproliferation. *Autoimmunity Reviews.* 2007; 7(2): 132–6.

42 Monini P, Colombini S, Sturzl M et al. Reactivation and persistence of human herpesvirus-8 infection in B cells and monocytes by Th-1 cytokines increased in Kaposi's sarcoma. *Blood.* 1999; 93(12): 4044–58.

43 Bestawros A, Boulassel MR, Michel RP et al. HHV-8 linked to Kaposi's sarcoma, Castleman's disease and primary effusion lymphoma in a HIV-1-infected man. *Journal of Clinical Virology.* 2008; 42(2): 179–81.

44 A commonly-used alternate name is Kaposi's sarcoma.

45 Caponetti G, Dezube BJ, Restrepo CS et al. Kaposi sarcoma of the musculoskeletal system: A review of 66 patients. *Cancer.* 2007; 109(6): 1040–52.

46 Pantanowitz L, Dezube BJ. Kaposi sarcoma in unusual locations. *BMC Cancer.* 2008; 8: 190.

47 "Sarcoma" refers to a cancer of mesenchymal (or connective) tissue, such as cartilage, fat, muscle, or bone. Sarcomas can develop in the endothelial lining of blood and lymph vessels.
48 Grayson W, Pantanowitz L. Histological variants of cutaneous Kaposi sarcoma. *Diagnostic Pathology.* 2008; 3: 31.
49 Haubrich WS. Kaposi of Kaposi's sarcoma. *Gastroenterology.* 2003; 125(2): 327.
50 Buonaguro FM, Tornesello ML, Beth-Giraldo E et al. Herpesvirus-like DNA sequences detected in endemic, classic, iatrogenic and epidemic Kaposi's sarcoma (KS) biopsies. *International Journal of Cancer.* 1996; 65(1): 25–8.
51 Antman K, Chang Y. Kaposi's sarcoma. *New England Journal of Medicine.* 2000; 342(14): 1027–38.
52 Iscovich J, Boffetta P, Franceschi S et al. Classic kaposi sarcoma: epidemiology and risk factors. *Cancer.* 2000; 88(3): 500–17.
53 Di Lorenzo G. Update on classic Kaposi sarcoma therapy: new look at an old disease. *Critical Reviews in Oncology/Hematology.* 2008; 68(3): 242–9.
54 Hiatt KM, Nelson AM, Lichy JH et al. Classic Kaposi Sarcoma in the United States over the last two decades: A clinicopathologic and molecular study of 438 non-HIV-related Kaposi Sarcoma patients with comparison to HIV-related Kaposi Sarcoma. *Modern Pathology.* 2008; 21(5): 572–82.
55 Pellet C, Kerob D, Dupuy A et al. Kaposi's sarcoma-associated herpesvirus viremia is associated with the progression of classic and endemic Kaposi's sarcoma. *Journal of Investigative Dermatology.* 2006; 126(3): 621–7.
56 Lebbe C, Legendre C, Frances C. Kaposi sarcoma in transplantation. *Transplantation Reviews.* 2008; 22(4): 252–61.
57 Boshoff C, Weiss RA. Epidemiology and pathogenesis of Kaposi's sarcoma-associated herpesvirus. *Philosophical Transactions of the Royal Society of London. Series B, Biological Sciences.* 2001; 356(1408): 517–34.
58 Duprez R, Kassa-Kelembho E, Plancoulaine S et al. Human herpesvirus 8 serological markers and viral load in patients with AIDS-associated Kaposi's sarcoma in Central African Republic. *Journal of Clinical Microbiology.* 2005; 43(9): 4840–3.
59 Nawar E, Mbulaiteye SM, Gallant JE et al. Risk factors for Kaposi's sarcoma among HHV-8 seropositive homosexual men with AIDS. *International Journal of Cancer.* 2005; 115(2): 296–300.
60 Restrepo CS, Martinez S, Lemos JA et al. Imaging manifestations of Kaposi sarcoma. *Radiographics.* 2006; 26(4): 1169–85.
61 Caceres CF, Konda K, Segura ER et al. Epidemiology of male same-sex behaviour and associated sexual health indicators in low- and middle-income countries: 2003–2007 estimates. *Sexually Transmitted Infections.* 2008; 84(suppl 1): i49–i56.
62 Mbulaiteye SM, Goedert JJ. Transmission of Kaposi sarcoma-associated herpesvirus in sub-Saharan Africa. *AIDS.* 2008; 22(4): 535–7.
63 Bhaduri-McIntosh S. Human herpesvirus-8: clinical features of an emerging viral pathogen. *Pediatric Infectious Disease Journal.* 2005; 24(1): 81–2.
64 Ganem D. KSHV infection and the pathogenesis of Kaposi's sarcoma. *Annual Review of Pathology.* 2006; 1: 273–96.
65 Renne R, Zhong W, Herndier B et al. Lytic growth of Kaposi's sarcoma-associated herpesvirus (human herpesvirus 8) in culture. *Nature Medicine.* 1996; 2(3): 342–6.

66 Cannon MJ, Dollard SC, Black JB et al. Risk factors for Kaposi's sarcoma in men seropositive for both human herpesvirus 8 and human immunodeficiency virus. *AIDS.* 2003; 17(2): 215–22.
67 Colman R, Blackbourn DJ. Risk factors in the development of Kaposi's sarcoma. *AIDS.* 2008; 22(13): 1629–32.
68 Simonart T. Role of environmental factors in the pathogenesis of classic and African-endemic Kaposi sarcoma. *Cancer Letters.* 2006; 244(1): 1–7.
69 Ganem D. KSHV infection and the pathogenesis of Kaposi's sarcoma. *Annual Review of Pathology.* 2006; 1: 273–96.
70 Zeng Y, Zhang X, Huang Z et al. Intracellular Tat of human immunodeficiency virus type 1 activates lytic cycle replication of Kaposi's sarcoma-associated herpesvirus: role of JAK/STAT signaling. *Journal of Virology.* 2007; 81(5): 2401–17.
71 Greene W, Kuhne K, Ye F et al. Molecular biology of KSHV in relation to AIDS-associated oncogenesis. *Cancer Treatment and Research.* 2007; 133: 69–127.
72 Boshoff C, Weiss RA. Epidemiology and pathogenesis of Kaposi's sarcoma-associated herpesvirus. *Philosophical Transactions of the Royal Society of London. Series B, Biological Sciences.* 2001; 356(1408): 517–34.
73 Viejo-Borbolla A, Schulz TF. Kaposi's sarcoma-associated herpesvirus (KSHV/HHV8): key aspects of epidemiology and pathogenesis. *AIDS reviews.* 2003; 5(4): 222–9.
74 Hansen A, Boshoff C, Lagos D. Kaposi sarcoma as a model of oncogenesis and cancer treatment. *Expert Review of Anticancer Therapy.* 2007; 7(2): 211–20.
75 Schwartz RA. Kaposi's sarcoma: an update. *Journal of Surgical Oncology.* 2004; 87(3): 146–51.
76 Gessain A, Duprez R. Spindle cells and their role in Kaposi's sarcoma. *International Journal of Biochemistry & Cell Biology.* 2005; 37(12): 2457–65.
77 Douglas JL, Gustin JK, Dezube B et al. Kaposi's sarcoma: a model of both malignancy and chronic inflammation. *Panminerva Medica.* 2007; 49(3): 119–38.
78 Pyakurel P, Pak F, Mwakigonja AR et al. Lymphatic and vascular origin of Kaposi's sarcoma spindle cells during tumor development. *International Journal of Cancer.* 2006; 119(6): 1262–7.
79 Schmid H, Zietz C. Human herpesvirus 8 and angiosarcoma: analysis of 40 cases and review of the literature. *Pathology.* 2005; 37(4): 284–7.
80 Teo CG. Conceptual emergence of human herpesvirus 8 (Kapsi's sarcoma-associated herpesvirus) as an oral herpesvirus. *Advances in Dental Research.* 2006; 19(1): 85–90.
81 Ensoli B, Sturzl M. Kaposi's sarcoma: a result of the interplay among inflammatory cytokines, angiogenic factors and viral agents. *Cytokine Growth Factor Reviews.* 1998; 9(1): 63–83.
82 Duprez R, Lacoste V, Briere J et al. Evidence for a multiclonal origin of multicentric advanced lesions of Kaposi sarcoma. *Journal of the National Cancer Institute.* 2007; 99(14): 1086–94.
83 Wood NH, Feller L. The malignant potential of HIV-associated Kaposi sarcoma. *Cancer Cell International.* 2008; 8(1): 14.
84 Dham A, Peterson BA. Castleman disease. *Current Opinion in Hematology.* 2007; 14(4): 354–9.
85 Collins LS, Fowler A, Tong CY et al. Multicentric Castleman's disease in HIV infection. *International Journal of STD & AIDS.* 2006; 17(1): 19–24.

86 Rafaniello Raviele P, Pruneri G, Maiorano E. Plasmablastic lymphoma: a review. *Oral Diseases.* 2009; 15(1): 38–45.
87 Effusion refers to a collection of fluid in a body cavity, usually between two adjacent tissues.
88 Ascoli V, Lo Coco F, Torelli G et al. Human herpesvirus 8-associated primary effusion lymphoma in HIV—patients: A clinicoepidemiologic variant resembling classic Kaposi's sarcoma. *Haematologica.* 2002; 87(4): 339–43.
89 Chen YB, Rahemtullah A, Hochberg E. Primary effusion lymphoma. *Oncologist.* 2007; 12(5): 569–76.
90 Hengge UR, Ruzicka T, Tyring SK et al. Update on Kaposi's sarcoma and other HHV8 associated diseases. Part 2: pathogenesis, Castleman's disease, and pleural effusion lymphoma. *Lancet Infectious Diseases.* 2002; 2(6): 344–52.
91 Gerard L, Agbalika F, Sheldon J et al. No increased human herpesvirus 8 seroprevalence in patients with HIV-associated non-Hodgkin's lymphoma. *Journal of Acquired Immune Deficiency Syndromes.* 2001; 26(2): 182–4.
92 Ascoli V, Lo-Coco F. Body cavity lymphoma. *Current Opinion in Pulmonary Medicine.* 2002; 8(4): 317–22.
93 Paner GP, Jensen J, Foreman KE et al. HIV and HHV-8 negative primary effusion lymphoma in a patient with hepatitis C virus-related liver cirrhosis. *Leukemia & Lymphoma.* 2003; 44(10): 1811–4.
94 Ascoli V, Lo-Coco F. Body cavity lymphoma. *Current Opinion in Pulmonary Medicine.* 2002; 8(4): 317–22.
95 Carbone A, Gloghini A. KSHV/HHV8-associated lymphomas. *British Journal of Haematology.* 2008; 140(1): 13–24.
96 Geraminejad P, Memar O, Aronson I et al. Kaposi's sarcoma and other manifestations of human herpesvirus 8. *Journal of the American Academy of Dermatology.* 2002; 47(5): 641–55.
97 Jenkins FJ, Hayes RB, Jackson A et al. Human herpesvirus 8 seroprevalence among prostate cancer case patients and control subjects. *Journal of Infectious Diseases.* 2007; 196(2): 208–11.
98 Malnati MS, Dagna L, Ponzoni M et al. Human herpesvirus 8 (HHV-8/KSHV) and hematologic malignancies. *Reviews in Clinical and Experimental Hematology.* 2003; 7(4): 375–405.
99 Dupin N, Fisher C, Kellam P et al. Distribution of human herpesvirus-8 latently infected cells in Kaposi's sarcoma, multicentric Castleman's disease, and primary effusion lymphoma. *Proceedings of the National Academy of Sciences of the United States of America.* 1999; 96(8): 4546–51.
100 Deloose ST, Smit LA, Pals FT et al. High incidence of Kaposi sarcoma-associated herpesvirus infection in HIV-related solid immunoblastic/plasmablastic diffuse large B-cell lymphoma. *Leukemia.* 2005; 19(5): 851–5.
101 Carbone A, Gloghini A, Vaccher E et al. Kaposi's sarcoma-associated herpesvirus/human herpesvirus type 8-positive solid lymphomas: a tissue-based variant of primary effusion lymphoma. *Journal of Molecular Diagnostics.* 2005; 7(1): 17–27.
102 Boulanger E, Meignin V, Afonso PV et al. Extracavitary tumor after primary effusion lymphoma: relapse or second distinct lymphoma? *Haematologica.* 2007; 92(9): 1275–6.
103 Yates JA, Zakai NA, Griffith RC et al. Multicentric Castleman disease, Kaposi sarcoma, hemophagocytic syndrome, and a novel HHV8-lymphoproliferative disorder. *AIDS Reader.* 2007; 17(12): 596–8, 601.

104 Seliem RM, Griffith RC, Harris NL et al. HHV-8+, EBV+ multicentric plasmablastic microlymphoma in an HIV+ Man: the spectrum of HHV-8+ lymphoproliferative disorders expands. *American Journal of Surgical Pathology.* 2007; 31(9): 1439–45.

105 Liu W, Lacouture ME, Jiang J et al. KSHV/HHV8-associated primary cutaneous plasmablastic lymphoma in a patient with Castleman's disease and Kaposi's sarcoma. *Journal of Cutaneous Pathology.* 2006; 33(suppl 2): 46–51.

106 Trento E, Castilletti C, Ferraro C et al. Human herpesvirus 8 infection in patients with cutaneous lymphoproliferative diseases. *Archives of Dermatology.* 2005; 141(10): 1235–42.

107 Du MQ, Diss TC, Liu H et al. KSHV- and EBV-associated germinotropic lymphoproliferative disorder. *Blood.* 2002; 100(9): 3415–8.

108 Pica F, Volpi A. Transmission of human herpesvirus 8: an update. *Current Opinion in Infectious Diseases.* 2007; 20(2): 152–6.

109 Martin JN. Diagnosis and epidemiology of human herpesvirus 8 infection. *Seminars in Hematology.* 2003; 40(2): 133–42.

110 Drago F, Rebora A. Human herpesvirus as a sexually transmitted agent. *The Lancet.* 2001; 357(9252): 307.

111 Teo CG. Conceptual emergence of human herpesvirus 8 (Kaposi's sarcoma-associated herpesvirus) as an oral herpesvirus. *Advances in Dental Research.* 2006; 19(1): 85–90.

112 O'Leary JJ, Kennedy M, Luttich K et al. Localisation of HHV-8 in AIDS related lymphadenopathy. *Molecular Pathology.* 2000; 53(1): 43–7.

113 Duus KM, Lentchitsky V, Wagenaar T et al. Wild-type Kaposi's sarcoma-associated herpesvirus isolated from the oropharynx of immune-competent individuals has tropism for cultured oral epithelial cells. *Journal of Virology.* 2004; 78(8): 4074–84.

114 Pica F, Volpi A. Transmission of human herpesvirus 8: an update. *Current Opinion in Infectious Diseases.* 2007; 20(2): 152–6.

115 Martin JN. Diagnosis and epidemiology of human herpesvirus 8 infection. *Seminars in Hematology.* 2003; 40(2): 133–42.

116 Al-Otaibi LM, Ngui SL, Scully CM et al. Salivary human herpesvirus 8 shedding in renal allograft recipients with Kaposi's sarcoma. *Journal of Medical Virology.* 2007; 79(9): 1357–65.

117 Widmer IC, Erb P, Grob H et al. Human herpesvirus 8 oral shedding in HIV-infected men with and without Kaposi sarcoma. *Journal of Acquired Immune Deficiency Syndromes.* 2006; 42(4): 420–5.

118 Yoshii N, Kanekura T, Eizuru Y et al. Transcripts of the human herpesvirus 8 genome in skin lesions and peripheral blood mononuclear cells of a patient with classic Kaposi's sarcoma. *Clinical and Experimental Dermatology.* 2006; 31(1): 125–7.

119 Bagasra O, Patel D, Bobroski L et al. Localization of human herpesvirus type 8 in human sperms by in situ PCR. *Journal of Molecular Histology.* 2005; 36(6–7): 401–12.

120 Martro E, Esteve A, Schulz TF et al. Risk factors for human Herpesvirus 8 infection and AIDS-associated Kaposi's sarcoma among men who have sex with men in a European multicentre study. *International Journal of Cancer.* 2007; 120(5): 1129–35.

121 Huang YQ, Li JJ, Poiesz BJ et al. Detection of the herpesvirus-like DNA sequences in matched specimens of semen and blood from patients with

AIDS-related Kaposi's sarcoma by polymerase chain reaction in situ hybridization. *American Journal of Pathology.* 1997; 150(1): 147–53.
122. Harrington WJ, Jr., Bagasra O, Sosa CE et al. Human herpesvirus type 8 DNA sequences in cell-free plasma and mononuclear cells of Kaposi's sarcoma patients. *Journal of Infectious Diseases.* 1996; 174(5): 1101–5.
123. Casper C, Krantz E, Selke S et al. Frequent and asymptomatic oropharyngeal shedding of human herpesvirus 8 among immunocompetent men. *Journal of Infectious Diseases.* 2007; 195(1): 30–6.
124. Pauk J, Huang ML, Brodie SJ et al. Mucosal shedding of human herpesvirus 8 in men. *New England Journal of Medicine.* 2000; 343(19): 1369–77.
125. Widmer IC, Erb P, Grob H et al. Human herpesvirus 8 oral shedding in HIV-infected men with and without Kaposi sarcoma. *Journal of Acquired Immune Deficiency Syndromes.* 2006; 42(4): 420–5.
126. Harrington WJ, Jr., Bagasra O, Sosa CE et al. Human herpesvirus type 8 DNA sequences in cell-free plasma and mononuclear cells of Kaposi's sarcoma patients. *Journal of Infectious Diseases.* 1996; 174(5): 1101–5.
127. Dourmishev LA, Dourmishev AL, Palmeri D et al. Molecular genetics of Kaposi's sarcoma-associated herpesvirus (human herpesvirus-8) epidemiology and pathogenesis. *Microbiology and Molecular Biology Reviews.* 2003; 67(2): 175–212.
128. Pellett PE, Wright DJ, Engels EA et al. Multicenter comparison of serologic assays and estimation of human herpesvirus 8 seroprevalence among US blood donors. *Transfusion.* 2003; 43(9): 1260–8.
129. Hudnall SD, Chen T, Rady P et al. Human herpesvirus 8 seroprevalence and viral load in healthy adult blood donors. *Transfusion.* 2003; 43(1): 85–90.
130. Angeletti PC, Zhang L, Wood C. The viral etiology of AIDS-associated malignancies. *Advances in Pharmacology.* 2008; 56: 509–57.
131. Engels EA, Eastman H, Ablashi DV et al. Risk of transfusion-associated transmission of human herpesvirus 8. *Journal of the National Cancer Institute.* 1999; 91(20): 1773–5.
132. Dollard SC, Nelson KE, Ness PM et al. Possible transmission of human herpesvirus-8 by blood transfusion in a historical United States cohort. *Transfusion.* 2005; 45(4): 500–3.
133. Stein L, Carrara H, Norman R et al. Antibodies against human herpesvirus 8 in South African renal transplant recipients and blood donors. *Transplant Infectious Disease.* 2004; 6(2): 69–73.
134. Pica F, Volpi A. Transmission of human herpesvirus 8: an update. *Current Opinion in Infectious Diseases.* 2007; 20(2): 152–6.
135. Enbom M, Urassa W, Massambu C et al. Detection of human herpesvirus 8 DNA in serum from blood donors with HHV-8 antibodies indicates possible bloodborne virus transmission. *Journal of Medical Virology.* 2002; 68(2): 264–7.
136. Hladik W, Dollard SC, Mermin J et al. Transmission of human herpesvirus 8 by blood transfusion. *New England Journal of Medicine.* 2006; 355(13): 1331–8.
137. Cottoni F, Santarelli R, Gentile G et al. High rate of human herpesvirus-8 seroprevalence in thalassemic patients in Italy. *Journal of Clinical Virology.* 2004; 30(1): 106–9.
138. Cathomas G. Kaposi's sarcoma-associated herpesvirus (KSHV)/human herpesvirus 8 (HHV-8) as a tumour virus. *Herpes.* 2003; 10(3): 72–7.

139 Cannon MJ, Dollard SC, Smith DK et al. Blood-borne and sexual transmission of human herpesvirus 8 in women with or at risk for human immunodeficiency virus infection. *New England Journal of Medicine.* 2001; 344(9): 637–43.

140 Sosa C, Benetucci J, Hanna C et al. Human herpesvirus 8 can be transmitted through blood in drug addicts. *Medicina.* 2001; 61(3): 291–4.

141 Renwick N, Dukers NH, Weverling GJ et al. Risk factors for human herpesvirus 8 infection in a cohort of drug users in the Netherlands, 1985–1996. *Journal of Infectious Diseases.* 2002; 185(12): 1808–12.

142 Lin CW, Chang CP, Wu FY et al. Comparative prevalence of plasma human herpesvirus 8 DNA in sexual contact and intravenous injection routes of HIV transmission. *FEMS Immunology and Medical Microbiology.* 2008; 52(3): 428–30.

143 Viejo-Borbolla A, Schulz TF. Kaposi's sarcoma-associated herpesvirus (KSHV/HHV8): key aspects of epidemiology and pathogenesis. *AIDS Reviews.* 2003; 5(4): 222–9.

144 Pellett PE, Spira TJ, Bagasra O et al. Multicenter comparison of PCR assays for detection of human herpesvirus 8 DNA in semen. *Journal of Clinical Microbiology.* 1999; 37(5): 1298–301.

145 Malope BI, MacPhail P, Mbisa G et al. No evidence of sexual transmission of Kaposi's sarcoma herpes virus in a heterosexual South African population. *AIDS.* 2008; 22(4): 519–26.

146 Pica F, Volpi A. Transmission of human herpesvirus 8: an update. *Current Opinion in Infectious Diseases.* 2007; 20(2): 152–6.

147 Ljungman P, de la Camara R, Cordonnier C et al. Management of CMV, HHV-6, HHV-7 and Kaposi-sarcoma herpesvirus (HHV-8) infections in patients with hematological malignancies and after SCT. *Bone Marrow Transplantation.* 2008; 42(4): 227–40.

148 Alkharsah KR, Dedicoat M, Blasczyk R et al. Influence of HLA alleles on shedding of Kaposi sarcoma-associated herpesvirus in saliva in an African population. *Journal of Infectious Diseases.* 2007; 195(6): 809–16.

149 Johnson AS, Maronian N, Vieira J. Activation of Kaposi's sarcoma-associated herpesvirus lytic gene expression during epithelial differentiation. *Journal of Virology.* 2005; 79(21): 13769–77.

150 Sadagopan S, Sharma-Walia N, Veettil MV et al. Kaposi's sarcoma-associated herpesvirus induces sustained NF-kappaB activation during de novo infection of primary human dermal microvascular endothelial cells that is essential for viral gene expression. *Journal of Virology.* 2007; 81(8): 3949–68.

151 Guttman-Yassky E, Kra-Oz Z, Dubnov J et al. Infection with Kaposi's sarcoma-associated herpesvirus among families of patients with classic Kaposi's sarcoma. *Archives of Dermatology.* 2005; 141(11): 1429–34.

152 Malope BI, Pfeiffer RM, Mbisa G et al. Transmission of Kaposi sarcoma-associated herpesvirus between mothers and children in a South African population. *Journal of Acquired Immune Deficiency Syndromes.* 2007; 44(3): 351–5.

153 Casper C, Carrell D, Miller KG et al. HIV serodiscordant sex partners and the prevalence of human herpesvirus 8 infection among HIV negative men who have sex with men: baseline data from the EXPLORE Study. *Sexually Transmitted Infections.* 2006; 82(3): 229–35.

154 Butler LM, Osmond DH, Jones AG et al. Use of saliva as a lubricant in anal sexual practices among homosexual men. *Journal of Acquired Immune Deficiency Syndromes*. 2009; 50(2): 162–7.
155 Cannon MJ, Dollard SC, Smith DK et al. Blood-borne and sexual transmission of human herpesvirus 8 in women with or at risk for human immunodeficiency virus infection. *New England Journal of Medicine*. 2001; 344(9): 637–43.
156 Sosa C, Klaskala W, Chandran B et al. Human herpesvirus 8 as a potential sexually transmitted agent in Honduras. *Journal of Infectious Diseases*. 1998; 178(2): 547–51.
157 Casper C, Meier AS, Wald A et al. Human herpesvirus 8 infection among adolescents in the REACH cohort. *Archives of Pediatrics & Adolescent Medicine*. 2006; 160(9): 937–42.
158 Caselli E, Galvan M, Cassai E et al. Human herpesvirus 8 enhances human immunodeficiency virus replication in acutely infected cells and induces reactivation in latently infected cells. *Blood*. 2005; 106(8): 2790–7.
159 Simonart T. Role of environmental factors in the pathogenesis of classic and African-endemic Kaposi sarcoma. *Cancer Letters*. 2006; 244(1): 1–7.
160 Webster-Cyriaque J, Duus K, Cooper C et al. Oral EBV and KSHV infection in HIV. *Advances in Dental Research*. 2006; 19(1): 91–5.
161 Henke-Gendo C, Schulz TF. Transmission and disease association of Kaposi's sarcoma-associated herpesvirus: recent developments. *Current Opinion in Infectious Diseases*. 2004; 17(1): 53–7.
162 Cathomas G. Kaposi's sarcoma-associated herpesvirus (KSHV)/human herpesvirus 8 (HHV-8) as a tumour virus. *Herpes*. 2003; 10(3): 72–7.
163 Sarmati L. HHV-8 infection in African children. *Herpes*. 2004; 11(2): 50–3.
164 Delorme S, Houde I, Deschenes L. Seroprevalence of antibodies against human herpesvirus 8 in a population of renal transplant recipients at Hotel-Dieu de Quebec Hospital. *Journal of Clinical Microbiology*. 2003; 41(11): 5207–8.
165 Mohanna S, Maco V, Bravo F et al. Epidemiology and clinical characteristics of classic Kaposi's sarcoma, seroprevalence, and variants of human herpesvirus 8 in South America: a critical review of an old disease. *International Journal of Infectious Diseases*. 2005; 9(5): 239–50.
166 de Souza VA, Sumita LM, Nascimento MC et al. Human herpesvirus-8 infection and oral shedding in Amerindian and non-Amerindian populations in the Brazilian Amazon region. *Journal of Infectious Diseases*. 2007; 196(6): 844–52.
167 Dukers NH, Rezza G. Human herpesvirus 8 epidemiology: what we do and do not know. *AIDS*. 2003; 17(12): 1717–30.
168 Plancoulaine S, Abel L, van Beveren M et al. Human herpesvirus 8 transmission from mother to child and between siblings in an endemic population. *The Lancet*. 2000; 356(9235): 1062–5.
169 Mbulaiteye S, Marshall V, Bagni RK et al. Molecular evidence for mother-to-child transmission of Kaposi sarcoma-associated herpesvirus in Uganda and K1 gene evolution within the host. *Journal of Infectious Diseases*. 2006; 193(9): 1250–7.
170 Hladik W, Dollard SC, Mermin J et al. Transmission of human herpesvirus 8 by blood transfusion. *New England Journal of Medicine*. 2006; 355(13): 1331–8.

171 Viejo-Borbolla A, Schulz TF. Kaposi's sarcoma-associated herpesvirus (KSHV/HHV8): key aspects of epidemiology and pathogenesis. *AIDS Reviews*. 2003; 5(4): 222-9.
172 Plancoulaine S, Abel L, van Beveren M et al. Human herpesvirus 8 transmission from mother to child and between siblings in an endemic population. *The Lancet*. 2000; 356(9235): 1062-5.
173 Mantina H, Kankasa C, Klaskala W et al. Vertical transmission of Kaposi's sarcoma-associated herpesvirus. *International Journal of Cancer*. 2001; 94(5): 749-52.
174 Martin JN. Diagnosis and epidemiology of human herpesvirus 8 infection. *Seminars in Hematology*. 2003; 40(2): 133-42.
175 Antman K, Chang Y. Kaposi's sarcoma. *New England Journal of Medicine*. 2000; 342(14): 1027-38.
176 Casper C, Carrell D, Miller KG et al. HIV serodiscordant sex partners and the prevalence of human herpesvirus 8 infection among HIV negative men who have sex with men: baseline data from the EXPLORE Study. *Sexually Transmitted Infections*. 2006; 82(3): 229-35.
177 Casper C. Defining a role for antiviral drugs in the treatment of persons with HHV-8 infection. *Herpes*. 2006; 13(2): 42-7.
178 Parkin DM. The global health burden of infection-associated cancers in the year 2002. *International Journal of Cancer*. 2006; 118(12): 3030-44.
179 Rouhani P, Fletcher CD, Devesa SS et al. Cutaneous soft tissue sarcoma incidence patterns in the U.S.: an analysis of 12,114 cases. *Cancer*. 2008; 113(3): 616-27.
180 Bahl S, Theis B, Nishri D et al. Changing incidence of AIDS-related Kaposi sarcoma and non-Hodgkin lymphoma in Ontario, Canada. *Cancer Causes & Control*. 2008; 19(10): 1251-8.
181 Franceschi S, Maso LD, Rickenbach M et al. Kaposi sarcoma incidence in the Swiss HIV Cohort Study before and after highly active antiretroviral therapy. *British Journal of Cancer*. 2008; 99(5): 800-4.
182 Pica F, Volpi A. Transmission of human herpesvirus 8: an update. *Current Opinion in Infectious Diseases*. 2007; 20(2): 152-6.
183 Viejo-Borbolla A, Schulz TF. Kaposi's sarcoma-associated herpesvirus (KSHV/HHV8): key aspects of epidemiology and pathogenesis. *AIDS Reviews*. 2003; 5(4): 222-9.
184 Whitby D, Marshall VA, Bagni RK et al. Reactivation of Kaposi's sarcoma-associated herpesvirus by natural products from Kaposi's sarcoma endemic regions. *International Journal of Cancer*. 2007; 120(2): 321-8.
185 Tanzi E, Zappa A, Caramaschi F et al. Human herpesvirus type 8 infection in an area of Northern Italy with high incidence of classical Kaposi's sarcoma. *Journal of Medical Virology*. 2005; 76(4): 571-5.
186 Mbulaiteye SM, Biggar RJ, Pfeiffer RM et al. Water, socioeconomic factors, and human herpesvirus 8 infection in Ugandan children and their mothers. *Journal of Acquired Immune Deficiency Syndromes*. 2005; 38(4): 474-9.
187 Simonart T. Role of environmental factors in the pathogenesis of classic and African-endemic Kaposi sarcoma. *Cancer Letters*. 2006; 244(1): 1-7.
188 Coluzzi M, Manno D, Guzzinati S et al. The bloodsucking arthropod bite as possible cofactor in the transmission of human herpesvirus-8 infection and in the expression of Kaposi's sarcoma disease. *Parassitologia*. 2002; 44(1-2): 123-9.

189 Ascoli V, Facchinelli L, Valerio L et al. Kaposi's sarcoma, human herpesvirus 8 infection and the potential role of promoter-arthropod bites in northern Sweden. *Journal of Medical Virology.* 2006; 78(11): 1452–5.
190 Ascoli V, Facchinelli L, Valerio L et al. Distribution of mosquito species in areas with high and low incidence of classic Kaposi's sarcoma and seroprevalence for HHV-8. *Medical and Veterinary Entomology.* 2006; 20(2): 198–208.
191 Greene W, Kuhne K, Ye F et al. Molecular biology of KSHV in relation to AIDS-associated oncogenesis. *Cancer Treatment and Research.* 2007; 133: 69–127.
192 Biggar RJ, Engels EA, Whitby D et al. Antibody reactivity to latent and lytic antigens to human herpesvirus-8 in longitudinally followed homosexual men. *Journal of Infectious Diseases.* 2003; 187(1): 12–8.
193 Lambert M, Gannage M, Karras A et al. Differences in the frequency and function of HHV8-specific CD8 T cells between asymptomatic HHV8 infection and Kaposi sarcoma. *Blood.* 2006; 108(12): 3871–80.
194 Feller L, Wood NH, Lemmer J. HIV-associated Kaposi sarcoma: pathogenic mechanisms. *Oral Surgery, Oral Medicine, Oral Pathology, Oral Radiology, and Endodontics.* 2007; 104(4): 521–9.
195 Guihot A, Dupin N, Marcelin AG et al. Low T cell responses to human herpesvirus 8 in patients with AIDS-related and classic Kaposi sarcoma. *Journal of Infectious Diseases.* 2006; 194(8): 1078–88.
196 Ensoli B, Sturzl M, Monini P. Reactivation and role of HHV-8 in Kaposi's sarcoma initiation. *Advances in Cancer Research.* 2001; 81: 161–200.
197 Sturzl M, Zietz C, Monini P et al. Human herpesvirus-8 and Kaposi's sarcoma: relationship with the multistep concept of tumorigenesis. *Advances in Cancer Research.* 2001; 81: 125–59.
198 Pyakurel P, Pak F, Mwakigonja AR et al. KSHV/HHV-8 and HIV infection in Kaposi's sarcoma development. *Infectious Agents and Cancer.* 2007; 2: 4.
199 Della Bella S, Taddeo A, Calabro ML et al. Peripheral blood endothelial progenitors as potential reservoirs of Kaposi's sarcoma-associated herpesvirus. *PLoS ONE.* 2008; 3(1): e1520.
200 Naranatt PP, Krishnan HH, Svojanovsky SR et al. Host gene induction and transcriptional reprogramming in Kaposi's sarcoma-associated herpesvirus (KSHV/HHV-8)-infected endothelial, fibroblast, and B cells: insights into modulation events early during infection. *Cancer Research.* 2004; 64(1): 72–84.
201 Xu Y, Ganem D. Induction of chemokine production by latent Kaposi's sarcoma-associated herpesvirus infection of endothelial cells. *Journal of General Virology.* 2007; 88(Pt 1): 46–50.
202 Bubman D, Cesarman E. Pathogenesis of Kaposi's sarcoma. *Hematology/Oncology Clinics of North America.* 2003; 17(3): 717–45.
203 Gessain A, Duprez R. Spindle cells and their role in Kaposi's sarcoma. *International Journal of Biochemistry & Cell Biology.* 2005; 37(12): 2457–65.
204 Stebbing J, Portsmouth S, Bower M. Insights into the molecular biology and sero-epidemiology of Kaposi's sarcoma. *Current Opinion in Infectious Diseases.* 2003; 16(1): 25–31.
205 Schulz TF. The pleiotropic effects of Kaposi's sarcoma herpesvirus. *Journal of Pathology.* 2006; 208(2): 187–98.

206 Cathomas G. Kaposi's sarcoma-associated herpesvirus (KSHV)/human herpesvirus 8 (HHV-8) as a tumour virus. *Herpes.* 2003; 10(3): 72–7.
207 Ensoli B, Sturzl M, Monini P. Reactivation and role of HHV-8 in Kaposi's sarcoma initiation. *Advances in Cancer Research.* 2001; 81: 161–200.
208 Zeng Y, Zhang X, Huang Z et al. Intracellular Tat of human immunodeficiency virus type 1 activates lytic cycle replication of Kaposi's sarcoma-associated herpesvirus: role of JAK/STAT signaling. *Journal of Virology.* 2007; 81(5): 2401–17.
209 Dezube BJ. AIDS-related Kaposi sarcoma: the role of local therapy for a systemic disease. *Archives of Dermatology.* 2000; 136(12): 1554–6.
210 Matzen K, Dirkx AE, oude Egbrink MG et al. HIV-1 Tat increases the adhesion of monocytes and T-cells to the endothelium in vitro and in vivo: implications for AIDS-associated vasculopathy. *Virus Research.* 2004; 104(2): 145–55.
211 Douglas JL, Gustin JK, Dezube B et al. Kaposi's sarcoma: a model of both malignancy and chronic inflammation. *Panminerva Medica.* 2007; 49(3): 119–38.
212 Goedert JJ, Cote TR, Virgo P et al. Spectrum of AIDS-associated malignant disorders. *The Lancet.* 1998; 351(9119): 1833–9.
213 Haverkos HW. Viruses, chemicals and co-carcinogenesis. *Oncogene.* 2004; 23(38): 6492–9.
214 Szajerka T, Jablecki J. Kaposi's sarcoma revisited. *AIDS Reviews.* 2007; 9(4): 230–6.
215 Colman R, Blackbourn DJ. Risk factors in the development of Kaposi's sarcoma. *AIDS.* 2008; 22(13): 1629–32.
216 Haverkos HW. Viruses, chemicals and co-carcinogenesis. *Oncogene.* 2004; 23(38): 6492–9.
217 Yu F, Harada JN, Brown HJ et al. Systematic identification of cellular signals reactivating Kaposi sarcoma-associated herpesvirus. *PLoS Pathogens.* 2007; 3(3): e44.
218 Lu C, Zeng Y, Huang Z et al. Human herpesvirus 6 activates lytic cycle replication of Kaposi's sarcoma-associated herpesvirus. *American Journal of Pathology.* 2005; 166(1): 173–83.
219 Qin D, Zeng Y, Qian C et al. Induction of lytic cycle replication of Kaposi's sarcoma-associated herpesvirus by herpes simplex virus type 1: involvement of IL-10 and IL-4. *Cellular Microbiology.* 2008; 10(3): 713–28.
220 Vieira J, O'Hearn P, Kimball L et al. Activation of Kaposi's sarcoma-associated herpesvirus (human herpesvirus 8) lytic replication by human cytomegalovirus. *Journal of Virology.* 2001; 75(3): 1378–86.
221 Ablashi DV, Chatlynne LG, Whitman JE, Jr. et al. Spectrum of Kaposi's sarcoma-associated herpesvirus, or human herpesvirus 8, diseases. *Clinical Microbiology Reviews.* 2002; 15(3): 439–64.
222 Tedeschi R, Dillner J, De Paoli P. Laboratory diagnosis of human herpesvirus 8 infection in humans. *European Journal of Clinical Microbiology & Infectious Diseases.* 2002; 21(12): 831–44.
223 Ljungman P, de la Camara R, Cordonnier C et al. Management of CMV, HHV-6, HHV-7 and Kaposi-sarcoma herpesvirus (HHV-8) infections in patients with hematological malignancies and after SCT. *Bone Marrow Transplantation.* 2008; 42(4): 227–40.
224 Nsubuga MM, Biggar RJ, Combs S et al. Human herpesvirus 8 load and progression of AIDS-related Kaposi sarcoma lesions. *Cancer Letters.* 2008; 263(2): 182–8.

225 Biggar RJ, Engels EA, Whitby D et al. Antibody reactivity to latent and lytic antigens to human herpesvirus-8 in longitudinally followed homosexual men. *Journal of Infectious Diseases.* 2003; 187(1): 12–8.
226 Other herpesviruses: HHV-6, HHV-7, HHV-8, HSV-1 and -2, VZV. *American Journal of Transplantation.* 2004; 4(suppl 10): 66–71.
227 Lorenzen T, Albrecht D, Paech V et al. HHV-8 DNA in blood and the development of HIV-associated Kaposi's sarcoma in the era of HAART—a prospective evaluation. *European Journal of Medical Research.* 2002; 7(6): 283–6.
228 Lebbe C, Legendre C, Frances C. Kaposi sarcoma in transplantation. *Transplantation Reviews.* 2008; 22(4): 252–61.
229 Nascimento MC, de Souza VA, Sumita LM et al. Comparative study of Kaposi's sarcoma-associated herpesvirus serological assays using clinically and serologically defined reference standards and latent class analysis. *Journal of Clinical Microbiology.* 2007; 45(3): 715–20.
230 Sergerie Y, Abed Y, Roy J et al. Comparative evaluation of three serological methods for detection of human herpesvirus 8-specific antibodies in Canadian allogeneic stem cell transplant recipients. *Journal of Clinical Microbiology.* 2004; 42(6): 2663–7.
231 de Souza VA, Pierrotti LC, Sumita LM et al. Seroreactivity to Kaposi's sarcoma-associated herpesvirus (human herpesvirus 8) latent nuclear antigen in AIDS-associated Kaposi's sarcoma patients depends on CD4+ T-cell count. *Journal of Medical Virology.* 2007; 79(10): 1562–8.
232 Albrecht D, Meyer T, Lorenzen T et al. Epidemiology of HHV-8 infection in HIV-positive patients with and without Kaposi sarcoma: diagnostic relevance of serology and PCR. *Journal of Clinical Virology.* 2004; 30(2): 145–9.
233 Lonard BM, Sester M, Sester U et al. Estimation of human herpesvirus 8 prevalence in high-risk patients by analysis of humoral and cellular immunity. *Transplantation.* 2007; 84(1): 40–5.
234 Laney AS, Peters JS, Manzi SM et al. Use of a multiantigen detection algorithm for diagnosis of Kaposi's sarcoma-associated herpesvirus infection. *Journal of Clinical Microbiology.* 2006; 44(10): 3734–41.
235 Perez C, Tous M, Benetucci J et al. Correlations between synthetic peptide-based enzyme immunoassays and immunofluorescence assay for detection of human herpesvirus 8 antibodies in different Argentine populations. *Journal of Medical Virology.* 2006; 78(6): 806–13.
236 Wada K, Kubota N, Ito Y et al. Simultaneous quantification of Epstein-Barr virus, cytomegalovirus, and human herpesvirus 6 DNA in samples from transplant recipients by multiplex real-time PCR assay. *Journal of Clinical Microbiology.* 2007; 45(5): 1426–32.
237 Nishiwaki M, Fujimuro M, Teishikata Y et al. Epidemiology of Epstein-Barr virus, cytomegalovirus, and Kaposi's sarcoma-associated herpesvirus infections in peripheral blood leukocytes revealed by a multiplex PCR assay. *Journal of Medical Virology.* 2006; 78(12): 1635–42.
238 Fujimuro M, Nakaso K, Nakashima K et al. Multiplex PCR-based DNA array for simultaneous detection of three human herpesviruses, EVB, CMV and KSHV. *Experimental and Molecular Pathology.* 2006; 80(2): 124–31.
239 Phillips AM, Jones AG, Osmond DH et al. Awareness of Kaposi's sarcoma-associated herpesvirus among men who have sex with men. *Sexually Transmitted Diseases.* 2008; 35(12): 1011–4.

240 Martin JN, Osmond DH. Invited commentary: determining specific sexual practices associated with human herpesvirus 8 transmission. *American Journal of Epidemiology.* 2000; 151(3): 225–9.

241 Miller CS, Avdiushko SA, Kryscio RJ et al. Effect of prophylactic valacyclovir on the presence of human herpesvirus DNA in saliva of healthy individuals after dental treatment. *Journal of Clinical Microbiology.* 2005; 43(5): 2173–80.

242 Pellett PE, Wright DJ, Engels EA et al. Multicenter comparison of serologic assays and estimation of human herpesvirus 8 seroprevalence among US blood donors. *Transfusion.* 2003; 43(9): 1260–8.

243 Stein L, Carrara H, Norman R et al. Antibodies against human herpesvirus 8 in South African renal transplant recipients and blood donors. *Transplant Infectious Disease.* 2004; 6(2): 69–73.

244 Blajchman MA, Vamvakas EC. The continuing risk of transfusion-transmitted infections. *New England Journal of Medicine.* 2006; 355(13): 1303–5.

245 Barbara JA. The rationale for pathogen-inactivation treatment of blood components. *International Journal of Hematology.* 2004; 80(4): 311–6.

246 Marcelin AG, Calvez V, Dussaix E. KSHV after an organ transplant: should we screen? *Current Topics in Microbiology and Immunology.* 2007; 312: 245–62.

247 Michaels MG, Jenkins FJ. Human herpesvirus 8: is it time for routine surveillance in pediatric solid organ transplant recipients to prevent the development of Kaposi's sarcoma? *Pediatric Transplantation.* 2003; 7(1): 1–3.

248 Luppi M, Barozzi P, Rasini V et al. HHV-8 infection in the transplantation setting: a concern only for solid organ transplant patients? *Leukemia & Lymphoma.* 2002; 43(3): 517–22.

249 Vider-Shalit T, Fishbain V, Raffaeli S et al. Phase-dependent immune evasion of herpesviruses. *Journal of Virology.* 2007; 81(17): 9536–45.

250 Stebbing J, Powles T, Nelson M et al. Significance of Variation Within HIV, EBV, and KSHV Subtypes. *Journal of the International Association of Physicians in AIDS Care.* 2006; 5(3): 93–102.

251 Yoshikawa T. Significance of human herpesviruses to transplant recipients. *Current Opinion in Infectious Diseases.* 2003; 16(6): 601–6.

252 Chaturvedi AK, Mbulaiteye SM, Engels EA. Underestimation of relative risks by standardized incidence ratios for AIDS-related cancers. *Annals of Epidemiology.* 2008; 18(3): 230–4.

253 Johnson WD, Diaz RM, Flanders WD et al. Behavioral interventions to reduce risk for sexual transmission of HIV among men who have sex with men. *Cochrane Database of Systematic Reviews.* 2008.

254 Stebbing J, Portsmouth S, Gazzard B. How does HAART lead to the resolution of Kaposi's sarcoma? *Journal of Antimicrobial Chemotherapy.* 2003; 51(5): 1095–8.

255 Mocroft A, Kirk O, Clumeck N et al. The changing pattern of Kaposi sarcoma in patients with HIV, 1994–2003: the EuroSIDA Study. *Cancer.* 2004; 100(12): 2644–54.

256 Jacobson LP, Yamashita TE, Detels R et al. Impact of potent antiretroviral therapy on the incidence of Kaposi's sarcoma and non-Hodgkin's lymphomas among HIV-1-infected individuals. Multicenter AIDS Cohort Study. *Journal of Acquired Immune Deficiency Syndromes.* 1999; 21(suppl 1): S34–41.

257 Eltom MA, Jemal A, Mbulaiteye SM et al. Trends in Kaposi's sarcoma and non-Hodgkin's lymphoma incidence in the United States from 1973 through 1998. *Journal of the National Cancer Institute.* 2002; 94(16): 1204–10.
258 Schleiss MR. Vertically transmitted herpesvirus infections. *Herpes.* 2003; 10(1): 4–11.
259 Cannon MJ, Laney AS, Pellett PE. Human herpesvirus 8: current issues. *Clinical Infectious Diseases.* 2003; 37(1): 82–7.
260 Andres A. Cancer incidence after immunosuppressive treatment following kidney transplantation. *Critical Reviews in Oncology/Hematology.* 2005; 56(1): 71–85.
261 Schwartz RA, Micali G, Nasca MR et al. Kaposi sarcoma: a continuing conundrum. *Journal of the American Academy of Dermatology.* 2008; 59(2): 179–206.
262 Coluzzi M, Calabro ML, Manno D et al. Reduced seroprevalence of Kaposi's sarcoma-associated herpesvirus (KSHV), human herpesvirus 8 (HHV8), related to suppression of Anopheles density in Italy. *Medical and Veterinary Entomology.* 2003; 17(4): 461–4.
263 Simonart T. Iron: a target for the management of Kaposi's sarcoma? *BMC Cancer.* 2004; 4: 1.
264 Bihl F, Mosam A, Henry LN et al. Kaposi's sarcoma-associated herpesvirus-specific immune reconstitution and antiviral effect of combined HAART/chemotherapy in HIV clade C-infected individuals with Kaposi's sarcoma. *AIDS.* 2007; 21(10): 1245–52.
265 Schwartz RA, Micali G, Nasca MR et al. Kaposi sarcoma: a continuing conundrum. *Journal of the American Academy of Dermatology.* 2008; 59(2): 179–206.
266 Stebbing J, Gazzard B, Patterson S et al. Antibody-targeted MHC complex-directed expansion of HIV-1- and KSHV-specific CD8+ lymphocytes: a new approach to therapeutic vaccination. *Blood.* 2004; 103(5): 1791–5.
267 Yoshikawa T. Significance of human herpesviruses to transplant recipients. *Current Opinion in Infectious Diseases.* 2003; 16(6): 601–6.
268 Aldenhoven M, Barlo NP, Sanders CJ. Therapeutic strategies for epidemic Kaposi's sarcoma. *International Journal of STD & AIDS.* 2006; 17(9): 571–8.
269 Casper C, Krantz EM, Corey L et al. Valganciclovir for suppression of human herpesvirus-8 replication: a randomized, double-blind, placebo-controlled, crossover trial. *Journal of Infectious Diseases.* 2008; 198(1): 23–30.
270 Mwakigonja AR, Pyakurel P, Kokhaei P et al. Human herpesvirus-8 (HHV-8) sero-detection and HIV association in Kaposi's sarcoma (KS), non-KS tumors and non-neoplastic conditions. *Infectious Agents and Cancer.* 2008; 3: 10.
271 Stebbing J, Bower M, Srivastava P. Kaposi's sarcoma as a model for cancer immunotherapy. *Trends in Molecular Medicine.* 2004; 10(4): 187–93.
272 Klass CM, Offermann MK. Targeting human herpesvirus-8 for treatment of Kaposi's sarcoma and primary effusion lymphoma. *Current Opinion in Oncology.* 2005; 17(5): 447–55.
273 Noguchi K, Fukazawa H, Murakami Y et al. Gamma-herpesviruses and cellular signaling in AIDS-associated malignancies. *Cancer Science.* 2007; 98(9): 1288–96.

274 Dittmer DP, Krown SE. Targeted therapy for Kaposi's sarcoma and Kaposi's sarcoma-associated herpesvirus. *Current Opinion in Oncology.* 2007; 19(5): 452–7.
275 Godfrey A, Laman H, Boshoff C. RNA interference: a potential tool against Kaposi's sarcoma-associated herpesvirus. *Current Opinion in Infectious Diseases.* 2003; 16(6): 593–600.
276 Schwartz RA, Micali G, Nasca MR et al. Kaposi sarcoma: a continuing conundrum. *Journal of the American Academy of Dermatology.* 2008; 59(2): 179–206.
277 Dezube BJ, Pantanowitz L, Aboulafia DM. Management of AIDS-related Kaposi sarcoma: advances in target discovery and treatment. *AIDS Reader.* 2004; 14(5): 236–8, 43–4, 51–3.
278 Gasperini P, Sakakibara S, Tosato G. Contribution of viral and cellular cytokines to Kaposi's sarcoma-associated herpesvirus pathogenesis. *Journal of Leukocyte Biology.* 2008; 84(4): 994–1000.
279 Casper C, Wald A. The use of antiviral drugs in the prevention and treatment of Kaposi sarcoma, multicentric Castleman disease and primary effusion lymphoma. *Current Topics in Microbiology and Immunology.* 2007; 312: 289–307.
280 Pantanowitz L, Dezube BJ. Advances in the pathobiology and treatment of Kaposi sarcoma. *Current Opinion in Oncology.* 2004; 16(5): 443–9.
281 Baccaglini L, Atkinson JC, Patton LL et al. Management of oral lesions in HIV-positive patients. *Oral Surgery, Oral Medicine, Oral Pathology, Oral Radiology, and Endodontics.* 2007; 103(suppl): S50.e1–23.
282 *Final report and recommendations from the National Notifiable Diseases Working Group.* 2006. Public Health Agency of Canada. Available at www.phac-aspc.gc.ca/publicat/ccdr-rmtc/06vol32/dr3219ea.html. Accessed December 2007.
283 Cathomas G. Kaposi's sarcoma-associated herpesvirus (KSHV)/human herpesvirus 8 (HHV-8) as a tumour virus. *Herpes.* 2003; 10(3): 72–7.
284 Petersen PE. Oral cancer prevention and control—the approach of the World Health Organization. *Oral Oncology.* 2009; 45(4–5): 454–60.

12

HUMAN T-CELL LYMPHOTROPIC VIRUS TYPE 1

Although the precise mechanism of leukemogenesis in [adult T-cell leukemia] remains unclear, recent progress provides important clues in oncogenesis by HTLV-I.[1]

INTRODUCTION

Human T-cell lymphotropic virus type 1 (HTLV-1)[2] was the first human retrovirus to be discovered, and still the only one with a proven direct role in malignancy.[3,4] The genetic component of retroviruses is RNA. While the involvement of retroviruses in humans and human cancer is a relatively recent discovery, their scientific history is much longer. Studies of avian Rous sarcoma virus (RSV) that began 100 years ago eventually led to the discovery of the viral oncogene known as Src; this was followed by the identification of other viral oncogenes in retroviruses of mammals, including rodents, cats, and monkeys.[5,6]

The most famous member of the retrovirus family is human immunodeficiency virus (HIV). Like HIV, HTLV-1 is thought to have emerged in humans following simian-to-human transmission.[7-9] In fact, some researchers think of HTLV-1 as merely the human subtype of a more general category known as primate T-cell lymphotropic virus type 1, or PTLV-1.[10,11] Transferability between species has allowed for development of experimental cell lines and animal models within which to study HTLV-1 infection and related disease. In short, the virus has become valuable as a paradigm for basic oncological research.[12,13]

An estimated 10–20 million people worldwide are currently infected with HTLV-1.[14] The geographic distribution of the virus is highly variable. For instance, Japan is a well-known focus of endemic infection (accounting for 5–10% of total global prevalence). However, the largest absolute number of carriers in the world may actually be in Brazil.[15,16]

The evidence associating HTLV-1 infection with adult T-cell leukemia (ATL), also commonly known as adult T-cell leukemia/lymphoma (ATLL), led the International Agency for Research on Cancer (IARC) to classify the virus as a carcinogen in 1996.[17] HTLV-1 has also been connected to the development of HTLV-1-associated myelopathy/tropical spastic paraparesis (HAM/TSP), a neurodegenerative disease characterized by demyelination of the brain and spinal cord.[18,19] Several other diseases have also been associated with the virus.[20,21]

Most infected individuals remain asymptomatic throughout life, with only 1–5% developing ATL, and an even smaller fraction experiencing HAM/TSP.[22,23] Nonetheless, ATL patients usually die within 1–2 years of diagnosis, typically due to opportunistic infections or hypercalcemia and other bone involvements.[24] As little progress has been made on successful therapies for treating ATL (and/or HTLV-1 infection), developing a strategy for preventing the occurrence of infections becomes all the more important.[25,26]

THE VIRUS

Although HTLV-1 has infected humans for thousands of years, the virus was not discovered until 1980.[27,28] Two years following the description of viral type 1, HTLV-2 was identified.[29] The two viruses share a similar genetic organization, and a clear tropism for T lymphocytes (especially in cell cultures).[30,31] HTLV-2 has been connected to neurologic disease akin to HAM/TSP, as well as to variant hairy cell leukemia, though the evidence is not extensive.[32,33] The equivocal indications of a cancer linkage led IARC to conclude over a decade ago that there was inadequate support for a carcinogenic effect of HTLV-2 in humans.[34] This continues to be the consensus of researchers, but, of course, further assessment may lead to a different conclusion.[35] For instance, researchers have recently suggested that HTLV-2 may be involved with certain forms of cutaneous T-cell lymphoma (CTCL).[36]

A phenomenon of ongoing interest is the observed protective effect of HTLV-2 against progression to acquired immunodeficiency syndrome

(AIDS) in patients coinfected with HIV.[37-39] By contrast, some studies suggest that HTLV-1 infection promotes the development of AIDS. One biological mechanism that may explain the different effects is the tropism of HTLV-1 for CD4+ T-cells (the key cellular type involved with AIDS); HTLV-2, on the other hand, prefers CD8+ cells.[40]

Two other genetic types, designated as HTLV-3 and -4, have subsequently been identified in Africa, but their disease associations also remain unclear.[41-43]

Collectively, the retroviruses are classified under the family Retroviridae, which comprises a number of genera. HTLV-1 belongs to the genus *Deltaretrovirus*, which also includes a viral type that infects cattle.[44] The classic molecular feature of retroviruses is the use of the reverse transcriptase enzyme to convert their single-stranded RNA into DNA, which is then integrated into the host cell genome in order to facilitate both latent and productive infections.[45] Sometimes this genetic material ends up as a permanent part of the host DNA, suggesting some ancient process of host–virus co-evolution.[46] The investigation of these so-called "endogenous retroviruses," and of their possible impact on human diseases such as cancer, is still at an early stage.[47] The only other known RNA-based tumor virus outside of the retroviruses is hepatitis C.

The capsid of HTLV-1 and other retroviruses demonstrates an icosahedral symmetry; as another characteristic feature, the capsid is surrounded by a lipid-containing envelope. The genetic structure of the virus is complex, consisting of promoter, structural, enzymatic, regulatory, and accessory coding regions. The genome of HTLV-1 is very stable compared to, for instance, HIV.[48-50] As well as being evolutionarily conservative, transmission is often vertical (i.e., mother-to-infant), so that infections become endemic in close-knit ethnic groups; this means that the virus can be used as a marker for some human populations.[51,52]

The tracing of HTLV-1 (and HTLV-2) genetic subtypes is a fascinating study in its own right. Since the discovery of the viruses, researchers have been matching the identified variants against the known regions of endemic infection.[53] Six subtypes of HTLV-1 have been well-characterized, classified as Melanesian/Australian, Japanese, Transcontinental, and three African forms. The classic subtypes appear to have arisen from different interspecies transfer events.[54] The various African strains have been associated with the viral genetic pattern seen in South American and Caribbean populations, a phenomenon that is possibly explained by the forced "migrations" related to the slave trade.[55,56]

A modern extension of the migration theme is the preponderance of HTLV-1 infections in the United Kingdom and parts of the United States, a pattern attributable to the influx of Caribbean peoples.[57,58] Likewise, the majority of HTLV-1 infections in Israel are found in immigrants from a known endemic area in Iran.[59] Another example of more ancient migrations is suggested by the common HTLV-1 subtype found among circumpolar populations, such as the Inuit in Canada and the Nivki of Eastern Russia.[60]

This combination of genetic facts has led researchers to track the distribution of HTLV-1 in terms of both "the anthropological backgrounds of the virus-possessing populations as well as spatial contact between them."[61] In other words, as seen with other agents in this book, HTLV-1 provides valuable information on the origins of various human populations and their settlement patterns.

EVIDENCE OF ASSOCIATED CANCERS

Depending on the ultimate oncogenic status applied to HIV (see the "Introduction" to this book), HTLV-1 is the only human retrovirus known to be a direct etiologic agent in carcinogenesis.[62] An association between the virus and ATL was established more than 25 years ago, based on immunological and other evidence.[63] Corroboration of HTLV-1 as the causative agent of ATL has been provided by detection of the virus in the target T-cells prior to transformation, and by the ability of the virus to immortalize those cells in vitro.[64,65] As a necessary cause, and one that is an integral part of the diagnosis of the cancer, the attributable fraction of HTLV-1 in ATL is, by definition, 100%.[66]

The involvement of HTLV-1 in other hematologic malignancies is controversial. The virus has been intensively investigated in the context of CTCL. Of particular interest are mycosis fungoides (MF), the most common form of CTCL, and its leukemic variant, Sèzary syndrome.[67-70] Recently, evidence of HTLV-2 involvement in these conditions has emerged.[71] One of the complexities of such research is the fact that cutaneous forms of ATL are sometimes indistinguishable from other T-cell lymphomas localized in the skin.[72] In order to guide etiologic research and clinical responses, these ambiguous cases require careful molecular analysis.[73] While most patients with CTCL are negative for antibodies to the structural proteins of HTLV-1, the oncogenic Tax sequence from the viral genome is usually found in the peripheral blood mononuclear cells collected from these individuals.[74-76] This suggests that, even if HTLV-1 is not directly associated with CTCL, a close viral homologue may yet be identified as the true etiologic agent.[77,78]

Other blood disorders have also been of interest, including T-cell large granular lymphocyte leukemia and T-cell prolymphocytic leukemia.

However, the evidence of HTLV-1 involvement has been equivocal.[79,80] Once again, a novel homologous virus may ultimately be identified and implicated in these diseases.[81]

The role of HTLV-1 in other types of cancer remains inconclusive. Importantly, the virus does not appear to increase an individual's overall risk of cancer, which may be explained by an apparent protective effect against gastric cancer.[82,83] Although HTLV-1 has been associated with excess cervical and lung tumors, no clear weight of evidence for such a relationship has been established, and some research has provided contrary evidence.[84,85] Neurofibromas, mammary carcinomas, and adrenal medullary tumors have all been found in transgenic mice and rats carrying the crucial HTLV-1 Tax gene noted above.[86]

Beyond the well-established association with neurologic disorders (notably HAM/TSP), the virus has also been connected to a number of nonmalignant inflammatory diseases, including pediatric infectious dermatitis, uveitis and other ocular diseases, bronchiolitis, and some cases of arthropathy and polymyositis.[87-94] Other autoimmune manifestations of HTLV-1 infection are also suspected, including Graves disease, inflammatory thyroiditis, Sjögren's syndrome, and even diabetes mellitus type I. One of the most interesting potential autoimmune associations of HTLV-1 is with multiple sclerosis (MS); though largely discounted in some recent research, new supportive evidence emerged in a 2007 study of Aboriginal MS patients in British Columbia, Canada.[95]

TRANSMISSION AND OCCURRENCE OF THE AGENT

Transmission of HTLV-1 occurs from mother to child, probably via breastfeeding. Other modes of person-to-person transmission include contaminated blood (e.g., blood transfusions, sharing infected needles), and heterosexual intercourse.[96,97] Of the possible viral reservoirs, breast milk and blood have both been well-established by researchers; blood appears to be the most efficient medium of infection. Older studies have demonstrated seroconversion (i.e., detectable antibody) rates of 44% for patients receiving HTLV-1-positive blood, and 25% for infants fed infected breast milk.[98,99]

The literature is unclear regarding the precise means of transfer in the case of sexual intercourse. Because the male-to-female direction dominates, it is natural to suggest semen as the vehicle. However, carefully tracing the citation trail reveals that this discussion has rested on the analysis of one male ejaculate sample from 1984![100] To explain how seminal transmission might work, a recent reviewer has speculated about "infected cells that are phagocytosized by vaginal macrophages."[101]

Because of the feasibility of prevention strategies, the most intensely studied route of HTLV-1 spread continues to be vertical transmission through breastfeeding.

There is some evidence that the actual route of infection may determine disease development. Breastfeeding (i.e., oral/mucosal exposure) and transmission by blood have been preferentially correlated with ATL and HAM/TSP, respectively.[102,103] In fact, ATL has not been reported following a blood transfusion, except in cases of concurrent immunodeficiency. As newborns have immature immune systems, this may partly account for the observed connection of breastfeeding with leukemogenesis.[104] Chronic immunodeficiency has in fact been suggested as a necessary cofactor for the development of ATL following infection.[105] Studies have further identified reduced Tax-specific immunoreactivity as the risk factor of concern in ATL development.[106,107]

Research has indicated that the probability of an infected mother transmitting HTLV-1 to her child is about 20%, with the risk in any specific case being influenced by antibody titres, proviral load,[108] and protracted breastfeeding.[109] Transmission through the placenta has been reported, albeit infrequently.[110] Since infection rates tend to be higher among family members and others in close social contact, various environmental factors are thought to play a role. Studies in both endemic and nonendemic regions have linked low socioeconomic status to increased risk of transmission.[111-113] In developed countries, HTLV-2 infection has been especially associated with injection drug use.[114-116] Driven by this transmission modality, more than half of potential blood donors in the United States who screen positive for HTLV are actually infected with type 2 virus.[117]

It appears that transmission involving cell-free virus particles is not as efficient as passing HTLV-1 by means of live infected cells.[118,119] This would explain why transfusion of cell-free, HTLV-1-infected plasma has sometimes not led to seroconversion.[120] Investigating the molecular aspects of retrovirus transmission through cell-to-cell contact has emerged as a fascinating area of biological and clinical study.[121] Recently, infection of immune system cells known as dendritic cells has been investigated as an important step in the process of HTLV-1 reaching its ultimate target cell, CD4+ T-lymphocytes.[122]

One of the characteristics of both HTLV-1 and -2 is endemicity that tends to be highly localized in geographic regions and/or ethnic groups. HTLV-1 is endemic in southwestern Japan, central Africa, South America, and the Caribbean.[123] Within these regions, there is a further "unexplained predilection for coastal areas."[124] There are additional focal points of HTLV-1 infection, for example, areas within Iran and other countries that are near the Caspian Sea.[125,126] A notable concentration of infection is also found among Aboriginal people groups in the Americas.[127] It is important to recognize that the seroprevalence found in endemic locations can still vary widely, from 0.1% to 30% of adults.[128]

In developed countries, infection is primarily found among immigrants from endemic regions (and their children and sexual partners), sex workers, and injection drug users.[129] These categories suggest that epidemiologic data obtained from screening in blood donation programs may underestimate the true prevalence of HTLV-1 in North America and Europe. This is because people are only permitted to participate in blood donor clinics if they are already screened to be at low risk of "parenterally transmissible" infections.[130] Blood donation testing data do generally suggest that the HTLV-1 rate in developed countries is relatively low, about 10 per 100,000.[131,132] However, seroprevalence among pregnant women, an important risk group in terms of vertical transmission, has sometimes been shown to be much higher. For example, a review of European countries reported rates ranging from 7 to over 100 per 100,000 pregnant women.[133]

In Canada, reports of HTLV-1 infection are generally very rare. Since 1990, the Canadian Blood Services has detected an average of 1.25–1.50 positive HTLV-1 tests per 100,000 annual blood donations.[134] By comparison, blood donor seroprevalence data from a 7-year period in Northern Alberta, Canada, was published in 2007. The rate of HTLV infection (about 7 per 100,000) was somewhat higher than expected by Canadian standards.[135]

A helpful statistic used in the evaluation of blood donation safety is estimated residual risk (ERR); in the present context, ERR refers to the probability of an HTLV-1 infection going undetected in a blood donation.[136] In the Canadian context, the ERR over the 1990–2000 time period was 0.095 per 100,000 blood donations.[137] By 2000–2005, further improvements in testing had reduced the number to 0.023 (95% CI 0.004–0.083).[138]

Since the early 1990s, data have been obtained on HTLV-1 seroprevalence among Aboriginal clients at substance abuse treatment centers in British Columbia, Canada. Overall, 11 out of 1,953 (563 per 100,000) subjects were positive for HTLV-1 infection, 50 times the rate expected in a developed country.[139] As well, the first four cases of HTLV-1-related disease (specifically HAM/TSP) ever reported among Canadian Aboriginals were identified in that context. Even higher infection rates have been detected in a specific coastal tribe in British Columbia

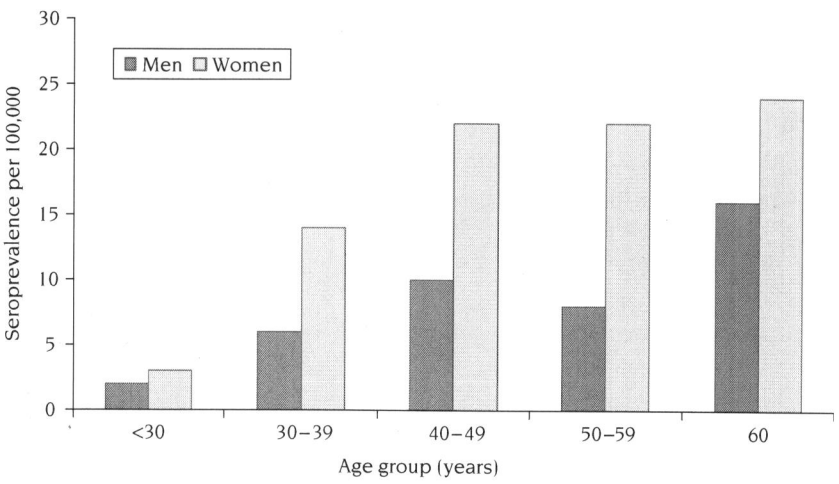

Figure 12.1. Seroprevalence of HTLV-1 in blood donors by age and gender, United States, 1991–1995. Source: Murphy et al., Journal of Infectious Disease, 1999.

(i.e., 2.8% or 2,800 per 100,000).[140] A more modest but still disconcerting occurrence of HTLV-1 infection was reported among the Inuit in Canada's northern territory of Nunavut at the end of 2005.[141] A follow-up survey among this population ultimately discovered a seroprevalence rate of 370 per 100,000, high enough to mandate targeted public health interventions.[142]

As shown in Figure 12.1, HTLV-1 seroprevalence by gender and age groups among blood donors in the United States indicates higher infection rates in females and a general increase in prevalence with age.[143] Greater efficiencies in viral transmission from male to female during the years of highest sexual activity may account for the gender differential.[144]

DISEASE MECHANISM AND PROCESSES

The two diseases most often associated with HTLV-1 have already been introduced, namely, a malignancy (ATL) and a nonmalignant neurologic disorder (HAM/TSP). The links between the virus and the two disparate diseases (which almost never occur together) in turn point to multiple pathogenetic mechanisms.[145] Consistent with the cancer focus of the book, this section will concentrate on HTLV-1-related malignancy. Specifically, the pathogenesis of ATL will be briefly reviewed.

ATL is normally divided into four clinical subtypes, though other classifications have been proposed.[146] While HTLV-1 manifests in different ways in the various disease entities, the main themes of viral involvement are common to all forms of ATL. Thus, even though it seems that HTLV-1 can infect a variety of cells, ultimately it exhibits a tropism for CD4 + T-lymphocytes; these cells eventually become the malignant locus of ATL development in a small subset of infected patients.[147] Recently, research has confirmed that the T-cell insufficiency seen in ATL is a result of infection prior to disease onset, rather than a consequence of the disease itself.[148] HTLV-2 differs in its specific cellular target, demonstrating a tropism for CD8 + T-lymphocytes.[149]

Importantly, oncogenic animal retroviruses can be divided into two groups: acute transforming retroviruses and a nonacute form. The first category includes viruses that are typically "replication defective," and tend to induce tumors rapidly due to early expression of their oncogenes. Nonacute retroviruses are "replication competent," and they induce tumors with longer latencies.[150] HTLV-1 seems to fit the second category.

The latent phase of HTLV-1 infection commonly lasts for decades; consequently, ATL rarely develops in children.[151] Conversely, the risk of ATL may be greatest among those who become infected with HTLV-1 in childhood.[152] One childhood manifestation of infection that can lead to HAM/TSP or even ATL is known as infective dermatitis associated with HTLV-1, or IDH.[153]

After entry into the target cells, viral RNA is reverse-transcribed into DNA that integrates into the genetic material of the host cell.[154] The passing of the alien genome from parent to daughter cells by mitosis appears to be the main route of HTLV-1 expansion.[155] In fact, one of the important risk factors for ATL development is the elevated proviral load that results from this multiplication.[156] Further refinement of the molecular mechanisms and related disease risks continues to be of great research interest.

The leukemogenic process related to HTLV-1 is being gradually elucidated by researchers. A vital breakthrough was the identification of the nonstructural viral protein called Tax.[157] It appears to be a necessary factor in cellular proliferation, particularly in the preleukemic stages of disease. The critical functions of Tax have been established through many molecular studies, in vitro cell cultures, and animal models.[158,159] Notably, these include disruption of components of normal cell cycle regulation and tumor suppression. In fact, Tax appears to be involved from the very start of the disease process, that is, in facilitating the unique cell-to-cell viral genome transmission that is characteristic of retroviruses such as HTLV and HIV.[160]

Tax involvement does not end with facilitating transmission. In terms of its impact on target cells in the host, the viral protein has been characterized as a "hyper-tasker."[161] The Tax protein reprograms several cellular processes, including transcription, cell cycle regulation, DNA repair, and apoptosis.[162–165] These mechanisms are all part of the multistep carcinogenesis process that contributes to the long latency before leukemia emerges.[166] In particular, Tax prevents cell cycle arrest and apoptosis that would otherwise be the consequence of unrepaired DNA damage.[167] The protein is also responsible for inhibiting DNA repair. The resulting accumulation of mutations is a key element of the leukemogenic process.[168]

Given its multiple direct roles in carcinogenesis, Tax is properly characterized as an oncoprotein. It is important to note that the different features of the parallel oncoprotein (sometimes called Tax2) found in HTLV-2 may also account for its specific disease properties.[169]

Many mysteries remain concerning HTLV-1 and ATL.[170] For instance, Tax is often suppressed in tumor cells; in fact, its expression is not consistently detected in primary leukemic cells.[171] Recently, another gene, HTLV-I basic leucine zipper factor (HBZ), which is expressed in all ATL cells, has been suspected of playing a key role in the cancer process.[172–174]

Only 2–3% of individuals infected with HTLV-1 develop ATL, so the virus cannot be considered to be a sufficient cause of disease.[175] As is commonly found in carcinogenesis, host genetic factors influence the onset of ATL.[176] A very limited range of modifiable, exogenous cofactors have also been identified and/or investigated. Coinfections have been the main focus in this regard. Human herpesvirus type 6 and the nematode worm *Strongyloides stercoralis* have been proposed as promoters of HTLV-1-related infection and disease.[177–179] While the evidence remains limited, the involvement of *S. stercoralis* is of particular interest, because the worm affects 30–100 million people in the regions where HTLV-1 is also endemic.[180] Recently, Epstein-Barr virus has been investigated as a coinfection that may promote more aggressive skin and lymph node involvement in the progression of ATL.[181]

It is no surprise that a sister retrovirus, HIV, has generated substantial attention among researchers. In fact, in the last 10 years, HTLV/HIV coinfection has emerged as a worldwide concern.[182] However, given the differential health burden, the greatest attention seems to be focused on how HTLV-1 or -2 impacts HIV-related disease progression, rather than the reverse.[183]

Whatever the range of etiologic factors and progression steps, the current prognosis of ATL patients is very poor. Apart from the general resistance to chemotherapy, the direct and indirect contributors to morbidity and mortality include the compromising effects of HTLV-1 on the host immune system (leading to opportunistic infections and sepsis), pulmonary complications, and uncontrolled hypercalcemia.[184,185] Remission may be achieved, but relapses invariably follow, and finally death within 1–2 years of diagnosis.[186] This dire outcome naturally motivates prevention efforts.

VIRAL DETECTION METHODS

Given the complexity of hematologic cancers, and the necessary etiologic connection of HTLV-1 to ATL, detecting viral infection is of increasing importance in disease diagnosis.[187] There are direct implications for secondary prevention and treatment, but detection is also potentially important in primary prevention. Molecular screening of blood and tissue donors is an obvious prevention application. As well, HTLV-1 testing can be used in prenatal screening of pregnant women who are planning to breastfeed their infants.[188]

Infection can be detected by the presence of HTLV-1-specific antibodies in blood serum. In the case of microbes that are routinely cleared by the host immune system, it is important to clarify that the presence of antibodies does not distinguish between past and present infections. But HTLV-1 tends to persist in the host for life, so serodetection becomes more relevant. Nonetheless, more direct confirmation of the virus is sometimes required. The most specific and sensitive way to detect HTLV-1 is by identifying viral genome in host cells by means of polymerase chain reaction (PCR).[189–192] One U.S. study showed that PCR methods revealed HTLV-1 and -2 prevalence at twice the level suggested by serology alone.[193] In the arena of blood and tissue donor screening, a parallel development has involved the introduction of nucleic acid-amplification testing.[194]

PREVENTION APPROACHES

Following the book's usual pattern, each of the six prevention categories will now be reviewed with respect to HTLV-1.

Avoiding Exposure	Preventing Infection	Prophylactic Eradication	Preventing Cofactor	Therapeutic Eradication	Interrupting Transformation

1. Avoiding Exposure to the Agent

As always, the earliest stage of protection against an infection emerges from knowledge about routes of transmission, and avoidance of exposure to these routes where possible. Maneuvers to prevent HTLV-1 infection may be possible, as transmission has been better characterized compared with other viruses.[195] As described earlier, the two main transfer media are breast milk and blood, with semen being another possibility.[196] Saliva has also been suggested as an infection reservoir,[197] but breastfeeding, parenteral exposure through transfusions and injections, and male-to-female transfer by sexual intercourse seem to be the predominant means of transmission. As a consequence, the approaches to interrupting exposure are on the surface relatively straightforward, though inevitable challenges occur in real-world applications. It should be noted that, for all of the methods in this section, implementation would be more difficult than the targetted public health response that is possible with an "outbreak" in a smaller population such as that reported in Nunavut, Canada.[198]

First, screening pregnant women and discouraging those who are infected with HTLV-1 from breastfeeding can substantially reduce HTLV-1 prevalence and the occurrence of ATL, even in endemic areas such as Japan.[199] Mothers with high HTLV-1 antibody titres and proviral loads have a higher likelihood of passing the virus to their children, which underlines the importance of more intensive surveillance strategies for such risk groups.[200,201] Simply shifting to alternate feeding methods in all cases of maternal infection would seem to make the most sense, unless there are practical or cultural barriers to implementing such a strategy. Even such commonsense measures must always be carefully evaluated, as financial and other costs related to prenatal screening and bottlefeeding may be important.[202] A specific countervailing factor is the well-known protective immunological effects of breast milk on infants.[203] Clinicians have been understandably motivated to find alternatives to eliminating breast milk altogether; promising options that have been discussed to balance benefit and safety include reducing the overall period that an infant is breastfed, and applying measures (e.g., freeze-thawing) to expressed maternal milk in order to inactivate any HTLV infection.[204,205]

Second, screening blood donations has provided an effective means for preventing HTLV-1 transmission.[206] Such a program has been in place for 20 years in Japan; several other countries have established similar screening strategies.[207,208] These measures lead to an ERR of transmission by transfusion that is exceedingly small.[209,210] While the value of screening in countries of high endemicity seems evident, the issue of cost-effectiveness remains an important consideration in other jurisdictions. A report from the 1990s on universal HTLV-1 screening in the United Kingdom estimated that it would cost the blood donation program £1.3 million per disease case averted.[211] Similarly, a Norwegian study calculated that the cost of saving a life when screening for HTLV-1 could be as high as U.S.$1.2 million.[212] Unfortunately, HTLV-1-positive donors do not always exhibit risk factors, so selecting high risk individuals for basic screening does not seem a feasible alternative. Another challenge is establishing when and where even more stringent (and more expensive) screening tests may be justified.

Since injection drug use involving contaminated needles is another known risk factor for parenteral transmission, treatment and support programs, needle exchanges, safe injection sites, and similar measures may be important in areas of high HTLV-1 prevalence. Of course, as with healthy sexual practices, there are compelling reasons to pursue these strategies that extend far beyond the threat of HTLV-1 infection.

In turning to the third area of reducing the transmission of HTLV-1, that is, sexual activity, it may be assumed that the same techniques are applicable as are used with any sexually transmitted infection; notably, this would include condom use and limiting the number of sexual partners. In fact, modest evidence does exist indicating that condom use reduces HTLV-1 transmission.[213]

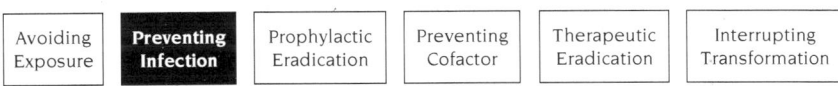

2. Preventing Infection after Exposure to the Agent

As with most infections that seriously threaten human health, vaccination for HTLV-1 represents the "holy grail" for public health planners. The interest in such a measure is greatest in regions of high endemicity, where exposure prevention is difficult to establish.[214,215] The relative lack of urgency in most developed countries may account for the fact that a vaccine has not yet been produced.[216] Shuh and Beilke recently summed up recent progress in the following terms: "Despite enthusiasm about developing an effective HTLV-1 vaccine, interest in advancing candidate vaccine into clinical trials has not been realized."[217]

The HTLV-1 vaccine substrates under consideration include peptide, recombinant protein, DNA, and viral vectors.[218] Potential targets for prophylactic and/or therapeutic vaccines are still being characterized.[219] In this regard, the genetic stability of the virus is an important and positive part of the development equation.[220]

Successful HTLV-1 introduction into animal models has enhanced the potential for testing experimental vaccines.[221] Both primates and rodents are already being used in such studies, with encouraging results.[222,223]

| Avoiding Exposure | Preventing Infection | **Prophylactic Eradication** | Preventing Cofactor | Therapeutic Eradication | Interrupting Transformation |

3. Prophylactic Eradication or Suppression

Methods for prophylactic suppression of HTLV-1 are not available. Unlike hepatitis B, effectiveness of immunoglobulin prophylaxis against HTLV-1 has not been established in the clinical setting. Again, animal studies have generated promising results. For example, studies in Japan demonstrated the protective effect of passive HTLV-1 immunization in rabbits and macaques.[224,225] One intriguing result, also emerging from Japan, has been the effect of reimmunizing with HTLV-1 cells in a rat model; immune responsiveness has been increased and proviral loads reduced.[226] It should be recalled that proviral load is a known clinical risk factor for the development of ATL.

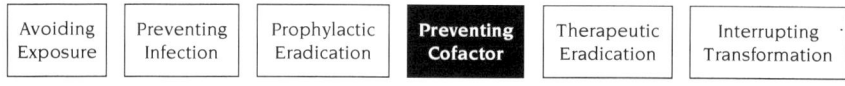

4. Cofactor Prevention

Modifiable cofactors contributing to ATL development have not been well-characterized, limiting prevention opportunities. Coinfection with the nematode worm *S. stercoralis* continues to generate some interest, partly because it is controllable.[227] A recent Canadian review pointed out the potential surveillance implications related to immigration policy. Before 1961, census data suggested that about 5% of immigrants to the country came from *S. stercoralis*-endemic regions; by 1991–2001, the figure was approaching 80%.[228] Screening for HTLV-1 in individuals coinfected with the worm may be advisable.

Other apparent cofactors tend to fall away on closer analysis. For example, the fact that ATL is relatively common in transplant patients suggests paying attention to immunosuppression issues. However, it seems that, at least in the case of renal transplantation, the increased risk actually may be traced to HTLV-1 transmission through hemodialysis blood transfusions.[229] This transforms the discussion into a subset of exposure prevention (specifically, blood donation screening) rather than cofactor control.

Finally, the expected prevention opportunity related to HIV coinfection also has not materialized. While highly active antiretroviral therapy

(HAART) is certainly effective in controlling HIV-related disease, it seems to have little impact on HTLV-1/2 pathogenesis.[230]

| Avoiding Exposure | Preventing Infection | Prophylactic Eradication | Preventing Cofactor | **Therapeutic Eradication** | Interrupting Transformation |

5. Therapeutic Eradication or Suppression

As noted earlier, the proviral load of HTLV-1 in an individual has been identified as a key risk factor for ATL development. As such, there may be a potential preventive benefit in reducing that load, if not completely removing the virus from the human body. The literature on this topic is scarce. One case report in the literature has described a teenage boy who was HTLV-1-positive and underwent a bone marrow transplant (for congenital pure red-cell anemia); viral genome sequences gradually disappeared in blood and bone-marrow samples, and became undetectable after 60 months.[231] On another front, animal studies have begun to demonstrate the potential of therapeutic vaccines.[232] Some researchers have suggested that the focus should be on reducing the expression of oncogenic factors (such as Tax) rather than on proviral load per se.[233] This theme will be briefly discussed in the next section.

Some of the therapeutic interventions under investigation lie on the borderline of the present prevention category. The reality is that the experimental drugs and procedures targeting HTLV-1 infection have been tested primarily in patients already with ATL. Thus, most of the potential therapies are beyond the scope of cancer primary prevention per se. This sort of distinction is important in terms of hematopoietic stem cell transplantation (HSCT), which has been tested in patient series as a potential ATL therapy.[234]

Two encouraging results have emerged in the investigation of HSCT. First, the method appears to be effective as a cure for ATL. This has been confirmed in multiple patients using bone marrow from both related and unrelated donors.[235,236] The first successful treatment was followed for a total of 12 years, with favorable outcomes maintained.[237] These results have prompted calls for a full, phase II clinical trial of HSCT for ATL.[238] The second encouraging result is that often the HTLV-1 proviral load became undetectable in treated patients. The Tax protein is implicated in this outcome, as it is a major target antigen of reactivated cytotoxic T-lymphocyte responses following HSCT.[239] A recent study suggested that, even when HTLV-1-positive cells are detected after transplantation to treat ATL, they may be due to contamination in the donated tissue rather than being a persistent reservoir in the host.[240]

Another possibility is that HSCT only returns the infection to the latent or carrier state. In this sense, the therapy should beconsidered a control of progression rather than a cure (and thus properly belonging to the next section).[241] Whatever the final assessment of HSCT, it still firmly resides in the world of secondary or tertiary prevention following leukemia development, rather than a prevention modality directed at HTLV-1 infection per se. The only relevant public health question would be: is there a subset of infected individuals at high-risk for ATL development where transplantation as a preventive step would ever be justifiable?

| Avoiding Exposure | Preventing Infection | Prophylactic Eradication | Preventing Cofactor | Therapeutic Eradication | **Interrupting Transformation** |

6. Interrupting Transformation Related to Infection

There are a number of important features marking the effort to arrest disease processes related to HTLV-1. First, a growing understanding of the molecular pathway of infection and carcinogenesis has generated a number of potential therapeutic targets.[242–245] Given the extraordinary role of Tax in the function of HTLV-1, it is not surprising that experimental approaches are being directed toward that protein.[246,247] Also, as seen in other prevention categories, the unique access to different animal models in which HTLV-1 or similar viruses can be activated allows for powerful methods of experimental study. Finally, the intense focus on HIV/AIDS treatments has prompted a "spill-over effect" on clinical strategies for other retroviruses, including HTLV-1.[248] Despite these advantages, progress has been slow in developing measures to modify HTLV-1 disease processes and prevent ATL.[249,250]

A multidimensional treatment approach to HTLV-1 infection has potential for success (similar to HAART for HIV patients); however, specific antiretroviral drugs have not yet been established.[251,252] Finally, a possible preventive application may still emerge from ATL-specific therapies; this ideally would involve a drug proven to be successful in controlling or even curing the leukemia, but which is also effective at an earlier, premalignant stage of the disease process.

CONCLUSION

Because of the evidence of low seroprevalence, HTLV-1 does not appear to be a substantial public health concern in North America. Moreover, only a small fraction of individuals who are infected will ultimately develop ATL. Researchers and health authorities in the developed world have concluded that combating HTLV-1 infections is a low-priority objective relative to the long list of other disease burdens.[253] Even endemic regions such as South America have many other healthcare demands that may be more pressing.[254] Overall, this could explain the relatively low slow progress to date with regard to potential treatments. The one exception to this rule would be Japan, where financial resources and research interest match the sense of urgency about HTLV-1 control.[255]

Areas experiencing substantial immigration from endemic regions of the world (such as the United Kingdom in reference to Caribbean populations) may need to reposition HTLV-1 as a higher priority. There certainly are areas of Ontario, Canada, where a similar stance may be required in response to Caribbean immigrants. This was reinforced through the recent report of an HTLV-1-positive man who immigrated to Canada from the Virgin Islands; interestingly, he was also infected with a known cofactor for ATL, the nematode worm *S. stercoralis*.[256] In the contemporary "global community," international travel to high-risk locations represents a related source of concern. Countries also need to be watchful for any new developments (including emerging endemicities) within current populations, as has recently been seen in Canada's North.

Fortunately, the first line of prevention that can be deployed in every setting actually generates multiple public health benefits, so the relatively low impact of HTLV-1 should not be an impediment to taking up such measures. Included here would be programs that facilitate the use of sterile needles during injection drug use and any intervention that encourages safer sex practices. Measures with multiple advantages will likely be the ones most commonly pursued in most societies, with prevention of HTLV-1 exposure occurring as a collateral benefit to programs addressing ore urgent health concerns.

While some jurisdictions are actively considering all the various forms of exposure protection, other countries may question the necessity.[257] The critical question is: when are universal HTLV-1 interventions warranted? Canada is a curious example of mixed policies. Interestingly, the country established blood donation screening for HTLV-1 as far back as 1988.[258] In 2007, HTLV-1 was also confirmed as part of the national protocol to ensure the safety of transplanted tissues.[259] However, the infection is not nationally reportable, nor is universal prenatal screening of pregnant women required in every province/territory.[260] And the infrastructure to treat breast milk or subsidize alternatives to breast-feeding is not under consideration, let alone established. Several of the preceding interventions, while plausible and even evidence-based, can be quite costly relative to the predicted benefits in a population.

Finally, while the low disease burden of HTLV-1 may not yet be compelling a strong preventive response in the developed world, the virus continues to be of interest at a research level. On a key front, the virus has had an impact on the taxonomy of disease. The discipline of disease classification has taken a new turn with HTLV-1, in the sense that confirmation of infection is now an essential part of the definition of the pathology caused by the virus. It will be interesting to see if other instances of microbial cancer etiology shape cancer taxonomy in similar ways in the future.

NOTES

1. Yasunaga J, Matsuoka M. Human T-cell leukemia virus type I induces adult T-cell leukemia: from clinical aspects to molecular mechanisms. *Cancer Control.* 2007; 14(2): 133–40.
2. Scientific literature searches are complicated by heterogeneous labels for the virus. Other terms for HTLV include human T-cell lymphoma virus, human T-cell leukemia virus, and even human T-cell leukemia/lymphoma virus; in each case, the proposed name simply reflects one the many terms for the cancer caused by the virus. A more superficial variation relates to spelling; for example, the alternate form "leukaemia" is widely used in medicine. Note that there are also variations on the name adopted in this chapter. For example, "human T-lymphotropic virus" may be found in some academic papers. As well, lymphotropic is sometimes spelled "lymphotrophic." In the acronym, a Roman numeral "I" is occasionally used to mark the viral type, rather than the Arabic "1."
3. Shuh M, Beilke M. The human T-cell leukemia virus type 1 (HTLV-1): new insights into the clinical aspects and molecular pathogenesis of adult T-cell leukemia/lymphoma (ATLL) and tropical spastic paraparesis/HTLV-associated myelopathy (TSP/HAM). *Microscopy Research and Technique.* 2005; 68(3–4): 176–96.
4. Matsuoka M, Jeang KT. Human T-cell leukaemia virus type 1 (HTLV-1) infectivity and cellular transformation. *Nature Reviews. Cancer.* 2007; 7(4): 270–80.
5. Martin GS. The road to Src. *Oncogene.* 2004; 23(48): 7910–7.
6. Maeda N, Fan H, Yoshikai Y. Oncogenesis by retroviruses: old and new paradigms. *Reviews in Medical Virology.* 2008; 18(6): 387–405.
7. Slattery JP, Franchini G, Gessain A. Genomic evolution, patterns of global dissemination, and interspecies transmission of human and simian T-cell leukemia/lymphotropic viruses. *Genome Research.* 1999; 9(6): 525–40.
8. Azran I, Schavinsky-Khrapunsky Y, Priel E et al. Implications of the evolution pattern of human T-cell leukemia retroviruses on their pathogenic virulence (Review). *International Journal of Molecular Medicine.* 2004; 14(5): 909–15, Jarrett RF. Viruses and lymphoma/leukaemia. *Journal of Pathology.* 2006; 208(2): 176–86.

9   Etenna SL, Caron M, Besson G et al. New insights into prevalence, genetic diversity, and proviral load of human T-cell leukemia virus types 1 and 2 in pregnant women in Gabon in equatorial central Africa. *Journal of Clinical Microbiology.* 2008; 46(11): 3607–14.

10 Goubau P, Vandamme AM, Desmyter J. Questions on the evolution of primate T-lymphotropic viruses raised by molecular and epidemiological studies of divergent strains. *Journal of Acquired Immune Deficiency Syndromes and Human Retrovirology.* 1996; 13(suppl 1): S242–7.

11 Azran I, Schavinsky-Khrapunsky Y, Priel E et al. Implications of the evolution pattern of human T-cell leukemia retroviruses on their pathogenic virulence (Review). *International Journal of Molecular Medicine.* 2004; 14(5): 909–15.

12 Lairmore MD, Silverman L, Ratner L. Animal models for human T-lymphotropic virus type 1 (HTLV-1) infection and transformation. *Oncogene.* 2005; 24(39): 6005–15.

13 Sperka T, Miklossy G, Tie Y et al. Bovine leukemia virus protease: comparison with human T-lymphotropic virus and human immunodeficiency virus proteases. *Journal of General Virology.* 2007; 88(Pt 7): 2052–63.

14 Edlich RF, Hill LG, Williams FM. Global epidemic of human T-cell lymphotrophic virus type-I (HTLV-I): an update. *Journal of Long-Term Effects of Medical Implants.* 2003; 13(2): 127–40.

15 Takatsuki K. Discovery of adult T-cell leukemia. *Retrovirology.* 2005; 2: 16.

16 Nobre V, Guedes AC, Proietti FA et al. Increased prevalence of human T cell lymphotropic virus type 1 in patients attending a Brazilian dermatology clinic. *Intervirology.* 2007; 50(4): 316–8.

17 *Human Immunodeficiency Viruses and Human T-Cell Lymphotropic Viruses*, Vol. 67. 1996. IARC Monographs on the Evaluation of Carcinogenic Risks to Humans. Available at http://monographs.iarc.fr/ENG/Monographs/vol67/volume67.pdf. Accessed December 2007.

18 Barmak K, Harhaj E, Grant C et al. Human T cell leukemia virus type I-induced disease: pathways to cancer and neurodegeneration. *Virology.* 2003; 308(1): 1–12.

19 Nose H, Saito M, Usuku K et al. Clinical symptoms and the odds of human T-cell lymphotropic virus type 1-associated myelopathy/ tropical spastic paraparesis (HAM/TSP) in healthy virus carriers: application of best-fit logistic regression equation based on host genotype, age, and provirus load. *Journal of Neurovirology.* 2006; 12(3): 171–7.

20 Ohshima K. Pathological features of diseases associated with human T-cell leukemia virus type I. *Cancer Science.* 2007; 98(6): 772–8.

21 Araujo AQ, Silva MT. The HTLV-1 neurological complex. *Lancet Neurology.* 2006; 5(12): 1068–76.

22 Nicot C. Current views in HTLV-I-associated adult T-cell leukemia/lymphoma. *American Journal of Hematology.* 2005; 78(3): 232–9.

23 Kannagi M, Harashima N, Kurihara K et al. Tumor immunity against adult T-cell leukemia. *Cancer Science.* 2005; 96(5): 249–55.

24 Jarrett RF. Viruses and lymphoma/leukaemia. *Journal of Pathology.* 2006; 208(2): 176–86.

25 Greer JP. Therapy of peripheral T/NK neoplasms. *Hematology. American Society of Hematology. Education Program.* 2006: 331–7.

26 Proietti FA, Carneiro-Proietti AB, Catalan-Soares BC et al. Global epidemiology of HTLV-I infection and associated diseases. *Oncogene.* 2005; 24(39): 6058–68.
27 Gallo RC. History of the discoveries of the first human retroviruses: HTLV-1 and HTLV-2. *Oncogene.* 2005; 24(39): 5926–30.
28 Verdonck K, Gonzalez E, Van Dooren S et al. Human T-lymphotropic virus 1: recent knowledge about an ancient infection. *Lancet Infectious Diseases.* 2007; 7(4): 266–81.
29 Gallo RC. History of the discoveries of the first human retroviruses: HTLV-1 and HTLV-2. *Oncogene.* 2005; 24(39): 5926–30.
30 Sieburg M, Tripp A, Ma JW et al. Human T-cell leukemia virus type 1 (HTLV-1) and HTLV-2 tax oncoproteins modulate cell cycle progression and apoptosis. *Journal of Virology.* 2004; 78(19): 10399–409.
31 Ferreira OC, Jr., Planelles V, Rosenblatt JD. Human T-cell leukemia viruses: epidemiology, biology, and pathogenesis. *Blood Reviews.* 1997; 11(2): 91–104.
32 Roucoux DF, Murphy EL. The epidemiology and disease outcomes of human T-lymphotropic virus type II. *AIDS Reviews.* 2004; 6(3): 144–54.
33 Araujo A, Hall WW. Human T-lymphotropic virus type II and neurological disease. *Annals of Neurology.* 2004; 56(1): 10–9.
34 *Human Immunodeficiency Viruses and Human T-Cell Lymphotropic Viruses, Vol. 67.* 1996. IARC Monographs on the Evaluation of Carcinogenic Risks to Humans. Available at http://monographs.iarc.fr/ENG/Monographs/vol67/volume67.pdf. Accessed December 2007.
35 Feuer G, Green PL. Comparative biology of human T-cell lymphotropic virus type 1 (HTLV-1) and HTLV-2. *Oncogene.* 2005; 24(39): 5996–6004.
36 Zendri E, Pilotti E, Perez M et al. The HTLV tax-like sequences in cutaneous T-cell lymphoma patients. *Journal of Investigative Dermatology.* 2008; 128(2): 489–92.
37 Bassani S, Lopez M, Toro C et al. Influence of human T cell lymphotropic virus type 2 coinfection on virological and immunological parameters in HIV type 1-infected patients. *Clinical Infectious Diseases.* 2007; 44(1): 105–10.
38 Turci M, Pilotti E, Ronzi P et al. Coinfection with HIV-1 and human T-Cell lymphotropic virus type II in intravenous drug users is associated with delayed progression to AIDS. *Journal of Acquired Immune Deficiency Syndromes.* 2006; 41(1): 100–6.
39 Pilotti E, Elviri L, Vicenzi E et al. Postgenomic up-regulation of CCL3L1 expression in HTLV-2-infected persons curtails HIV-1 replication. *Blood.* 2007; 109(5): 1850–6.
40 Casoli C, Pilotti E, Bertazzoni U. Molecular and cellular interactions of HIV-1/HTLV coinfection and impact on AIDS progression. *AIDS Reviews.* 2007; 9(3): 140–9.
41 Switzer WM, Qari SH, Wolfe ND et al. Ancient origin and molecular features of the novel human T-lymphotropic virus type 3 revealed by complete genome analysis. *Journal of Virology.* 2006; 80(15): 7427–38.
42 Calattini S, Chevalier SA, Duprez R et al. Human T-cell lymphotropic virus type 3: complete nucleotide sequence and characterization of the human tax3 protein. *Journal of Virology.* 2006; 80(19): 9876–88.

43 Wolfe ND, Heneine W, Carr JK et al. Emergence of unique primate T-lymphotropic viruses among central African bushmeat hunters. *Proceedings of the National Academy of Sciences of the United States of America*. 2005; 102(22): 7994–9.

44 Gillet N, Florins A, Boxus M et al. Mechanisms of leukemogenesis induced by bovine leukemia virus: prospects for novel anti-retroviral therapies in human. *Retrovirology*. 2007; 4: 18.

45 Yasunaga J, Matsuoka M. Human T-cell leukemia virus type I induces adult T-cell leukemia: from clinical aspects to molecular mechanisms. *Cancer Control*. 2007; 14(2): 133–40.

46 Griffiths DJ. Endogenous retroviruses in the human genome sequence. *Genome Biology*. 2001; 2(6): REVIEWS1017.

47 Moyes D, Griffiths DJ, Venables PJ. Insertional polymorphisms: a new lease of life for endogenous retroviruses in human disease. *Trends in Genetics*. 2007; 23(7): 326–33.

48 Lemey P, Van Dooren S, Vandamme AM. Evolutionary dynamics of human retroviruses investigated through full-genome scanning. *Molecular Biology and Evolution*. 2005; 22(4): 942–51.

49 Van Dooren S, Pybus OG, Salemi M et al. The low evolutionary rate of human T-cell lymphotropic virus type-1 confirmed by analysis of vertical transmission chains. *Molecular Biology and Evolution*. 2004; 21(3): 603–11.

50 Karpas A. Human retroviruses in leukaemia and AIDS: reflections on their discovery, biology and epidemiology. *Biological Reviews of the Cambridge Philosophical Society*. 2004; 79(4): 911–33.

51 Vandamme AM, Salemi M, Desmyter J. The simian origins of the pathogenic human T-cell lymphotropic virus type I. *Trends in Microbiology*. 1998; 6(12): 477–83.

52 Kashima S, Alcantara LC, Takayanagui OM et al. Distribution of human T cell lymphotropic virus type 1 (HTLV-1) subtypes in Brazil: genetic characterization of LTR and tax region. *AIDS Research and Human Retroviruses*. 2006; 22(10): 953–9.

53 Gessain A, de The G. What is the situation of human T cell lymphotropic virus type II (HTLV-II) in Africa? Origin and dissemination of genomic subtypes. *Journal of Acquired Immune Deficiency Syndromes and Human Retrovirology*. 1996; 13(suppl 1): S228–35.

54 Gessain A, Mahieux R, de The G. Genetic variability and molecular epidemiology of human and simian T cell leukemia/lymphoma virus type I. *Journal of Acquired Immune Deficiency Syndromes and Human Retrovirology*. 1996; 13(suppl 1): S132–45.

55 Pouliquen JF, Hardy L, Lavergne A et al. High seroprevalence of human T-cell lymphotropic virus type 1 in blood donors in Guyana and molecular and phylogenetic analysis of new strains in the Guyana shelf (Guyana, Suriname, and French Guiana). *Journal of Clinical Microbiology*. 2004; 42(5): 2020–6.

56 Mota AC, Van Dooren S, Fernandes FM et al. The close relationship between South African and Latin American HTLV type 1 strains corroborated in a molecular epidemiological study of the HTLV type 1 isolates from a blood donor cohort. *AIDS Research and Human Retroviruses*. 2007; 23(4): 503–7.

57 Payne LJ, Tosswill JH, Taylor GP et al. In the shadow of HIV-HTLV infection in England and Wales, 1987–2001. *Communicable Disease and Public Health*. 2004; 7(3): 200–6.

58 Levine PH, Dosik H, Joseph EM et al. A study of adult T-cell leukemia/lymphoma incidence in central Brooklyn. *International Journal of Cancer.* 1999; 80(5): 662–6.
59 Miller M, Achiron A, Shaklai M et al. Ethnic cluster of HTLV-I infection in Israel among the Mashhadi Jewish population. *Journal of Medical Virology.* 1998; 56(3): 269–74.
60 Fahim S, Prokopetz R, Jackson R et al. Human T-cell lymphotropic virus type 1-associated adult T-cell leukemia/lymphoma in the Inuit people of Nunavut. *Canadian Medical Association Journal.* 2006; 175(6): 579.
61 Yamashita M, Ido E, Miura T et al. Molecular epidemiology of HTLV-I in the world. *Journal of Acquired Immune Deficiency Syndromes and Human Retrovirology.* 1996; 13(suppl 1): S124–31.
62 Johnson JM, Harrod R, Franchini G. Molecular biology and pathogenesis of the human T-cell leukaemia/lymphotropic virus Type-1 (HTLV-1). *International Journal of Experimental Pathology.* 2001; 82(3): 135–47.
63 Yoshida M. Discovery of HTLV-1, the first human retrovirus, its unique regulatory mechanisms, and insights into pathogenesis. *Oncogene.* 2005; 24(39): 5931–7.
64 Yoshida M, Seiki M, Yamaguchi K et al. Monoclonal integration of human T-cell leukemia provirus in all primary tumors of adult T-cell leukemia suggests causative role of human T-cell leukemia virus in the disease. *Proceedings of the National Academy of Sciences of the United States of America.* 1984; 81(8): 2534–7.
65 Gallo RC. Human retroviruses after 20 years: a perspective from the past and prospects for their future control. *Immunological Reviews.* 2002; 185: 236–65.
66 Yamaguchi K, Watanabe T. Human T lymphotropic virus type-I and adult T-cell leukemia in Japan. *International Journal of Hematology.* 2002; 76(suppl 2): 240–5.
67 Sakamoto FH, Colleoni GW, Teixeira SP et al. Cutaneous T-cell lymphoma with HTLV-I infection: clinical overlap with adult T-cell leukemia/lymphoma. *International Journal of Dermatology.* 2006; 45(4): 447–9.
68 Shohat M, Shohat B, Mimouni D et al. Human T-cell lymphotropic virus type 1 provirus and phylogenetic analysis in patients with mycosis fungoides and their family relatives. *British Journal of Dermatology.* 2006; 155(2): 372–8.
69 Fouchard N, Mahe A, Huerre M et al. Cutaneous T cell lymphomas: mycosis fungoides, Sezary syndrome and HTLV-I-associated adult T cell leukemia (ATL) in Mali, West Africa: a clinical, pathological and immunovirological study of 14 cases and a review of the African ATL cases. *Leukemia.* 1998; 12(4): 578–85.
70 Pancake BA, Zucker-Franklin D, Coutavas EE. The cutaneous T cell lymphoma, mycosis fungoides, is a human T cell lymphotropic virus-associated disease. A study of 50 patients. *Journal of Clinical Investigation.* 1995; 95(2): 547–54.
71 Zendri E, Pilotti E, Perez M et al. The HTLV tax-like sequences in cutaneous T-cell lymphoma patients. *Journal of Investigative Dermatology.* 2008; 128(2): 489–92.
72 Yagi H, Takigawa M, Hashizume H. Cutaneous type of adult T cell leukemia/lymphoma: a new entity among cutaneous lymphomas. *Journal of Dermatology.* 2003; 30(9): 641–3.

73 Sakamoto FH, Colleoni GW, Teixeira SP et al. Cutaneous T-cell lymphoma with HTLV-I infection: clinical overlap with adult T-cell leukemia/lymphoma. *International Journal of Dermatology.* 2006; 45(4): 447–9.
74 Pawlaczyk M, Filas V, Sobieska M et al. No evidence of HTLV-I infection in patients with mycosis fungoides and Sezary syndrome. *Neoplasma.* 2005; 52(1): 52–5.
75 Zucker-Franklin D. The role of human T cell lymphotropic virus type I tax in the development of cutaneous T cell lymphoma. *Annals of the New York Academy of Sciences.* 2001; 941: 86–96.
76 Morozov VA, Syrtsev AV, Ellerbrok H et al. Mycosis fungoides in European Russia: no antibodies to human T cell leukemia virus type I structural proteins, but virus-like sequences in blood and saliva. *Intervirology.* 2005; 48(6): 362–71.
77 Bazarbachi A, Saal F, Laroche L et al. HTLV-1-like particles and HTLV-1-related DNA sequences in an unambiguous case of Sezary syndrome. *Leukemia.* 1994; 8(1): 201–7.
78 Ghosh SK, Abrams JT, Terunuma H et al. Human T-cell leukemia virus type I tax/rex DNA and RNA in cutaneous T-cell lymphoma. *Blood.* 1994; 84(8): 2663–71.
79 Pawson R, Schulz TF, Matutes E et al. The human T-cell lymphotropic viruses types I/II are not involved in T prolymphocytic leukemia and large granular lymphocytic leukemia. *Leukemia.* 1997; 11(8): 1305–11.
80 Kojima K, Hara M, Sawada T et al. Human T-lymphotropic virus type I provirus and T-cell prolymphocytic leukemia. *Leukemia and Lymphoma.* 2000; 38(3–4): 381–6.
81 Lamy T, Loughran TP, Jr. Current concepts: large granular lymphocyte leukemia. *Blood Reviews.* 1999; 13(4): 230–40.
82 Arisawa K, Soda M, Akahoshi M et al. Human T-cell lymphotropic virus type-1 infection and risk of cancer: 15.4 year longitudinal study among atomic bomb survivors in Nagasaki, Japan. *Cancer Science.* 2006; 97(6): 535–9.
83 Hirata T, Nakamoto M, Nakamura M et al. Low prevalence of human T cell lymphotropic virus type 1 infection in patients with gastric cancer. *Journal of Gastroenterology and Hepatology.* 2007; 22(12): 2238–41.
84 Blattner WA. Human retroviruses: their role in cancer. *Proceedings of the Association of American Physicians.* 1999; 111(6): 563–72.
85 Castle PE, Escoffery C, Schachter J et al. Chlamydia trachomatis, herpes simplex virus 2, and human T-cell lymphotrophic virus type 1 are not associated with grade of cervical neoplasia in Jamaican colposcopy patients. *Sexually Transmitted Diseases.* 2003; 30(7): 575–80.
86 Arisawa K, Soda M, Akahoshi M et al. Human T-cell lymphotropic virus type-1 infection and risk of cancer: 15.4 year longitudinal study among atomic bomb survivors in Nagasaki, Japan. *Cancer Science.* 2006; 97(6): 535–9.
87 Nagai M, Osame M. Human T-cell lymphotropic virus type I and neurological diseases. *Journal of Neurovirology.* 2003; 9(2): 228–35.
88 Primo JR, Brites C, Oliveira Mde F et al. Infective dermatitis and human T cell lymphotropic virus type 1-associated myelopathy/tropical spastic paraparesis in childhood and adolescence. *Clinical Infectious Diseases.* 2005; 41(4): 535–41.
89 Pinheiro SR, Martins-Filho OA, Ribas JG et al. Immunologic markers, uveitis, and keratoconjunctivitis sicca associated with human T-cell lymphotropic virus type 1. *American Journal of Ophthalmology.* 2006; 142(5): 811–15.

90 Buggage RR. Ocular manifestations of human T-cell lymphotropic virus type 1 infection. *Current Opinion in Ophthalmology.* 2003; 14(6): 420–5.
91 Yamamoto M, Matsuyama W, Oonakahara K et al. Influence of human T lymphotrophic virus type I on diffuse pan-bronchiolitis. *Clinical and Experimental Immunology.* 2004; 136(3): 513–20.
92 Kadota J, Mukae H, Fujii T et al. Clinical similarities and differences between human T-cell lymphotropic virus type 1-associated bronchiolitis and diffuse panbronchiolitis. *Chest.* 2004; 125(4): 1239–47.
93 Kato T, Asahara H, Kurokawa MS et al. HTLV-I env protein acts as a major antigen in patients with HTLV-I-associated arthropathy. *Clinical Rheumatology.* 2004; 23(5): 400–9.
94 Gilbert DT, Morgan O, Smikle MF et al. HTLV-1 associated polymyositis in Jamaica. *Acta Neurologica Scandinavica.* 2001; 104(2): 101–4.
95 Oger J. HTLV-1 infection and the viral etiology of multiple sclerosis. *Journal of the Neurological Sciences.* 2007; 262(1–2): 100–4.
96 Edlich RF, Arnette JA, Williams FM. Global epidemic of human T-cell lymphotropic virus type-I (HTLV-I). *Journal of Emergency Medicine.* 2000; 18(1): 109–19.
97 Iga M, Okayama A, Stuver S et al. Genetic evidence of transmission of human T cell lymphotropic virus type 1 between spouses. *Journal of Infectious Diseases.* 2002; 185(5): 691–5.
98 Manns A, Wilks RJ, Murphy EL et al. A prospective study of transmission by transfusion of HTLV-I and risk factors associated with seroconversion. *International Journal of Cancer.* 1992; 51(6): 886–91.
99 Oki T, Yoshinaga M, Otsuka H et al. A sero-epidemiological study on mother-to-child transmission of HTLV-I in southern Kyushu, Japan. *Asia-Oceania Journal of Obstetrics and Gynaecology.* 1992; 18(4): 371–7.
100 Nakano S, Ando Y, Ichijo M et al. Search for possible routes of vertical and horizontal transmission of adult T-cell leukemia virus. *Gann.* 1984; 75(12): 1044–5.
101 Karpas A. Human retroviruses in leukaemia and AIDS: Reflections on their discovery, biology and epidemiology. *Biological Reviews of the Cambridge Philosophical Society.* 2004; 79(4): 911–33.
102 Barmak K, Harhaj E, Grant C et al. Human T cell leukemia virus type I-induced disease: pathways to cancer and neurodegeneration. *Virology.* 2003; 308(1): 1–12.
103 Ratner L. Human T cell lymphotropic virus-associated leukemia/lymphoma. *Current Opinion in Oncology.* 2005; 17(5): 469–73.
104 Bartholomew C, Jack N, Edwards J et al. HTLV-I serostatus of mothers of patients with adult T-cell leukemia and HTLV-I-associated myelopathy/tropical spastic paraparesis. *Journal of Human Virology.* 1998; 1(4): 302–5.
105 Kurihara K, Shimizu Y, Takamori A et al. Human T-cell leukemia virus type-I (HTLV-I)-specific T-cell responses detected using three-divided glutathione-S-transferase (GST)-Tax fusion proteins. *Journal of Immunological Methods.* 2006; 313(1–2): 61–73.
106 Hisada M, Okayama A, Shioiri S et al. Risk factors for adult T-cell leukemia among carriers of human T-lymphotropic virus type I. *Blood.* 1998; 92(10): 3557–61.

107 Akimoto M, Kozako T, Sawada T et al. Anti-HTLV-1 tax antibody and tax-specific cytotoxic T lymphocyte are associated with a reduction in HTLV-1 proviral load in asymptomatic carriers. *Journal of Medical Virology.* 2007; 79(7): 977–86.

108 A provirus is the latent form of the viral genome that is incorporated into the DNA of the host cell, and which is capable of replication.

109 Proietti FA, Carneiro-Proietti AB, Catalan-Soares BC et al. Global epidemiology of HTLV-I infection and associated diseases. *Oncogene.* 2005; 24(39): 6058–68.

110 Ravandi F, Kantarjian H, Jones D et al. Mature T-cell leukemias. *Cancer.* 2005; 104(9): 1808–18.

111 Proietti FA, Carneiro-Proietti AB. HTLV in the Americas. *Pan American Journal of Public Health.* 2006; 19(1): 7–8.

112 Manns A, Hisada M, La Grenade L. Human T-lymphotropic virus type I infection. *The Lancet.* 1999; 353(9168): 1951–8.

113 Sanchez-Palacios C, Gotuzzo E, Vandamme AM et al. Seroprevalence and risk factors for human T-cell lymphotropic virus (HTLV-I) infection among ethnically and geographically diverse Peruvian women. *International Journal of Infectious Diseases.* 2003; 7(2): 132–7.

114 de la Fuente L, Toro C, Soriano V et al. HTLV infection among young injection and non-injection heroin users in Spain: prevalence and correlates. *Journal of Clinical Virology.* 2006; 35(3): 244–9.

115 Giuliani M, Rezza G, Lepri AC et al. Risk factors for HTLV-I and II in individuals attending a clinic for sexually transmitted diseases. *Sexually Transmitted Diseases.* 2000; 27(2): 87–92.

116 Murphy EL, Watanabe K, Nass CC et al. Evidence among blood donors for a 30-year-old epidemic of human T lymphotropic virus type II infection in the United States. *Journal of Infectious Diseases.* 1999; 180(6): 1777–83.

117 Courouce AM, Pillonel J, Lemaire JM et al. HTLV testing in blood transfusion. *Vox Sanguinis.* 1998; 74(suppl 2): 165–9.

118 Bangham CR. The immune control and cell-to-cell spread of human T-lymphotropic virus type 1. *Journal of General Virology.* 2003; 84(Pt 12): 3177–89.

119 Takatsuki K. Adult T-cell leukemia. *Internal Medicine.* 1995; 34(10): 947–52.

120 Karpas A. Human retroviruses in leukaemia and AIDS: reflections on their discovery, biology and epidemiology. *Biological Reviews of the Cambridge Philosophical Society.* 2004; 79(4): 911–33.

121 Jolly C, Sattentau QJ. Retroviral spread by induction of virological synapses. *Traffic.* 2004; 5(9): 643–50.

122 Jones KS, Petrow-Sadowski C, Huang YK et al. Cell-free HTLV-1 infects dendritic cells leading to transmission and transformation of CD4(+) T cells. *Nature Medicine.* 2008; 14(4): 429–36.

123 Verdonck K, Gonzalez E, Van Dooren S et al. Human T-lymphotropic virus 1: recent knowledge about an ancient infection. *Lancet Infectious Diseases.* 2007; 7(4): 266–81.

124 Bangham CR. HTLV-1 infections. *Journal of Clinical Pathology.* 2000; 53(8): 581–6.

125 Abbaszadegan MR, Gholamin M, Tabatabaee A et al. Prevalence of human T-lymphotropic virus type 1 among blood donors from Mashhad, Iran. *Journal of Clinical Microbiology.* 2003; 41(6): 2593–5.
126 Senyuta N, Syrtsev A, Yamashita M et al. Sero-epidemiologic and phylogenetic studies of HTLV-I infection in 2 countries of the Caspian Sea region. *International Journal of Cancer.* 1998; 77(4): 488–93.
127 Vrielink H, Reesink HW. HTLV-I/II prevalence in different geographic locations. *Transfusion Medicine Reviews.* 2004; 18(1): 46–57.
128 Bangham CR. HTLV-1 infections. *Journal of Clinical Pathology.* 2000; 53(8): 581–6.
129 Proietti FA, Carneiro-Proietti AB, Catalan-Soares BC et al. Global epidemiology of HTLV-I infection and associated diseases. *Oncogene.* 2005; 24(39): 6058–68.
130 Taylor GP. The epidemiology of HTLV-I in Europe. *Journal of Acquired Immune Deficiency Syndromes and Human Retrovirology.* 1996; 13(suppl 1): S8–14.
131 Carneiro-Proietti AB, Catalan-Soares BC, Castro-Costa CM et al. HTLV in the Americas: challenges and perspectives. *Pan American Journal of Public Health.* 2006; 19(1): 44–53.
132 Nicot C. Current views in HTLV-I-associated adult T-cell leukemia/lymphoma. *American Journal of Hematology.* 2005; 78(3): 232–9.
133 Taylor GP, Bodeus M, Courtois F et al. The seroepidemiology of human T-lymphotropic viruses: types I and II in Europe: a prospective study of pregnant women. *Journal of Acquired Immune Deficiency Syndromes.* 2005; 38(1): 104–9.
134 Figures adapted from Sibbald B. HTLV-1 virus detected in Nunavut. *Canadian Medical Association Journal.* 2006; 174(2): 150–1.
135 Zahariadis G, Plitt SS, O'Brien S et al. Prevalence and estimated incidence of blood-borne viral pathogen infection in organ and tissue donors from northern Alberta. *American Journal of Transplantation.* 2007; 7(1): 226–34.
136 More precisely, residual risk is the chance of a contaminated donation escaping the window period of laboratory detection (i.e., the time between first infection and when the viral load becomes detectable).
137 Chiavetta JA, Escobar M, Newman A et al. Incidence and estimated rates of residual risk for HIV, hepatitis C, hepatitis B and human T-cell lymphotropic viruses in blood donors in Canada, 1990–2000. *Canadian Medical Association Journal.* 2003; 169(8): 767–73.
138 O'Brien SF, Yi QL, Fan W et al. Current incidence and estimated residual risk of transfusion-transmitted infections in donations made to Canadian Blood Services. *Transfusion.* 2007; 47(2): 316–25.
139 Martin JD, Mathias RG, Sarin C et al. Human T-lymphotropic virus type I and II infections in First Nations alcohol and drug treatment centres in British Columbia, Canada, 1992–2000. *International Journal of Circumpolar Health.* 2002; 61(2): 98–103.
140 Peters AA, Coulthart MB, Oger JJ et al. HTLV type I/II in British Columbia Amerindians: a seroprevalence study and sequence characterization of an HTLV type IIa isolate. *AIDS Research and Human Retroviruses.* 2000; 16(9): 883–92.

141 Fahim S, Prokopetz R, Jackson R et al. Human T-cell lymphotropic virus type 1-associated adult T-cell leukemia/lymphoma in the Inuit people of Nunavut. *Canadian Medical Association Journal*. 2006; 175(6): 579.

142 CBC News item on the Nunavut Department of Health and Social Services report. Available at http://www.cbc.ca/health/story/2007/08/07/nu-virus.html. Accessed January 2008.

143 Murphy EL, Watanabe K, Nass CC et al. Evidence among blood donors for a 30-year-old epidemic of human T lymphotropic virus type II infection in the United States. *Journal of Infectious Diseases*. 1999; 180(6): 1777–83.

144 Manns A, Hisada M, La Grenade L. Human T-lymphotropic virus type I infection. *The Lancet*. 1999; 353(9168): 1951–8.

145 Ferreira OC, Jr., Planelles V, Rosenblatt JD. Human T-cell leukemia viruses: epidemiology, biology, and pathogenesis. *Blood Reviews*. 1997; 11(2): 91–104.

146 Amano M, Kurokawa M, Ogata K et al. New entity, definition and diagnostic criteria of cutaneous adult T-cell leukemia/lymphoma: human T-lymphotropic virus type 1 proviral DNA load can distinguish between cutaneous and smoldering types. *Journal of Dermatology*. 2008; 35(5): 270–5.

147 Manel N, Battini JL, Taylor N et al. HTLV-1 tropism and envelope receptor. *Oncogene*. 2005; 24(39): 6016–25.

148 Shimizu Y, Takamori A, Utsunomiya A et al. Impaired Tax-specific T-cell responses with insufficient control of HTLV-1 in a subgroup of individuals at asymptomatic and smoldering stages. *Cancer Science*. 2009; 100(3): 481–9.

149 Wang TG, Ye J, Lairmore MD et al. In vitro cellular tropism of human T cell leukemia virus type 2. *AIDS Research and Human Retroviruses*. 2000; 16(16): 1661–8.

150 Maeda N, Fan H, Yoshikai Y. Oncogenesis by retroviruses: old and new paradigms. *Reviews in Medical Virology*. 2008; 18(6): 387–405.

151 Ravandi F, Kantarjian H, Jones D et al. Mature T-cell leukemias. *Cancer*. 2005; 104(9): 1808–18.

152 Proietti FA, Carneiro-Proietti AB, Catalan-Soares BC et al. Global epidemiology of HTLV-I infection and associated diseases. *Oncogene*. 2005; 24(39): 6058–68.

153 Bittencourt AL, Primo J, Oliveira MF. Manifestations of the human T-cell lymphotropic virus type I infection in childhood and adolescence. *Jornal de Pediatria*. 2006; 82(6): 411–20.

154 Derse D, Heidecker G, Mitchell M et al. Infectious transmission and replication of human T-cell leukemia virus type 1. *Frontiers in Bioscience*. 2004; 9: 2495–9.

155 Jarrett RF. Viruses and lymphoma/leukaemia. *Journal of Pathology*. 2006; 208(2): 176–86.

156 Komori K, Hasegawa A, Kurihara K et al. Reduction of human T-cell leukemia virus type 1 (HTLV-1) proviral loads in rats orally infected with HTLV-1 by reimmunization with HTLV-1-infected cells. *Journal of Virology*. 2006; 80(15): 7375–81.

157 Peloponese JM, Jr., Kinjo T, Jeang KT. Human T-cell leukemia virus type 1 Tax and cellular transformation. *International Journal of Hematology*. 2007; 86(2): 101–6.

158 Satou Y, Matsuoka M. Implication of the HTLV-I bZIP factor gene in the leukemogenesis of adult T-cell leukemia. *International Journal of Hematology*. 2007; 86(2): 107–12.
159 Giam CZ, Jeang KT. HTLV-1 Tax and adult T-cell leukemia. *Frontiers in Bioscience*. 2007; 12: 1496–507.
160 Nejmeddine M, Barnard AL, Tanaka Y et al. Human T-lymphotropic virus, type 1, tax protein triggers microtubule reorientation in the virological synapse. *Journal of Biological Chemistry*. 2005; 280(33): 29653–60.
161 Wycuff DR, Marriott SJ. The HTLV-I Tax oncoprotein: hyper-tasking at the molecular level. *Frontiers in Bioscience*. 2005; 10: 620–42.
162 Marriott SJ, Semmes OJ. Impact of HTLV-I Tax on cell cycle progression and the cellular DNA damage repair response. *Oncogene*. 2005; 24(39): 5986–95.
163 Tabakin-Fix Y, Azran I, Schavinky-Khrapunsky Y et al. Functional inactivation of p53 by human T-cell leukemia virus type 1 Tax protein: mechanisms and clinical implications. *Carcinogenesis*. 2006; 27(4): 673–81.
164 Pumfery A, de la Fuente C, Kashanchi F. HTLV-1 Tax: centrosome amplification and cancer. *Retrovirology*. 2006; 3: 50.
165 Chen J, Petrus M, Bryant BR et al. Induction of the IL-9 gene by HTLV-I Tax stimulates the spontaneous proliferation of primary adult T-cell leukemia cells by a paracrine mechanism. *Blood*. 2008; 111(10): 5163–72.
166 Grassmann R, Aboud M, Jeang KT. Molecular mechanisms of cellular transformation by HTLV-1 Tax. *Oncogene*. 2005; 24(39): 5976–85.
167 Taylor JM, Nicot C. HTLV-1 and apoptosis: role in cellular transformation and recent advances in therapeutic approaches. *Apoptosis*. 2008; 13(6): 733–47.
168 Azran I, Schavinsky-Khrapunsky Y, Aboud M. Role of Tax protein in human T-cell leukemia virus type-I leukemogenicity. *Retrovirology*. 2004; 1: 20.
169 Sieburg M, Tripp A, Ma JW et al. Human T-cell leukemia virus type 1 (HTLV-1) and HTLV-2 tax oncoproteins modulate cell cycle progression and apoptosis. *Journal of Virology*. 2004; 78(19): 10399–409.
170 Yasunaga J, Matsuoka M. Leukaemogenic mechanism of human T-cell leukaemia virus type I. *Reviews in Medical Virology*. 2007; 17(5): 301–11.
171 Barbeau B, Mesnard JM. Does the HBZ Gene Represent a New Potential Target for the Treatment of Adult T-Cell Leukemia? *International Reviews of Immunology*. 2007; 26(5–6): 283–304.
172 Mesnard JM, Barbeau B, Devaux C. HBZ, a new important player in the mystery of adult T-cell leukemia. *Blood*. 2006; 108(13): 3979–82.
173 Satou Y, Yasunaga J, Yoshida M et al. HTLV-I basic leucine zipper factor gene mRNA supports proliferation of adult T cell leukemia cells. *Proceedings of the National Academy of Sciences of the United States of America*. 2006; 103(3): 720–5.
174 Murata K, Yamada Y. The state of the art in the pathogenesis of ATL and new potential targets associated with HTLV-1 and ATL. *International Reviews of Immunology*. 2007; 26(5–6): 249–68.
175 Vose JM. Peripheral T-cell non-Hodgkin's lymphoma. *Hematology/Oncology Clinics of North America*. 2008; 22(5): 997–1005.
176 Yasunaga J, Matsuoka M. Leukaemogenic mechanism of human T-cell leukaemia virus type I. *Reviews in Medical Virology*. 2007; 17(5): 301–11.

177 Mori S, Sugahara K, Uemura A et al. Usefulness of a comprehensive PCR-based assay for human herpes viral DNA in blood mononuclear cell samples. *Laboratory Hematology.* 2005; 11(3): 163–70.

178 Courouble G, Rouet F, Herrmann-Storck C et al. Epidemiologic study of the association between human T-cell lymphotropic virus type 1 and Strongyloides stercoralis infection in female blood donors (Guadeloupe, French West Indies). *West Indian Medical Journal.* 2004; 53(1): 3–6.

179 Carvalho EM, Da Fonseca Porto A. Epidemiological and clinical interaction between HTLV-1 and Strongyloides stercoralis. *Parasite Immunology.* 2004; 26(11–12): 487–97.

180 Lim S, Katz K, Krajden S et al. Complicated and fatal Strongyloides infection in Canadians: risk factors, diagnosis and management. *Canadian Medical Association Journal.* 2004; 171(5): 479–84.

181 Ueda S, Maeda Y, Yamaguchi T et al. Influence of Epstein-Barr virus infection in adult T-cell leukemia. *Hematology.* 2008; 13(3): 154–62.

182 Casoli C, Pilotti E, Bertazzoni U. Molecular and cellular interactions of HIV-1/HTLV coinfection and impact on AIDS progression. *AIDS Reviews.* 2007; 9(3): 140–9.

183 Shuh M, Beilke M. The human T-cell leukemia virus type 1 (HTLV-1): new insights into the clinical aspects and molecular pathogenesis of adult T-cell leukemia/lymphoma (ATLL) and tropical spastic paraparesis/HTLV-associated myelopathy (TSP/HAM). *Microscopy Research and Technique.* 2005; 68(3–4): 176–96.

184 Matsuoka M. Human T-cell leukemia virus type I (HTLV-I) infection and the onset of adult T-cell leukemia (ATL). *Retrovirology.* 2005; 2(1): 27.

185 Bazarbachi A, Ghez D, Lepelletier Y et al. New therapeutic approaches for adult T-cell leukaemia. *Lancet Oncology.* 2004; 5(11): 664–72.

186 Jarrett RF. Viruses and lymphoma/leukaemia. *Journal of Pathology.* 2006; 208(2): 176–86.

187 Thorstensson R, Albert J, Andersson S. Strategies for diagnosis of HTLV-I and -II. *Transfusion.* 2002; 42(6): 780–91.

188 Ades AE, Parker S, Walker J et al. Human T cell leukaemia/lymphoma virus infection in pregnant women in the United Kingdom: population study. *British Medical Journal.* 2000; 320(7248): 1497–501.

189 Poiesz BJ, Poiesz MJ, Choi D. The human T-cell lymphoma/leukaemia viruses. *Cancer Investigation.* 2003; 21(2): 253–77.

190 Davidson F, Lycett C, Jarvis LM et al. Detection of HTLV-I and -II in Scottish blood donor samples and archive donations. *Vox Sanguinis.* 2006; 91(3): 231–6.

191 Berini CA, Pando MA, Bautista CT et al. HTLV-1/2 among high-risk groups in Argentina: molecular diagnosis and prevalence of different sexual transmitted infections. *Journal of Medical Virology.* 2007; 79(12): 1914–20.

192 Lee TH, Chafets DM, Busch MP et al. Quantitation of HTLV-I and II proviral load using real-time quantitative PCR with SYBR Green chemistry. *Journal of Clinical Virology.* 2004; 31(4): 275–82.

193 Pancake BA, Zucker-Franklin D, Marmor M et al. Determination of the true prevalence of infection with the human T-cell lymphotropic viruses (HTLV-I/II) may require a combination of biomolecular and serological analyses. *Proceedings of the Association of American Physicians.* 1996; 108(6): 444–8.

194 Zou S, Dodd RY, Stramer SL et al. Probability of viremia with HBV, HCV, HIV, and HTLV among tissue donors in the United States. *New England Journal of Medicine*. 2004; 351(8): 751–9.
195 Taylor GP, Matsuoka M. Natural history of adult T-cell leukemia/lymphoma and approaches to therapy. *Oncogene*. 2005; 24(39): 6047–57.
196 Tajima K, Cartier L. Epidemiological features of HTLV-I and adult T cell leukemia. *Intervirology*. 1995; 38(3–4): 238–46.
197 Achiron A, Pinhas-Hamiel O, Barak Y et al. Detection of proviral human T-cell lymphotrophic virus type I DNA in mouthwash samples of HAM/TSP patients and HTLV-I carriers. *Archives of Virology*. 1996; 141(1): 147–53.
198 Sobol I, Palacios C, Osborne G et al. Initial management of an outbreak of the HTLV-1 virus in Nunavut, Canada. *Alaska Medicine*. 2007; 49(2 suppl): 204–6.
199 Kashiwagi K, Furusyo N, Nakashima H et al. A decrease in mother-to-child transmission of human T lymphotropic virus type I (HTLV-I) in Okinawa, Japan. *American Journal of Tropical Medicine and Hygiene*. 2004; 70(2): 158–63.
200 Li HC, Biggar RJ, Miley WJ et al. Provirus load in breast milk and risk of mother-to-child transmission of human T lymphotropic virus type I. *Journal of Infectious Diseases*. 2004; 190(7): 1275–8.
201 Ureta-Vidal A, Angelin-Duclos C, Tortevoye P et al. Mother-to-child transmission of human T-cell-leukemia/lymphoma virus type I: implication of high antiviral antibody titer and high proviral load in carrier mothers. *International Journal of Cancer*. 1999; 82(6): 832–6.
202 Ades AE, Parker S, Walker J et al. Human T cell leukaemia/lymphoma virus infection in pregnant women in the United Kingdom: population study. *British Medical Journal*. 2000; 320(7248): 1497–501.
203 Carneiro-Proietti AB, Catalan-Soares BC, Castro-Costa CM et al. HTLV in the Americas: challenges and perspectives. *Pan American Journal of Public Health*. 2006; 19(1): 44–53.
204 Wiktor SZ, Pate EJ, Rosenberg PS et al. Mother-to-child transmission of human T-cell lymphotropic virus type I associated with prolonged breast-feeding. *Journal of Human Virology*. 1997; 1(1): 37–44.
205 Ando Y, Ekuni Y, Matsumoto Y et al. Long-term serological outcome of infants who received frozen-thawed milk from human T-lymphotropic virus type-I positive mothers. *Journal of Obstetrics and Gynaecology Research*. 2004; 30(6): 436–8.
206 Proietti FA, Carneiro-Proietti AB, Catalan-Soares BC et al. Global epidemiology of HTLV-I infection and associated diseases. *Oncogene*. 2005; 24(39): 6058–68.
207 Inaba S, Okochi K, Sato H et al. Efficacy of donor screening for HTLV-I and the natural history of transfusion-transmitted infection. *Transfusion*. 1999; 39(10): 1104–10.
208 Thorstensson R, Albert J, Andersson S. Strategies for diagnosis of HTLV-I and -II. *Transfusion*. 2002; 42(6): 780–91.
209 Seed CR, Kiely P, Keller AJ. Residual risk of transfusion transmitted human immunodeficiency virus, hepatitis B virus, hepatitis C virus and human T lymphotrophic virus. *Internal Medicine Journal*. 2005; 35(10): 592–8.

210 Schreiber GB, Busch MP, Kleinman SH et al. The risk of transfusion-transmitted viral infections. The Retrovirus Epidemiology Donor Study. *New England Journal of Medicine*. 1996; 334(26): 1685–90.
211 Pagliuca A, Pawson R, Mufti GJ. HTLV-I screening in Britain. *British Medical Journal*. 1995; 311(7016): 1313–4.
212 Stigum H, Magnus P, Samdal HH et al. Human T-cell lymphotropic virus testing of blood donors in Norway: A cost-effect model. *International Journal of Epidemiology*. 2000; 29(6): 1076–84.
213 Trujillo L, Munoz D, Gotuzzo E et al. Sexual practices and prevalence of HIV, HTLV-I/II, and Treponema pallidum among clandestine female sex workers in Lima, Peru. *Sexually Transmitted Diseases*. 1999; 26(2): 115–8.
214 Bazarbachi A, Ghez D, Lepelletier Y et al. New therapeutic approaches for adult T-cell leukaemia. *Lancet Oncology*. 2004; 5(11): 664–72.
215 Daisley H, Charles WP, Swanston W. Role of HTLV-1 co-infection in the AIDS epidemic in the Caribbean: a cause for concern. *International Journal of STD and AIDS*. 1999; 10(7): 487–9.
216 Gallo RC. Human retroviruses after 20 years: a perspective from the past and prospects for their future control. *Immunological Reviews*. 2002; 185: 236–65.
217 Shuh M, Beilke M. The human T-cell leukemia virus type 1 (HTLV-1): new insights into the clinical aspects and molecular pathogenesis of adult T-cell leukemia/lymphoma (ATLL) and tropical spastic paraparesis/HTLV-associated myelopathy (TSP/HAM). *Microscopy Research and Technique*. 2005; 68(3–4): 176–96.
218 Lynch MP, Kaumaya PT. Advances in HTLV-1 peptide vaccines and therapeutics. *Current Protein and Peptide Science*. 2006; 7(2): 137–45.
219 Kurihara K, Shimizu Y, Takamori A et al. Human T-cell leukemia virus type-I (HTLV-I)-specific T-cell responses detected using three-divided glutathione-S-transferase (GST)-Tax fusion proteins. *Journal of Immunological Methods*. 2006; 313(1–2): 61–73.
220 Kubota R, Hanada K, Furukawa Y et al. Genetic stability of human T lymphotropic virus type I despite antiviral pressures by CTLs. *Journal of Immunology*. 2007; 178(9): 5966–72.
221 Lairmore MD, Silverman L, Ratner L. Animal models for human T-lymphotropic virus type 1 (HTLV-1) infection and transformation. *Oncogene*. 2005; 24(39): 6005–15.
222 Kazanji M, Heraud JM, Merien F et al. Chimeric peptide vaccine composed of B- and T-cell epitopes of human T-cell leukemia virus type 1 induces humoral and cellular immune responses and reduces the proviral load in immunized squirrel monkeys (Saimiri sciureus). *Journal of General Virology*. 2006; 87(Pt 5): 1331–7.
223 Sundaram R, Lynch MP, Rawale S et al. Protective efficacy of multiepitope human leukocyte antigen-A*0201 restricted cytotoxic T-lymphocyte peptide construct against challenge with human T-cell lymphotropic virus type 1 Tax recombinant vaccinia virus. *Journal of Acquired Immune Deficiency Syndromes*. 2004; 37(3): 1329–39.
224 Tanaka Y, Ishii K, Sawada T et al. Prophylaxis against a Melanesian variant of human T-lymphotropic virus type I (HTLV-I) in rabbits using HTLV-I immune globulin from asymptomatically infected Japanese carriers. *Blood*. 1993; 82(12): 3664–7.

225 Murata N, Hakoda E, Machida H et al. Prevention of human T cell lymphotropic virus type I infection in Japanese macaques by passive immunization. *Leukemia*. 1996; 10(12): 1971–4.
226 Komori K, Hasegawa A, Kurihara K et al. Reduction of human T-cell leukemia virus type 1 (HTLV-1) proviral loads in rats orally infected with HTLV-1 by reimmunization with HTLV-1-infected cells. *Journal of Virology*. 2006; 80(15): 7375–81.
227 Satoh M, Kokaze A. Treatment strategies in controlling strongyloidiasis. *Expert Opinion on Pharmacotherapy*. 2004; 5(11): 2293–301.
228 Lim S, Katz K, Krajden S et al. Complicated and fatal Strongyloides infection in Canadians: risk factors, diagnosis and management. *Canadian Medical Association Journal*. 2004; 171(5): 479–84.
229 Hoshida Y, Li T, Dong Z et al. Lymphoproliferative disorders in renal transplant patients in Japan. *International Journal of Cancer*. 2001; 91(6): 869–75.
230 Casoli C, Pilotti E, Bertazzoni U. Molecular and cellular interactions of HIV-1/HTLV coinfection and impact on AIDS progression. *AIDS Reviews*. 2007; 9(3): 140–9.
231 Kawa K, Nishiuchi R, Okamura T et al. Eradication of human T-lymphotropic virus type 1 by allogeneic bone-marrow transplantation. *The Lancet*. 1998; 352(9133): 1034–5.
232 Kazanji M, Heraud JM, Merien F et al. Chimeric peptide vaccine composed of B- and T-cell epitopes of human T-cell leukemia virus type 1 induces humoral and cellular immune responses and reduces the proviral load in immunized squirrel monkeys (Saimiri sciureus). *Journal of General Virology*. 2006; 87(Pt 5): 1331–7.
233 Asquith B, Mosley AJ, Heaps A et al. Quantification of the virus-host interaction in human T lymphotropic virus I infection. *Retrovirology*. 2005; 2: 75.
234 Shiratori S, Yasumoto A, Tanaka J et al. A retrospective analysis of allogeneic hematopoietic stem cell transplantation for adult T cell leukemia/lymphoma (ATL): clinical impact of graft-versus-leukemia/lymphoma effect. *Biology of Blood and Marrow Transplantation*. 2008; 14(7): 817–23.
235 Okamura J, Utsunomiya A, Tanosaki R et al. Allogeneic stem-cell transplantation with reduced conditioning intensity as a novel immunotherapy and antiviral therapy for adult T-cell leukemia/lymphoma. *Blood*. 2005; 105(10): 4143–5.
236 Kato K, Kanda Y, Eto T et al. Allogeneic bone marrow transplantation from unrelated human T-cell leukemia virus-I-negative donors for adult T-cell leukemia/ lymphoma: retrospective analysis of data from the Japan Marrow Donor Program. *Biology of Blood and Marrow Transplantation*. 2007; 13(1): 90–9.
237 Tholouli E, Liu Yin JA. Successful treatment of HTLV-1-associated acute adult T-cell leukemia lymphoma by allogeneic bone marrow transplantation: a 12 year follow-up. *Leukemia and Lymphoma*. 2006; 47(8): 1691–2.
238 Fukushima T, Miyazaki Y, Honda S et al. Allogeneic hematopoietic stem cell transplantation provides sustained long-term survival for patients with adult T-cell leukemia/lymphoma. *Leukemia*. 2005; 19(5): 829–34.
239 Kannagi M. Immunologic control of human T-cell leukemia virus type I and adult T-cell leukemia. *International Journal of Hematology*. 2007; 86(2): 113–7.

240 Yamasaki R, Miyazaki Y, Moriuchi Y et al. Small number of HTLV-1-positive cells frequently remains during complete remission after allogeneic hematopoietic stem cell transplantation that are heterogeneous in origin among cases with adult T-cell leukemia/lymphoma. *Leukemia.* 2007; 21(6): 1212–7.

241 Tajima K, Amakawa R, Uehira K et al. Adult T-cell leukemia successfully treated with allogeneic bone marrow transplantation. *International Journal of Hematology.* 2000; 71(3): 290–3.

242 Murata K, Yamada Y. The state of the art in the pathogenesis of ATL and new potential targets associated with HTLV-1 and ATL. *International Reviews of Immunology.* 2007; 26(5–6): 249–68.

243 Ohsugi T, Koito A. Current topics in prevention of human T-cell leukemia virus type i infection: NF-kappa B inhibitors and APOBEC3. *International Reviews of Immunology.* 2008; 27(4): 225–53.

244 Horie R. NF-kappaB in pathogenesis and treatment of adult T-cell leukemia/lymphoma. *International Reviews of Immunology.* 2007; 26(5–6): 269–81.

245 Faris M. Potential for molecular targeted therapy for adult T-cell leukemia/lymphoma. *International Reviews of Immunology.* 2008; 27(1–2): 71–8.

246 Kannagi M, Harashima N, Kurihara K et al. Adult T-cell leukemia: future prophylaxis and immunotherapy. *Expert Review of Anticancer Therapy.* 2004; 4(3): 369–76.

247 Kobayashi H, Ngato T, Sato K et al. In vitro peptide immunization of target tax protein human T-cell leukemia virus type 1-specific CD4+ helper T lymphocytes. *Clinical Cancer Research.* 2006; 12(12): 3814–22.

248 Tozser J, Weber IT. The protease of human T-cell leukemia virus type-1 is a potential therapeutic target. *Current Pharmaceutical Design.* 2007; 13(12): 1285–94.

249 Lynch MP, Kaumaya PT. Advances in HTLV-1 peptide vaccines and therapeutics. *Current Protein and Peptide Science.* 2006; 7(2): 137–45.

250 Ravandi F, Kantarjian H, Jones D et al. Mature T-cell leukemias. *Cancer.* 2005; 104(9): 1808–18.

251 Bazarbachi A, Ghez D, Lepelletier Y et al. New therapeutic approaches for adult T-cell leukaemia. *Lancet Oncology.* 2004; 5(11): 664–72.

252 Hill SA, Lloyd PA, McDonald S et al. Susceptibility of human T cell leukemia virus type I to nucleoside reverse transcriptase inhibitors. *Journal of Infectious Diseases.* 2003; 188(3): 424–7.

253 Sibbald B. HTLV-1 virus detected in Nunavut. *Canadian Medical Association Journal.* 2006; 174(2): 150–1.

254 Carneiro-Proietti AB, Catalan-Soares BC, Castro-Costa CM et al. HTLV in the Americas: challenges and perspectives. *Pan American Journal of Public Health.* 2006; 19(1): 44–53.

255 Yamada Y, Tomonaga M. The current status of therapy for adult T-cell leukaemia-lymphoma in Japan. *Leukemia and Lymphoma.* 2003; 44(4): 611–8.

256 Lagace-Wiens PR, Harding GK. A Canadian immigrant with coinfection of Strongyloides stercoralis and human T-lymphotropic virus 1. *Canadian Medical Association Journal.* 2007; 177(5): 451–3.

257 Alarcon JO, Friedman HB, Montano SM et al. High endemicity of human T-cell lymphotropic virus type 1 among pregnant women in peru. *Journal of Acquired Immune Deficiency Syndromes.* 2006; 42(5): 604–9.

258 Thorstensson R, Albert J, Andersson S. Strategies for diagnosis of HTLV-I and -II. *Transfusion*. 2002; 42(6): 780–91.
259 *Guidance Document: Cells, Tissues and Organs (CTO) for Transplantation*. Available at http://www.hc-sc.gc.ca/dhp-mps/alt_formats/hpfb-dgpsa/pdf/brgtherap/cto_draft_gd-cto_ebauche_ld_e.pdf. Accessed January 2008.
260 Final Report and Recommendations from the National Notifiable Diseases Working Group. Available at http://www.phac-aspc.gc.ca/publicat/ccdr-rmtc/06vol32/dr3219ea.html. Accessed January 2008.

13

CONCLUSION—INFECTION AND CANCER: A PARADIGM SHIFT

> The fact that the etiologic burden [of infectious agents of cancer] may be much greater than generally perceived needs more emphasis in cancer prevention and control efforts.[1]

The term "paradigm shift" was coined by Thomas Kuhn in 1962 to describe a fundamental change in basic assumptions and interpretations within an area of science. Kuhn could not have known how the publication of his now-famous book, *The Structure of Scientific Revolutions*, would so aptly coincide with the beginning of a remarkable era in cancer research and clinical practice. The idea of a paradigm shift, first introduced in that book, may be aptly applied to the developments that are well underway in the realm of infectious agents and cancers. The emerging information continues to prompt substantial responses from practitioners, patients, and researchers alike.

Since the discovery in the 1960s of the role of viruses in both a rare lymphoma (i.e., Burkitt lymphoma) and a much more common nonhematologic cancer (i.e., hepatocellular carcinoma), the number of infectious agents implicated in malignancies has steadily expanded. The infectious agents now confirmed or suspected of causing cancer range from bacteria to protozoa to microscopic flatworms. Viruses dominate the inventory, which is consistent with their fundamental ability to affect the genetic integrity and alter regular functions of host cells. Cancer is essentially a disease marked by uncontrolled genetic instability that finally leads to uncontrolled cell growth.[2,3] As will be summarized below, viruses are remarkably attuned to interact in this process.

Given such a noteworthy development in biology and pathology, it is natural to ask: what are the practical implications? The project that inspired and sponsored the development of this book in fact had three application agendas:

1. Increase the profile of this subject among cancer prevention leaders, with a focus on selected infectious agents
2. Lay out the biology and prevention possibilities related to those agents
3. Consider future research and policy directions

In this chapter, the contents of the book will be considered in light of each of these project aims.

SUBSTANTIAL SUBJECT

The first objective involved raising the consciousness of key players in cancer prevention about the importance of and potential for decreasing cancer incidence by addressing direct infectious causes. Knowledge of the role of infectious agents in cancer causation is only beginning to take hold among the media and the general public. The gradual increase in awareness belies the fact that current estimates of global cancer cases attributable to infectious agents approach 20%.[4] By any measure, this is a burden that is worthy of significant public health attention, especially if it can be demonstrated that incidence and/or mortality could be reduced by feasible prevention strategies.

The oncogenic agents in this book have mostly been covered on their own terms, apart from noting the interactions that arise in a case of coinfection and a few observations on the similarities and contrasts between the agents. Some reviewers have gone further, especially identifying functional patterns across the largest group of oncogenic agents, the DNA tumor viruses. For example, there are important differences between smaller (e.g., HPV) and larger (e.g., EBV, HHV-8) tumor viruses, as outlined in Table 13.1.[5]

There are two infectious agents covered in this book that have received significant attention from health care leaders and, to a lesser degree, from the public. First, a safe and effective hepatitis B virus vaccine has been available for over 25 years, and has been used widely since the 1990s.[6] Hepatitis B vaccination, however, is not consistently framed as a cancer prevention

Table 13.1. Comparison of DNA Cancer-Causing Viruses

	Smaller Viral Size	Larger Viral Size
Example	Human papillomavirus	Human herpesvirus
Replication mechanism	Co-opts the host machinery to achieve viral replication	Encodes its own DNA polymerase
Viral DNA location in neoplasia	Generally integrates into host DNA	Episomal, i.e., maintained separately, but tethered to host chromosome by distinctive viral latent proteins
Transformation genes	Generally a small number, e.g., two in HPV (E6, E7)	Encode several transforming genes
Transformation targets	Limited host cell tropism	Causes cancer in many cell types

measure. Its role in protecting against *nonmalignant* forms of liver disease often overshadows consideration of hepatocellular carcinoma.

However, a second agent, the human papillomavirus (HPV), finally put the role of infection in cancer etiology squarely on the health care agenda. Cancer prevention leaders, health care planners, funding providers, and the general public have become increasingly aware that persistent infection is strongly implicated in cervical cancer (indeed, acting as a *necessary* cause), and that prevention of both infection and the related malignancy is a real possibility. In the case of HPV, basic science has driven successful prevention innovation, which in turn has stimulated even more scientific investigation. The avalanche of published studies seen in recent years, as well as the importance of cancer of the cervix globally, helps to explain the disproportionate attention paid to HPV in this book.

The rising interest in HPV-related primary cancer prevention has resulted from the confluence of three forces: (1) the development and licensing of a vaccine against specific HPV types, with demonstrated protection against cervical cancer precursors, (2) the intense marketing campaign by the company that designed the first product, and (3) the fact that the main cancer being addressed, cervical cancer, occupies an important position in the spectrum of malignancies. Thus, cervical cancer is well known to women in the developed world because of the medical and personal burden attached to diagnosis, and the high-profile and successful efforts related to screening and early detection over many decades. Furthermore, in the developing world, cervical cancer is the female malignancy with the second highest incidence. Above all, the availability of a vaccine is considered to be the "holy grail" when dealing with an infection, and generally perceived as more attractive than, for example, exposure avoidance measures. The advent of efficacious prophylactic vaccines means that the attention being paid to HPV is currently unmatched by any other infectious agent of cancer. But the collateral interest inspired by HPV has certainly been broader; and because of scientific publishing, new vaccination programs, and media coverage, both the professional and popular appreciation of the entire field of infections and malignancy has forever been changed.

One of the implicit arguments of this book is that the scientific discussion and preventive response to infectious agents should be expanded beyond the current focus, which mainly is on HPV (and, to a lesser extent, HBV).[7,8] While HPV is very important, accounting for almost a third of infection-related cancers in the world, a full accounting of this subject requires a more comprehensive view. This book has been aimed at stimulating such an inclusive agenda. As Table 13.2 outlines, the agents covered in this book generate 98% of the known infection-related cancer cases in the world.

The information in Table 13.2 also underlines the fact that the relative burden sometimes shifts between developed and developing countries. For example, the percentage of cancer cases attributable to *Helicobacter pylori* in developed countries (i.e., 3.9%) is higher than that for any other infectious agent (and actually accounts for half of the attributable risk related to infection), whereas in developing countries the bacteria comes in third (at 7.0%) behind both Hepatitis B/C viruses (8.2%) and HPV (7.7%). This variation will likely have implications for the distribution of resources to both research and prevention efforts in different jurisdictions.[9]

Table 13.2. Key Infections and Cancer Burden

Infectious Agent	Estimated Proportion of 2002 Cancer Cases Attributable to Infection		
	Global (%)	Developed (%)	Developing (%)
Human papillomaviruses	5.2	2.2	7.7
Hepatitis B and C	4.9	1.0	8.2
Helicobacter pylori	5.5	3.9	7.0
Epstein-Barr virus	1.0	0.4	1.6
Human T-cell lymphotropic virus type I	0.03	0.01	0.05
Human herpesvirus type 8	0.9	0.1	1.1
Other	0.3	0.1	0.7
Total	17.8	7.7	26.3

Source: Parkin, *International Journal of Cancer*, 2006.

Conclusion—Infection and Cancer   509

PREVENTION POSSIBILITIES

An important component of the review of the main infectious agents covered in this book has been an inventory of existing and emerging prevention measures. Indeed, many sections of each chapter, including those dealing with transmission, disease mechanisms, and even techniques of microbe detection, were ultimately intended to serve the prevention cause.

As outlined in the introductory chapter, the scoping of the prevention theme in this book may be considered from two different perspectives. First, from a traditional vantage point, *primary prevention with respect to the cancer* focuses on groups of individuals who have not yet developed a frank cancer and omits the classic secondary prevention measures, including screening, early detection, and treatment of premalignancy or occult malignancy.

Changing the perspective from the cancer to the underlying infection actually requires a further shift in thinking and action based on asking whether or not an infection has already taken hold and been detected. In these terms, it is perhaps appropriate to think of two overarching categories of intervention. The first refers to preventive measures that are applied before an infection takes hold, and the second to interventions appropriate after an infection has been detected. These two categories were further divided, ultimately generating six types of prevention (Figure 13.1).

There are various ways in which this grid proved useful to the authors of this book:

1. Reinforcing the biological connection underlying preventive interventions and infection-related carcinogenesis
2. Allowing for comparisons of the established and emerging prevention efforts across different infectious agents
3. Motivating planners to consider prevention options both before and after infection and thereby guiding a comprehensive approach to preventing associated cancer

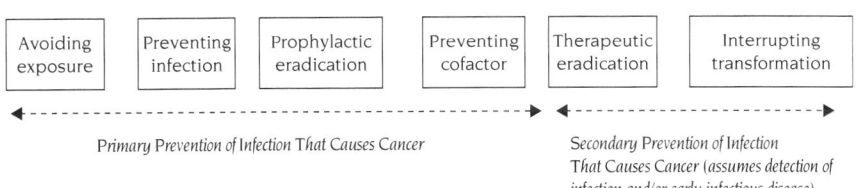

Figure 13.1. Prevention options in infection-related carcinogenesis.

It might be perceived that the category "Preventing Cofactor" does not directly address the infectious agent. However, dealing with cofactor(s) does qualify as a set of interventions that can occur before (and after) an infection becomes established. Furthermore, as seen in a number of instances, a cofactor of interest may itself be an infectious agent (e.g., HIV in HHV-8-caused Kaposi sarcoma; malaria protozoa in EBV-caused Burkitt lymphoma).

In summary, the second aim of this project was to provide an up-to-date, accessible presentation of the biology and prevention options related to infectious agents, with this information being categorized according to the typology in Figure 13.1.

Table 13.3 summarizes the key prevention options for each of the agents detailed in this book. The interventions include both established and emerging/investigational options, and were mostly selected according to applicability in the developed world.

The information in Table 13.3, combined with the full commentary in each chapter, suggests that the majority of the interventions are still at an investigational stage, or of unproven efficacy. Only a few approaches are well-established, and thus bear the promise of substantial benefit in reducing incidence and mortality of cancer. These include vaccination to prevent HBV, use of immunoglobulin for the same agent, and vaccination for HPV. This relatively weak preventive repertoire might be more alarming were it not for the fact that the infectious agents with the highest cancer burden are the ones being targeted. However, this comforting perspective certainly does not obviate the need for more research effort directed toward expanding the prevention armamentarium.

FUTURE FOCUS

The third objective of this book was to suggest directions for future research, practice, and policy. These suggested directions were aimed primarily at the sponsors of the project that led to this book, namely, the National Infectious Agents Committee (NIAC), part of the Primary Prevention Action Group of the Canadian Partnership Against Cancer, and the National Cancer Institute of Canada (NCIC), part of the Canadian Cancer Society. However, many of the activities of these agencies are representative of the efforts of any number of countries seeking to develop a program that will prevent infections that cause cancer.

Table 13.3. Preventing Infection and Related Cancer in the Developed World Established and Investigational Interventions

Infectious Agent	Prevention Category					
	1. Avoiding Exposure	2. Preventing Infection	3. Prophylactic Eradication	4. Preventing Cofactor	5. Therapeutic Eradication	6. Interrupting Transformation
Human papillomavirus	Sexual health behaviors	Vaccine		Sexual health behaviors	Vaccine	Interferon; intrabodies
Hepatitis B virus		Vaccine	Immunoglobulin for infants born to infected women	Alcohol intake and obesity as synergistic factors		
Hepatitis C virus	Injection drug safety behaviors; sexual health behaviors			Alcohol intake and obesity as synergistic factors	Interventions in category 6 can clear some cases of HCV	Interferon; nucleoside and nucleotide analogues
Helicobacter pylori	Sanitation; hygiene		Note: policy debated	Limit salt intake; not smoking	Antibiotics	Chemoprevention

(Continued)

Table 13.3. (Continued)

Infectious Agent	Prevention Category					
	1. Avoiding Exposure	2. Preventing Infection	3. Prophylactic Eradication	4. Preventing Cofactor	5. Therapeutic Eradication	6. Interrupting Transformation
Epstein-Barr virus	Socioeconomic improvement	Vaccine	Infusion of cytotoxic T lymphocytes	Limit salted fish intake; control coinfections; safer pretransplant agents	Antilatency medications	Antitranscription medications
Human herpesvirus type 8	Sexual health behaviors			**Highly active antiretroviral therapy among the HIV-positive**		Antiviral medications
Human lymphotropic virus type 1	**Infected mothers not breastfeeding; screening blood donations**	Vaccine	Immunoglobulin	Control of *S. stercoralis* infection	Vaccine; stem cell transplants	Therapies counteracting the Tax protein mechanisms in HTLV-1 infection

Established intervention | Investigational intervention

At least four areas of potential interest have emerged that could help shape just such a national program. In this final major section of the book, future directions will be discussed in the following areas:

1. Basic investigation of cancer
2. Translational research
3. Prevention research and policy development
4. New partnerships and knowledge dissemination

Basic Investigation of Cancer

Some of the most exciting developments in the prevention of infection-related cancers, including initiatives involving vaccines, have been informed by scientific investigations of the natural history of infection and the mechanisms of disease. While not becoming overly weighted with information about molecular biology, the various chapters of this book have underlined the prevention implications of understanding fundamental aspects of infectious agents and host cells.

Apart from illuminating potential prevention targets, the tumor-causing mechanisms of infections provide invaluable collateral knowledge about cancer in general. Viruses especially may be regarded as toolkits to aid in the understanding of cancer; this is equally true of RNA- and DNA-based viruses.[10] Undoubtedly, future progress in prevention will require ongoing commitment to basic scientific research into the disease mechanisms of oncogenic infections.

Retroviruses. Retroviruses have generated important insights about cancer. Investigations of human T-cell lymphotropic virus type 1 (HTLV-1) has been particularly useful in helping researchers understand human carcinogenesis, even though it is responsible for only a very small percentage of the global cancer burden.

As described in Chapter 12, retroviruses reverse transcribe their RNA into DNA for integration into the host's genome. Studies of RNA tumor viruses in animals led to the seminal concept of the oncogene (plus its product, the oncoprotein).[11] Oncogenes are mutated forms of normal genes (called proto-oncogenes) that control healthy cell functions.

A fascinating specialty research area related to retroviruses is the endogenous retrovirus. Endogenous retroviruses are essentially formed from ancient foreign DNA that has been integrated permanently into the genetic code of human beings.[12] Most retroviruses, including HIV, infect regular body cells (known as somatic cells), but some can also infect the germline cells, ensuring that the viral genetic material becomes transmitted to the next generation. When this occurs, the genetic segment introduced into the organism is termed an endogenous retrovirus. The possible oncogenic role of endogenous retroviruses is being investigated through animal studies.[13,14]

DNA viruses. The DNA viruses, such as HPV and EBV, have been very fruitful as a source of information about carcinogenesis.[15,16] For example, researchers have focused on the ability of DNA viruses to control telomere length in the host genome,[17] as well as on viral involvement in the ubiquitin system in the cells of AIDS-related cancer.[18] Perhaps the most important contribution to cancer research from the study of DNA viruses has been identifying the role of the famous tumor suppressor proteins p53 and Rb.[19]

Comparing viruses, distinguishing cancer mechanisms. There are well-understood indirect ways for infectious agents to influence cancer development, such as inducing immunosuppression or immune/inflammatory responses in the host.[20–23] The criteria to distinguish direct and indirect carcinogenesis are themselves debatable. Some authorities restrict infectious direct carcinogens to those that are "functionally linked in maintaining a transformed phenotype."[24] In this book, the definition has been more expansive, encompassing any infectious agent that directly influences the components or functions of a host cell so that cancer is eventually initiated in that cell and/or the opportunity for malignant transformation is increased. This allows agents to be included that are no longer detectable in neoplastic tissue, but created conditions for transformation at some previous point in host cells.

The distinction between direct and indirect etiology can create controversy about how to classify the oncogenic role of agents, such as HIV and *H. pylori*, that mainly seem to operate by indirect pathways.[25,26] In terms of prevention potential, it may be important to distinguish infectious direct carcinogens from infections that act as cofactors or promoters alongside other factors that are the true cancer initiators. For example, the xenotropic murine leukemia related virus may play a role in the development of prostate cancer, but only via its effect on inflammatory pathways.[27] As direct etiologic agents have been the main focus of the present book, this virus would not qualify for inclusion.

In contrast, it is clear based on the chosen definition of this book that viruses can function in two basic ways to directly cause malignancy:

1. Introducing mutations into the host genome, which in turn affect cellular processes
2. Interfering with cellular processes through viral gene products

Understanding both types of influence sheds light on the fundamental aberrant processes that lead to cancer. The mechanisms are especially being investigated in the context of oncogenes (and their related product) that have a pleiotropic effect on cellular processes; for example, the Tax protein of HTLV-1 and the LANA protein of HHV-8 each bind with about 100 proteins in the host cell. Interestingly, there is evidence that different viruses interact with the *same* cellular proteins to bring about cancer and other diseases.[28] This has been shown, for instance, with Tax and an investigational oncogene in adenoviruses. Such discoveries may multiply insights about how cancer processes occur in cells.

Genetic instability. The first category of carcinogenic impact on host cells, that is, induction of genetic changes, has been an intense focus of recent research. HTLV-1 in particular has provided a window on the fundamental mechanisms of chromosomal instability.[29] Again, some intriguing overlaps between viruses have emerged. For example, recognizing the similar functions of Tax in HTLV-1 and the E7 oncogene in HPV has offered insights about the early steps in carcinogenesis related to genetic instability.[30]

Disrupted cellular processes. Insight has been provided by Hanahan and Weinberg on the second category of cancer induction, that is, directly influencing cellular processes. They described six hallmarks of cancer that arise as a result of genetic aberrations.[31] Importantly, half of the cancer-inducing mechanisms actually match well-known viral manipulations of cellular processes[32]; these include the following:

1. Promoting cellular proliferation in the absence of environmental growth cues
2. Inhibiting cellular responses to antigrowth signals
3. Providing resistance to apoptosis or programmed cell death

Recognition of the functional parallels between viral infection and steps in carcinogenesis explains why interaction of viruses with host cells can offer a window on carcinogenesis in general. It also suggests that some tumor viruses can act as a type of substitute for one or more of the events that result in complete cellular transformation.[33,34]

Research agenda. Having overviewed advances in the basic understanding of cancer derived from investigation of oncogenic infections, it is natural to ask what the future research trends might be in developed countries. Several possibilities are outlined below.

- An area of great interest and potential importance involves the association between so-called polymicrobial infections and cancer.

Several examples of this phenomenon have been described in the book, and many more may emerge as microbial detection methods improve. A motivator of this type of research is the simple fact that multiple infections are routinely found in individuals in both the developed and developing world. While this scenario is especially common when the infections share a transmission route (e.g., sexual activity), interest is also high when more than one route is involved. Multiple pathways of coinfections may both complicate and expand the opportunities to reduce cancer through exposure control.

- Demonstrating proof of interactions between coinfections in the development of cancer is an important area of investigation for epidemiologists and molecular biologists alike. While intriguing results have begun to emerge concerning what one researcher referred to as the "dangerous liaison"[35] between coinfections in the development of cancer, research in this area has only just begun.
- The carcinogenic mechanisms related to coinfection with HIV are not fully elucidated. The preponderance of evidence reinforces the traditional status of the virus as an indirect factor in carcinogenesis, through its immunosuppressive effects. However, the emerging understanding of a more direct mechanism of HIV on cancer promotion is worthy of further investigation. The interaction of the characteristic Tat protein of HIV with the oncoproteins of other viruses has been a special focus.[36,37] If a direct role of HIV in carcinogenesis were to be confirmed and more fully described in the future, it would be a very significant development given the global impact of the AIDS epidemic.
- Some subtopics related to coinfections have resonance across the world, for example, the potential molecular interaction of HPV and HHV-8 in oral cancers.[38] Other examples have dominant applications in the developing world, but still cry out for developed world investment as an expression of compassion and social justice. The latter includes the potential "triple threat" of EBV, malaria, and arboviruses in the genesis of Burkitt lymphoma.
- Pursuing new insights about the transmission of infectious agents known to cause cancer remains a high priority in light of the critical importance for exposure prevention. There are several infectious agents where important knowledge gaps remain concerning transmission.
- The emergence of agent-based definitions of hematologic cancer highlights the possibility that more and more agents may be deemed *necessary* causes of cancer. Examples include HTLV-1

and adult T-cell leukemia, and HHV-8 and a certain variation of primary effusion lymphoma. The importance of the designation "necessary cause" is that it concentrates prevention initiatives for a cancer on the pertinent infection. By preventing all cases of the oncogenic infection, it is theoretically possible to avoid all incident cases of the related cancer. Continuing to refine the very definition of cancers based on necessary infectious causes is a research area with exciting preventive potential.
- Finally, the substantial inventory of investigational agents summarized in the "Introduction" to the book generates its own research agenda. The list has been reproduced in Table 13.6 at the end of this chapter, with added details concerning the proposed cancer associations and selected scientific sources. Of course, the weight of evidence surrounding these agents is not equal—some are much more well established as cancer agents (e.g., the polyomaviruses, cytomegalovirus[39,40]), whereas others have only been examined in the most cursory way for their oncogenicity. It is highly likely that, as detection methods and research budgets allow, the candidate list of direct agents will grow. The implications of confirming more infectious agents are not trivial. In 1999, pioneer researcher H. zur Hausen predicted that the proportion of cancers attributable to microbes would *double* from the then understood level of 15%, particularly "if other cancers currently associated with specific virus infections are proved to be caused by such agents."[41]

Translational Research

The basic scientific information about cancer and infections must be translated into real-world applications. Such applications need to be adapted to different settings, in particular recognizing the difference between developed and developing countries. As indicated in Table 13.2, over a quarter of the cancer burden in the developing world may be attributed to an infectious cause. The cancer burden attached to each of the agents examined in this book is 2–10 times higher there than in a developed country such as Canada. This is one of the proposed explanations of the fact that the cancer burden is rising in the developing world, and at a faster rate than seen in developed settings.[42,43] If there are delays in implementing effective measures (such as vaccination) against infection-related cancers in the developing world, it is likely that current health disparities will increase.[44]

There is a clear "big three" among infectious agents that potentially represent the highest public health concern in terms of cancer prevention: HPV, hepatitis viruses, and *H. pylori*. Interestingly, this is true whether the focus is on developed or developing countries, suggesting the potential for global benefit even if the resources of developed countries are directed mostly toward their domestic cancer priorities. What is learned in the United States and Canada and Europe about prevention modalities may be translatable to Africa and less developed areas of Asia.

Even while developed countries strive to make a difference on the global stage, there are certainly translational issues to be pursued on the home front as well. This agenda is not limited to looking at infections with substantial prevalence in the national population and/or those that lead to a substantial burden of cancer. First, it must be recognized that the concept of burden is not always straightforward. For example, while HPV infection is prevalent in Canada, cervical cancer incidence and mortality are not. On the other hand, even when cancer mortality is small relative to other malignancies, heavy investment in secondary prevention is often the real concern in terms of health economics. This situation certainly pertains to cervical cancer, partly explaining the intensive effort to understand the role of HPV in carcinogenesis and to possibly improve primary prevention.

A further consideration is the reality of immigration. For example, Canada is characterized by one of the highest immigration rates in the world. Inevitably, this means that people may arrive from regions where a cancer-causing infection is endemic, for example HPV infection and cervical cancer.[45,46]

Furthermore, specific viruses may manifest themselves in diverse ways among different ethnic groups. For example, while HPV-16 clearly is the dominant viral type in terms of cancer causation in all parts of the world, the prevalence of other HPV variants may be quite different from region to region. For instance, while HPV-18 remains a very important etiologic agent in most settings, some Chinese groups present with rival prevention candidates (e.g., HPV-52 and -58). Such phenomena raise questions about the real-world effectiveness of a vaccine targeting HPV-16 and 18 both among multicultural communities in Canada, the United States, and Europe, and in developing countries. Additional unique characteristics of ethnic populations also may require a targeted response. For instance, an unusual spike in HPV prevalence after middle-age among Mexican women has been of interest to U.S. authorities; this may be one explanation for the elevated cervical cancer incidence in the United States–Mexico border region.[47]

Immigrants to the United States and Canada also tend to fit, at least temporarily, under the umbrella of a "vulnerable population" due to lower access to health care services. Such groups need to be monitored to assure that they are not being underserved on primary and/or secondary prevention fronts. Also, special attention should be paid to the prevention needs implied by any unique epidemiological patterns. Examples of other vulnerable populations relevant to the United States and Canadian contexts include Kaposi sarcoma (caused by HHV-8) among persons with AIDS, and the recent outbreaks of HTLV-1 among Inuit groups. Research based on ongoing surveillance of infection and cancer rates may be important.

The fact that there has been such a high success rate among developed countries in reducing incidence and mortality from cervical cancer means that new programs possibly should be targeted at vulnerable or at-risk groups in order to generate the best public health returns. Research on both targets and interventions should be on an ongoing priority. Learning may be successfully transferred between agents. For example, the history of efforts to target HIV prevention interventions may contain lessons for HPV control.

Many translational research questions may arise in the context of HPV prevention in coming years. Several issues were identified in Chapter 7 directly related to the implementation of new HPV vaccines. A dominant question involves the real-world effectiveness of any vaccine, as opposed to the efficacy results from experimental trials; but many other direct and tangential questions would benefit from a translational research focus. For example, how can current cervical screening programs both be enhanced and modified in a postvaccination era marked by increasingly sophisticated molecular detection technologies? Given that current HPV vaccines target about 70% of cancer-causing HPV infections, screening programs will need to be maintained in the long run to prevent the other 30% of cervical cancers. This is in addition to the screening needs among older women who will not be vaccinated or who are already infected by one of the HPV types covered in the vaccine.

Some public health care providers have expressed concerns about the practical gaps and opportunity costs when the prevention emphasis for an agent such as HPV is shifted from current public health maneuvers to elementary school immunizations. For instance, will individuals be as available for the booster dose that may be required in their early 20s, a period that also happens to coincide with increased mobility and increased sexual activity and therefore higher exposure to HPV? Will the groups of younger and middle-aged women who are now at risk for missing Pap smears and various follow-up interventions also neglect to take full advantage of a vaccine program?

Perhaps most importantly, if Pap smear testing declines because it seems less necessary in a postvaccine era, what will be the ultimate effect on cervical cancer rates? And what will be the collateral impact of reduced counseling and testing for other sexually transmitted infections (STIs) that sometimes occur at routine Pap appointments? The latter question becomes more urgent given the role of STIs as cofactors with HPV in the development of precursor lesions and malignancies. These questions and others could drive various monitoring and evaluation projects.

The following list outlines additional research issues with practical implications, again mostly in the context of HPV infection:

- While cervical, anogenital, and head and neck cancers certainly remain areas of strong interest in terms of avoidable morbidity and mortality, any evidence of a possible role of HPV (or other infectious agent) in the more prevalent cancers (lung, female breast, etc.) would change the prevention agenda dramatically.
- More needs to be understood about the impact of vertical transmission and the possibility of cancer being caused by latent infections first contracted in infancy or perhaps in a family setting. Such data may influence projections concerning, for example, HPV vaccine effectiveness (since efficacy data are only applicable in females naive to the HPV types covered by the vaccine).
- In the case of nonsystemic infections such as HPV, what tissues need to be tested for the presence of current or past infections? For instance, does more attention need to be paid to the role of HPV in preventing cancers of the skin?
- Which cofactors (genetic, behavioral, or environmental) play key roles in the progress from established infection in the target tissue to malignant transformation? Understanding such risk profiles allows cofactor control to occupy its proper place among prevention priorities. This is especially important when considering whether, for instance, novel (and usually expensive) genetic screening is cost-effective in identification of high-risk groups.

Prevention Research and Policy Development

One of the most important emphases in translational research is the development of specific prevention measures, followed by robust evaluation. An exciting aspect of understanding the importance of infectious causes of cancer is that infection control is already a well-accepted and well-studied priority in public health. Engaging the traditions and resources of public health in the potential for cancer reduction is an encouraging prospect. Moreover, a prevention focus on infectious agents may even enjoy an advantage over traditional cancer risk factor control, as suggested in a recent comment by Tokudome and colleagues[48]:

> Because of the possibility of applying prophylactic vaccination and immunoglobulin therapy or prescribing antibiotics, infection-related malignancies would appear to be more controllable than tobacco-associated malignant tumors and much more readily preventable than aging- and lifestyle-related cancers.

Indeed, it is debatable whether enough attention is currently being paid by health care planners to the infection–cancer connection. The primary prevention measures for some infections covered in this book seem to only be at an early stage of consideration and implementation. This is an area of policy development that could occupy the attention of national cancer organizations for years to come. The typology of prevention categories devised for this book may be helpful in focusing energy on prevention opportunities that are not being explored or exploited.

There are three broad strategic areas to consider in devising new prevention measures and integrating them into an overall cancer control policy.

The infection-related cancer burden must be refined. It is important to develop a clear understanding of the proportion of cancers attributable to an infectious cause, and how this attributable risk compares to other causal factors. An aspect of this research involves understanding the prevalence of oncogenic infections in particular geographical areas; pursuing such a project, as illustrated in the Caribbean context (Table 13.4), could help to guide prevention priorities.[49]

The next step in an accounting of disease burden and priority targets for prevention involves combining the relative risk of cancer for each infectious agent with its established prevalence in a population. This allows for the calculation of what is known as the attributable risk for a cancer type

Table 13.4. Cancer-Associated Viral Infections, Caribbean Region

Virus	Prevalence (%)
EBV	92.2
HPV	57.5
HBV	9.4
HHV-8	4.5
HTLV-1	1.0
HCV	0.4

Source: Ragin et al., *Cancer Investigation*, 2008. Used by permission.

with respect to a cause, such as an infectious agent. Table 13.5 provides an example of this exercise, recently carried out for the Netherlands.[50]

Interestingly, the percentage of the total cancer incidence attributable to the listed infections is less than half of the figure estimated for developed countries as a whole (Table 13.2). Among other benefits, the information in Table 13.5 demonstrates that the infection-focused structure of this book can be usefully reoriented to highlight the cancers involved, which in turn reflects the ultimate target of any cancer prevention project.

The prevention priorities must be refined. The theoretical efficacy of a prevention measure must ultimately be tested against real-world effectiveness, which takes into consideration feasibility, uptake rates, etc. Timing is also a critical factor. There are currently infected populations that urgently need effective preventive interventions; exposure avoidance and other approaches at the early end of the prevention spectrum understandably are of little interest to people already infected with an agent. On the other hand, the interests of future generations will always

Table 13.5. Cancer Cases Attributable to Infection, by Cancer Type, The Netherlands, 2003

Cancer Type	Infectious Agent	Attributable Risk (%)	Cases Caused by Agent	Total Cancer Incidence (%)
Liver	HBV	23	72	0.10
	HCV	20	61	0.08
Cervix	HPV	100	584	0.80
Stomach: Noncardia	H. pylori	74	1070	1.46
Kaposi sarcoma	HHV-8	100	38	0.05
Non-Hodgkin's lymphoma				
MALT lymphoma (stomach)	H. pylori	74	90	0.12
Burkitt lymphoma	EBV	25	7	0.01
Adult T-cell leukemia	HTLV-1	n/a	9	0.01
Anogenital				
Penis	HPV	40	40	0.05
Vulva/vagina	HPV	40	121	0.17
Anus	HPV	90	113	0.15
Nasopharynx	EBV	90	67	0.09
Mouth	HPV	3	25	0.03
Oropharynx	HPV	12	39	0.05
Hodgkin's lymphoma	EBV	20–70	159	0.22
All cancer			2495	3.39

Source: van Lier et al., *Cancer Letters*, 2008. Used by permission.

Conclusion—Infection and Cancer

elevate the importance of primary prevention efforts; changing the risk profile in an endemic region requires robust exposure prevention and/or vaccination programs.

The fundamental question for some agents is: are there any current, nonvaccine strategies that are effective in reducing the incidence (and, eventually, prevalence) of infection in a population? A follow-up question would be: what are the best emerging prevention options to see further gains in terms of overall cancer burden? In other words, what will be the best high-leverage strategies in the future, selected from the following list[51-58]:

1. New approaches to exposure prevention that overcome the usual resistance to sociobehavioral interventions
2. Second generation vaccines, as well as new vaccines for agents not yet covered
3. Reduction of cofactors (such as salted food intake, smoking, HIV infection, etc.)
4. Innovative antimicrobial treatments (such as radioimmunotherapy) that promise to retard, reverse, and even prevent cancers altogether

The economic analysis must be refined. Once real-world effectiveness of a prevention intervention is known, it is also important to understand the cost-effectiveness of the intervention. This is especially important when different prevention methods, with varying levels of effectiveness, are available. Cost-effectiveness is one tool that can assist planners in making decisions about the best way to configure a prevention program. One of the interesting parallels between many of the infectious agents covered in this book is their involvement in both a distinctive cancer and substantial benign disease. Thus, an essential component of any economic analysis is the collateral benefit in the control of nonmalignant disease when oncogenic infection is reduced. In short, there is interest in understanding the role of chronic infections well beyond cancer.[59]

New Partnerships and Knowledge Dissemination

A new approach to cancer control calls for new partnerships. Section "Prevention Research and Policy Development" already implied that cancer prevention specialists need to work closely with vaccine scientists. The importance of collaboration between leaders from developed and developing regions has also been suggested.

National organizations working toward cancer control such as the Canadian Partnership Against Cancer, the U.S. National Institutes of Health, and others have a valuable role to play in bringing together researchers and planners from disparate fields. Infection-related cancer calls for partnership among leaders in oncology, epidemiology, health economics, public health, cancer advocacy, communicable diseases, and vaccine development. Contributions are required from laboratories, academics, government, clinicians, health planners, cancer education groups, the media, and industry. Dialogue and cooperation among new colleagues will enhance understanding and response in the area of infections and cancer.

There is also much work to be done in educating the general public about the important arena of infection and cancer. The challenge that remains was brought home in a news article at the end of April 2008. The remarkable fact is that the following sentence was written by a reporter specializing in health care who had recently written a major series on HPV and vaccination: "The problem with cancer is that unlike many diseases, it has no alien source—no infection or bacteria towards which treatment can be directed."[60] If a well-read member of the media is not informed about the evidence concerning infectious agents and cancer, it only reinforces the need to disseminate knowledge much more widely.

Finally, the United States and Canada, along with other wealthy countries, should be concerned with supporting progress on the cancer front in less-developed regions. Developed countries have a role to play in exploring the costs and cultural appropriateness of options for prevention in low-resource settings. The challenge is to conduct both basic science and prevention research to enable improvements in cancer incidence in developing nations.

There is every sign that the topic and target of infectious agents of cancer is only going to expand in importance. A 2007 review of the established oncogenic infections offered the following assessment[61]:

> Many other viral agents have been classified as possibly carcinogenic to humans and others have been occasionally found in human tumors suggesting...an underestimation of virus involvement in the etiology of human cancer. Prevention and control of infection by these agents could dramatically reduce the incidence of some prevalent cancers and, consequently, have a great impact on public health.

The hope is that the current book will spur on knowledge translation, inform the planning of prevention efforts, and motivate further research that would continue to advance a paradigm shift in the global response to infectious causes of cancer.

Table 13.6. Investigational Infectious Agents in Human Cancer

Infectious Agent	Cancer	Reference: Lead Author (Year)
Viruses		
Herpesviridae/ Simplexvirus		
Human herpesvirus 1	Nonmelanoma skin cancer	Leite (2005)
	Primary cutaneous plasmacytoma	Zendri (2005)
	Oral squamous cell carcinoma	Yang (2004)
Human herpesvirus 2	Cervical cancer	McDougall (1984)
Herpesviridae/Cytomegalovirus		
Human cytomegalovirus	Glioblastoma multiforme (glioma)	Mitchell (2008)
	Nonmelanoma skin cancer	Zafiropoulos (2003)
	Adenocarcinomas of the prostate and colon	Doniger (1999)
	Cervical carcinomas	Doniger (1999)
Herpesviridae/ Roseolovirus		
Human herpesvirus 6	Angioimmunoblastic T-cell lymphoma	Zhou (2007)
	Nonmelanoma skin cancer	Leite (2005)
	Lymphomas (Hodgkin's disease, Burkitt's lymphoma)	Daibata (2000)
	Lymphoid malignancies	Doniger (1999)
Adenoviridae/ Mastadenovirus		
Adenovirus	Brain tumors (glioblastomas, oligodendrogliomas, ependymomas)	Kosulin (2007)
	Small-cell lung cancer	Kuwano (1997)
	Pediatric acute lymphoblastic leukaemia	Gustafsson (2007)
Human adenovirus 5	Ewing's sarcoma	West (2000)
Polyomaviridae/ Polyomavirus		
BK polyomavirus	Prostate cancer	Balis (2007)
	Adrenal cancer	Barzon (2007)
	Renal cell carcinomas	Narayanan (2007)
	Colorectal cancer	Casini (2005)
	Glial tumors, meningiomas	Delbue (2005)

(Continued)

Table 13.6. *(Continued)*

Infectious Agent	Cancer	Reference: Lead Author (Year)
	Cervical carcinoma	Martini (2004)
	Genital tumors	Martini (2004)
	Kaposi's sarcoma	Monini (1996)
	Bone cancer	De Mattei (1995)
	Urinary tract tumors	Monini (1995)
	Insulinoma (adenoma of the pancreatic islets)	Corallini (1987)
JC polyomavirus	Lung cancer	Zheng (2007)
	Colorectal cancer	Casini (2005)
	Esophageal carcinoma	Del Valle (2005)
	Glial tumors, meningiomas	Delbue (2005)
Merkel cell polyomavirus	Merkel cell carcinoma	Feng (2008)
Simian virus 40	Breast carcinomas	Hachana (2009)
	Diffuse large B-cell lymphomas	Amara (2007)
	Adrenal cancer	Barzon (2007)
	Mesothelioma	Comar (2007)
	Lung cancer (bronchopulmonary carcinomas)	Giuliani (2007)
	Brain cancer	Vilchez (2003)
	Bone cancer (osteosarcoma)	Vilchez (2003)
	Non-Hodgkin's lymphoma	Vilchez (2002)
Parvoviridae/ Erythrovirus		
B19 virus	Papillary thyroid carcinoma	Wang (2008)
	Lymphoblastic and myeloblastic leukemia	Kerr (2003)
Retroviridae/ Betaretrovirus		
Human mammary tumour virus	Breast cancer	Melana (2007)
Melanoma-associated retrovirus	Melanoma	Hengge (2008)
Mouse mammary tumor virus	Breast cancer	Lawson (2006)
	Lymphomas	Cotterchio (2002)
Retroviridae/ Deltaretrovirus		
Human T-cell lymphotropic virus 2	Variant hairy cell leukemia	Feuer (2005)
Arenaviridae/Deltavirus		
Hepatitis delta virus	Hepatocellular carcinoma	Kurbanov (2007)

Paramyxoviridae/
  Morbillivirus
   Measles virus   Hodgkin's disease   Benharroch (2004)
Circoviridae/Anellovirus
   Torque teno virus   Hepatocellular carcinoma   Tokita (2002)
                                  Lung cancer   Bando (2008)

Bacteria
Spriochaetaceae
   Borrelia burgdorferi   Primary cutaneous B-cell   Bogle (2005)
                                lymphoma (MALT
                                lymphoma)

Campylobacteraceae
   Campylobacter jejuni   Immunoproliferative small Lecuit (2004)
                                intestine disease (MALT
                                lymphoma)

Helicobacteraceae
   Helicobacter bilis   Gallbladder cancer   Matsukura (2002)
                                Biliary tract cancer   Murata (2004)
   Helicobacter   Gastric MALT lymphoma   Joo (2007)
    heimannii
   Helicobacter hepaticus   Gallbladder cancer   Pradhan (2004)
   Helicobacter spp.   Primary liver carcinoma   Nilsson (2000)
Enterobacteriaceae
   Eschericihia coli   Colon cancer   Travaglione (2008)
   Salmonella typhi   Gallbladder cancer   Lazcano-Ponce
                                                                 (2001)

Desulfovibrionaceae
   Lawsonia   Colorectal cancer   Lax (2002)
    intracellularis
Bartonellacaea
   Bartonella spp.   Vascular tumors   Dehio (2005)
Chlamydiaceae
   Chlamydia   Cholesteatoma   Ronchetti (2003)
    pneumoniae   Lung cancer   Littman (2004)
   Chlamydia psittaci   Ocular adnexal lymphoma Ferreri (2004)
                                (MALT lymphoma)
   Chlamydia   Cervical squamous cell   Madeleine (2007)
    trachomatis   carcinomas
Mycoplasmataceae
   Mycoplasma spp.   Gastric cancer   Kwon (2004)
Mycobacteriaceae
   Mycobacterium   Lung cancer   Ardies (2003)
    tuberculosis
Streptococcaceae
   Streptococcus infan-   Colon cancer   Biarc (2004)
    tarius (or bovis)

(Continued)

Table 13.6. (Continued)

Infectious Agent	Cancer	Reference: Lead Author (Year)
Fungi		
Arthrodermatoceae		
Epidermophyton floccosum	Reticulum cell sarcoma	Levene (1973)
Microsporum canis	Lung cancer	Nakachi (1999)
Herpotrichiellaceae		
Fonsecaea pedrosoi	Acral lentiginous melanoma	dos Santos Gon (2006)
Protozoa		
Plasmodiidae		
Plasmodium spp. (Malaria)	Burkitt lymphoma	Eze (1990)
Trichomonadida		
Trichomonas vaginalis	Cervical cancer	Khurana (2005)
Cryptosporidiidae		
Cryptosporidium parvum	Colic adenocarcinoma	Certad (2007)
Sarcocystidae		
Toxoplasma gondii	Pituitary adenoma	Zhang (2002)
	Primary ocular tumors, meningioma, leukemia and lymphoma	Khurana (2005)
Worms and Flukes		
Opisthorchiidae		
Clonorchis sinensis	Cholangiocarcinoma	Choi (2004)
Opisthorchis felineus	Cholangiocarcinoma	Sripa (2007)
Opisthorchis viverrini	Cholangiocarcinoma	Sripa (2007)
	Liver cancer	Khurana (2005)
Schistosomatidae		
Schistosoma haematobium	Bladder cancer	Sripa (2007)
Schistosoma japonicum	Colorectal cancer	Yosry (2006)
	Hepatocellular carcinomas	Yosry (2006)
Schistosoma mansoni	Hepatocellular carcinomas	Khurana (2005)
Schistosoma spp.	Fallopian tube carcinoma	Beadles (2007)
Strongyloididae		
Strongyloides stercoralis	Adult T-cell leukemia	Carvalho (2004)
	Cholangiocarcinoma	Hirata (2007)
Taeniidae		
Taenia solium	Cerebral glioma	Del Brutto (1997)

BIBLIOGRAPHY FOR TABLE 13.6

Amara K, Trimeche M, Ziadi S et al. Presence of simian virus 40 DNA sequences in diffuse large B-cell lymphomas in Tunisia correlates with aberrant promoter hypermethylation of multiple tumor suppressor genes. *International Journal of Cancer.* 2007; 121(12): 2693–702.

Ardies CM. Inflammation as cause for scar cancers of the lung. *Integrative Cancer Therapies.* 2003; 2(3): 238–46.

Balis V, Sourvinos G, Soulitzis N et al. Prevalence of BK virus and human papillomavirus in human prostate cancer. *International Journal of Biological Markers.* 2007; 22(4): 245–51.

Bando M, Takahashi M, Ohno S et al. Torque teno virus DNA titre elevated in idiopathic pulmonary fibrosis with primary lung cancer. *Respirology.* 2008; 13(2): 263–9.

Barzon L, Trevisan M, Masi G et al. Detection of polyomaviruses and herpesviruses in human adrenal tumors. *Oncogene.* 2008; 27(6): 857–64.

Beadles W, Wilks D, Monaghan H. Fallopian tube carcinoma associated with schistosomiasis. *Journal of Infection.* 2007; 55(5): e121–3.

Benharroch D, Shemer-Avni Y, Myint YY et al. Measles virus: evidence of an association with Hodgkin's disease. *British Journal of Cancer.* 2004; 91(3): 572–9.

Biarc J, Nguyen IS, Pini A et al. Carcinogenic properties of proteins with pro-inflammatory activity from Streptococcus infantarius (formerly S.bovis). *Carcinogenesis.* 2004; 25(8): 1477–84.

Bogle MA, Riddle CC, Triana EM et al. Primary cutaneous B-cell lymphoma. *Journal of the American Academy of Dermatology.* 2005; 53(3): 479–84.

Carvalho EM, Da Fonseca Porto A. Epidemiological and clinical interaction between HTLV-1 and Strongyloides stercoralis. *Parasite Immunology.* 2004; 26(11–12): 487–97.

Casini B, Borgese L, Del Nonno F et al. Presence and incidence of DNA sequences of human polyomaviruses BKV and JCV in colorectal tumor tissues. *Anticancer Research.* 2005; 25(2A): 1079–85.

Certad G, Ngouanesavanh T, Guyot K et al. Cryptosporidium parvum, a potential cause of colic adenocarcinoma. *Infectious Agents and Cancer.* 2007; 2: 22.

Choi BI, Han JK, Hong ST et al. Clonorchiasis and cholangiocarcinoma: etiologic relationship and imaging diagnosis. *Clinical Microbiology Reviews.* 2004; 17(3): 540–52.

Comar M, Rizzardi C, de Zotti R et al. SV40 multiple tissue infection and asbestos exposure in a hyperendemic area for malignant mesothelioma. *Cancer Research.* 2007; 67(18): 8456–9.

Corallini A, Pagnani M, Viadana P et al. Association of BK virus with human brain tumors and tumors of pancreatic islets. *International Journal of Cancer.* 1987; 39(1): 60–7.

Cotterchio M, Nadalin V, Sauer M. Human breast cancer and lymphomas may share a common aetiology involving Mouse Mammary Tumour Virus (MMTV). *Medical Hypotheses.* 2002; 59(4): 492–4.

Daibata M. Human herpesvirus 6(HHV-6) and HHV-8 in malignant lymphoma. *Nippon Rinsho.* 2000; 58(3): 560–6.

De Mattei M, Martini F, Corallini A et al. High incidence of BK virus large-T-antigen-coding sequences in normal human tissues and tumors of different histotypes. *International Journal of Cancer*. 1995; 61(6): 756–60.

Dehio C. Bartonella-host-cell interactions and vascular tumour formation. *Nature Reviews Microbiology*. 2005; 3(8): 621–31.

Del Brutto OH, Castillo PR, Mena IX et al. Neurocysticercosis among patients with cerebral gliomas. *Archives of Neurology*. 1997; 54(9): 1125–8.

Del Valle L, White MK, Enam S et al. Detection of JC virus DNA sequences and expression of viral T antigen and agnoprotein in esophageal carcinoma. *Cancer*. 2005; 103(3): 516–27.

Delbue S, Pagani E, Guerini FR et al. Distribution, characterization and significance of polyomavirus genomic sequences in tumors of the brain and its covering. *Journal of Medical Virology*. 2005; 77(3): 447–54.

Doniger J, Muralidhar S, Rosenthal LJ. Human cytomegalovirus and human herpesvirus 6 genes that transform and transactivate. *Clinical Microbiology Reviews*. 1999; 12(3): 367–82.

dos Santos Gon A, Minelli L. Melanoma in a long-standing lesion of chromoblastomycosis. *International Journal of Dermatology*. 2006; 45(11): 1331–3.

Eze MO, Hunting DJ, Ogan AU. Reactive oxygen production against malaria—a potential cancer risk factor. *Medical Hypotheses*. 1990; 32(2): 121–3.

Feng H, Shuda M, Chang Y et al. Clonal integration of a polyomavirus in human Merkel cell carcinoma. *Science*. 2008; 319(5866): 1096–100.

Ferreri AJ, Guidoboni M, Ponzoni M et al. Evidence for an association between Chlamydia psittaci and ocular adnexal lymphomas. *Journal of the National Cancer Institute*. 2004; 96(8): 586–94.

Feuer G, Green PL. Comparative biology of human T-cell lymphotropic virus type 1 (HTLV-1) and HTLV-2. *Oncogene*. 2005; 24(39): 5996–6004.

Giuliani L, Jaxmar T, Casadio C et al. Detection of oncogenic viruses SV40, BKV, JCV, HCMV, HPV and p53 codon 72 polymorphism in lung carcinoma. *Lung Cancer* 2007; 57(3): 273–81.

Gustafsson B, Huang W, Bogdanovic G et al. Adenovirus DNA is detected at increased frequency in Guthrie cards from children who develop acute lymphoblastic leukaemia. *British Journal of Cancer*. 2007; 97(7): 992–4.

Hachana M, Trimeche M, Ziadi S et al. Evidence for a role of the Simian Virus 40 in human breast carcinomas. *Breast Cancer Research and Treatment*. 2009; 113(1): 43–58.

Hengge UR. Role of viruses in the development of squamous cell cancer and melanoma. *Advances in Experimental Medicine and Biology*. 2008; 624: 179–86.

Hirata T, Kishimoto K, Kinjo N et al. Association between Strongyloides stercoralis infection and biliary tract cancer. *Parasitology Research*. 2007; 101(5): 1345–8.

Joo M, Kwak JE, Chang SH et al. Helicobacter heilmannii-associated gastritis: clinicopathologic findings and comparison with Helicobacter pylori-associated gastritis. *Journal of Korean Medical Science*. 2007; 22(1): 63–9.

Kerr JR, Barah F, Cunniffe VS et al. Association of acute parvovirus B19 infection with new onset of acute lymphoblastic and myeloblastic leukaemia. *Journal of Clinical Pathology*. 2003; 56(11): 873–5.

Khurana S, Dubey ML, Malla N. Association of parasitic infections and cancers. *Indian Journal of Medical Microbiology*. 2005; 23(2): 74–9.

Kosulin K, Haberler C, Hainfellner JA et al. Investigation of adenovirus occurrence in pediatric tumor entities. *Journal of Virology.* 2007; 81(14): 7629–35.

Kurbanov F, Tanaka Y, Elkady A et al. Tracing hepatitis C and Delta viruses to estimate their contribution in HCC rates in Mongolia. *Journal of Viral Hepatitis.* 2007; 14(9): 667–74.

Kuwano K, Kawasaki M, Kunitake R et al. Detection of group C adenovirus DNA in small-cell lung cancer with the nested polymerase chain reaction. *Journal of Cancer Research and Clinical Oncology.* 1997; 123(7): 377–82.

Kwon HJ, Kang JO, Cho SH et al. Presence of human mycoplasma DNA in gastric tissue samples from Korean chronic gastritis patients. *Cancer Science.* 2004; 95(4): 311–5.

Lawson JS, Gunzburg WH, Whitaker NJ. Viruses and human breast cancer. *Future Microbiology.* 2006; 1: 33–51.

Lax AJ, Thomas W. How bacteria could cause cancer: one step at a time. *Trends in Microbiology.* 2002; 10(6): 293–9.

Lazcano-Ponce EC, Miquel JF, Munoz N et al. Epidemiology and molecular pathology of gallbladder cancer. *Cancer Journal for Clinicians.* 2001; 51(6): 349–64.

Lecuit M, Abachin E, Martin A et al. Immunoproliferative small intestinal disease associated with Campylobacter jejuni. *New England Journal of Medicine.* 2004; 350(3): 239–48.

Leite JL, Stolf HO, Reis NA et al. Human herpesvirus type 6 and type 1 infection increases susceptibility to nonmelanoma skin tumors. *Cancer Letters.* 2005; 224(2): 213–9.

Levene GM. Chronic fungal infection (E. floccosum), erythroderma, immune deficiency and lymphoma. *Proceedings of the Royal Society of Medicine.* 1973; 66(8): 745–6.

Littman AJ, White E, Jackson LA et al. Chlamydia pneumoniae infection and risk of lung cancer. *Cancer Epidemiology, Biomarkers and Prevention.* 2004; 13(10): 1624–30.

Madeleine MM, Anttila T, Schwartz SM et al. Risk of cervical cancer associated with Chlamydia trachomatis antibodies by histology, HPV type and HPV cofactors. *International Journal of Cancer.* 2007; 120(3): 650–5.

Martini F, Iaccheri L, Martinelli M et al. Papilloma and polyoma DNA tumor virus sequences in female genital tumors. *Cancer Investigation.* 2004; 22(5): 697–705.

Matsukura N, Yokomuro S, Yamada S et al. Association between Helicobacter bilis in bile and biliary tract malignancies: H. bilis in bile from Japanese and Thai patients with benign and malignant diseases in the biliary tract. *Japanese Journal of Cancer Research.* 2002; 93(7): 842–7.

McDougall JK, Nelson JA, Myerson D et al. HSV, CMV, and HPV in human neoplasia. *Journal of Investigative Dermatology.* 1984; 83(1 suppl): 72s–6s.

Melana SM, Nepomnaschy I, Sakalian M et al. Characterization of viral particles isolated from primary cultures of human breast cancer cells. *Cancer Research.* 2007; 67(18): 8960–5.

Mitchell DA, Xie W, Schmittling R et al. Sensitive detection of human cytomegalovirus in tumors and peripheral blood of patients diagnosed with glioblastoma. *Neuro-Oncology.* 2008; 10(1): 10–8.

Monini P, Rotola A, de Lellis L et al. Latent BK virus infection and Kaposi's sarcoma pathogenesis. *International Journal of Cancer.* 1996; 66(6): 717–22.

Monini P, Rotola A, Di Luca D et al. DNA rearrangements impairing BK virus productive infection in urinary tract tumors. *Virology.* 1995; 214(1): 273–9.

Murata H, Tsuji S, Tsujii M et al. Helicobacter bilis infection in biliary tract cancer. *Alimentary Pharmacology and Therapeutics.* 2004; 20(suppl 1): 90–4.

Nakachi K, Limtrakul P, Sonklin P et al. Risk factors for lung cancer among Northern Thai women: epidemiological, nutritional, serological, and bacteriological surveys of residents in high- and low-incidence areas. *Japanese Journal of Cancer Research.* 1999; 90(11): 1187–95.

Narayanan M, Szymanski J, Slavcheva E et al. BK virus associated renal cell carcinoma: case presentation with optimized PCR and other diagnostic tests. *American Journal of Transplantation.* 2007; 7(6): 1666–71.

Nilsson HO, Taneera J, Castedal M et al. Identification of Helicobacter pylori and other Helicobacter species by PCR, hybridization, and partial DNA sequencing in human liver samples from patients with primary sclerosing cholangitis or primary biliary cirrhosis. *Journal of Clinical Microbiology.* 2000; 38(3): 1072–6.

Pradhan SB, Dali S. Relation between gallbladder neoplasm and Helicobacter hepaticus infection. *Kathmandu University Medical Journal.* 2004; 2(4): 331–5.

Ronchetti F, Ronchetti R, Guglielmi F et al. Detection of Chlamydia pneumoniae in cholesteatoma tissue: any pathogenetic role? *Otology and Neurotology.* 2003; 24(3): 353–7.

Sripa B, Kaewkes S, Sithithaworn P et al. Liver fluke induces cholangiocarcinoma. *PLoS Medicine.* 2007; 4(7): e201.

Tokita H, Murai S, Kamitsukasa H et al. High TT virus load as an independent factor associated with the occurrence of hepatocellular carcinoma among patients with hepatitis C virus-related chronic liver disease. *Journal of Medical Virology.* 2002; 67(4): 501–9.

Travaglione S, Fabbri A, Fiorentini C. The Rho-activating CNF1 toxin from pathogenic E. coli: a risk factor for human cancer development? *Infectious Agents and Cancer.* 2008; 3: 4.

Vilchez RA, Kozinetz CA, Arrington AS et al. Simian virus 40 in human cancers. *American Journal of Medicine.* 2003; 114(8): 675–84.

Vilchez RA, Madden CR, Kozinetz CA et al. Association between simian virus 40 and non-Hodgkin lymphoma. *The Lancet.* 2002; 359(9309): 817–23.

Wang JH, Zhang WP, Liu HX et al. Detection of human parvovirus B19 in papillary thyroid carcinoma. *Br J Cancer.* 2008; 98(3): 611–8.

West DC. Ewing sarcoma family of tumors. *Current Opinion in Oncology.* 2000; 12(4): 323–9.

Yang YY, Koh LW, Tsai JH et al. Involvement of viral and chemical factors with oral cancer in Taiwan. *Japanese Journal of Clinical Oncology.* 2004; 34(4): 176–83.

Yosry A. Schistosomiasis and neoplasia. *Contributions to Microbiology.* 2006; 13: 81–100.

Zafiropoulos A, Tsentelierou E, Billiri K et al. Human herpes viruses in non-melanoma skin cancers. *Cancer Letters.* 2003; 198(1): 77–81.

Zendri E, Venturi C, Ricci R et al. Primary cutaneous plasmacytoma: a role for a triggering stimulus? *Clinical and Experimental Dermatology.* 2005; 30(3): 229–31.

Zhang X, Li Q, Hu P et al. Two case reports of pituitary adenoma associated with Toxoplasma gondii infection. *Journal of Clinical Pathology.* 2002; 55(12): 965–6.

Zheng H, Abdel Aziz HO, Nakanishi Y et al. Oncogenic role of JC virus in lung cancer. *Journal of Pathology.* 2007; 212(3): 306–15.

Zhou Y, Attygalle AD, Chuang SS et al. Angioimmunoblastic T-cell lymphoma: histological progression associates with EBV and HHV6B viral load. *British Journal of Haematology.* 2007; 138(1): 44–53.

NOTES

1 Tokudome S, Suzuki S, Kojima M et al. Is the proportion of infection-related cancers much greater than generally appreciated? *International Journal of Cancer.* 2005; 113(3): 509.

2 Ciro M, Bracken AP, Helin K. Profiling cancer. *Current Opinion in Cell Biology.* 2003; 15(2): 213–20.

3 Bignold LP. Initiation of genetic instability and tumour formation: A review and hypothesis of a nongenotoxic mechanism. *Cellular and Molecular Life Sciences.* 2003; 60(6): 1107–17.

4 Parkin DM. The global health burden of infection-associated cancers in the year 2002. *International Journal of Cancer.* 2006; 118(12): 3030–44.

5 Adapted from Damania B. DNA tumor viruses and human cancer. *Trends in Microbiology.* 2007; 15(1): 38–44.

6 Lavanchy D. Hepatitis B virus epidemiology, disease burden, treatment, and current and emerging prevention and control measures. *Journal of Viral Hepatitis.* 2004; 11(2): 97–107.

7 Strong K, Mathers C, Epping-Jordan J et al. Preventing cancer through tobacco and infection control: how many lives can we save in the next 10 years? *European Journal of Cancer Prevention.* 2008; 17(2): 153–61.

8 Frieden TR, Myers JE, Krauskopf MS et al. A public health approach to winning the war against cancer. *Oncologist.* 2008; 13(12): 1306–13.

9 Sitas F, Parkin DM, Chirenje M et al. Part II: cancer in indigenous Africans—causes and control. *Lancet Oncology.* 2008; 9(8): 786–95.

10 Javier RT, Butel JS. The history of tumor virology. *Cancer Research.* 2008; 68(19): 7693–706.

11 Javier RT. Cell polarity proteins: common targets for tumorigenic human viruses. *Oncogene.* 2008; 27(55): 7031–46.

12 Barros Kanzaki LI. Hypothetical HTLV-I induction by ionizing radiation. *Medical Hypotheses.* 2006; 67(1): 177–82.

13 Zhang F, Da R, Song W et al. Pathogenic risk of endogenous retrovirus infection in immunodeficient hosts. *Virus Research.* 2008; 132(1–2): 237–41.

14 Oricchio E, Sciamanna I, Beraldi R et al. Distinct roles for LINE-1 and HERV-K retroelements in cell proliferation, differentiation and tumor progression. *Oncogene.* 2007; 26(29): 4226–33.

15 Damania B. DNA tumor viruses and human cancer. *Trends in Microbiology.* 2007; 15(1): 38–44.

16 Elgui de Oliveira D. DNA viruses in human cancer: an integrated overview on fundamental mechanisms of viral carcinogenesis. *Cancer Letters.* 2007; 247(2): 182–96.
17 Thus, "elevation of telomerase transcription and/or activity can be used as mechanisms to bypass replicative senescence and to increase proliferative capacity, and these mechanisms, in turn, increase the cumulative risk of genetic alterations." Bellon M, Nicot C. Regulation of telomerase and telomeres: human tumor viruses take control. *Journal of the National Cancer Institute.* 2008; 100(2): 98–108.
18 Shackelford J, Pagano JS. Role of the ubiquitin system and tumor viruses in AIDS-related cancer. *BioMedCentral Biochemistry.* 2007; 8(suppl 1): S8.
19 Javier RT. Cell polarity proteins: common targets for tumorigenic human viruses. *Oncogene.* 2008; 27(55): 7031–46.
20 Grogg KL, Miller RF, Dogan A. HIV infection and lymphoma. *Journal of Clinical Pathology.* 2007; 60(12): 1365–72.
21 Kundu JK, Surh YJ. Inflammation: gearing the journey to cancer. *Mutation Research.* 2008; 659(1–2): 15–30.
22 Goswami B, Rajappa M, Sharma M et al. Inflammation: its role and interplay in the development of cancer, with special focus on gynecological malignancies. *International Journal of Gynecological Cancer.* 2008; 18(4): 591–9.
23 Sansoni P, Vescovini R, Fagnoni F et al. The immune system in extreme longevity. *Experimental Gerontology.* 2008; 43(2): 61–5.
24 Nindl I, Rosl F. Molecular concepts of virus infections causing skin cancer in organ transplant recipients. *American Journal of Transplantation.* 2008; 8(11): 2199–204.
25 Lim ST, Levine AM. Non-AIDS-defining cancers and HIV infection. *Current HIV/AIDS Reports.* 2005; 2(3): 146–53.
26 Farinati F, Cardin R, Cassaro M et al. Helicobacter pylori, inflammation, oxidative damage and gastric cancer: a morphological, biological and molecular pathway. *European Journal of Cancer Prevention.* 2008; 17(3): 195–200.
27 Klein EA, Silverman R. Inflammation, infection, and prostate cancer. *Current Opinion in Urology.* 2008; 18(3): 315–9.
28 Boxus M, Twizere JC, Legros S et al. The HTLV-1 Tax interactome. *Retrovirology.* 2008; 5: 76.
29 Pumfery A, de la Fuente C, Kashanchi F. HTLV-1 Tax: centrosome amplification and cancer. *Retrovirology.* 2006; 3: 50.
30 Nitta T, Kanai M, Sugihara E et al. Centrosome amplification in adult T-cell leukemia and human T-cell leukemia virus type 1 Tax-induced human T cells. *Cancer Science.* 2006; 97(9): 836–41.
31 Hanahan D, Weinberg RA. The hallmarks of cancer. *Cell.* 2000; 100(1): 57–70.
32 Dayaram T, Marriott SJ. Effect of transforming viruses on molecular mechanisms associated with cancer. *Journal of Cellular Physiology.* 2008; 216(2): 309–14.
33 Damania B. DNA tumor viruses and human cancer. *Trends in Microbiology.* 2007; 15(1): 38–44.
34 Vousden KH, Farrell PJ. Viruses and human cancer. *British Medical Bulletin.* 1994; 50(3): 560–81.

35 Elgui de Oliveira D. DNA viruses in human cancer: an integrated overview on fundamental mechanisms of viral carcinogenesis. *Cancer Letters.* 2007; 247(2): 182–96.
36 Aoki Y, Tosato G. Interactions between HIV-1 Tat and KSHV. *Current Topics in Microbiology and Immunology.* 2007; 312: 309–26.
37 Zeng Y, Zhang X, Huang Z et al. Intracellular Tat of human immunodeficiency virus type 1 activates lytic cycle replication of Kaposi's sarcoma-associated herpesvirus: role of JAK/STAT signaling. *Journal of Virology.* 2007; 81(5): 2401–17.
38 Underbrink MP, Hoskins SL, Pou AM et al. Viral interaction: a possible contributing factor in head and neck cancer progression. *Acta Oto-laryngologica.* 2008; 128(12): 1361–9.
39 Moens U, Van Ghelue M, Johannessen M. Oncogenic potentials of the human polyomavirus regulatory proteins. *Cellular and Molecular Life Sciences.* 2007; 64(13): 1656–78.
40 Soderberg-Naucler C. HCMV microinfections in inflammatory diseases and cancer. *Journal of Clinical Virology.* 2008; 41(3): 218–23.
41 zur Hausen H. Viral oncogenesis. In: *Microbes and Malignancy. Infection as a Cause of Human Cancer.* Parsonnet J, ed. New York: Oxford University Press, 1999, pp 107–130.
42 Kanavos P. The rising burden of cancer in the developing world. *Annals of Oncology.* 2006; 17(suppl 8): viii15–viii23.
43 Jones SB. Cancer in the developing world: a call to action. *British Medical Journal.* 1999; 319(7208): 505–8.
44 Franco EL. Commentary: health inequity could increase in poor countries if universal HPV vaccination is not adopted. *British Medical Journal.* 2007; 335(7616): 378–9.
45 Azerkan F, Zendehdel K, Tillgren P et al. Risk of cervical cancer among immigrants by age at immigration and follow-up time in Sweden, from 1968 to 2004. *International Journal of Cancer.* 2008; 123(11): 2664–70.
46 Bosch FX, Burchell AN, Schiffman M et al. Epidemiology and natural history of human papillomavirus infections and type-specific implications in cervical neoplasia. *Vaccine.* 2008; 26(suppl 10): K1–16.
47 Coughlin SS, Richards TB, Nasseri K et al. Cervical cancer incidence in the United States in the US-Mexico border region, 1998–2003. *Cancer.* 2008; 113(suppl 10): 2964–73.
48 Tokudome S, Suzuki S, Kojima M et al. Is the proportion of infection-related cancers much greater than generally appreciated? *International Journal of Cancer.* 2005; 113(3): 509.
49 Ragin C, Edwards R, Heron DE et al. Prevalence of cancer-associated viral infections in healthy afro-Caribbean populations: a review of the literature. *Cancer Investigation.* 2008; 26(9): 936–47.
50 van Lier EA, van Kranen HJ, van Vliet JA et al. Estimated number of new cancer cases attributable to infection in the Netherlands in 2003. *Cancer Letters.* 2008; 272(2): 226–31.
51 Drain PK, Halperin DT, Hughes JP et al. Male circumcision, religion, and infectious diseases: an ecologic analysis of 118 developing countries. *BioMed Central Infectious Diseases.* 2006; 6: 172.

52 Howett MK, Kuhl JP. Microbicides for prevention of transmission of sexually transmitted diseases. *Current Pharmaceutical Design*. 2005; 11(29): 3731–46.
53 Frazer IH, Lowy DR, Schiller JT. Prevention of cancer through immunization: prospects and challenges for the 21st century. *European Journal of Immunology*. 2007; 37(suppl 1): S148–55.
54 Bao YP, Li N, Smith JS et al. Human papillomavirus type distribution in women from Asia: a meta-analysis. *International Journal of Gynecological Cancer*. 2008; 18(1): 71–9.
55 Potts M, Halperin DT, Kirby D et al. Reassessing HIV Prevention. *Science*. 2008; 320: 749–50.
56 Gingues S, Gill MJ. The impact of highly active antiretroviral therapy on the incidence and outcomes of AIDS-defining cancers in Southern Alberta. *HIV Medicine*. 2006; 7(6): 369–77.
57 Wang XG, Revskaya E, Bryan RA et al. Treating cancer as an infectious disease—viral antigens as novel targets for treatment and potential prevention of tumors of viral etiology. *Public Library of Science ONE*. 2007; 2(10): e1114.
58 Dadachova E, Wang XG, Casadevall A. Targeting the virus with radioimmunotherapy in virus-associated cancers. *Cancer Biotherapy and Radiopharmaceuticals*. 2007; 22(3): 303–8.
59 Hadley C. The infection connection. Helicobacter pylori is more than just the cause of gastric ulcers—it offers an unprecedented opportunity to study changes in human microecology and the nature of chronic disease. *European Molecular Biology Organization Reports*. 2006; 7(5): 470–3.
60 Gram K. Sleeper cell. *Vancouver Sun*. April 28, 2008.
61 Boccardo E, Villa LL. Viral origins of human cancer. *Current Medicinal Chemistry*. 2007; 14(24): 2526–39.

INDEX

Note: Page numbers in bold and *italics* refer to figures and tables, respectively.

AAV. *See* Adeno-associated virus
Acute lymphoblastic leukemia (ALL). *See also* Leukemia
   EBV infection and, 393
Adeno-associated virus (AAV), 106
Adult T-cell leukemia (ATL). *See also* Leukemia
   EBV infection and, 480
   HHV-6 infection and, 480
   HTLV-1 infection and, 474, 476, 479–80
Aflatoxin
   risk factor for liver cancer, 304
AIDS. *See HIV/AIDS*
AIN. *See* Anal intraepithelial neoplasia
ALL. *See* Acute lymphoblastic leukemia
Anal cancer, 143–46, *144*, *See also* Cancer
Anal intraepithelial neoplasia (AIN), 143, 145
Anogenital cancers, 130–39, *See also* Cancer
Anogenital warts. *See* Genital warts; Warts

ATL. *See* Adult T-cell leukemia
Aural cancer, 159, *See also* Cancer

Biomarkers, for HPV disease detection, 232–33, *234*
BL. *See* Burkitt lymphoma
Bladder cancer. *See* Urinary bladder cancer
Blood donation
   HTLV-1 transmission and, **478**, 482–83
BLPD. *See* B-lymphoproliferative disease
B-lymphoproliferative disease (BLPD)
   EBV infection and, 401
Bowen's disease, 163, 168
Breast cancer, 161, *See also* Cancer
Breastfeeding
   HTLV-1 transmission and, 482
Bronchial cancer, 158–59, *See also* Cancer
Burkitt lymphoma (BL). *See also* Lymphoma
   characteristics of, *388*
   EBV infection and, 388–89, 401

Cancer
  anal, 143–46, *144*
  aural, 159
  breast, 161
  bronchial, 158–59
  cervical. *See* Cervical cancer
  colorectal, 160
  esophageal, 157
  genital, 130–39
  head and neck, 148–60
  laryngeal, 155–56
  leukemia. *See* Leukemia
  liver, 291–96, **292**
  lung, 159
  lymphoma. *See* Lymphoma
  nasopharyngeal, 158
  non-melanoma skin, 163, 165
  ocular surface, 158
  oral cavity, 151–53
  oropharyngeal, 153
  ovarian, 160
  penile, 136–39, *138*
  prostate, 160
  renal, 160
  second primary. *See* Second primary cancer
  sinonasal, 156–57
  skin, 161–68, **164**, *165*, *167*
  tonsillar, 154–55, *155*
  urinary bladder, 161
  vaginal, 134–35
  vulvar, 130–34, *132*
Cervarix™ vaccine, 265, 266, 267, 268, 278
Cervical cancer. *See also* Cancer
  AAV and, 106
  aboriginal groups, 86–88
  age and other risk correlates, 99–100
  burden of, 81–88, **88**
    global variation, *81*, **82**, **83**
  C. trachomatis and, 105
  diet and obesity, 107
  disease cofactors, 100–106
  genetic factors, 101–2
  global, 81
  HIV and, 105–6
  HPV and, 79–108
    genotyping, clinical utility of, 98–99
    geographical variation of viral involvement, 93–97, **94**, *95*
    high-risk viral types, 89–91, **90**, *91*
    multiple viral types, 92–93
    subtypes and variants, 97–98
    tumor histology and viral type, 91–92
  HSV and, 105
  oral contraceptives, 103–5
  Pap smear for, 92
  parity, 103–5
  public health implications, 107–8
  screening disparities, 219–21, *228*
  smoking and, 273
  target groups and specific populations, 82, 83–86, **84**, **85**
  trends, 83–86, **84**
  United States and Canada, 81–88
Cervical intraepithelial neoplasia (CIN), 22, 89, 93, 97, 103, 133, 135, 141, 216, 225, 273
  HPV DNA testing for, 98, 222, 225
Children
  HPV infection in, 42–45
Chlamydia trachomatis (*C. trachomatis*)
  and cervical cancer, 105
Cholangiocarcinoma, 293, *See also* Cancer
CIN. *See* Cervical intraepithelial neoplasia
Circumcision
  effect on HPV infection, 139–41
CMV. *See* Cytomegalovirus
Colorectal cancer, 160, *See also* Cancer
Cornification. *See* Keratin and keratinization

Cowden syndrome, *167*
CTCL. *See* Cutaneous T-cell lymphoma
Cutaneous T-cell lymphoma (CTCL). *See also* Lymphoma
  HTLV-1 infection and, 474
  HTLV-2 infection and, 474
Cytomegalovirus (CMV), 431, 525

EBV. *See* Epstein-Barr virus
Epidermodysplasia verruciformis (EV), 158, 165–66
Epstein-Barr virus (EBV), 4–5, 157, 385–411, *392*, *405*, 429, 438
  associated with acute lymphoblastic leukemia, 393
  associated with adult T-cell leukemia, 480
  associated with Burkitt lymphoma, 388–89, 401
  associated with Hodgkin's disease, 389
  associated with lymphoepithelioma-like carcinoma, 391
  associated with nasopharyngeal carcinoma, 398, 401
  associated with non-Hodgkin's lymphoma, 389
  associated with post-transplant lymphoproliferative disorder, 390, 402
  associated with primary effusion lymphoma, 389
  characteristics of, *388*
  detection methods, 398–99, *398*
  disease mechanism, 393–98
    carcinogenesis, 397
    infection pathways and latency, 394–96
    prevention opportunities, 397–98
    reactivation, replication and lysis, 396–97
    tissue targets, 393–94
  hemophagocytic syndrome and, 403
  history of discovery, 386–87
  prevention approaches
    after exposure, 400
    avoiding exposure, 399–400
    cofactor prevention, 400–402
    prophylactic eradication or suppression, 400
    therapeutic eradication or suppression, 402
    transformation, interrupting, 403
  transmission and occurrence of, 392–93
Esophageal cancer, 157, *See also* Cancer

Fanconi anemia, *167*

Gardasil™ vaccine, 265, *266*, 268–69, 278
Gastric cancer. *See also* Cancer
  atrophic gastritis and, 347, 355
  cardia and non-cardia sites, 346–47
  H. pylori and, 345–48
  necessary cause, 345–46
  reflux disease and, 342, 346
  risk factors, *347*
Genital warts, 22, 23, 27, 32–33, 43, 89, 148, *See also* Warts
  in pre-pubescent girls, 43–44

H. pylori. See *Helicobacter pylori*
HAART. *See* Highly active antiretroviral therapy
Hailey-Hailey disease, *167*
HAM/TSP. *See* HTLV-1-associated myelopathy/tropical spastic paraparesis
HBIG. *See* Hepatitis B immune globulin
HBV. *See* Hepatitis B virus

HCC. *See* Hepatocellular carcinoma
HCV. *See* Hepatitis C virus
HD. *See* Hodgkin's disease
Head and neck cancers, 148–60, *See also* Cancer
  transformation in, 150–51
  transmission of, 149–50
Helicobacter pylori (*H. pylori*), 341–62
  associated with gastric adenocarcinoma, 345–48
  associated with mucosa-associated lymphoid tissue (MALT) lymphoma of the stomach, 344–45
  associated with non-gastric digestive system cancers, 348
  characteristics of, 352
  detection methods, 353–55
  disease mechanism, 352–53
  history of discovery, 343–44
  prevention approaches, 355–61
    after exposure, 356
    avoiding exposure, 356
    cofactor prevention, 358–59
    prophylactic eradication or suppression, 357–58
    therapeutic eradication or suppression, 359–60
    transformation, interrupting, 360–61
  protective role in esophageal adenocarcinoma, 348
  risk factors, 353
  transmission and occurrence of, 349–51
Helicobacter species
  biliary tract cancer and, 348
  liver cancer and, 348
Hemophagocytic syndrome (HPS), 403
Hepatitis B immune globulin (HBIG), 312
Hepatitis B vaccination, 506, *See also* Vaccination

Hepatitis B virus (HBV), 289–90
  associated with liver cancer, 291–94
  associated with non-Hodgkin's lymphoma, 344
  characteristics of, 295
  detection methods, 305–6
  disease mechanism, 301–3
  disease risk factors, 303–5
  genotypes, 289–90
  history of discovery, 302, **303**
  prevention approaches
    after exposure, 308–11
    avoiding exposure, 307–8
    cofactor prevention, 314–15
    prophylactic eradication or suppression, 311–13
    therapeutic eradication or suppression, 315–16
    transformation, interrupting, 316–18
  transmission and occurrence of, 296–99, *298*
Hepatitis C virus (HCV), 290–91
  associated with B-cell lymphoma, 293
  associated with glomerulonephritis, 294
  associated with liver cancer, 293, 294–96
  associated with mixed cryoglobulinemia, 294
  associated with mucosa-associated lymphoid tissue (MALT) lymphoma, 295
  associated with non-Hodgkin's lymphoma, 293, 344
  associated with Sjögren's syndrome, 294–95
  autoimmunity, 294
  characteristics of, 303
  detection methods, 305–6
  disease mechanism, 303
  disease risk factors, 303–5
  genotypes, 290–91

history of discovery, 288
prevention approaches
   after exposure, 308–11
   avoiding exposure, 307–8
   cofactor prevention, 314–15
   prophylactic eradication or
      suppression, 313–14
   therapeutic eradication or
      suppression, 315–16
   transformation, interrupting,
      316–18
second primary cancer and, 295
transmission and occurrence of,
   299–301
Hepatitis viruses, 287–319
   classification, 289, See also
      Hepatitis B virus; Hepatitis C
      virus
Hepatocellular carcinoma (HCC),
   287, **292**, 301, See also Liver
   cancer
Herpes simplex virus (HSV), 525
   and cervical cancer, 105
Herpes simplex virus type 1
   (HSV-1), 446
Herpes simplex virus type 2 (HSV-2),
   35
   associated with vulvar cancer,
      134
Herpesviruses. See Human
   herpesviruses
HHV-3. See Human herpesvirus 3
HHV-4. See Epstein-Barr virus
HHV-6. See Human herpesvirus 6
HHV-8. See Human herpesvirus 8
Highly active antiretroviral therapy
   (HAART), 485
   for Kaposi sarcoma, 443, 449
   for non-Hodgkin's lymphoma,
      449–50
HIV/AIDS, 12–13, 105–6, 277,
   299, 388, 429, 433, 435–36,
   472–73, 480, 486
   HHV-8 infection and, 519
Hodgkin's disease (HD)

EBV infection and, 389
HPS. See Hemophagocytic syndrome
HPV. See Human papillomavirus *and
   entries for individual HPV
   types and subtopics (below)*
HPV and related disease detection,
   213–33
   biomarkers for, 232–33, *234*
   head and neck surveillance,
      231–32
   HPV DNA testing. See HPV DNA
      testing
   in men, 230–31
   liquid-based cytology (LBC),
      217–18, 223
   Pap smear
      anal, 227–30
      cervical, 216–21, **221**
   prevention approaches, **260**
   serum antibody testing, 225–26
   visual screening, 226–27
HPV DNA testing, 27, 34–35,
   43–44, 70, 91, 93, 98, 131,
   135, 136, 147, 151, 152, 154,
   156, 157, 158, 215, 216,
   222–25, **223**, 275
   compared with Pap smear, 215,
      218, 223
   for evaluation of treatment, 222
   in HIV-positive populations,
      223–24
   sampling and collection issues,
      224–25
HPV-1, 43
   associated with skin cancer, 165
HPV-2, 43
   associated with skin cancer, 164, 165
HPV-5
   associated with skin cancer, 165
HPV-6, 23, 27, 33, 43
   associated with genital warts, 23
   associated with head and neck
      cancers, 148
   associated with juvenile recurrent
      respiratory papillomatosis, 43

HPV-6 (*Contd.*)
   associated with laryngeal cancer, 156
   associated with ocular surface cancer, 158
   associated with penile cancer, 137
   associated with skin cancer, 163
HPV-7
   associated with skin cancer, 164
HPV-8
   associated with penile cancer, 137
   associated with skin cancer, 165
HPV-9
   associated with skin cancer, 165
HPV-10
   associated with skin cancer, 164
HPV-11, 23, 27, 43
   associated with esophageal cancer, 157
   associated with genital warts, 23
   associated with juvenile recurrent respiratory papillomatosis, 43
   associated with laryngeal cancer, 156
   associated with ocular surface cancer, 158
   associated with penile cancer, 137
HPV-12, 28
HPV-14
   associated with skin cancer, 165
HPV-16, 22, 23, 24, 27, 33, 40, 42, 44, 45, 62, 70
   associated with cervical cancer, 90, 91, 93, 94, 98, 102
   associated with esophageal cancer, 157
   associated with head and neck cancers, 148, 149, 150
   associated with laryngeal cancer, 156
   associated with ocular surface cancer, 158
   associated with oral cavity cancer, 152
   associated with oropharyngeal cancer, 153
   associated with ovarian carcinoma, 160
   associated with penile cancer, 137, 139
   associated with second primary cancer, 147
   associated with sinonasal cancer, 156, 157
   associated with skin cancer, 163, 166–68
   associated with tonsillar cancer, 155
   associated with vaginal cancer, 134, 135
   associated with vulvar cancer, 131, 132
   infection in males, 142
HPV-18, 22, 23, 24, 27, 42, 44, 62
   associated with cervical cancer, 90, 91–92, 93, 94, 98, 99
   associated with head and neck cancers, 148
   associated with laryngeal cancer, 156
   associated with ocular surface cancer, 158
   associated with oral cavity cancer, 152
   associated with penile cancer, 137
   associated with sinonasal cancer, 156, 157
   associated with vaginal cancer, 134, 135
   associated with vulvar cancer, 131, 132
HPV-23
   associated with skin cancer, 165
HPV-24
   associated with skin cancer, 165
HPV-25
   associated with skin cancer, 165

HPV-31
    associated with cervical cancer, 90, 97, 98
    associated with nasopharyngeal carcinoma, 158
HPV-32
    associated with oral cavity cancer, 152
HPV-33
    associated with cervical cancer, 90
    associated with vulvar cancer, 132
HPV-35
    associated with cervical cancer, 90
HPV-45
    associated with cervical cancer, 90
HPV-52, 40
    associated with cervical cancer, 90, 94, 97
HPV-53, 33
HPV-58, 40
    associated with cervical cancer, 90, 94, 97
HPV-59
    associated with cervical cancer, 90
HPV-73, 33
HPV-84, 33
HPV-101
    associated with skin cancer, 164
HPV-103
    associated with skin cancer, 164
HSV-1. *See* Herpes simplex virus type 1
HSV-2. *See* Herpes simplex virus type 2
HTLV-1. *See* Human T-cell lymphotropic virus type 1
HTLV-1-associated myelopathy/ tropical spastic paraparesis (HAM/TSP)
    HTLV-1 infection and, 475
HTLV-2. *See* Human T-cell lymphotropic virus type 2
HTLV-3. *See* Human T-cell lymphotropic virus type 3
HTLV-4. *See* Human T-cell lymphotropic virus type 4
Human herpesvirus 3 (HHV-3), 430, 432
Human herpesvirus 4 (HHV-4). *See* Epstein-Barr virus
Human herpesvirus 6 (HHV-6), 525
    associated with adult T-cell leukemia, 480
Human herpesvirus 8 (HHV-8), 429–53
    associated with head and neck cancers, 149
    associated with Kaposi sarcoma, 433–37
    associated with multi-centric Castleman disease, 437
    associated with plasmablastic lymphomas, 437
    associated with primary effusion lymphoma, 437–38
    detection methods, 446–47
    disease mechanism, 444–46
    geographic location of subtypes, *432*
    history of discovery, 430–33
    prevention approaches, 447–51
        after exposure, 448–49
        avoiding exposure, 447–48
        cofactor prevention, 449–50
        prophylactic eradication or suppression, 449
        therapeutic eradication or suppression, 450–51
        transformation, interrupting, 451
    transmission and occurrence of, 438–44
Human herpesviruses. *See also entries for individual herpesviruses, including* Cytomegalovirus *and* Herpes simplex virus
    classification, *431*
Human immunodeficiency virus (HIV). *See* HIV/AIDS

Human papillomavirus (HPV), 21,
      66–71, 507–8
   associated with cervical cancer.
      See Cervical cancer
   associated with non-cervical
      cancer, 129–68
   characteristics of, 32
   classification, 26, *See also entries
      for individual HPV types*
   detection. *See* HPV and related
      disease detection; HPV DNA
      testing
   disease characteristics of, 31
   disease mechanism
      immune evasion, 63–66
      keratinization as mark and
         marker, 68–69
      malignant transformation,
         69–71
      productive infection and virion
         release, 69
      proliferation phase, 66–67
   history of discovery, 25–27
   infection in infants and children,
      42–45, *44, 45*
   infection in males, 141–43
   lesions, 27–31, *29*
   occurrence of, 35–42
      age-specific, 41–42, **41**
      time trends, 40–41
      type-specific, 38–40, *38*
   prevention approaches, 259–78, *261*
      after exposure, 264–72
      avoiding exposure, 261–64
      cofactor prevention, 273–74
      prophylactic eradication or
         suppression, 272
      therapeutic eradication or
         suppression, 274–76
      transformation, interrupting,
         276–77
   susceptible sites and target tissues,
      57–62
   transmission of, 32–35
   types, *29*
   type-specific occurrence, *39*
Human T-cell lymphotropic virus
      type 1 (HTLV-1), 7–8, 105,
      471–88
   associated with adult T-cell
      leukemia, 474, 476, 479–80
   associated with cutaneous T-cell
      lymphoma, 474
   associated with HAM/TSP, 475
   associated with mycosis
      fungoides, 474
   associated with Sèzary
      syndrome, 474
   associated with skin cancer, 162
   characteristics of, 476
   classification, 473
   detection methods, 481
   disease mechanism, 478–81
   history of discovery, 472–74
   infective dermatitis associated
      with, 479
   prevention approaches, 481–86
      after exposure, 483–84
      avoiding exposure, 482–83
      cofactor prevention, 484–85
      prophylatic eradication or
         supression, 484
      therapeutic eradication or
         supression, 485–86
      transformation, interrupting, 486
   transmission and occurrence of,
      475–78
Human T-cell lymphotropic
      virus type 2 (HTLV-2),
      472–73, 476
   associated with cutaneous T-cell
      lymphoma, 474
   characteristics of, 476
Human T-cell lymphotropic virus
      type 3 (HTLV-3), 473
Human T-cell lymphotropic virus
      type 4 (HTLV-4), 473

ICC. *See* Intrahepatic
      cholangiocarcinoma

Infectious agents, 3, 5, 6, 10, 11, 505–24, 507, 508, See also entries for individual infectious agents
  and cancer, overview, 3–16
  future research directions
    basic investigation of cancer, 513–17, 525
    new partnerships and knowledge dissemination, 523–24
    prevention research and policy development, 520–23, 521, 522,
    translational research, 517–20
  investigational agents, 517, 525
  practical implications, 506
  prevention paradigm and approaches, 509–10, 509, 511
Interferon-alpha, 317
Intrahepatic cholangiocarcinoma (ICC), 293

Juvenile recurrent respiratory papillomatosis (RRP), 42–43

Kaposi sarcoma (KS), 431, 433–37
  clinicoepidemiologic variants of, 434
  disease mechanism, 444–46
  HAART therapy for, 449
  incidence of, 444
Kaposi sarcoma-associated herpesvirus (KSHV). See Human herpesvirus 8
Keratin and keratinization, 58, 59, 60, 62
  as HPV disease marker, 68–69
Kidney cancer. See Renal cancer
Kissing disease, 441, See Mononucleosis
KS. See Kaposi sarcoma
KSHV. See Human herpesvirus 8

Laryngeal cancer, 155–56, See also Cancer

LBC. See Liquid-based cytology
LELC. See Lymphoepithelioma-like carcinoma
Leukemia
  acute lymphoblastic, 393
  adult T-cell, 474, 476, 479–80
Liquid-based cytology (LBC), 217–18, 223
Liver cancer, **292**, See also Cancer; Hepatocellular carcinoma
  hepatitis viruses and, 291–96
  risk factors, 303–5, 304
Lung cancer, 159, See also Cancer
Lymphoepithelioma-like carcinoma (LELC), 293, See also Cancer
Lymphoma
  Burkitt, 388–89, 401
  cutaneous T-cell, 474
  mucosa-associated lymphoid tissue (MALT), 295, 341, 344–45
  non-Hodgkin's, 293, 389, 449–50
  primary effusion, 389, 437–38

Males
  detection of HPV in, 230–31
  HPV infection in, 141–43
MALT. See Mucosa-associated lymphoid tissue lymphoma
MC. See Mixed cryoglobulinemia
MCD. See Multi-centric Castleman disease
Melanoma-associated retrovirus, 162
MF. See Mycosis fungoides
Mixed cryoglobulinemia (MC), 294
Mononucleosis
  and Epstein-Barr virus, 386
Mucosa-associated lymphoid tissue (MALT) lymphoma, 295, 341, See also Lymphoma
  H. pylori and, 344–45
  hepatitis C virus and, 295
Multi-centric Castleman disease (MCD), 437
Mycosis fungoides (MF)
  HTLV-1 and, 474

Nasopharyngeal carcinoma
    (NPC), 158
  EBV infection and, 390, 398, 401
Netherton syndrome, 167
NHL. See Non-Hodgkin's lymphoma
NMSC. See Non-melanoma skin
    cancer
Non-Hodgkin's lymphoma (NHL).
    See also Lymphoma
  EBV infection and, 389
  HAART therapy for, 449–50
  hepatitis viruses and, 293
Non-melanoma skin cancer (NMSC),
    163, 165, See also Cancer;
    Skin cancer
Non-steroidal anti-inflammatory
    drugs (NSAIDs)
  and *H. pylori* infection, 355,
    358–59, 361
  and HPV infection, 277
NPC. See Nasopharyngeal
    carcinoma

Ocular surface cancer, 158, See also
    Cancer
Oral cavity cancer, 151–53, See also
    Cancer
Oral contraceptives, 273–74
  and cervical cancer, 103–5
Oropharyngeal cancer, 153, See also
    Cancer
Ovarian cancer, 160, See also Cancer

p16(INK4a), 232–33
Pap smear, **223**
  anal, 227–30
  cervical, 92, 216–21
    innovations, 217–19
    screening diaparities, 219–21, **221**
    test accuracy, 216–17
PEL. See Primary effusion lymphoma
Penile cancer, 136–39, *138*, See also
    Cancer
Penile intraepithelial neoplasia (PIN),
    136, 139

Penis. See also Penile cancer
  circumcision, 131
  phimosis, 139–40
PIN. See Penile intraepithelial
    neoplasia
Polymerase chain reaction
    (PCR), 481
  for EBV infection, 399
Post-transplant lymphoproliferative
    disorder (PTLD)
  EBV infection and, 402
Prevention of infections that cause
    cancer. See entries for
    individual infectious agents
Primary effusion lymphoma (PEL).
    See also Lymphoma
  EBV infection and, 389
  human herpesvirus 8 and, 437–38
Primate T-cell lymphotropic virus
    type 1 (PTLV-1), 471
Prophylactic vaccines. See
    Vaccination; Vaccines
Prostate cancer, 160, See also Cancer
PTLD. See Post-transplant
    lymphoproliferative disorder
PTLV-1. See Primate T-cell
    lymphotropic virus type 1

Recurrent respiratory papillomatosis.
    See Juvenile recurrent
    respiratory papillomatosis
Renal cancer, 160, See also Cancer
Retroviruses. See HIV/AIDS; *entries
    for individual Human T-cell
    lymphotropic virus types*
RRP. See Juvenile recurrent
    respiratory papillomatosis

Schistosomiasis, 303–4
Second primary cancer (SPC), 133,
    146–48, 295, See also Cancer
Sèzary syndrome (SS)
  HTLV-1 infection and, 474
Sicca complex. See Sjögren's
    syndrome

Sinonasal cancer, 156–57, See also Cancer
Sjögren's syndrome, 294–95
Skin cancer, 161–68, See also Cancer
   due to UV radiation, 166–68
   future research on infectious causation, 168
   genetic syndromes and, *167*
   HPV and, 163–66, **164**, *165*
   HTLV-1 and, 162
   non-melanoma, 163
   solar keratosis, 162
Smoking
   risk factor for cervical cancer, 102–3
SPC. *See* Second primary cancer

Tat protein, 446
Tax protein
   HTLV-1 infection and, 479–80
Therapeutic vaccines. *See* Vaccination; Vaccines
Tonsillar cancer, 154–55, *155*, See also Cancer

Urinary bladder cancer, 161, See also Cancer
UV radiation
   and skin cancer, 166–68

Vaccination, **309**, See also Cervaris™ vaccine; Gardasil™ vaccine; Vaccines
   and cervical screening programs, 269–71
   for hepatitis B, 297, 303, 308–11, 506–7
   for HPV, 26, 39, *266*, 268–72, 275–76
   trial results, 261–62
Vaccines, 267, See also Cervaris™ vaccine; Gardasil™ vaccine; Vaccination
   chimeric, 265
   prophylactic, 26, 264, 265
   therapeutic, 26, 264–65
Vaginal cancer, 134–35, See also Cancer
Vaginal intraepithelial neoplasia (VaIN), 134
VaIN. *See* Vaginal intraepithelial neoplasia
Varicella-zoster virus (VZV). *See* Human herpesvirus 3
VIN. *See* Vulvar intraepithelial neoplasia
Vulvar cancer, 130–34, *132*, See also Cancer
Vulvar intraepithelial neoplasia (VIN), 131, *132*, 133, 141
VZV. *See* Human herpesvirus 3

Warts
   Butcher's, 28
   cutaneous, 43
   genital, 22, 23, 27, 32–33, 43–44, 89, 139, 148, 150, 268
   hand, 150

Xeroderma pigmentosum, *167*